Biopolymers for Medical Applications

Biopolymers for Medical Applications

Editors

Juan M. Ruso

Soft Matter and Molecular Biophysics Group
Department of Applied Physics
University of Santiago de Compostela
Santiago de Compostela
Spain

Paula V. Messina

Department of Chemistry
Universidad Nacional del Sur INQUISUR-CONICET
Bahía Blanca
Argentina

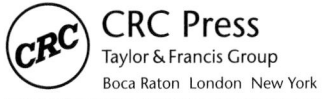

CRC Press
Taylor & Francis Group
Boca Raton London New York

CRC Press is an imprint of the
Taylor & Francis Group, an **informa** business

A SCIENCE PUBLISHERS BOOK

CRC Press
Taylor & Francis Group
6000 Broken Sound Parkway NW, Suite 300
Boca Raton, FL 33487-2742

First issued in paperback 2021

© 2017 by Taylor & Francis Group, LLC
CRC Press is an imprint of Taylor & Francis Group, an Informa business

No claim to original U.S. Government works

ISBN-13: 978-0-367-78270-2 (pbk)
ISBN-13: 978-1-4987-4496-6 (hbk)

Library of Congress Cataloging-in-Publication Data

Names: Ruso, Juan M. (Juan Manuel), editor. | Messina, Paula V., editor.
Title: Biopolymers for medical applications / editors, Juan M. Ruso, Paula V. Messina.
Description: Boca Raton, FL : CRC Press, 2016. | "A Science Publishers book."
| Includes bibliographical references and index.
Identifiers: LCCN 2016029027| ISBN 9781498744966 (hardback : alk. paper) |
ISBN 9781498744973 (e-book)
Subjects: | MESH: Biopolymers
Classification: LCC QP801.B69 | NLM QT 37.5.P7 | DDC 572/.33--dc23
LC record available at https://lccn.loc.gov/2016029027

Visit the Taylor & Francis Web site at
http://www.taylorandfrancis.com

and the CRC Press Web site at
http://www.crcpress.com

Preface

Owing to their higher chemical and impact resistance in addition to their superior mechanical and thermal properties, biopolymers have become "the material of choice" in healing therapies. A wide range of different polymers are available for multiple medical applications; so much so that it is expected that the use of glass and metals in therapeutic devices will decline over the next few years while the use of polymers will increase. Although this subject has long been an important area of research for biochemists and physicists, engineers, pharmacists and physicians are now taking a keen interest in it. Polymers' versatility and, the scientist's ability to engineer and customize their physical, chemical and biological properties to match the requirements of the varied and specific medical applications are the keys to their increasing use. Applications, just to name a few, include medical tubing, controlled drug delivery and wound management (e.g., adhesives, sutures, lubricants and surgical meshes), orthopedic devices (screws, pins, and rods), dental materials (filler after a tooth extraction) and tissue engineering.

This book has been devised so as to offer an overview of currently "hot" topics in this field. We, as editors of this book, have selected reputed scientists whose research and ideas have significantly contributed to progress in this area. Recognizing that there are different approaches to biopolymers is not enough. Experiments have been the centerpiece of the scientific method since Galileo. However, the power of modern computers has made computational approaches a key aspect in all kind of scientific research. This diversity needs to be preserved and promoted. Given that different approaches emphasize different aspects and offer different perspectives allows us to have a fuller, more balanced understanding of the complex entity called biopolymers. Especially in the long term, a discipline that contains a variety of different approaches can cope with a changing world better than others characterized by only a single way. For this reason, in this book, we have made special emphasis to both disciplines are reflected.

The different classes of advanced materials based on biopolymer systems including biopolymer nano-fibers and nano-tubes, smart nano-assemblies for drug and gene delivery, ordered supramolecular systems as well as novel composite materials based on nanoparticles and biopolymers, are covered in the book. In the first nine chapters of this monograph a detailed account of the present status of biopolymers it is provided and highlighted the recent developments made by leading research groups.

Since the requirements of medical applications are variable, there is no ideal biopolymer. Therefore, new materials are developed based on the desired properties for very specific purposes. This means that in addition to materials, processing techniques and computational tools are inherent in this process. Thus, the book is completed with five chapters featuring concepts of modeling and simulation of biological systems, drug-target interaction analysis via perturbation theory, guided self-assembly by structural DNA nanotechnology, dynamic examination of molecular drug-protein binding and selective imprinted xerogels. In chapters ranging from 10 to 14, the recent advances of mathematical and theoretical models, applied to find an accurate representation of the complexity of biological systems, have been highlighted. It shows how reasonably simple mathematics can be combined with different models to draw exciting conclusions. Interconnections are made between diverse biological examples and a variety of discrete and continuous equation models. On the other hand, the constant progresses in both computer power and algorithm design, makes highly promising the future of computer-aided drug design; thus, with every passing day molecular dynamics simulations, the science of simulating the motions of a system of particles, play an increasingly important role. The three final chapters of this book discusses the atomistic computer simulations of biopolymers (i.e., a protein), receptors and their associated small-molecule ligands that can act in drug discovery, including the identification of cryptic or allosteric binding sites, the enhancement of traditional virtual-screening methodologies, and the direct prediction of small-molecule binding energies. The limitations of current simulation methodologies, comprising the high computational costs and approximations of molecular forces required were also discussed.

The variety of topics covered in this book aims to provide a comprehensive overview of the field of biopolymers for medical applications. Besides its usefulness for academics and industrial researchers, the book is of humanistic inspiration, revealing the special sensitivity of authors who have made a great effort to uproot the palisades that traditionally separate advanced professionals from those unfamiliar with these subjects. Indeed, we hope to convince the latter of the many new research opportunities in this field.

Last, but not least, the fact that we are writing this preface is, without any doubt, due to the cooperation, support, and understanding of all the contributors who invested a considerable amount of time in helping this book to reach fruition. We have been privileged to coordinate the efforts of many talented scientists.

Juan M. Ruso and Paula V. Messina

Contents

Biopolymers in Regenerative Medicine: Overview, Current Advances and Future Trends

Juan M. Ruso[1] and *Paula V. Messina*[2,*]

Introduction

Overview

An ambition of regenerative medicine is the *in vivo* restoration or, alternatively, the *in vitro* generation of a complex functional organ consisting of a scaffold made out of synthetic or natural materials that has been loaded with living cells (Melek 2015, 2014; Terzic and Nelson 2010). Mammalian cells respond *in vivo* to the biological stimulus from the surrounding environment, which is structured by nanometer-scaled components. Consequently, materials intended for the reconstruction of the human body have to reproduce the correct signals that guide the cells towards a desirable behavior (Patel 2011), in this sense, polímeros are currently investigated. Exciting advances based on application of the self-assembled biocompatible polymeric scaffolds for regeneration of tissues and organs were systematically explored and described in detail in the literature (Niaounakis 2014; Kalia and Avérous 2011;

---

[1] Soft Matter and Molecular Biophysics Group, Department of Applied Physics, University of Santiago de Compostela, Santiago de Compostela, 15782, Spain.
[2] Department of Chemistry, Universidad Nacional del Sur, 8000, Bahía Blanca, Argentina. INQUISUR-CONICET.
* Corresponding author: pmessina@uns.edu.ar

Imam et al. 1999; Atala and Allickson 2014; Dutta and Dutta 2013). Their effectiveness in providing supports for cell growth and development in various tissues and enhancing or mimicking an extracellular matrix (ECM) has been carefully analyzed (Nedovic and Willaert 2013; Hunt and Grover 2010). Clinical results showing the benefits of such treatments, as well as their limitations are explored and novel polymer formulas, for coating implants, stents, and other medical devices, have been developed (Plackett 2011; Jagur-Grodzinski 2006; Tseng et al. 2002; Weber et al. 2006; Mani et al. 2007; Jung et al. 2009a; Jung et al. 2009b; De Vicente et al. 2010; Ferreira et al. 2009; Schwarz et al. 2009). Furthermore, the application of these polymeric materials in tissue engineering of cartilage and bones are explored (Stevens 2008; Bessa et al. 2008; Yilgor et al. 2010; Beltrán et al. 2013). An innovative and transiently evolving biotechnological subfield, the synthetic biology, attempts to insert enhanced functionality and response to biomaterials by the use of recombinant polymer biotechnology to include genetic units that are not typically present on them (Hammer and Kamat 2012). Consistently, synthetic membranes from bio-inspired block co-polypeptides developed into another emerging area of interest (Bellomo et al. 2004).

This chapter offers a structural synopsis of biopolymers and discusses their physicochemical characteristics, organization—properties relationship, applications, and limitations. The classification of polymers is briefly mentioned and their chemical structures are provided. Biopolymers that are hydrolytically labile and erode (biodegradable polymers) as well as those that are bio-inert and remain unchanged after implantation (non-degradable polymers) are considered. Some synthetic derivatives of natural materials are briefly discussed where appropriate. It is the authors' intention to provide a thorough general idea of the biopolymers' applications to regenerative medicine. This chapter tends to be a guide for further reading on most biopolymer classifications and properties.

The basics: biopolymer definition and classification

There is no a general consensus in literature and patents about the exact definition of the generic terms *degradable*, *biodegradable*, *bio-based*, *compostable*, *biopolymer*, and *bioplastic*; they appear to have multiple and overlapping meanings. We have presented here a brief description of each definition highlighting their differences. For more information consult Niaounakis (2014).

Degradable is a general term used to describe all polymeric materials that disintegrate by a range of physical and chemical processes, while *biodegradable* is a term focused on the polymer's functionality, that is, "biodegradability". This term is applied to those materials that will degrade, within a specific period of time and environment, under the action of microorganisms such as molds, fungi, and bacteria. According to the withdrawn standard ASTM D5488-94 (ASTM Internationa, 1994), the terms *biodegradable polymers* specifically refer to polymers that are "*capable of undergoing decomposition into carbon dioxide, methane, water, inorganic compounds, or biomass in which the predominant mechanism is the enzymatic action of microorganisms that can be measured by standard tests, over a specific period of time, reflecting available disposal conditions.*" On the other hand, the Japan Bioplastics Association

(JBPA) defines the term biodegradability as the characteristics of material that can be microbiologically degraded to the final products of carbon dioxide and water, which, in turn, are recycled in nature (Niaounakis 2014). *Biodegradation* should be differentiated from *disintegration*, which simply implies the breakdown of a material into small and separate fragments. Biodegradable polymers can be certified according to any of the following legally binding international standards: ISO 17088:2012, EN 13432:2000, EN 14995:2006, ASTM D6400-12 (Niaounakis 2014). As a consequence of this classification, a polymer may be *degradable* but not *biodegradable*.

Bio-based is a word focused on the origin of raw materials, and it's applied to polymers obtained from renewable resources. In practical terms, a bio-based polymer is not *per se* an ecological polymer; this is subjected to a variety of concerns, including the material origin, the production method, and finally how such material is disposed at the end of its useful life. Accordingly to these classifications, not every bio-based polymer is biodegradable, e.g., bio-based polyethylene or polyamide 11; and not every biodegradable polymer is bio-based, e.g., poly(ε-caprolactone) or poly(glycolic acid); nevertheless some polymers fall into both categories, such as polyhydroxyalkanoates (PHA)s. Currently, there are no standards to certify a "bio-based product". However, the bio-based content of a product can be quantify by measuring the bio-based content of materials via carbon isotope analysis, ASTM D6866-12 (ASTM International 2012b).

Compostable polymers were circumscribed to the ASTM D6002 (ASTM International 1996), that stated "*a plastic which is capable of undergoing biological decomposition in a compost site as part of an available program*". Nevertheless, this definition obtained considerable disapproval, and in January 2011, the ASTM removed the standard ASTM D6002 (ASTM International 1996) and substituted it for the standard ASTM D6002-96(2002) (ASTM International 2011a); posteriorly it was withdrawn, with no replacement. To be called compostable, a polymer should meet one of the following international standards: ASTM Standard D6400-12 (ASTM International 2012a) or CEN standard EN 14995:2006 (for compostable plastics), D6868-11 or EN 13432:2000 (for compostable packaging) (ASTM International 2011b), and ISO 17088:2012. The ISO-Standard not only refers to plastic packaging but to plastics in general. The biodegradation and/or disintegration rate, in addition to toxicity are the points that make the difference between *biodegradable* and *compostable* polymers. All compostable polymers are biodegradable by default, but not vice versa. Definitely, two different criteria point out the definition of a *biopolymer*: the source of the raw materials, and the biodegradability of the polymer. As a consequence, a biopolymer is a polymer derived from renewable resources, as well as a biological and fossil-based bio-degradable polymer (Niaounakis 2014). Based on its capacity to be chemically consumed by bacteria, fungi, or other biological means, biopolymers can be divided into two wide groups: *biodegradable* and *non-biodegradable* biopolymers. Alternatively, biopolymers can be classified on their origin as being either *bio-based* or *fossil fuel-based*. The central categories for distinguishing among the different types of biopolymers are mentioned below (Niaounakis 2014):

   i. Bio-based biodegradable biopolymers.
  ii. Non-Biodegradable bio-based biopolymers.
 iii. Biodegradable biopolymers made from fossil fuels.

The biopolymers belonging to (i) can be biologically generated by microorganisms, plants, and animals, or chemically synthesized from biological starting materials (e.g., corn, sugar, starch, etc.). Examples of biodegradable bio-based biopolymers are: (1) synthetic polymers from renewable resources such as poly(lactic acid) (PLA); (2) biopolymers produced by microorganisms, such as PHAs; (3) and those that are biosynthesized by various routes in the biosphere, such as starch or proteins. The biopolymers corresponding to (ii) can be produced either from biomass or from renewable resources and are non-biodegradable. Examples of non-biodegradable bio-based biopolymers are: (1) synthetic polymers from renewable resources such as specific polyamides from castor oil (polyamide 11), specific polyesters based on biopropanediol, biopolyethylene (bio-LDPE, bio-HDPE), biopolypropylene (bio-PP), or biopoly (vinyl chloride) (bio-PVC) based on bio-ethanol (e.g., from sugar cane), etc.; (2) naturally occurring biopolymers such as natural rubber or amber. The biopolymers of the last item (iii) are produced from fossil fuel, such as synthetic aliphatic polyesters made from crude oil or natural gas, and are formally biodegradable and compostable. Some examples of biodegradable biopolymers made from fossil fuels are: Poly(ε-caprolactone) (PCL), poly(butylene succinate) (PBS), and selected aliphatic-aromatic co-polyesters. All of them can be degraded by microorganisms (Niaounakis 2014).

Biopolymers and *bio-plastics* are often considered synonymous, while they are different materials. *Biopolymers* are polymers that fit the definition given above and the *bio-plastics* are the plastics that are created by using biopolymers. According to the European Bioplastics e.V., a plastic material is defined as a bio-plastic if it is either bio-based, biodegradable, or contains both properties (Niaounakis 2014). On the basis of this classification, a material is considered a bio-polymer if it is comprise of any biodegradable polymer (e.g., polymers of type i or iii) or of any bio-based polymers (e.g., polymers of type i or ii). A particular case is the bio-polyethylene derived from sugarcane, designated as "green polyethylene"; it is non-biodegradable, but emits less greenhouse gases when compared to fossil-based polyethylene, and accordingly, is classified as a biopolymer (Niaounakis 2013). In general, polymers can also be classified on basis of their response to heat as thermoplastics, thermosets, or elastomers (Raquez et al. 2010); and by their composition as blends (Paul 2012), composites (White et al. 2001; Saheb and Jog 1999), or laminates (Powell 2012); these classifications can be extended to biopolymers. Currently, the level of bio-based thermoset biopolymers exceeds the volume of bio-based thermoplastic biopolymers (Mohanty et al. 2005). Biopolymer blends are mixtures of polymers from different origins such as the commercial product Ecovio® (BASF AG), which is a blend of PLA and poly(butylene adipate-co-terephthalate) (PBAT) (Ecoflex®, BASF AG). An extra group is constituted by the bio-composites; these are biopolymers or synthetic polymers reinforced with natural fibers (Mohanty et al. 2005), such as sisal, flax, hemp, jute, banana, wood, and various grasses, and/or fillers and additives. Novel bio-composites are based on a biodegradable matrix polymer reinforced with natural fibers (Mohanty et al. 2005).

Biomaterials chronology and biopolymers

Originally, the selection of materials for their use as medical implants was dependent on those already available off the shelf (Hench and Polak 2002). Early implantable materials include metals such as gold that were used in dentistry over 2,000 years ago (Langer and Tirrell 2004). The term "biomaterials" was first introduced within the last 50 years (Atala et al. 2010). Practically at the same time, and aided by the hasty industrial expansions of polymer synthesis, the assessment of synthetic polymers for biomedical applications was initiated. Polymethylmethacrylate, PMMA, was used in dentistry in the 1930s and cellulose acetate was used in dialysis tubing in the 1940s. Dacron was used to make vascular grafts; polyether urethanes, the materials used in ladies' girdles, were used in artificial hearts; and PMMA and stainless steel were used in total hip replacements (Langer and Tirrell 2004). The elaboration of plastic contact lenses, utilizing primarily PMMA, started around 1936 (Efron 2010), and the first data on the use of nylon as a suture was reported in 1941 (Atala et al. 2010). At the end of World War II, a wide variety of polymeric materials were available to inspiring surgeons to break new grounds in replacing diseased or damaged body parts. Materials such as silicones, polyurethanes, Teflon, Nylon, methacrylates, blends with titanium, and stainless steel were available for surgeons to overcome medical problems. Inspired by the idea to restore lost organ or tissue functionality, health and dental experts, made use of minimal regulatory controls to elaborate and improvise replacements, bridges, conduits, and even organ systems based on such materials. Those early implants made from the available industrial materials were frequently incompatible with the host tissue, generally due to their insufficient purity.

From the beginning, alterations of the host tissue in reaction to the materials presence became ostensible. Additives such as plasticizers, un-polymerized reactants, and degradation products were evaluated as possible causes, leading to a conscious

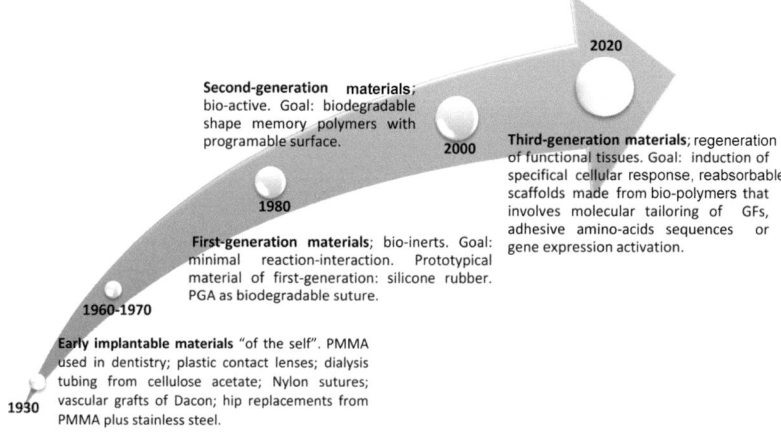

Fig. 1: Participation of biopolymer in the biomaterials evolution.

exploration of polymer features for biomedical applications and biocompatibility testing. With an emerging knowledge of the immunological system and the understanding of the possible foreign body reaction, a first generation of materials was developed during the 1960s and 1970s (Ratner et al. 2004). The first-generation materials were designed as bio-inert. The main objective was to create a material that would match the mechanical properties of the replaced tissue, and would not allow protein adsorption and cell adhesion, in order to reduce the possible immune response and rejection. The elastomeric polymer, silicone rubber was widely used as a prototypical material of the first generation (Teck Lim et al. 2013). In the early 1980s, research shifted from materials that exclusively exhibited a bio-inert tissue response to materials that actively interacted with their environment. The second-generation biomaterials are specifically designed to be "bioactive". This means they should elicit specific and desired cellular responses, like cell adhesion, proliferation and differentiation into a specific cell type, e.g., bone cells that will form a new bone tissue and thus integrate the implant strongly into the surrounding natural tissue (Hench and Polak 2002). The reaction of the cells should be controllable by the physical and chemical properties of the material surface. An additional advance in this second generation was the development of biodegradable materials that exhibited controllable chemical breakdown into non-toxic degradation products, which were either metabolized or directly eliminated. Biodegradable synthetic polymers were designed to resolve the interface problem, since the foreign material is ultimately replaced by regenerating tissues and eventually the regeneration site is histologically indistinguishable from the host tissue. Since the 1960s, a biodegradable suture composed of polyglycolic (PGA) acid has been in clinical use (Atala et al. 2010; Ratner et al. 2004). Many groups continue to search for biodegradable polymers with needed properties such as strength, flexibility, a chemical composition conducive to tissue development, and a degradation rate consistent with the specific application (Zhou et al. 2012; Shih and Lin 2012; Evans et al. 2004). Polymeric materials with novel properties such as shape-memory and programmable and interactive surfaces that control the cellular microenvironment are also under investigation (Han et al. 2014; Brosnan et al. 2013; McCloskey 2013). Other biopolymers' applications rapidly emerged, thus providing versatile technologies for regenerative medicine, for example, as fracture fixation assistances, as drug delivery devices or as transports of signaling molecules or genetic code information. Biopolymers-based systems can permit delivery of drugs, active proteins, and other macromolecules (Jonker et al. 2012; Pal et al. 2013; Estrada and Champion 2015; Srichana and Domb 2009) localized the site where the drug is needed. Despite considerable clinical success of bio-inert, bioactive, and resorbable implants, there is still a high long-term prostheses failure rate and need for revision surgery (Atala et al. 2010; Ratner et al. 2004). Artificial biomaterials cannot respond, unlike living tissue, to changing physiological loads or biochemical stimuli so improvements of first- and second-generation biomaterials have been incomplete. To overcome these limitations, a third generation of biomaterials that involves molecular tailoring of resorbable polymers for specific cellular responses is being developed. By immobilizing specific biomolecules, such as signaling molecules or cell-specific adhesion peptides or proteins, onto a material it is possible to mimic the extracellular matrix (ECM) environment and stimulate the specific response of cells at a molecular level and activate specific gene expression that regulates regeneration and the self-healing process. One of the most advanced strategies in the present research on tissue engineering is the construction of tridimensional (3D) porous scaffolds made of resorbable biopolymers that should be seeded with the patient's own cells or even stem cells (Weiss and Calvert 2000; Rezwan et al. 2006; Stoddart et al. 2009). Upon implantation into the body, the polymeric scaffolds will provide the cells the necessary support during self-healing process and should be gradually degraded, as they will be continuously replaced by new bone; finally it will disappear completely. Biomimetic surfaces prepared on basis of biopolymers are promising tools to control cell adhesion, implant integration, cell differentiation, and tissue development (Dalsin et al. 2003; Cheng et al. 2012; Kim et al. 2005). Constantly expanding knowledge of the basic biology of stem cell differentiation and the corresponding signaling pathways as well as tissue development provides the basis for novel molecular design of scaffolds. It is rather important that the engineered scaffold will be designed to be steadily remodeled *in vivo* and to resemble the histological and mechanical properties of the surrounding tissue. Due to this paradigm shift, mechanically labile hydrogels, especially injectable systems that can be used to directly encapsulate cells, have gained great importance as a basis for biomimetic cell carriers (Yu and Ding 2008; Nicodemus and Bryant 2008; Wu et al. 2008; Jiang et al. 2014). In spite of the great advances attained, in the case of polymer-based devices for bone tissue replacement, their potential use is still very limited due to their insufficient mechanical properties as load-bearing implants. These materials need further improvements, e.g., strong mechanically resistant reinforcement with fibrous or particulate component and loading with bioactive molecules which would accelerate the formation of regenerated, mineralized, and fully functional bone tissue. The subsequent sections will provide a synopsis on the biopolymers impact on the third-generation materials, focusing on their translational potential evidenced by preclinical studies outcomes.

The Role of Biopolymers in Translational Medicine

Novel tissue engineering (TE) strategies are developed with the aim to overcome the socio-economic and health burden of different tissues injuries and improve the life of patients worldwide (Ratner et al. 2004). In the last decades, a pool of multiple techniques and methodologies for biomaterials fabrication has been described in an attempt to address and explore the major functional architectural and compositional cues of native tissues (Atala and Allickson 2014; Chaikof et al. 2002; Song et al. 2010; Hook et al. 2010; Hassan et al. 2012b). The search for improved and tissue-oriented implantable units has extended the knowledge on biomaterials' potential and highlighted the interest for multimodal scaffolds with novel structures and physical-chemical features (Hassan et al. 2012a; Hassan et al. 2012b; Ruso et al. 2013; D'Elía et al. 2013; Gravina et al. 2014; Ruso et al. 2015). The multifunctional or multimodal properties of these scaffolds result from the combination of different topographies that are not typically available in a given material, increasing their potential role in regenerative medical strategies (Gravina et al. 2015; D'Elía et al. 2013; Gravina et al. 2014; Hassan et al. 2012a; Hassan et al. 2012b; M Ruso et al. 2015). Polymers play a pivotal role to the construction of 3D templates and to the attainment of synthetic ECM environments for tissue regeneration (Sartuqui et al. 2015; Stevens and George 2005; Hong and Stegemann 2008; Geckil et al. 2010; Tsang and Bhatia 2004).

Figure 2 shows the increasing interest in the study of polymeric materials and their application in tissue engineering; there is a particular emphasis on the development of musculoskeletal tissue's substitutes. Among the common materials applied to regenerative medicine, the interest on polymers in the last ten years corresponds to the 60% of the researchers' reports, Fig. 3. Biopolymers can be obtained from both synthetic and natural resources (Atala and Allickson 2014; Imam et al. 1999; Jagur-Grodzinski 2006; Kalia and Avérous 2011; Niaounakis 2013; Niaounakis 2014). Since each group possesses distinct advantages and limitations, a wide variety of composite materials and interpenetrating networks have been utilized to achieve desired results. Synthetic polymers are versatile to tailoring a wide range of degradation rates, structural features and mechanical properties, representing a reliable mine of new-fangled materials. The composition of the synthetic polymers can be designed to minimize the immune response and combine the best properties together. Synthetic polymers have been described by their degradation by hydrolysis of the ester bonds under physiological conditions and to avoid problems of immunogenicity, that are compelling arguments for achieving the purpose and pursuing the approaches of TE and regenerative medicine (Atala and Allickson 2014). Nevertheless, the majority of synthetic polymers are hydrophobic, which presents a major drawback for the migration of viable cells into the scaffold core. Examples of synthetic and popular

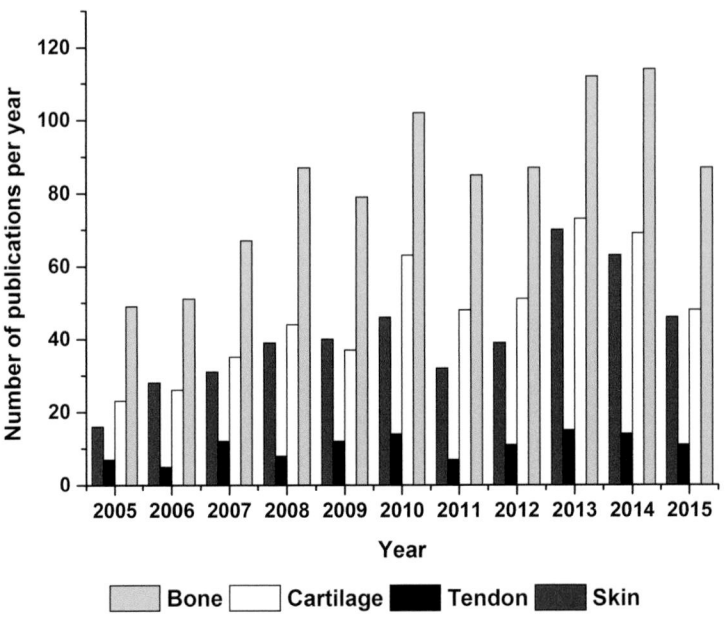

Fig. 2: Chronological evolution of investigations in biopolymers-based materials in the tissue engineering area. Data Base: Scopus, October 2015; search description: biopolymer, tissue engineering.

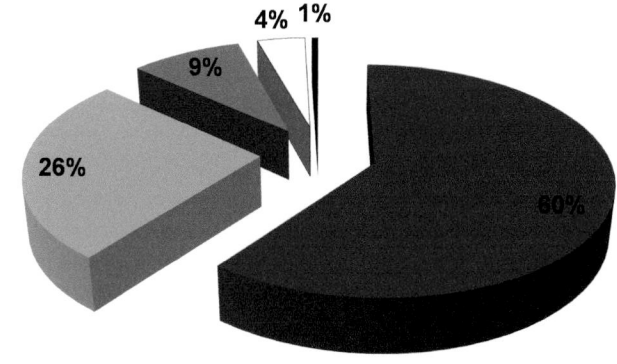

■ Polymers ■ Composites ■ Ceramics □ Bioactive Glass ■ Metallic Foams

Fig. 3: Application of different materials to regenerative medicine in the last 10 years. Data Base: Scopus, October 2015.

biodegradable synthetic polymers include poly(ethylene glycol) (PEG)/poly(ethylene oxide) (PEO), Poly(ethylene-covinylacetate) (EVA), poly(α-hydroxy acids), especially poly(lactic acid) (PLA), poly(glycolic acid) (PGA) and their co-polymers, poly(ε-caprolactone) (PLGA), poly(propylene fumarate), poly(dioxanone), polyorthoesters, polycarbonates, polyanhydrides, and polyphosphazenes. Particularly interesting are PLA and PGA polyesters which have been extensively used in biodegradable implants, tissue engineering, and drug delivery systems, see Tables 1 and 2. Natural polymers have been presented as an interesting option to the currently used synthetic materials due to a higher biodegradability rate and non-cytotoxicity (Atala and Allickson 2014). They are taken from native sources, exhibit similar properties to soft tissues; and their synthesis often involves enzyme-catalyzed, chain growth polymerization reactions of activated monomers, which are typically formed within cells by metabolic processes. Within this group are included collagen, gelatin, dextran, agarose/alginate, hyaluronic acid, cellulose, and fibrin gels (see Tables 1 and 2). Although they have to be purified to avoid foreign body response after implantation, natural polymers are widely used in regenerative medicine. They have a wide range of mechanical, chemical, and physical properties, are resistant to biochemical attack, and as a consequence of their versatility and flexibility they can be easily processed and shaped. Moreover, they are inert towards host tissues after implantation and are available at a reasonable cost.

Independent of their origin, polymers lack properties to stimulate biological functions, such as osteo-conductivity and cell bioactivity. As a consequence, hybrid variants of these materials have emerged through synthetic designs (Bourgeat-Lami et al. 2002) and genetic engineering of peptide-based biopolymers (Atala and Allickson 2014). Biodegradable polymers have been selected for the drug delivery system as they do not need surgery to be removed after releasing of the drugs and can be excreted by the body itself. Examples of biomedical applications using biopolymers include heart valves, vascular grafts, artificial hearts, breast implants, contact lenses, intraocular lenses, components of extracorporeal oxygenators, dialyzers and plasmapheresis

Table 1: Regular natural- and synthetic-based biopolymers involved in regenerative medicine.

Natural-Based Biopolymers

Name	Characteristics
Hyaluronic Acid	Hyaluronic acid (HA) is a glycosaminoglycan (GAG) present in all vertebrates. HA is a major component of connective tissues and plays an important role in lubrication, cell differentiation, and cell growth.

1 →4 linked β-D-mannuronic acid (M) and α-L-guluronic acid (G) residues

Name	Characteristics
Chitosan	Chitosan is a linear polysaccharide obtained from deacetylation of chitin (main component in the exoskeletons of crustaceans' shells) and is a material structurally similar to GAGs, being degradable by enzymes in humans.

Randomly distributed b-(1-4)-linked D-glucosamine and N-acetyl-D-glucosamine

Name	Characteristics
Alginic Acid/ Sodium Alginate	Alginic Acid or its sodium salt, Sodium Alginate, is an anionic polysaccharide disseminated in the cell walls of brown algae. G residues associate with divalent cations to form ionic crosslinks.

Carrageenan	γ – carrageenan β – carrageenan	It is extracted from red seaweeds; carrageenan displays close similarities with mammalian GAGs.
Agarose		Agarose is a natural-based polysaccharide obtained from agar.
Poly(hydroxyalkanoates) (PHAs) /	poly-(R)-3-hydroxybutyrate (P3HB)	PHAs are linear polyesters produced in nature by bacterial fermentation of sugar or lipids.
Collagen Monomeric and crosslinked 3D triple helical structures. Many types, type I consists of two identical α1 chains and one α2 chain		Collagen is the central structural protein in the extracellular space in animals' connective tissues; it is the most abundant protein in mammals, representing about 25%–35% of the whole-body protein content.
Gelatin		Gelatin is an irreversibly hydrolyzed form of collagen.

Table 1 cont....

Table 1 cont.

Natural-Based Biopolymers

Name	Characteristics
Elastin	Elastin is the elastic component in soft tissues that allows tissue to return to normal shape following stretch or pinch. Formed by crosslinking smaller tropoelastin polymers using lysyl oxidase to form mesh-like structures.
Fibrin It is a fibrous, non-globular protein involved in the clotting of blood	It is formed by the action of the protease thrombin that cleaves fibrinogen which causes the latter to polymerize, generating soft gels. Gelation kinetics is controlled by the ratio of thrombin to fibrinogen, calcium concentration, and temperature.
Fibronectin Glycoprotein secreted by fibroblasts	This binds integrins, transmits mechanical cues from the environment to the cell and binds other ECM proteins such as collagen and fibrin.
Keratin	Insoluble polymer found in non-mineralized tissues. Bundles form intermediate filaments that make up hair (α-keratins) and nails (β-keratins). Monomers form stable left-handed superhelical structures to form filaments.
Silk	Silk is a natural protein fiber mainly composed of fibroin and is extracted from the cocoons of the Bombyxmori silkworm. Foams, sponges, films, and hydrogels are formed from the silk solution.

Starch is a polysaccharide consisting of a large number of glucose units joined by glycosidic bonds and produced by green plants as an energy store. It is quite abundant in nature and is an almost unlimited source and low-cost associated raw material.

Table 1 cont....

Starch

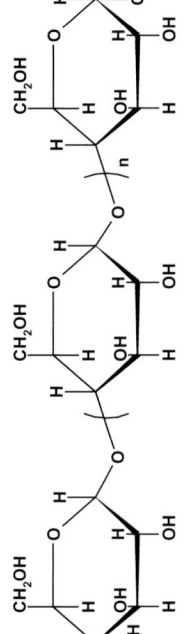

CH₂OH

n = 300 - 600

Table 1 cont.

Synthetic-Based Biopolymers

Name	Characteristics
Poly(ethylene glycol) (PEG)/Poly(ethylene oxide) (PEO)	PEG, PEO, or POE refers to an oligomer or polymer of ethylene oxide. The three names are chemically synonymous, but historically PEG is preferred in the biomedical field, whereas PEO is more prevalent in the field of polymer chemistry.
Poly(ethylene-covinylacetate) (PEVA)	Poly(ethylene-covinylacetate) (PEVA) is the copolymer of ethylene and vinylacetate. It is a polymer that approaches elastomeric ("rubber-like") materials in softness and flexibility.
Poly(lactic acid) (PLA)	Polylactic acid (PLA) is thermoplastic, aliphatic polyester, produced from non-toxic renewable feedstock, naturally occurring organic acid, or made by fermentation of sugars obtained from renewable resources such as sugarcane.

Polyglycolic Acid (PGA)/Poly l-glycolic Acid (PLGA)

PGA and PLGA are synthesized by means of ring-opening co-polymerization of two different monomers, the cyclic dimers (1,4-dioxane-2,5-diones) of glycolic acid and lactic acid.

Poly(ε-caprolactone) (PCL)

Polycaprolactone (PCL) is a biodegradable polyester with a low melting point of around 60°C and a glass transition temperature of about −60°C.

Poly(propylene fumarate) (PPF)

PPF can be cross-linked via radical polymerization by itself or with cross-linkers such as methylmethacrylate, N-vinyl pyrrolidinone (NVP), and biodegradable macromers of PPF-diacrylate or poly(ethylene glycol)-diacrylate.

Table 2: Applications of natural- and synthetic-based biopolymers to regenerative medicine.

Biopolymer	Properties	Biomaterial Form	Application	Example of Approved Clinical Product	
Hyaluronic Acid	Minimal immune response and chemotactic combined with the adequate agents. Osteo-inductive and angiogenesis in combination with GFs.	3D Scaffolds, hydrogels, electrospun fibers, nano-and micro-gels.	Keratynocytes encapsulation, bone and cartilage reparation, drug delivery, vocal fold and nerve regeneration, spinal cord injuries.	Hyalograft 3D ™	(Bressan et al. 2011; Stoppel et al. 2015; Prestwich 2011; Burdick and Prestwich 2011; Lee et al. 2009; Jia et al. 2006; Park et al. 2010; Horn et al. 2007)
Chitosan	Soluble, cationic in acidic conditions, and insoluble in neutral and basic conditions. Hemostatic stimulates osteo-conduction and wound healing. Shape-ability to fit the defect site, degradability.	3D Scaffolds, hydrogel, membrane, nano-particles.	Wound healing, orthopedics, cardiac repair, neural tissue engineering, cornea repair, drug and gene delivery.	Hemcon®	(Stoppel et al. 2015; Azad et al. 2004; Obara et al. 2003; Mi et al. 2001; Noel et al. 2010; Noel et al. 2008; Lu et al. 2008; Chien et al. 2012; Roy et al. 1999; Gustafson et al. 2007)
Alginic Acid/ Sodium Alginate	Degradation through ionic exchange with surrounding media. Variations in local mechanical properties controlled by concentration of calcium ions.	Soft gels, composite materials, electrospun fibers.	Wound healing, drug delivery, soft tissue engineering, cell delivery, *in vitro* stem cell maintenance.	DIABECELL® NTCELL® Xelma	(Bressan et al. 2011; Stoppel et al. 2015; Tan 2010; Vowden et al. 2006; Lee et al. 2009; Ghidoni et al. 2008; Sun and Tan 2013)
Agarose	Slow degradation profile and the low mechanical properties, 3D scaffolds exhibiting soft and flexible structure suitable for chondrocyte maintenance and MSC differentiation.	3D Scaffolds, hydrogels.	Skeletal tissues regeneration, efficient system for cartilage-like substitutes, islet, kidney and fibroblast encapsulation, nerve regeneration.		(Stokols et al. 2006; Stoppel et al. 2015; Elisseeff et al. 2005; Chen et al. 2006)
Carrageenan	Thermally, pH and cation concentration responsive material, in expensive and easy to manipulate. Effectiveness in maintaining the proliferative and chondrogenic potential of encapsulated cells.	Hydrogel	Skeletal tissues regeneration, cell delivery system.		(Popa et al. 2011; Popa et al. 2014; Mihaila et al. 2013)

Natural-Based

PHAs	Adequate substrate for bone cells growth. Scaffolds of brittle nature.	3D Scaffolds, HAp nano-composite, nano-particles.	Corneal epithelium repair, heart valves, bone tissue regeneration, drug delivery systems.	HCE	(Sodian et al. 2000; Sodian et al. 2002; Errico et al. 2009; Pielichowska and Blazewicz 2010)
Collagen Gelatin	Low immune response, good substrate for cell adhesion, chemotactic. Easily remodeled and degraded by cells. Chemical crosslinking decreases degradation and improves long-term mechanical properties. Many types available. Improper expression or mutation leads to disease.	Hydrogel, 3D scaffolds, membrane.	Fibroblast and keratinocytes encapsulation, wound healing, skin substitute, muscle repair, nerve regeneration, anti-aging, soft tissue reconstruction, bone repair.	Integra™ ApliGraft® ORCEL™ NeuroFlex® NeuroMatrix® NeuroMend® Dynamatrix® INFUSE®	(Bressan et al. 2011; Stoppel et al. 2015; Heimbach et al. 2003; Halim et al. 2010; Meek and Coert 2013; Nevins et al. 2010; McKay et al. 2007; Zhang et al. 2009a)
Elastin	Small tropoelastin polymers can be used to form composite materials. Easily remodeled by cells.	Films, gels 3D scaffolds, electrospun fibers.	Cardiac stent coatings, soft tissue reconstruction, orthopedics and cell encapsulation.		(Boland et al. 2004; Jordan et al. 2007; Schwartz and Wolff 1997; Salzberg 2006; Sell et al. 2006)
Fibrin	Stimulates cell migration, osteo-conduction and vascularization. Fibrinolytic inhibitors, like aprotinin or aminocaproic acid, reduce *in vitro* degradation rates.	3D scaffolds	Wound healing, lung and cardiac repair, *in vivo* cell delivery, bone defects reparation.	TachoSil® CASCADE® Autologous Platelet System	(Siemer et al. 2007; Anegg et al. 2007; Torio-Padron et al. 2007; Cherubino and Marra 2009; Christman et al. 2004; Wu et al. 2012)
Fibronectin	Improper regulation of expression leads to diseases such as cancer, fibrosis.	Grafted onto 2D and 3D surfaces to improve bio-compatibility.	Wound healing, stem cell differentiation, cardiac repair, bone regeneration.		(Grinnell 1984; Mosahebi et al. 2003; Prestwich 2011; Barker 2011; Stoppel et al. 2015)

Table 2 cont....

Table 2 cont.

Natural-Based

Biopolymer	Properties	Biomaterial Form	Application	Example of Approved Clinical Product	
Keratin	Structure attributed to disulfide bridges; more bridges yields lower elasticity. Classified as neutral-basic or acidic, dictating *in vivo* occurrence.	3D scaffold, hydrogel, films.	Cornea tissue engineering, wound healing, skin regeneration, cardiac repair, drug delivery, nerve repair, cell encapsulation.		(Apel et al. 2008; Elloumi-Hannachi et al. 2010; Satija et al. 2009; Reichl 2009; Nishida et al. 2004; Sierpinski et al. 2008)
Silk	Low enzymatic degradation rate controlled by crystallinity (β-sheet content), and some concerns arise on potential cytotoxic effects. Intrinsic mechanical properties. Mechanics tailored by modifying concentration, crystallization, molecular weight, and scaffold size.	3D Scaffolds, foams, films, sponges, hydrogels, electrospun fibers.	Tendon and skeletal tissues regeneration, cornea repair, drug delivery.		(Zhang et al. 2009b; Kundu 2014; Stoppel et al. 2015; Meinel et al. 2005)
Starch	Thermoplastic behavior, promotes cell adhesion, non-cytotoxic and biocompatible.	3D scaffold	Bone and cartilage regeneration, spinal cord injury treatment.		(Salgado et al. 2004; Martins et al. 2009; Gomes et al. 2006; Sá-Lima et al. 2010; Salgado et al. 2009)
PEG/PEO	Versatility of the PEG macromer chemistry and excellent biocompatibility.	3D Scaffold, hydrogels, micelles.	Fibroblast and keratinocytes encapsulation, ulcers wound healing, drug and gene delivery.	PolyActive™ Xelma	(Bressan et al. 2011; Lin and Anseth 2009a; Park et al. 2004; Salinas et al. 2007; Elisseeff et al. 1999; Mahoney and Anseth 2006; Osada et al. 2009; Lin and Anseth 2009a)

	Properties	Form	Applications	Product	References
Synthetic-Based					
PEVA	It has low-temperature toughness, stress-crack resistance, hot-melt adhesive waterproof properties, and resistance to UV radiation.	Micro/nano-fibre layers, nano-composite scaffolds.	Drug delivery system, cardiovascular stents.		(Sultana et al. 2015; Alhusein et al. 2012; Strohbach and Busch 2015)
PLA	Degradation by hydrolysis. They can present some problems regarding cytotoxicity.	3D scaffold, electrospun fibers, micro-spheres.	Fibroblast and keratynocytes encapsulation, macromolecules immobilization, bone, cartilage and nerve regeneration.	DermaGraft™	(Bressan et al. 2011; Hart et al. 2012; Zhu et al. 2004; Kim et al. 2006; Evans et al. 2002; Kang et al. 2005; Uematsu et al. 2005)
PGA/PLGA	Biodegradable and thermoplastic polymer.	3D scaffolds, fibers, membranes.	Drug release, stents, stem cell encapsulation and differentiation, cartilage and bone regeneration, facial nerve defects regeneration.		(Crow et al. 2005; Tammela and Talja 2003; Kotsar et al. 2008; Zare-Mehrjardi et al. 2011; Mouthuy et al. 2013; Nassif and El Sabban 2011; Zhu and Lou 2014)
PCL	Low chemical versatility and slow degradation by hydrolysis or bulk erosion. Difficulties for withstanding mechanical loads.	3D scaffolds, nano-composites, micelles, electrospun fibers, vesicles.	Bone regeneration, drug delivery, cell encapsulation, skin regeneration.		(Williams et al. 2005; Fujihara et al. 2005; Allen et al. 2000; Reneker et al. 2002; Jagur-Grodzinski 2006; Cao et al. 2003; Dai et al. 2004)
PPF	Satisfactory biological results, mechanical properties inferior to those of PGA, PLGA.	Hydrogel, 3D scaffold, nano-composite.	Cartilage and bone regeneration, cell encapsulation, nerve regeneration.		(Liao et al. 2007; Lee et al. 2011; Kim et al. 2009; Wang et al. 2009; Tan and Marra 2010; Lee et al. 2008)

units, coatings for pharmaceutical tablets and capsules, sutures, adhesives, and blood substitutes, kidney, liver, pancreas, bladder, bone cement, catheters, external and internal ear repairs, cardiac assist devices, implantable pumps, joint replacements, pacemaker, encapsulations, soft-tissue replacement, artificial blood vessels, artificial skin, dentistry, drug delivery, and targeting sites of inflammation or tumors and bags for the transport of blood plasma (Langer and Tirrell 2004; Mani et al. 2007; Melek 2015; Meyers et al. 2008; Niaounakis 2014; Patel 2011; Rathenow et al. 2004; Ratner et al. 2004; Stevens 2008; Teck Lim et al. 2013; Terzic and Nelson 2010; Tseng et al. 2002; Weiss and Calvert 2000; White et al. 2001; Yu and Ding 2008; Zhou et al. 2012; Zilla et al. 2007); some selected examples are summarized in Table 2.

Building Biomimetic Materials on the Basis of Biopolymers: along Physic, Chemistry, Biology, and Materials Science

The investigation of biopolymers has been reserved to biochemists and molecular biologists for over half a century. Nevertheless, during the last decade, the soft matter physics, chemical, and material science's community has been seized to this research field (Chassenieux et al. 2013). The earliest multidisciplinary "bioengineering" collaborations were born sometime in the 1970s–1980s. Those teams of physicians, chemists and engineers not only noted the necessity of regulating the composition, purity, and physical properties of the materials they were using, but also recognized the need for new materials with innovative and superior properties (Ratner et al. 2004). This inspired the expansion of many original materials, starting from the 1970s. Novel materials were designed and fabricated specifically for medical use, such as biodegradable polymers, "*medical grade*" silicones, pyrolytic carbon, and bioactive glasses and ceramics. Others were derived from existing materials that were then manufactured using new technologies, such as polyester fibers that were knitted or woven in the form of tubes for use as vascular grafts or cellulose acetate plastic that was processed as bundles of hollow fibers for use in artificial kidney dialysers (Ratner et al. 2004). Further materials were specifically modified to provide special biological properties, resembling one of the earliest "*bioengineered*" biomaterials involving the immobilization of heparin to create anticoagulant surfaces (Ratner et al. 2004). Biopolymers become the new building blocks from the point of view of macromolecular chemistry; the models and the tools provided by the soft matter physical-chemical community resulted in a better understanding of the mechanisms involved during their assembly to perform analogous task of the biological molecular machines (Kay et al. 2007). For example, cells, muscles, and connective tissue owe their remarkable mechanical properties to the complex biological macromolecular assemblies that are predominantly made from mixtures of stiff biopolymers (Kroy 2006; Meyers et al. 2008). As the hardness of these biopolymers, and the resulting anisotropic networks leading to its smart mechanical and dynamic properties, are far from being understood, a better comprehension of their incessant assembly, disassembly, restructuring, active and passive mechanical deformation can be achieved by physical-chemical theoretical modeling (Dobrynin and Carrillo 2010; Pritchard et al. 2014). Moreover, molecular biologists can create accurate mutations of specific groups at precise points along the chain for understanding, for example, the influence of a particular residue on the folding–unfolding process; its stimulus on biopolymer mechanical properties can be directly obtained by atomic force microscopy (AFM) measurements (Alessandrini and Facci 2005). It should be noted that some implants and devices, such as artificial heart valves, are comprised of more than one class of biomaterial. Bio-nanocomposites is a fascinating and interdisciplinary topic that constitutes a great area of interest for biomedical technologies such as tissue engineering (Zhang et al. 2008), medical implants (Negroiu et al. 2008; Rathenow et al. 2004; Kidane et al. 2009), dental applications (Chen 2010), and controlled drug delivery (Morgan et al. 2008; Ke et al. 2011). Biopolymer nano-composites are the result of the precise combination of biopolymers and inorganic/organic units that interact at the nanometer scale. The extraordinary versatility of these new materials that comes from the large range of biopolymers and fillers available, such as clays, cellulose whiskers, and metal nanoparticles, can be tailored only by the correct confluence of multidisciplinary methodologies (Chassenieux et al. 2013). An extremely valuable tool for various applications in the science of biomaterials (Sionkowska 2011) is the use of hybrid polymer systems composed of natural and synthetic macromolecules. The goal of bio-artificial blending is to produce man-made assortments that confer unique structural and mechanical properties on the base of the individual properties of natural polymers and synthetic polymers. Biopolymer's blends are well known to exhibit a very rich and applicable phase behaviors (Chapman et al. 2012; Sionkowska 2011) and the miscibility of their components is an important aspect in determining the properties of the blend. The understanding of the underlying physics of these phase behaviors and of the rheology–morphology relationships of the resulting phases constitutes an interesting and important challenge for their optimal applications (Chassenieux et al. 2013). Actually, biomaterials scientists and engineers have developed a growing interest in natural tissues and biopolymers in combination with living cells. This is particularly evident in the field of tissue engineering, which focuses on the repair or regeneration of natural tissues and organs (Ratner et al. 2004). This interest has stimulated the development of novel technologies for the isolation, purification, and application of many different natural materials, including de-cellularized natural tissues and spider silk.

Biopolymers for Hard and Soft Tissue Regenerations

Although the reconstruction of small or moderate sized tissue imperfections are technically feasible, thanks to the natural ability of the body to repair itself, larger volume defects remain problematic. The state-of-the-art of medical and surgical therapies continues to be suboptimal, in part because of a lack of replacement biological parts (Bressan et al. 2011). In this sense, many natural biomaterials based on biopolymers have been widely considered for hard and soft tissue reconstruction. They can be used alone or combined with other synthetic or inorganic constituents. The main properties of these tissue engineered materials are the special dressing, nursing care, and the reduced time in grafting. Regardless of their mechanical fragility and high cost, many recent *in vivo* investigations contributed to the FDA approval of new biomaterials for clinical use based on natural biopolymers as matrices for cell delivery and as scaffolds for cell-free support of native tissues. Some selected examples are summarized in Table 2.

Biopolymers gels for cell encapsulation

Mammalian cells encapsulation on biopolymer gels becomes an increasing area of interest in regenerative medicine (Hunt and Grover 2010). The application these strategies to TE can be split into two main categories (Nedovic and Willaert 2013): (i) the replacement of the biochemical function or (ii) the replacement of the structurally functional tissue. Cell encapsulation in biopolymer hydrogels was originally explored for immuno isolation of cells producing therapeutic proteins for treatment of diseases. In such strategy it is required the chemical communication in the scaffold (i.e., diffusion of molecules),so it is possible to deliver cells encapsulated in an immuno isolatory nanoporous polymer membrane. The membranes are constructed in a way that their pores have to be large enough to allow nutrients, waste, and bioactive factors to diffuse but not so large as to allow immune cells to attack the cells inside (Nedovic and Willaert 2013). This strategy has mainly been employed to temporarily or permanently replace biochemical functions of the liver pancreas, and provide local protein delivery in neurological disorders. More recently, encapsulation of mammalian cells has been used in the regeneration of an array of different tissues. This second major strategy involves entrapping cells on a micro- or macro-porous polymer scaffold and promoting the formation of a new tissue that is structurally and functionally integrated with the surrounding tissue. The scaffold is constructed with a biocompatible material that it will degrade over time to leave only the integrated tissue in its place. A variety of naturally derived and synthetic biopolymers that can be processed into many different physical forms and geometries are used for cell encapsulation. The biomaterial component of these therapies must provide the appropriate mass transport properties, membrane or scaffold stability, and desirable cellular interactions depending on the location and desired function of the implant. Some of these studies are summarized in Table 2.

Stimuli responsive hydrogels based on biopolymers

Intelligent hydrogels based on biopolymers which can change their swelling behavior and other properties in response to chemical and physical stimuli such as pH, metabolites or/and ionic factors, temperature and electric fields, have attracted great interest. These "smart" hydrogels, in addition to their biocompatibility, biodegradability, and biological functions, exhibit single or multiple stimuli-responsive characters which could be used in biomedical applications, ranging from controlled drug delivery systems and cell adhesion mediators to controllers of enzyme function and gene expression in bioengineering or tissue engineering. Among them, temperature- and pH-responsive hydrogels have been the most widely studied, because these two factors have physiological significance (Oh et al. 2009; Chilkoti et al. 2006; Prabaharan and Mano 2006; Alarcon et al. 2005). Biopolymers having a lower critical solution temperature (LCST) below human body temperature have a potential for injectable depot systems in therapeutic delivery systems and in tissue engineering. A number of polysaccharides have been considered to be combined with the thermo-responsive materials including chitosan, alginate, cellulose, and dextran. Due to the pH-sensitive character of chitosan or alginate, combination of these polymers with a thermoresponsive material will produce dual-stimuli-responsive polymeric gels to be used as delivery vehicles that respond to localized conditions of pH and temperature in the human body (Prabaharan and Mano 2006). Control over the function of a therapeutic biopolymer can be obtained by polymer–biopolymer conjugate chemistry. Responsive polymer–biopolymer conjugates have been extensively studied by Hoffman, Stayton, and co-workers (Hoffman 2013; Pack et al. 2005). They reported a temperature and photochemically switchable endoglucanase that displayed varying and opposite activities depending whether temperature or UV–Vis illumination was used as the switch (Shimoboji et al. 2002). Regarding synthetic polymers, Poly(N-isopropylacrylamide) (PNIPAm) is the most studied. It undergoes a sharp coil–globule transition in water at 32°C, changing from a hydrophilic to a hydrophobic state below this temperature. Surface modification of materials can be used to control and modulate cellular-material interactions, for example, to promote bone and skin cell interaction with the implant, and to prevent the adhesion of unwanted cells. Okano and co-workers have extensively used thermoresponsive PNIPAm-based polymers as surface mediators of biopolymer and cell attachment (Okano and Winnik 2010; Peppas et al. 2010). Human skin fibroblasts have been shown to attach to and proliferate at the surface of thermoresponsive hydrogels of ethylene glycol vinyl ether and butyl vinyl ether co-polymers. Cultured cells were readily detached from the polymer surface by lowering the incubation temperature from 37°C to 10°C for 30 min. Incorporation of Arg-Gly-Asp (RGD) peptides at the surfaces resulted in higher values of cell proliferation in the initial stage (Gümüşderelioğlu and Karakeçili 2003). Stile and Healy, extended this concept by the preparation of PNIPAm–RGD conjugates and manipulated osteoblast adhesion (Stile et al. 2003).

3D bio-printed scaffolds

In order to permit cell morphogenesis associated with living tissue function, there is a need to supply the cells with appropriate stimuli within their physical 3D support structure. As it was mentioned in previous sections, biomimetic hydrogel scaffolds can be easily designed using natural ECM components, including collagen or fibrin. However, the range of physical properties, such as stiffness and mesh size—which can be controlled by the gelation process of the purified proteins—is relatively narrow. In addition, these materials are not typically available in large quantities and suffer from batch-to batch variations. Several attempts were made to improve the properties of protein hydrogel scaffolds by the introduction of covalent cross-linking, improving the self-assembly of the protein molecules or adding a coexistent polymer network (Zhu and Marchant 2011; Rajaram et al. 2015; Suo et al. 2014; Ahmed 2013). Because most of the conventional techniques for scaffold preparation are limited when it comes to the spatial control of porosity and pore size, computer-aided design (CAD) and advanced manufacturing techniques to improve scaffold development have been adopted by the tissue engineering community (Li et al. 2014; Bose et al. 2013). 3D bio-printing refers to the application of 3D printing technologies towards the development of precisely defined scaffolds for tissue regeneration. Although in the middle of 1990s the term was reserved only for inkjet-based approaches, nowadays it is collectively used for all additive manufacturing (AM) processes (Li et al. 2014; Gross et al. 2014). 3D printing strategies can be applied, in one way or another, to bio-printing; these include: stereolithography (SLA) (Dhariwala et al. 2004), selective laser sintering (SLS) (Chang et al. 2011), fused deposition modeling (FDM) (Mironov et al. 2008), syringe deposition (Zhang et al. 2015), two photon laser lithography (Müller et al. 2013), powder printing (Gbureck et al. 2007), 3D inkjet printing (Xu et al. 2006), and organ printing (Mironov et al. 2009). All of these AM technologies have in common the capability to build a scaffold or tissue construct with complicated 3D geometries, without the necessity of tooling, directly from CAD files and using chloroform for binding polylactic acid (PLA) and polyglycolic acid (PGA) powders in a powder binding approach. Chloroform was used for selective solvation of the polymeric particles, resulting in particle adhesion upon chloroform evaporation (Li et al. 2014). Engineers and clinicians arrived to a widespread consensus that 3D bio-printing will permit the manufacturing of much more complex and intricate scaffolds for tissue regeneration, mainly because of the opportunities it presents for customizing scaffold shape, structural complexity, and cellular organization. Selected examples are summarized in Table 2.

"Engineered" peptide-based biopolymers in biomedicine and biotechnology

In the 1950s, the fundamental polypeptides structural features were elucidated. Forty years later, Ghadiri (Ghadiri et al. 1993) and Zhang (Zhang et al. 1993) demonstrated that these rules can be exploited and adapted to produce supramolecular peptide based materials (Zelzer and Ulijn 2010). A fresh class of biomaterials becomes known due to the exceptional chemical, physical, and biological properties of the "engineered" peptide-based biopolymers. The expansion of peptide-based biomaterials was motivated by the convergence of protein engineering and macromolecular self-assembly (Chow et al. 2008). Prototypical examples of engineered peptide-based biomaterials include poly-amino acids, elastin-like polypeptides, silk-like proteins, coiled-coil domains, tropoelastin-based peptides, leucinezipper-based peptides, peptide amphiphiles, beta-sheet forming ionic oligopeptides, and beta-hairpin peptides (Chow et al. 2008). In addition, biopolymers can be easily functionalized to enhance their interactions with cells and provide an optimal platform for cellular activities and tissue functions. In this section, we will discuss two main classes of peptide-based biopolymers in tissue engineering: self-assembling polypeptides that form gels by environmental stimuli and polypeptides that form gels via chemical crosslinking.

The first class of hydrogels is based on naturally occurring fibrin, which is spontaneously formed by the polymerization of fibrinogen in the presence of thrombin and further cross-linked by the transglutaminase activity of factor XIIIa (Ehrbar et al. 2005; Schmoekel et al. 2005; Park et al. 2009; Sakiyama et al. 1999; Lee et al. 2010;

Nettles et al. 2008; McHale et al. 2005). Gel formulations prepared from fibrin glue plus matrix-bound vascular endothelial growth factors (VEGFs) are also promising candidate substrates for expansion or transplantation of endothelial progenitor cells (EPCs). Ehrbar et al. studied three variant forms (VEGF121), formulated within fibrin matrices, each with differential susceptibility to local cellular proteolytic activity (Ehrbar et al. 2005). Fibrin matrices were also successfully improved with bone morphogenetic protein-2 (BMP-2) to promote bone growth and healing (Schmoekel et al. 2005; Park et al. 2009) and with heparin-binding proteins to promote neuritis extension (Sakiyama et al. 1999; Lee et al. 2010). Elastin-like polypeptides (ELP) are useful for thermally sensitive injectable hydrogels because they undergo an inverse temperature phase transition and can be designed at the molecular level. The study of ELPs was pioneered by Dan Urry (Urry 1984), who synthesized a large number of polypeptides over the course of three decades and studied their biophysical properties in solution and as cross-linked elastomeric materials. ELPs have been investigated as an alternative scaffold for cartilage repair (McHale et al. 2005; Nettles et al. 2008). To emulate the triple helical structure of collagen, peptide-amphiphiles (PAs) consisting of a collagen sequence Gly-Val-Lys-Gly-Asp-Lys-Gly-Asn-Pro-Gly-Trp-Pro-Gly-Ala-Pro connected to a long-chain mono- or di-alkyl ester lipid, have been synthesized by Fields, Tirrell and coworkers (Yu et al. 1999). Neither the peptide nor the tail alone produced significant adhesion of melanoma cells; however, the self-assembled triple helical structure of the PA significantly promoted cell adhesion (Fields et al. 1998).

In the second class of hydrogels, chemically cross-linked 3D networks are formed by Michael-type addition reactions between thiol-bearing bioactive peptides and conjugated unsaturations on single- or multi-armed poly(ethylene glycol) (PEG) chains end functionalized with vinyl sulfone (Hubbell 2003). ELP are also good candidates for chemical crosslinking, because it is easy to incorporate chemically active amino acids at the guest residue position in the elastin-based repeat unit, Val-Pro-Gly-Xaa-Gly and in addition, because ELPs can be designed at the molecular level and genetically synthesized, unique properties can be introduced by incorporating other biologically active peptide sequences. Examples can be found of ELP hydrogels that are formed by irradiation (Annabi et al. 2009a), photo-initiation (Almany and Seliktar 2005), amine-reactive chemical crosslinking (Annabi et al. 2009b), and enzymatic crosslinking by tissue transglutaminase (McHale et al. 2005; Davis et al. 2010; Collighan and Griffin 2009). The hydrogels have been successfully used for cartilage and intervertebral disc tissue repair, small-diameter vascular grafts, urinary bladders, stem cell matrices, neural guides, stem cell sheets, and post-surgical wound treatment (Simnick et al. 2007; Chow et al. 2008; Lim 2007). The application of chemically cross-linked ELP hydrogels for *in situ* gelation by chemical crosslinking has been limited by poor solubility in water, concerns about toxicity, lack of biocompatible crosslinking reagents and by products, or slow gelation kinetics. Even though peptide-based biomaterials have become increasingly significant materials in regenerative medicine, their use has restrictions, related to their short shelf life and thermal instability. Many of these limitations can be addressed by emerging technologies, thus further expanding the uses of peptide-based biomaterials into applications for which they are currently impractical.

Perspectives and Outlooks

Biomaterial design and its application to regenerative medicine have made great strides in the past decades and holds tremendous impact for future clinical applications. Sustained growth of this field centers in part on the development of novel materials and improved scaffold processing techniques. The specificities of the biopolymer block in terms of bioactivity, biocompatibility, and biodegradability allow specific application over the bio-medical fields. Polymer–biopolymer interactions can increasingly be designed as well as selected, and so their intervention in cellular dysfunctions may be possible and lead to more powerful, specific, and potent therapies. Moreover, a deeper comprehension of the underlying mechanisms of tissue regeneration would contribute invaluably to tailoring scaffold properties in a more representative manner of the native environment. Currently, the focus has been on addressing biomimetic surface topography for influencing cell behavior, controlled delivery of bioactive signals to stimulate regeneration, bone construct vascularization, articular cartilage zonal architecture, and osteochondral interface integration. Polymer chains can be prepared with individual segments that respond to pH, temperature, ionic strength, UV irradiation and electric fields, affording truly multifunctional materials. 'Chemically-responsive' systems, such as the glucose-sensitive polymers, are also becoming accessible. Structure–function relationships previously only obtainable for biomacromolecules can now be deduced for wholly synthetic materials owing to the degree of control accessible through living polymerisation methodologies, while biopolymer synthesis and activity can be manipulated through molecular biology approaches. This convergence of synthetic and natural macromolecular chemistry inherently leads to biomedical applications, as the ability to control polymer structure leads to the ability to manipulate functionality. Bio-printers can automate the assembly process and permit pre-programmed and complex manipulation of biopolymers—from the macromolecular to the living cell level—to achieve architectural and biochemical complexity that was never before possible and produce tissue and organ substitutes that precisely mimic their natural counterparts. It is expected that these diverse methodologies for regenerative medicine will translate from 'bench to bedside' in the future.

Acknowledgements

The authors acknowledge Universidad Nacional del Sur (PGI 24/Q064), Concejo Nacional de Investigaciones Científicas y Técnicas de la República Argentina (CONICET, PIP—11220130100100CO) and Fundación Ramón Areces. PVM is an independent researcher of CONICET.

References

2014. Advancing regenerative medicine. Nat. Med. 20: 795–795.
Ahmed, E. M. 2013. Hydrogel: preparation, characterization, and applications. A review. Journal of Advanced Research 6: 105–121.

Alarcon, C. D. L. H., S. Pennadam and C. Alexander. 2005. Stimuli responsive polymers for biomedical applications. Chemical Society Reviews 34: 276–285.

Alessandrini, A. and P. Facci. 2005. AFM: a versatile tool in biophysics. Measurement Science and Technology 16: R65.

Alhusein, N., I. S. Blagbrough and A. Paul. 2012. Electrospun matrices for localised controlled drug delivery: release of tetracycline hydrochloride from layers of polycaprolactone and poly (ethylene-co-vinyl acetate). Drug Delivery and Translational Research 2: 477–488.

Allen, C., J. Han, Y. Yu, D. Maysinger and A. Eisenberg. 2000. Polycaprolactone–b-poly (ethylene oxide) copolymer micelles as a delivery vehicle for dihydrotestosterone. Journal of Controlled Release 63: 275–286.

Almany, L. and D. Seliktar. 2005. Biosynthetic hydrogel scaffolds made from fibrinogen and polyethylene glycol for 3D cell cultures. Biomaterials 26: 2467–2477.

Anegg, U., J. Lindenmann, V. Matzi, J. Smolle, A. Maier and F. Smolle-Jüttner. 2007. Efficiency of fleece-bound sealing (TachoSil®) of air leaks in lung surgery: a prospective randomised trial. European Journal of Cardio-Thoracic Surgery 31: 198–202.

Annabi, N., S. M. Mithieux, E. A. Boughton, A. J. Ruys, A. S. Weiss and F. Dehghani. 2009a. Synthesis of highly porous crosslinked elastin hydrogels and their interaction with fibroblasts *in vitro*. Biomaterials 30: 4550–4557.

Annabi, N., S. M. Mithieux, A. S. Weiss and F. Dehghani. 2009b. The fabrication of elastin-based hydrogels using high pressure CO_2. Biomaterials 30: 1–7.

Apel, P. J., J. P. Garrett, P. Sierpinski, J. Ma, A. Atala, T. L. Smith, L. A. Koman and M. E. Van Dyke. 2008. Peripheral nerve regeneration using a keratin-based scaffold: long-term functional and histological outcomes in a mouse model. The Journal of Hand Surgery 33: 1541–1547.

Astm International, W. C., PA. 1994. ASTM D5488-94de1, Standard Terminology of Environmental Labeling of Packaging Materials and Packages, www.astm.org.

Astm International, W. C., PA. 1996. ASTM D6002-96, Standard Guide for Assessing the Compostability of Environmentally Degradable Plastics, www.astm.org.

Astm International, W. C., PA. 2011a. ASTM D6002-96(2002)e1, Standard Guide for Assessing the Compostability of Environmentally Degradable Plastics (Withdrawn 2011), www.astm.org.

Astm International, W. C., PA. 2011b. ASTM D6868-11, Standard Specification for Labeling of End Items that Incorporate Plastics and Polymers as Coatings or Additives with Paper and Other Substrates Designed to be Aerobically Composted in Municipal or Industrial Facilities, www.astm.org.

Astm International, W. C., PA. 2012a. ASTM D6400-12, Standard Specification for Labeling of Plastics Designed to be Aerobically Composted in Municipal or Industrial Facilities, www.astm.org.

Astm International, W. C., PA. 2012b. ASTM D6866-12, Standard Test Methods for Determining the Biobased Content of Solid, Liquid, and Gaseous Samples Using Radiocarbon Analysis, www.astm.org.

Atala, A., R. Lanza, J. A. Thomson and R. Nerem. 2010. Principles of Regenerative Medicine. Academic Press, London NW1 7BY, UK; Burlington, MA 01803, USA and San Diego, CA 92101-4495, USA.

Atala, A. and J. Allickson. 2014. Translational Regenerative Medicine. Academic Press, London NW1 7BY, UK; Burlington, MA 01803, USA and San Diego, CA 92101-4495, USA.

Azad, A. K., N. Sermsintham, S. Chandrkrachang and W. F. Stevens. 2004. Chitosan membrane as a wound-healing dressing: characterization and clinical application. Journal of Biomedical Materials Research Part B: Applied Biomaterials 69: 216–222.

Barker, T. H. 2011. The role of ECM proteins and protein fragments in guiding cell behavior in regenerative medicine. Biomaterials 32: 4211–4214.

Bellomo, E. G., M. D. Wyrsta, L. Pakstis, D. J. Pochan and T. J. Deming. 2004. Stimuli-responsive polypeptide vesicles by conformation-specific assembly. Nature Materials 3: 244–248.

Beltrán, V., A. Matthijs, E. Borie, R. Fuentes, I. Valdivia-Gandur, W. Engelke et al. 2013. Bone healing in transverse maxillary defects with different surgical procedures using anorganic bovine bone in humans. International Journal of Morphology 31: 75–81.

Bessa, P. C., M. Casal and R. Reis. 2008. Bone morphogenetic proteins in tissue engineering: the road from laboratory to the clinic, part II (BMP delivery). Journal of Tissue Engineering and Regenerative Medicine 2: 81–96.

Boland, E. D., J. A. Matthews, K. J. Pawlowski, D. G. Simpson, G. E. Wnek and G. L. Bowlin. 2004. Electrospinning collagen and elastin: preliminary vascular tissue engineering. Front Biosci. 9: C1432.

Bose, S., S. Vahabzadeh and A. Bandyopadhyay. 2013. Bone tissue engineering using 3D printing. Materials Today 16: 496–504.

Bourgeat-Lami, E., I. Tissot and F. Lefebvre. 2002. Synthesis and characterization of SiOH-functionalized polymer latexes using methacryloxy propyl trimethoxysilane in emulsion polymerization. Macromolecules 35: 6185–6191.

Bressan, E., V. Favero, C. Gardin, L. Ferroni, L. Iacobellis, L. Favero et al. 2011. Biopolymers for hard and soft engineered tissues: application in odontoiatric and plastic surgery field. Polymers 3: 509–526.

Brosnan, S. M., A. H. Brown and V. S. Ashby. 2013. It is the outside that counts: chemical and physical control of dynamic surfaces. Journal of the American Chemical Society 135: 3067–3072.

Burdick, J. A. and G. D. Prestwich. 2011. Hyaluronic acid hydrogels for biomedical applications. Advanced Materials 23: H41–H56.

Cao, T., K.-H. Ho and S.-H. Teoh. 2003. Scaffold design and *in vitro* study of osteochondral coculture in a three-dimensional porous polycaprolactone scaffold fabricated by fused deposition modeling. Tissue Engineering 9: 103–112.

Chaikof, E. L., H. Matthew, J. Kohn, A. G. Mikos, G. D. Prestwich and C. M. Yip. 2002. Biomaterials and scaffolds in reparative medicine. Annals of the New York Academy of Sciences 961: 96–105.

Chang, C. C., E. D. Boland, S. K. Williams and J. B. Hoying. 2011. Direct-write bioprinting three-dimensional biohybrid systems for future regenerative therapies. Journal of Biomedical Materials Research Part B: Applied Biomaterials 98: 160–170.

Chapman, C. D., S. Shanbhag, D. E. Smith and R. M. Robertson-Anderson. 2012. Complex effects of molecular topology on diffusion in entangled biopolymer blends. Soft Matter 8: 9177–9182.

Chassenieux, C., D. Durand, P. Jyotishkumar and S. Thomas. 2013. Biopolymers: state of the art, new challenges, and opportunities. pp. 1–6. *In*: Thomas, S., D. Durand, C. Chassenieux and P. Jyotishkumar (eds.). Handbook of Biopolymer-Based Materials: From Blends and Composites to Gels and Complex Networks, Wiley-VCH Verlag GmbH & Co. KGaA.

Chen, F. H., K. T. Rousche and R. S. Tuan. 2006. Technology Insight: adult stem cells in cartilage regeneration and tissue engineering. Nature Clinical Practice Rheumatology 2: 373–382.

Chen, M.-H. 2010. Update on dental nanocomposites. Journal of Dental Research 89: 549–560.

Cheng, C., S. Li, S. Nie, W. Zhao, H. Yang, S. Sun et al. 2012. General and biomimetic approach to biopolymer-functionalized graphene oxide nanosheet through adhesive dopamine. Biomacromolecules 13: 4236–4246.

Cherubino, M. and K. G. Marra. 2009. Adipose-derived stem cells for soft tissue reconstruction. Regenerative Medicine 4: 109–117.

Chien, Y., Y.-W. Liao, D.-M. Liu, H.-L. Lin, S.-J. Chen, H.-L. Chen et al. 2012. Corneal repair by human corneal keratocyte-reprogrammed iPSCs and amphiphatic carboxymethyl-hexanoyl chitosan hydrogel. Biomaterials 33: 8003–8016.

Chilkoti, A., T. Christensen and J. A. Mackay. 2006. Stimulus responsive elastin biopolymers: applications in medicine and biotechnology. Current Opinion in Chemical Biology 10: 652–657.

Chow, D., M. L. Nunalee, D. W. Lim, A. J. Simnick and A. Chilkoti. 2008. Peptide-based biopolymers in biomedicine and biotechnology. Materials Science and Engineering: R: Reports 62: 125–155.

Christman, K. L., H. H. Fok, R. E. Sievers, Q. Fang and R. J. Lee. 2004. Fibrin glue alone and skeletal myoblasts in a fibrin scaffold preserve cardiac function after myocardial infarction. Tissue Engineering 10: 403–409.

Collighan, R. and M. Griffin. 2009. Transglutaminase 2 cross-linking of matrix proteins: biological significance and medical applications. Amino Acids 36: 659–670.

Crow, B., A. Borneman, D. Hawkins, G. Smith and K. Nelson. 2005. Evaluation of *in vitro* drug release, pH change, and molecular weight degradation of poly (L-lactic acid) and poly (D, L-lactide-co-glycolide) fibers. Tissue Engineering 11: 1077–1084.

D'elía, N. L., A. N. Gravina, J. M. Ruso, J. A. Laiuppa, G. E. Santillán and P. V. Messina. 2013. Manipulating the bioactivity of hydroxyapatite nano-rods structured networks: effects on mineral coating morphology and growth kinetic. Biochimica et Biophysica Acta (BBA)-General Subjects 1830: 5014–5026.

Dai, N.-T., M. Williamson, N. Khammo, E. Adams and A. Coombes. 2004. Composite cell support membranes based on collagen and polycaprolactone for tissue engineering of skin. Biomaterials 25: 4263–4271.

Dalsin, J. L., B.-H. Hu, B. P. Lee and P. B. Messersmith. 2003. Mussel adhesive protein mimetic polymers for the preparation of nonfouling surfaces. Journal of the American Chemical Society 125: 4253–4258.

Davis, N. E., S. Ding, R. E. Forster, D. M. Pinkas and A. E. Barron. 2010. Modular enzymatically crosslinked protein polymer hydrogels for *in situ* gelation. Biomaterials 31: 7288–7297.

De Vicente, J. C., G. Hernández-Vallejo, P. Braña-Abascal and I. Peña. 2010. Maxillary sinus augmentation with autologous bone harvested from the lateral maxillary wall combined with bovine-derived hydroxyapatite: clinical and histologic observations. Clinical Oral Implants Research 21: 430–438.

Dhariwala, B., E. Hunt and T. Boland. 2004. Rapid prototyping of tissue engineering constructs, using photopolymerizable hydrogels and stereolithography. Tissue Engineering 10: 1316–1322.

Dobrynin, A. V. and J.-M. Y. Carrillo. 2010. Universality in nonlinear elasticity of biological and polymeric networks and gels. Macromolecules 44: 140–146.

Dutta, P. K. and J. Dutta. 2013. Multifaceted Development and Application of Biopolymers for Biology, Biomedicine and Nanotechnology. Springer-Verlag, Berlin-Heidelberg.

Efron, N. 2010. Contact Lens Practice. Elsevier Health Sciences, United Kingdom.

Ehrbar, M., A. Metters, P. Zammaretti, J. A. Hubbell and A. H. Zisch. 2005. Endothelial cell proliferation and progenitor maturation by fibrin-bound VEGF variants with differential susceptibilities to local cellular activity. Journal of Controlled Release 101: 93–109.

Elisseeff, J., K. Anseth, D. Sims, W. Mcintosh, M. Randolph, M. Yaremchuk et al. 1999. Transdermal photopolymerization of poly (ethylene oxide)-based injectable hydrogels for tissue-engineered cartilage. Plastic and Reconstructive Surgery 104: 1014–1022.

Elisseeff, J., C. Puleo, F. Yang and B. Sharma. 2005. Advances in skeletal tissue engineering with hydrogels. Orthodontics & Craniofacial Research 8: 150–161.

Elloumi-Hannachi, I., M. Yamato and T. Okano. 2010. Cell sheet engineering: a unique nanotechnology for scaffold-free tissue reconstruction with clinical applications in regenerative medicine. Journal of Internal Medicine 267: 54–70.

Errico, C., C. Bartoli, F. Chiellini and E. Chiellini. 2009. Poly (hydroxyalkanoates)-based polymeric nanoparticles for drug delivery. BioMed. Research International.

Estrada, L. H. and J. Champion. 2015. Protein nanoparticles for therapeutic protein delivery. Biomaterials Science 3: 787–799.

Evans, D. G., J. C. Kelly and T. M. Dewitt. 2004. Resorbable structure for treating and healing of tissue defects. US Patent 20040006146 A1.

Evans, G. R., K. Brandt, S. Katz, P. Chauvin, L. Otto, M. Bogle et al. 2002. Bioactive poly (L-lactic acid) conduits seeded with Schwann cells for peripheral nerve regeneration. Biomaterials 23: 841–848.

Ferreira, C. E., A. B. Novaes, Jr., V. I. Haraszthy, M. Bittencourt, C. B. Martinelli and S. M. Luczyszyn. 2009. A clinical study of 406 sinus augmentations with 100% anorganic bovine bone. Journal of Periodontology 80: 1920–1927.

Fields, G. B., J. L. Lauer, Y. Dori, P. Forns, Y. C. Yu and M. Tirrell. 1998. Protein like molecular architecture: biomaterial applications for inducing cellular receptor binding and signal transduction. Peptide Science 47: 143–151.

Fujihara, K., M. Kotaki and S. Ramakrishna. 2005. Guided bone regeneration membrane made of polycaprolactone/calcium carbonate composite nano-fibers. Biomaterials 26: 4139–4147.

Gbureck, U., T. Hölzel, U. Klammert, K. Würzler, F. A. Müller and J. E. Barralet. 2007. Resorbable dicalcium phosphate bone substitutes prepared by 3D powder printing. Advanced Functional Materials 17: 3940–3945.

Geckil, H., F. Xu, X. Zhang, S. Moon and U. Demirci. 2010. Engineering hydrogels as extracellular matrix mimics. Nanomedicine 5: 469–484.

Ghadiri, M. R., J. R. Granja, R. A. Milligan, D. E. Mcree and N. Khazanovich. 1993. Self-assembling organic nanotubes based on a cyclic peptide architecture. Nature 366: 324–327.

Ghidoni, I., T. Chlapanidas, M. Bucco, F. Crovato, M. Marazzi, D. Vigo et al. 2008. Alginate cell encapsulation: new advances in reproduction and cartilage regenerative medicine. Cytotechnology 58: 49–56.

Gomes, M. E., H. L. Holtorf, R. L. Reis and A. G. Mikos. 2006. Influence of the porosity of starch-based fiber mesh scaffolds on the proliferation and osteogenic differentiation of bone marrow stromal cells cultured in a flow perfusion bioreactor. Tissue Engineering 12: 801–809.

Gravina, A. N., J. M. Ruso, J. A. Laiuppa, G. E. Santillán, J. L. Marco-Brown, N. L. D'Elia et al. 2014. Striped, bioactive Ce–TiO$_2$ materials with peroxynitrite-scavenging activity. Journal of Materials Chemistry B 2: 834–845.

Gravina, N., J. M. Ruso, D. A. Mbeh, L. H. Yahia, Y. Merhi, J. Sartuqui et al. 2015. Effect of ceria on the organization and bio-ability of anatase fullerene-like crystals. RSC Advances 5: 8077–8087.

Grinnell, F. 1984. Fibronectin and wound healing. Journal of Cellular Biochemistry 26: 107–116.

Gross, B. C., J. L. Erkal, S. Y. Lockwood, C. Chen and D. M. Spence. 2014. Evaluation of 3D printing and its potential impact on biotechnology and the chemical sciences. Analytical Chemistry 86: 3240–3253.

Gümüşderelioğlu, M. and A. G. Karakeçili. 2003. Uses of thermoresponsive and RGD/insulin-modified poly (vinyl ether)-based hydrogels in cell cultures. Journal of Biomaterials Science, Polymer Edition 14: 199–211.

Gustafson, S. B., P. Fulkerson, R. Bildfell, L. Aguilera and T. M. Hazzard. 2007. Chitosan dressing provides hemostasis in swine femoral arterial injury model. Prehospital Emergency Care 11: 172–178.

Halim, A. S., T. L. Khoo and S. J. M. Yussof. 2010. Biologic and synthetic skin substitutes: an overview. Indian journal of plastic surgery: official publication of the Association of Plastic Surgeons of India 43: S23.

Hammer, D. A. and N. P. Kamat. 2012. Towards an artificial cell. FEBS Letters 586: 2882–2890.

Han, Y., T. Bai and W. Liu. 2014. Controlled Heterogeneous Stem Cell Differentiation on a Shape Memory Hydrogel Surface. Scientific Reports 4.

Hart, C. E., A. Loewen-Rodriguez and J. Lessem. 2012. Dermagraft: use in the treatment of chronic wounds. Advances in Wound Care 1: 138–141.

Hassan, N., A. Soltero, D. Pozzo, P. V. Messina and J. M. Ruso. 2012a. Bioinspired templates for the synthesis of silica nanostructures. Soft Matter 8: 9553–9562.

Hassan, N., V. Verdinelli, J. M. Ruso and P. V. Messina. 2012b. Assessing structure and dynamics of fibrinogen films on silicon nanofibers: towards hemocompatibility devices. Soft Matter 8: 6582–6592.

Heimbach, D. M., G. D. Warden, A. Luterman, M. H. Jordan, N. Ozobia, C. M. Ryan et al. 2003. Multicenter postapproval clinical trial of Integra® dermal regeneration template for burn treatment. Journal of Burn Care & Research 24: 42–48.

Hench, L. L. and J. M. Polak. 2002. Third-generation biomedical materials. Science 295: 1014–1017.

Hoffman, A. S. 2013. Stimuli-responsive polymers: biomedical applications and challenges for clinical translation. Advanced Drug Delivery Reviews 65: 10–16.

Hong, H. and J. P. Stegemann. 2008. 2D and 3D collagen and fibrin biopolymers promote specific ECM and integrin gene expression by vascular smooth muscle cells. Journal of Biomaterials Science, Polymer Edition 19: 1279–1293.

Hook, A. L., D. G. Anderson, R. Langer, P. Williams, M. C. Davies and M. R. Alexander. 2010. High throughput methods applied in biomaterial development and discovery. Biomaterials 31: 187–198.

Horn, E. M., M. Beaumont, X. Z. Shu, A. Harvey, G. D. Prestwich, K. M. Horn et al. 2007. Influence of cross-linked hyaluronic acid hydrogels on neurite outgrowth and recovery from spinal cord injury. Journal of Neurosurgery: Spine 6: 133–140.

Hubbell, J. A. 2003. Materials as morphogenetic guides in tissue engineering. Current Opinion in Biotechnology 14: 551–558.

Hunt, N. C. and L. M. Grover. 2010. Cell encapsulation using biopolymer gels for regenerative medicine. Biotechnology Letters 32: 733–742.

Imam, S. H., R. V. Greene and B. R. Zaidi. 1999. Biopolymers: Utilizing Nature's Advanced Materials. American Chemical Society, Washington, DC.

Jagur-Grodzinski, J. 2006. Polymers for tissue engineering, medical devices, and regenerative medicine. Concise general review of recent studies. Polymers for Advanced Technologies 17: 395–418.

Jia, X., Y. Yeo, R. J. Clifton, T. Jiao, D. S. Kohane, J. B. Kobler et al. 2006. Hyaluronic acid-based microgels and microgel networks for vocal fold regeneration. Biomacromolecules 7: 3336–3344.

Jiang, Y., J. Chen, C. Deng, E. J. Suuronen and Z. Zhong. 2014. Click hydrogels, microgels and nanogels: emerging platforms for drug delivery and tissue engineering. Biomaterials 35: 4969–4985.

Jonker, A. M., D. W. LöWik and J. C. Van Hest. 2012. Peptide-and protein-based hydrogels. Chemistry of Materials 24: 759–773.

Jordan, S. W., C. A. Haller, R. E. Sallach, R. P. Apkarian, S. R. Hanson and E. L. Chaikof. 2007. The effect of a recombinant elastin-mimetic coating of an ePTFE prosthesis on acute thrombogenicity in a baboon arteriovenous shunt. Biomaterials 28: 1191–1197.

Jung, R. E., G. A. Hälg, D. S. Thoma and C. H. Hämmerle. 2009a. A randomized, controlled clinical trial to evaluate a new membrane for guided bone regeneration around dental implants. Clinical Oral Implants Research 20: 162–168.

Jung, R. E., S. I. Windisch, A. M. Eggenschwiler, D. S. Thoma, F. E. Weber and C. H. Hämmerle. 2009b. A randomized-controlled clinical trial evaluating clinical and radiological outcomes after 3 and 5 years of dental implants placed in bone regenerated by means of GBR techniques with or without the addition of BMP-2. Clinical Oral Implants Research 20: 660–666.

Kalia, S. and L. Avérous. 2011. Biopolymers: Biomedical and Environmental Applications. John Wiley & Sons. Scrivener Publishing 3 Winter Street, Suite 3 Salem, MA 01970.

Kang, S.-W., O. Jeon and B.-S. Kim. 2005. Poly (lactic-co-glycolic acid) microspheres as an injectable scaffold for cartilage tissue engineering. Tissue Engineering 11: 438–447.

Kay, E. R., D. A. Leigh and F. Zerbetto. 2007. Synthetic molecular motors and mechanical machines. Angewandte Chemie International Edition 46: 72–191.

Ke, F., Y.-P. Yuan, L.-G. Qiu, Y.-H. Shen, A.-J. Xie, J.-F. Zhu et al. 2011. Facile fabrication of magnetic metal–organic framework nanocomposites for potential targeted drug delivery. Journal of Materials Chemistry 21: 3843–3848.

Kidane, A. G., G. Burriesci, M. Edirisinghe, H. Ghanbari, P. Bonhoeffer and A. M. Seifalian. 2009. A novel nanocomposite polymer for development of synthetic heart valve leaflets. Acta Biomaterialia 5: 2409–2417.

Kim, H. W., H. H. Lee and J. Knowles. 2006. Electrospinning biomedical nanocomposite fibers of hydroxyapatite/poly (lactic acid) for bone regeneration. Journal of Biomedical Materials Research Part A 79: 643–649.

Kim, K., D. Dean, A. G. Mikos and J. P. Fisher. 2009. Effect of initial cell seeding density on early osteogenic signal expression of rat bone marrow stromal cells cultured on cross-linked poly (propylene fumarate) disks. Biomacromolecules 10: 1810–1817.

Kim, M. S., K. S. Seo, G. Khang and H. B. Lee. 2005. Preparation of a gradient biotinylated polyethylene surface to bind streptavidin-FITC. Bioconjugate Chemistry 16: 245–249.

Kotsar, A., T. Isotalo, J. Mikkonen, H. Juuti, P. M. Martikainen, M. Talja et al. 2008. A new biodegradable braided self-expandable PLGA prostatic stent: an experimental study in the rabbit. Journal of Endourology 22: 1065–1070.

Kroy, K. 2006. Elasticity, dynamics and relaxation in biopolymer networks. Current Opinion in Colloid & Interface Science 11: 56–64.

Kundu, S. 2014. Silk Biomaterials for Tissue Engineering and Regenerative Medicine. Elsevier, Sawston, Cambridge, CB22 3HJ, UK; Waltham, MA 02451, USA and Kidlington, OX5 1GB, UK.

Langer, R. and D. A. Tirrell. 2004. Designing materials for biology and medicine. Nature 428: 487–492.

Lee, J. W., K. S. Kang, S. H. Lee, J.-Y. Kim, B.-K. Lee and D.-W. Cho. 2011. Bone regeneration using a microstereolithography-produced customized poly (propylene fumarate)/diethyl fumarate photopolymer 3D scaffold incorporating BMP-2 loaded PLGA microspheres. Biomaterials 32: 744–752.

Lee, K.-W., S. Wang, M. J. Yaszemski and L. Lu. 2008. Physical properties and cellular responses to crosslinkable poly (propylene fumarate)/hydroxyapatite nanocomposites. Biomaterials 29: 2839–2848.

Lee, K. Y., L. Jeong, Y. O. Kang, S. J. Lee and W. H. Park. 2009. Electrospinning of polysaccharides for regenerative medicine. Advanced Drug Delivery Reviews 61: 1020–1032.

Lee, Y.-B., S. Polio, W. Lee, G. Dai, L. Menon, R. S. Carroll et al. 2010. Bio-printing of collagen and VEGF-releasing fibrin gel scaffolds for neural stem cell culture. Experimental Neurology 223: 645–652.

Li, X., R. Cui, L. Sun, K. E. Aifantis, Y. Fan, Q. Feng et al. 2014. 3D-printed biopolymers for tissue engineering application. International Journal of Polymer Science.

Liao, E., M. Yaszemski, P. Krebsbach and S. Hollister. 2007. Tissue-engineered cartilage constructs using composite hyaluronic acid/collagen I hydrogels and designed poly (propylene fumarate) scaffolds. Tissue Engineering 13: 537–550.

Lim, D. W. 2007. *In-situ* Crosslinkable and Self-assembling Elastin-like Polypeptide Block Copolymers for Cartilage Tissue Repair. ProQuest LLC, 789 E. Eisenhower Parkway PO Box 1346. Ann Arbor, MI 48106-1346.

Lin, C.-C. and K. Anseth. 2009a. PEG hydrogels for the controlled release of biomolecules in regenerative medicine. Pharmaceutical Research 26: 631–643.

Lu, W.-N., S.-H. Lü, H.-B. Wang, D.-X. Li, C.-M. Duan, Z.-Q. Liu et al. 2008. Functional improvement of infarcted heart by co-injection of embryonic stem cells with temperature-responsive chitosan hydrogel. Tissue Engineering Part A 15: 1437–1447.

Ruso, J. M., J. Sartuqui and P. V. Messina. 2015. Multiscale inorganic hierarchically materials: towards an improved orthopaedic regenerative medicine. Current Topics in Medicinal Chemistry 15: 2290–2305.

Mahoney, M. J. and K. S. Anseth. 2006. Three-dimensional growth and function of neural tissue in degradable polyethylene glycol hydrogels. Biomaterials 27: 2265–2274.

Mani, G., M. D. Feldman, D. Patel and C. M. Agrawal. 2007. Coronary stents: a materials perspective. Biomaterials 28: 1689–1710.

Martins, A., S. Chung, A. J. Pedro, R. A. Sousa, A. P. Marques, R. L. Reis et al. 2009. Hierarchical starch-based fibrous scaffold for bone tissue engineering applications. Journal of Tissue Engineering and Regenerative Medicine 3: 37–42.

Mccloskey, K. E. 2013. Biomimetic multiscale topography for cell alignment. pp. 471–483. *In*: Danquah, K.M. and I.R. Mahato (eds.). Emerging Trends in Cell and Gene Therapy, Humana Press, Totowa, NJ.

Mchale, M. K., L. A. Setton and A. Chilkoti. 2005. Synthesis and *in vitro* evaluation of enzymatically cross-linked elastin-like polypeptide gels for cartilaginous tissue repair. Tissue Engineering 11: 1768–1779.

Mckay, W. F., S. M. Peckham and J. M. Badura. 2007. A comprehensive clinical review of recombinant human bone morphogenetic protein-2 (INFUSE® Bone Graft). International Orthopaedics 31: 729–734.

Meek, M. F. and J. H. Coert. 2013. Recovery of two-point discrimination function after digital nerve repair in the hand using resorbable FDA-and CE-approved nerve conduits. Journal of Plastic, Reconstructive & Aesthetic Surgery 66: 1307–1315.

Meinel, L., R. Fajardo, S. Hofmann, R. Langer, J. Chen, B. Snyder et al. 2005. Silk implants for the healing of critical size bone defects. Bone 37: 688–698.

Melek, L. N. 2015. Tissue engineering in oral and maxillofacial reconstruction. Tanta Dental Journal 12: 211–223.

Meyers, M. A., P.-Y. Chen, A. Y.-M. Lin and Y. Seki. 2008. Biological materials: structure and mechanical properties. Progress in Materials Science 53: 1–206.

Mi, F.-L., S.-S. Shyu, Y.-B. Wu, S.-T. Lee, J.-Y. Shyong and R.-N. Huang. 2001. Fabrication and characterization of a sponge-like asymmetric chitosan membrane as a wound dressing. Biomaterials 22: 165–173.

Mihaila, S. M., A. K. Gaharwar, R. L. Reis, A. P. Marques, M. E. Gomes and A. Khademhosseini. 2013. Photocrosslinkable kappa-carrageenan hydrogels for tissue engineering applications. Advanced Healthcare Materials 2: 895–907.

Mironov, V., V. Kasyanov et al. 2007. Organ printing: promises and challenges. Regenerative Medicine 3(1): 93–103.

Mironov, V., R. P. Visconti, V. Kasyanov, G. Forgacs, C. J. Drake and R. R. Markwald. 2009. Organ printing: tissue spheroids as building blocks. Biomaterials 30: 2164–2174.

Mohanty, A. K., M. Misra and L. T. Drzal. 2005. Natural Fibers, Biopolymers, and Biocomposites. CRC Press, Boca Raton, FL.

Morgan, T. T., H. S. Muddana, E. I. Altinoglu, S. M. Rouse, A. Tabakovic, T. Tabouillot et al. 2008. Encapsulation of organic molecules in calcium phosphate nanocomposite particles for intracellular imaging and drug delivery. Nano Letters 8: 4108–4115.

Mosahebi, A., M. Wiberg and G. Terenghi. 2003. Addition of fibronectin to alginate matrix improves peripheral nerve regeneration in tissue-engineered conduits. Tissue Engineering 9: 209–218.

Mouthuy, P. A., Y. El-Sherbini, Z. Cui and H. Ye. 2016. Layering PLGA-based electrospun membranes and cell sheets for engineering cartilage–bone transition. Journal of Tissue Engineering and Regenerative Medicine 10: E263–E274.

Müller, M., J. Becher, M. Schnabelrauch and M. Zenobi-Wong. 2013. Printing thermoresponsive reverse molds for the creation of patterned two-component hydrogels for 3D cell culture. JoVE (Journal of Visualized Experiments) 77: e50632–e50632.

Nassif, L. and M. El Sabban. 2011. Mesenchymal stem cells in combination with scaffolds for bone tissue engineering. Materials 4: 1793–1804.

Nedovic, V. and R. Willaert. 2013. Fundamentals of Cell Immobilisation Biotechnology. Springer Science & Business Media, 233 Spring Street New York, NY 10013-1578, USA.

Negroiu, G., R. M. Piticescu, G. C. Chitanu, I. N. Mihailescu, L. Zdrentu and M. Miroiu. 2008. Biocompatibility evaluation of a novel hydroxyapatite-polymer coating for medical implants (*in vitro* tests). Journal of Materials Science: Materials in Medicine 19: 1537–1544.

Nettles, D. L., K. Kitaoka, N. A. Hanson, C. M. Flahiff, B. A. Mata, E. W. Hsu et al. 2008. *In situ* crosslinking elastin-like polypeptide gels for application to articular cartilage repair in a goat osteochondral defect model. Tissue Engineering Part A 14: 1133–1140.

Nevins, M., M. L. Nevins, M. Camelo, J. Camelo, P. Schupbach and D. M. Kim. 2010. The clinical efficacy of DynaMatrix extracellular membrane in augmenting keratinized tissue. The International Journal of Periodontics & Restorative Dentistry 30: 151–161.

Niaounakis, M. 2013. Biopolymers: Reuse, Recycling, and Disposal. William Andrew. William Andrew is an imprinted of Elsevier: kidlington, Oxford OXS, 1GB, UK and Waltham, MA 02451, USA.

Niaounakis, M. 2014. Biopolymers: Processing and Products. William Andrew. William Andrew is an imprinted of Elsevier: kidlington, Oxford OXS, 1GB, UK and Waltham, MA 02451, USA.

Nicodemus, G. D. and S. J. Bryant. 2008. Cell encapsulation in biodegradable hydrogels for tissue engineering applications. Tissue Engineering Part B: Reviews 14: 149–165.

Nishida, K., M. Yamato, Y. Hayashida, K. Watanabe, K. Yamamoto, E. Adachi et al. 2004. Corneal reconstruction with tissue-engineered cell sheets composed of autologous oral mucosal epithelium. New England Journal of Medicine 351: 1187–1196.

Noel, S. P., H. Courtney, J. D. Bumgardner and W. O. Haggard. 2008. Chitosan films: a potential local drug delivery system for antibiotics. Clinical Orthopaedics and Related Research 466: 1377–1382.

Noel, S. P., H. S. Courtney, J. D. Bumgardner and W. O. Haggard. 2010. Chitosan sponges to locally deliver amikacin and vancomycin: a pilot *in vitro* evaluation. Clinical Orthopaedics and Related Research® 468: 2074–2080.

Obara, K., M. Ishihara, T. Ishizuka, M. Fujita, Y. Ozeki, T. Maehara et al. 2003. Photocrosslinkable chitosan hydrogel containing fibroblast growth factor-2 stimulates wound healing in healing-impaired db/db mice. Biomaterials 24: 3437–3444.

Oh, J. K., D. I. Lee and J. M. Park. 2009. Biopolymer-based microgels/nanogels for drug delivery applications. Progress in Polymer Science 34: 1261–1282.

Okano, M. N. T. and F. M. Winnik. 2010. Poly (N isopropylacrylamide)-based Smart Surfaces for Cell Sheet Tissue Engineering. Material Matters 5: 56.

Osada, K., R. J. Christie and K. Kataoka. 2009. Polymeric micelles from poly (ethylene glycol)–poly (amino acid) block copolymer for drug and gene delivery. Journal of The Royal Society Interface, rsif. 2008.0547. focus.

Pack, D. W., A. S. Hoffman, S. Pun and P. S. Stayton. 2005. Design and development of polymers for gene delivery. Nature Reviews Drug Discovery 4: 581–593.

Pal, K., B. Behera, S. Roy, S. Sekhar Ray and G. Thakur. 2013. Chitosan based delivery systems on a length scale: Nano to macro. Soft Materials 11: 125–142.

Park, J., E. Lim, S. Back, H. Na, Y. Park and K. Sun. 2010. Nerve regeneration following spinal cord injury using matrix metalloproteinase-sensitive, hyaluronic acid-based biomimetic hydrogel scaffold containing brain-derived neurotrophic factor. Journal of Biomedical Materials Research Part A 93: 1091–1099.

Park, K.-H., H. Kim, S. Moon and K. Na. 2009. Bone morphogenic protein-2 (BMP-2) loaded nanoparticles mixed with human mesenchymal stem cell in fibrin hydrogel for bone tissue engineering. Journal of Bioscience and Bioengineering 108: 530–537.

Park, Y., M. P. Lutolf, J. A. Hubbell, E. B. Hunziker and M. Wong. 2004. Bovine primary chondrocyte culture in synthetic matrix metalloproteinase-sensitive poly (ethylene glycol)-based hydrogels as a scaffold for cartilage repair. Tissue Engineering 10: 515–522.

Patel, D. 2011. Regenerative medicine using nanotechnology: a review. International Journal of Pharmaceutical & Biological Archive 2(4).

Paul, D. R. 2012. Polymer Blends. Elsevier Academic Press, INC 111 Fifth Avenue, New York, New York, 10003.

Peppas, N. A., R. M. Ottenbrite, K. Park and T. Okano. 2010. Biomedical Applications of Hydrogels Handbook. Springer Science & Business Media. New York, Dordrecht, Heidelberg, London.

Pielichowska, K. and S. Blazewicz. 2010. Bioactive polymer/hydroxyapatite (nano) composites for bone tissue regeneration. Adv. Polym. Sci. 232: 97–207 DOI:10.1007/12_2010_50. Springer-Verlag Berlin Heidelberg.

Plackett, D. V. 2011. Biopolymers: New Materials for Sustainable Films and Coatings. John Wiley & Sons Ltd, West Sussex, PO19 8SQ, United Kingdom.

Popa, E. G., M. E. Gomes and R. L. Reis. 2011. Cell delivery systems using alginate–carrageenan hydrogel beads and fibers for regenerative medicine applications. Biomacromolecules 12: 3952–3961.

Popa, E. G., P. P. Carvalho, A. F. Dias, T. C. Santos, V. E. Santo, A. P. Marques et al. 2014. Evaluation of the *in vitro* and *in vivo* biocompatibility of carrageenan-based hydrogels. Journal of Biomedical Materials Research Part A 102: 4087–4097.

Powell, P. C. 2012. Engineering with Fibre-polymer Laminates. Springer Science & Business Media. New York, Dordrecht, Heidelberg, London.

Prabaharan, M. and J. F. Mano. 2006. Stimuli-responsive hydrogels based on polysaccharides incorporated with thermoresponsive polymers as novel biomaterials. Macromolecular Bioscience 6: 991–1008.

Prestwich, G. D. 2011. Hyaluronic acid-based clinical biomaterials derived for cell and molecule delivery in regenerative medicine. Journal of Controlled Release 155: 193–199.

Pritchard, R. H., Y. Y. S. Huang and E. M. Terentjev. 2014. Mechanics of biological networks: from the cell cytoskeleton to connective tissue. Soft Matter 10: 1864–1884.

Rajaram, A., D. J. Schreyer and D. X. Chen. 2015. Use of the polycation polyethyleneimine to improve the physical properties of alginate–hyaluronic acid hydrogel during fabrication of tissue repair scaffolds. Journal of Biomaterials Science, Polymer Edition 26: 433–445.

Raquez, J. M., M. Deléglise, M. F. Lacrampe and P. Krawczak. 2010. Thermosetting (bio)materials derived from renewable resources: A critical review. Progress in Polymer Science 35: 487–509.

Rathenow, J., A. Ban, J. Kunstmann, B. Mayer and S. Asgari. 2004. Biocompatibly coated medical implants. Google Patents.

Ratner, B. D., A. S. Hoffman, F. J. Schoen and J. E. Lemons. 2004. Biomaterials Science: An Introduction to Materials in Medicine. Academic Press, INC 111 Fifth Avenue, New York, New York, 10003.

Reichl, S. 2009. Films based on human hair keratin as substrates for cell culture and tissue engineering. Biomaterials 30: 6854–6866.

Reneker, D., W. Kataphinan, A. Theron, E. Zussman and A. Yarin. 2002. Nanofiber garlands of polycaprolactone by electrospinning. Polymer 43: 6785–6794.

Rezwan, K., Q. Chen, J. Blaker and A. R. Boccaccini. 2006. Biodegradable and bioactive porous polymer/inorganic composite scaffolds for bone tissue engineering. Biomaterials 27: 3413–3431.

Roy, K., H.-Q. Mao, S.-K. Huang and K. W. Leong. 1999. Oral gene delivery with chitosan–DNA nanoparticles generates immunologic protection in a murine model of peanut allergy. Nature Medicine 5: 387–391.

Ruso, J. M., V. Verdinelli, N. Hassan, O. Pieroni and P. V. Messina. 2013. Enhancing CaP Biomimetic Growth on TiO2 Cuboids Nanoparticles via Highly Reactive Facets. Langmuir 29: 2350–2358.

Sá-Lima, H., S. G. Caridade, J. F. Mano and R. L. Reis. 2010. Stimuli-responsive chitosan-starch injectable hydrogels combined with encapsulated adipose-derived stromal cells for articular cartilage regeneration. Soft Matter 6: 5184–5195.

Saheb, D. N. and J. Jog. 1999. Natural fiber polymer composites: a review. Advances in Polymer Technology 18: 351–363.

Sakiyama, S. E., J. C. Schensen and J. A. Hubbell. 1999. Incorporation of heparin-binding peptides into fibrin gels enhances neurite extension: an example of designer matrices in tissue engineering. The FASEB Journal 13: 2214–2224.

Salgado, A., O. Coutinho and R. Reis. 2004. Novel starch-based scaffolds for bone tissue engineering: cytotoxicity, cell culture, and protein expression. Tissue Engineering 10: 465–474.

Salgado, A., R. Sousa, J. Fraga, J. M. Pêgo, B. Silva, J. Malva et al. 2009. Effects of starch/polycaprolactone-based blends for spinal cord injury regeneration in neurons/glial cells viability and proliferation. Journal of Bioactive and Compatible Polymers 24: 235–248.

Salinas, C. N., B. B. Cole, A. M. Kasko and K. S. Anseth. 2007. Chondrogenic differentiation potential of human mesenchymal stem cells photoencapsulated within poly (ethylene glycol)-arginine-glycine-aspartic acid-serine thiol-methacrylate mixed-mode networks. Tissue Engineering 13: 1025–1034.

Salzberg, C. A. 2006. Nonexpansive immediate breast reconstruction using human a cellular tissue matrix graft (AlloDerm). Annals of Plastic Surgery 57: 1–5.

Sartuqui, J., N. D'elía, A. N. Gravina and P. V. Messina. 2015. Analyzing the hydrodynamic and crowding evolution of aqueous hydroxyapatite-gelatin networks: Digging deeper into bone scaffold design variables. Biopolymers 103: 393–405.

Satija, N. K., V. K. Singh, Y. K. Verma, P. Gupta, S. Sharma, F. Afrin, M. Sharma, P. Sharma, R. Tripathi and G. Gurudutta. 2009. Mesenchymal stem cell-based therapy: a new paradigm in regenerative medicine. Journal of Cellular and Molecular Medicine 13: 4385–4402.

Schmoekel, H. G., F. E. Weber, J. C. Schense, K. W. Grätz, P. Schawalder and J. A. Hubbell. 2005. Bone repair with a form of BMP-2 engineered for incorporation into fibrin cell in growth matrices. Biotechnology and Bioengineering 89: 253–262.

Schwartz, R. S. and R. G. Wolff. 1997. Molding and reacting a mixture of fibrin and elastin on a spacings-containing element; radially compressing to deliver to arterial lumens. Google Patents.

Schwarz, F., N. Sahm, K. Bieling and J. Becker. 2009. Surgical regenerative treatment of peri-implantitis lesions using a nanocrystalline hydroxyapatite or a natural bone mineral in combination with a collagen membrane: a four-year clinical follow-up report. Journal of Clinical Periodontology 36: 807–814.

Sell, S., M. J. Mcclure, C. P. Barnes, D. C. Knapp, B. H. Walpoth, D. G. Simpson and G. L. Bowlin. 2006. Electrospun polydioxanone–elastin blends: potential for bioresorbable vascular grafts. Biomedical Materials 1: 72.

Shih, H. and C.-C. Lin. 2012. Cross-linking and degradation of step-growth hydrogels formed by thiol–ene photoclick chemistry. Biomacromolecules 13: 2003–2012.

Shimoboji, T., E. Larenas, T. Fowler, S. Kulkarni, A. S. Hoffman and P. S. Stayton. 2002. Photoresponsive polymer–enzyme switches. Proceedings of the National Academy of Sciences 99: 16592–16596.

Siemer, S., S. Lahme, S. Altziebler, S. Machtens, W. Strohmaier, H.-W. Wechsel et al. 2007. Efficacy and safety of TachoSil® as haemostatic treatment versus standard suturing in kidney tumour resection: a randomised prospective study. European Urology 52: 1156–1163.

Sierpinski, P., J. Garrett, J. Ma, P. Apel, D. Klorig, T. Smith, L. A. Koman, A. Atala and M. Van Dyke. 2008. The use of keratin biomaterials derived from human hair for the promotion of rapid regeneration of peripheral nerves. Biomaterials 29: 118–128.

Simnick, A. J., D. W. Lim, D. Chow and A. Chilkoti. 2007. Biomedical and biotechnological applications of elastin-like polypeptides. Journal of Macromolecular Science, Part C: Polymer Reviews 47: 121–154.

Sionkowska, A. 2011. Current research on the blends of natural and synthetic polymers as new biomaterials: Review. Progress in Polymer Science 36: 1254–1276.

Sodian, R., S. P. Hoerstrup, J. S. Sperling, D. P. Martin, S. Daebritz, J. E. Mayer, Jr. and J. P. Vacanti. 2000. Evaluation of biodegradable, three-dimensional matrices for tissue engineering of heart valves. Asaio Journal 46: 107–110.

Sodian, R., M. Loebe, A. Hein, D. P. Martin, S. P. Hoerstrup, E. V. Potapov et al. 2002. Application of stereolithography for scaffold fabrication for tissue engineered heart valves. Asaio Journal 48: 12–16.

Song, W., A. C. Lima and J. F. Mano. 2010. Bioinspired methodology to fabricate hydrogel spheres for multi-applications using superhydrophobic substrates. Soft Matter 6: 5868–5871.

Srichana, T. and A. J. Domb. 2009. Polymeric biomaterials. pp. 83–119. In: Narayan R. (ed.). Biomedical Materials. Springer, New York.

Stevens, M. M. and J. H. George. 2005. Exploring and engineering the cell surface interface. Science 310: 1135–1138.

Stevens, M. M. 2008. Biomaterials for bone tissue engineering. Materials Today 11: 18–25.

Stile, R. A., K. R. Shull and K. E. Healy. 2003. Axisymmetric adhesion test to examine the interfacial interactions between biologically-modified networks and models of the extracellular matrix. Langmuir 19: 1853–1860.

Stoddart, M. J., S. Grad, D. Eglin and M. Alini. 2009. Cells and biomaterials in cartilage tissue engineering. Regenerative Medicine 4: 81–98.

Stokols, S., J. Sakamoto, C. Breckon, T. Holt, J. Weiss and M. H. Tuszynski. 2006. Templated agarose scaffolds support linear axonal regeneration. Tissue Engineering 12: 2777–2787.

Stoppel, W. L., C. E. Ghezzi, S. L. Mcnamara, L. D. Black III and D. L. Kaplan. 2015. Clinical applications of naturally derived biopolymer-based scaffolds for regenerative medicine. Annals of Biomedical Engineering 43: 657–680.

Strohbach, A. and R. Busch. 2015. Polymers for cardiovascular stent coatings. International Journal of Polymer Science.

Sultana, N., M. I. Hassan and M. M. Lim. 2015. Composite Synthetic Scaffolds for Tissue Engineering and Regenerative Medicine. Springer Cham, Heidelberg, New York, Dordrecht, London.

Sun, J. and H. Tan. 2013. Alginate-based biomaterials for regenerative medicine applications. Materials 6: 1285–1309.

Suo, H., K. Xu and X. Zheng. 2014. Using glucosamine to improve the properties of photocrosslinked gelatin scaffolds. Journal of Biomaterials Applications 0(0): 1–11.

Tammela, T. and M. Talja. 2003. Biodegradable urethral stents. BJU International 92: 843–850.

Tan, H. and K. G. Marra. 2010. Injectable, biodegradable hydrogels for tissue engineering applications. Materials 3: 1746–1767.

Tan, P. L. 2010. Company profile: tissue regeneration for diabetes and neurological diseases at living cell technologies. Regenerative Medicine 5: 181–187.

Teck Lim, G., S. A. Valente, C. R. Hart-Spicer, M. M. Evancho-Chapman, J. E. Puskas, W. I. Horne et al. 2013. New biomaterial as a promising alternative to silicone breast implants. Journal of the Mechanical Behavior of Biomedical Materials 21: 47–56.

Terzic, A. and T. J. Nelson. 2010. Regenerative medicine: advancing health care 2020. Journal of the American College of Cardiology 55: 2254–2257.

Torio-Padron, N., N. Baerlecken, A. Momeni, G. B. Stark and J. Borges. 2007. Engineering of adipose tissue by injection of human preadipocytes in fibrin. Aesthetic Plastic Surgery 31: 285–293.

Tsang, V. L. and S. N. Bhatia. 2004. Three-dimensional tissue fabrication. Advanced Drug Delivery Reviews 56: 1635–1647.

Tseng, D., W. Donahue and B. A. Parsons. 2002. Polymer coated stent. Google Patents.

Uematsu, K., K. Hattori, Y. Ishimoto, J. Yamauchi, T. Habata, Y. Takakura et al. 2005. Cartilage regeneration using mesenchymal stem cells and a three-dimensional poly-lactic-glycolic acid (PLGA) scaffold. Biomaterials 26: 4273–4279.

Urry, D. W. 1984. Protein elasticity based on conformations of sequential polypeptides: the biological elastic fiber. Journal of Protein Chemistry 3: 403–436.

Vowden, P., M. Romanelli, R. Peter, Å. Boström, A. Josefsson and H. Stege. 2006. The effect of amelogenins (Xelma™) on hard-to-heal venous leg ulcers. Wound Repair and Regeneration 14: 240–246.

Wang, S., M. J. Yaszemski, A. M. Knight, J. A. Gruetzmacher, A. J. Windebank and L. Lu. 2009. Photo-crosslinked poly (ε-caprolactone fumarate) networks for guided peripheral nerve regeneration: material properties and preliminary biological evaluations. Acta Biomaterialia 5: 1531–1542.

Weber, J., L. Atanasoska and T. Eidenschink. 2006. Corrosion resistant coatings for biodegradable metallic implants. Google Patents.

Weiss, L. E. and J. W. Calvert. 2000. Assembled scaffolds for three dimensional cell culturing and tissue generation. Google Patents.

White, S. R., N. Sottos, P. Geubelle, J. Moore, M. R. Kessler, S. Sriram et al. 2001. Autonomic healing of polymer composites. Nature 409: 794–797.

Williams, J. M., A. Adewunmi, R. M. Schek, C. L. Flanagan, P. H. Krebsbach, S. E. Feinberg et al. 2005. Bone tissue engineering using polycaprolactone scaffolds fabricated via selective laser sintering. Biomaterials 26: 4817–4827.

Wu, D.-Q., Y.-X. Sun, X.-D. Xu, S.-X. Cheng, X.-Z. Zhang and R.-X. Zhuo. 2008. Biodegradable and pH-sensitive hydrogels for cell encapsulation and controlled drug release. Biomacromolecules 9: 1155–1162.

Wu, X., J. Ren and J. Li. 2012. Fibrin glue as the cell-delivery vehicle for mesenchymal stromal cells in regenerative medicine. Cytotherapy 14: 555–562.

Xu, T., C. A. Gregory, P. Molnar, X. Cui, S. Jalota, S. B. Bhaduri et al. 2006. Viability and electrophysiology of neural cell structures generated by the inkjet printing method. Biomaterials 27: 3580–3588.

Yilgor, P., N. Hasirci and V. Hasirci. 2010. Sequential BMP-2/BMP-7 delivery from polyester nanocapsules. Journal of Biomedical Materials Research Part A 93: 528–536.

Yu, L. and J. Ding. 2008. Injectable hydrogels as unique biomedical materials. Chemical Society Reviews 37: 1473–1481.

Yu, Y.-C., V. Roontga, V. A. Daragan, K. H. Mayo, M. Tirrell and G. B. Fields. 1999. Structure and dynamics of peptide-amphiphiles incorporating triple-helical protein like molecular architecture. Biochemistry 38: 1659–1668.

Zare-Mehrjardi, N., M. Taghi Khorasani, K. Hemmesi, H. Mirzadeh, H. Azizi, B. Sadatnia et al. 2011. Differentiation of embryonic stem cells into neural cells on 3D poly (D, L-lactic acid) scaffolds versus 2D cultures. International Journal of Artificial Organs 34: 1012.

Zelzer, M. and R. V. Ulijn. 2010. Next-generation peptide nanomaterials: molecular networks, interfaces and supramolecular functionality. Chemical Society Reviews 39: 3351–3357.

Zhang, L. G., J. P. Fisher and K. Leong. 2015. 3D Bioprinting and Nanotechnology in Tissue Engineering and Regenerative Medicine. Academic Press, London NW1 7BY,UK.

Zhang, S., T. Holmes, C. Lockshin and A. Rich. 1993. Spontaneous assembly of a self-complementary oligopeptide to form a stable macroscopic membrane. Proceedings of the National Academy of Sciences 90: 3334–3338.

Zhang, S., Y. Huang, X. Yang, F. Mei, Q. Ma, G. Chen et al. 2009a. Gelatin nanofibrous membrane fabricated by electrospinning of aqueous gelatin solution for guided tissue regeneration. Journal of Biomedical Materials Research Part A 90: 671–679.

Zhang, X., M. R. Reagan and D. L. Kaplan. 2009b. Electrospun silk biomaterial scaffolds for regenerative medicine. Advanced Drug Delivery Reviews 61: 988–1006.

Zhang, Y., J. R. Venugopal, A. El-Turki, S. Ramakrishna, B. Su and C. T. Lim. 2008. Electrospun biomimetic nanocomposite nanofibers of hydroxyapatite/chitosan for bone tissue engineering. Biomaterials 29: 4314–4322.

Zhou, H., J. G. Lawrence and S. B. Bhaduri. 2012. Fabrication aspects of PLA-CaP/PLGA-CaP composites for orthopedic applications: a review. Acta Biomaterialia 8: 1999–2016.

Zhu, G. and W. Lou. 2014. Regeneration of facial nerve defects with xenogeneic acellular nerve grafts in a rat model. Head & Neck 36: 481–486.

Zhu, J. and R. E. Marchant. 2011. Design properties of hydrogel tissue engineering scaffolds. Expert Review of Medical Devices 8: 607–626.

Zhu, Y., C. Gao, X. Liu, T. He and J. Shen. 2004. Immobilization of biomacromolecules onto aminolyzed poly (L-lactic acid) toward acceleration of endothelium regeneration. Tissue Engineering 10: 53–61.

Zilla, P., D. Bezuidenhout and P. Human. 2007. Prosthetic vascular grafts: wrong models, wrong questions and no healing. Biomaterials 28: 5009–5027.

2

Application of Natural, Semi-synthetic, and Synthetic Biopolymers used in Drug Delivery Systems Design

Javier Sartuqui,[§] Noelia L. D'Elía,[§] A. Noel Gravina[§] and Luciano A. Benedini*

Introduction

Science and technology play a key role in the extended life expectancy. In this sense, a wide range of innovative techniques and new devices have been developed, resulting in a reduction of morbidity and mortality. The use of drug delivery systems to improve the efficacy of bioactive molecules remains essential strategy for achieving the treatment against diseases and the progress in this field has been essential. In this context, synthetic, semi-synthetic, or natural polymers are frequently used for developing drug delivery systems. Accordingly, their application goes from the generation of suspension with cyclodextrins to solubilize hydrophobic drugs to the formation of matrices which control, by means of their degradation, the release of drugs.

Departamento de Química, Universidad Nacional del Sur, INQUISUR-CONICET (8000) Bahía Blanca, Argentina.
* Corresponding author: lbenedini@uns.edu.ar
§ These authors contributed in the same way to this work.

There are relevant factors that should be evaluated when choosing a polymer for use as a drug carrier. One of the most important is the biocompatibility, which is related with the acceptance of the material by tissues. The problems encompassing this condition can include hypersensitivity reactions; since that the pharmaceutical formulation should be in contact with different tissues, some of them more sensitive than others, the long time by an increased time of carrier-tissue interaction may cause an alteration in drug biodisponibility due to changing biopharmaceutical parameters. Biodegradability is the timely degradation of the polymer in contact with the tissue; this is the other important feature that must be considered. Furthermore, the drug delivery system must be degraded and their components removed from the body to prevent their accumulation, and thus avoiding any potential toxicity.

In accordance with green chemistry, a solvent free processing to obtain the different drugs carriers is also important because the reduction of contaminant by-products is one of the biggest challenges for developing pharmaceutical products.

Frequently, natural polymers are synthetically modified to reinforce their positive features and to decrease the negative ones. These new compounds are named semi-synthetic derivatives. Sometimes positive characteristics can be improved, but negatives cannot be abolished. Hence, their advantages and disadvantages must be critically discussed, and the biocompatibility of these natural materials and their derivatives must be compared. Occasionally, availability from renewable resources is also considerate; and therefore, natural and semi-synthetic polymers are often advantageous compared to synthetic alternatives.

Finally, when active biomolecules are included into formulations based in polymers, their physicochemical features, and sensibility must be considered. Thus, some characteristics of the drugs such as charge and solubility, among others, could direct their inclusion into a polymeric matrix. On the other hand, sensitive drugs such as peptides, proteins, and nucleic acids are increasing their relevance and this effect is due to the fact that potential treatment options have a medical unmet demand which is not covered by classical drug therapies. For these active pharmaceutical ingredients (API), additional conditions must be taken into consideration.

Polysaccharides

Polysaccharides are polymeric biomaterials widely studied for drug delivery applications. These compounds can be produced by from microorganisms, animals, and plants; hence, they represent a renewable resource and are regarded as economical and environmentally favorable. Polysaccharides used for these applications combine several advantageous properties both clinical and physicochemical. Among the former can be mentioned low toxicity, good biocompatibility, and biodegradability, and among the latter, high stability and hydrophilicity. In addition, natural polysaccharides can be modified to improve, enhance, or avoid any molecular feature necessary to reach the ultimate objective. Thus, in this section we will focus on their main structural features and their importance in polysaccharides-based drug delivery systems.

Cyclodextrins

Cyclodextrins (CDs) are crystalline, non-hygroscopic, and cyclic oligosaccharides derived from starch. The first reference to a substance which later proved to be a CD, was published by Villiers, in 1891 (Villiers 1891) and was named "cellulosine" by Schardinger (Schardinger 1903). He also observed that two distinct crystalline "cellulosines" were formed, being probably α- and β-CDs. However, it wasn't until the 1960s when preparations of CDs, their structure, physical and chemical properties, as well as their inclusion complex forming properties were discovered (Szejtli 1998).

Chemically, CDs are cyclic oligosaccharides containing at least six D-(+)-glucopyranose units attached by α (1→4) glucoside bonds. The three natural cyclodextrins, α, β, and γ; differ in their ring size, solubility, and their content of glucose units, having 6, 7, or 8, respectively (Rowe et al. 2009). However, Endo et al. (1997) established an isolation and purification method for several kinds of large ring CDs and they also obtained a relatively large amount of δ-CD (Cyclomaltonose) with nine glucose units. Furthermore, both their molecular weight and their size cavity are increased from α to δ-CD. On the other hand, it must be considered that CDs can be modified to improve some of their physicochemical or toxicological features, and also to enhance physical and microbiological stability. From β-CD, numerous derivatives were obtained by chemical modification such as hydroxyethyl-β-CD, hydroxypropyl-β-CD, sulfobutylether-β-CD, methyl-β-CD among others.

Cyclodextrins have lipophilic inner cavities and hydrophilic outer surfaces, and are capable of interacting with a large variety of guest molecules to form non-covalent inclusion complexes. The lipophilicity of the cavity is due to the arrangement of hydroxyl groups within the molecule. They are chemically stable in neutral and basic conditions and undergo non-enzymatic hydrolysis in acidic conditions. According to the classification given by different pharmacopoeias, CDs are used as solubilizing and/ or stabilizing agents. CDs have been playing a very important role in formulation of poorly water-soluble drugs by improving apparent drug solubility and/or dissolution through inclusion complexation or solid dispersion (Tasić et al. 1992). In this context, the importance of CDs applications is found in the design of various novel delivery systems such as liposomes, microspheres, microcapsules, and nanoparticles (Challa et al. 2005). There are some factors influencing the formation and stability of inclusion complexes such as the presence of charge when the complexes drug-CDs are formed, temperature changes, addition of other co-polymers, and the preparation method of the formulation (Nagase et al. 2001; Mura et al. 1999).

β-cyclodextrins is the least expensive and therefore the most commonly used CD, even though it is the least soluble. Hence, it is primarily used in tablets and capsules formulations. In the case of parenteral formulations, α-CD is mainly used; however, resulting from having the smallest cavity among CDs, it can only form inclusion complexes with small-sized molecules. In contrast, γ-CD has the largest cavity and it can be used to form inclusion complexes with big molecules (Rowe et al. 2009). β-cyclodextrin may be used to develop an oral tablet formulation by means of wet-granulation and, on the other hand, by direct-compression processes. In parenteral formulations, CDs have been used to produce stable and soluble preparations of drugs that would otherwise have been formulated using a non-aqueous solvent.

In eye drops formulations, CDs form water-soluble complexes with lipophilic drugs such as corticosteroids and vitamin D2 (Palmieri et al. 1993). They can increase the water solubility of the drug, enhance drug absorption into the eye, improve aqueous stability, and reduce local irritation (Loftsson and Stefánsson 2002). CDs have also been used in the formulation of solutions (Prankerd et al. 1992), suppositories (Szente et al. 1984; Szente et al. 1985), and cosmetics (Amann and Dressnandt 1993; Buschmann and Schollmeyer 2002). In addition, other kind of drug delivery systems has been designed with CDs to carry sensitive drugs. In this context, it has been reported that their use as non-viral vectors for gene delivery induced an increment in the transfection efficiency, with high levels of reporter gene expression and also with low toxicity (Redenti et al. 2001; O'Neill et al. 2013; Lai 2014). Promising carriers for anti-cancer drug delivery in tumor therapy have been reported by Tan et al. (Tan et al. 2013). This research has shown greater control of drug release by incorporation of CDs into polymeric drug delivery systems. Here, 5-fluorouracil, doxorubicin, and vinblastine are carried into a complex built by a covalently linked reaction between chitosan and carboxylic acid group of CDs. These cyclic polysaccharides are able to have close cellular interactions, which make them a suitable option for carrying peptides, oligonucleotides, and proteins.

All toxicity studies have demonstrated that, when orally administered, CDs are practically non-toxic due to the lack of absorption in the gastrointestinal tract (Irie and Uekama 1997). However, lipophilic methylated CDs are surface active and they are, to some extent (~ 10%), absorbed in the gastrointestinal tract. Consequently only limited amounts of these lipophilic CD derivatives can be included in oral formulations and they are unsuitable for parenteral formulations. Furthermore, α, β, and methylated CDs are nephrotoxic and should not be used in parenteral formulations. In contrast, γ-CD, 2-hydroxypropyl-β-CD, sulfobutylether β-CD, sulfated β-CD, and maltosyl β-CD appear to be safe even when administered parenterally.

Cellulose and derivatives

Cellulose is the most abundant substance in the biosphere; it is the main molecule of cell walls of higher plants and it is also produced by some algae, fungi, protozoans, tunicates, and bacteria. The molecule is a linear polymer of D-anhydroglucopyranose units linked together by (1→4)-β-glycosidic bonds. The extensive intra- and intermolecular hydrogen bonding between the individual chains (Hinterstoisser and Salmén 2000) make it insoluble in water and most common solvents (Rowe et al. 2009). In order to improve water solubility, various cellulose derivatives have been synthesized by etherification of the hydroxyl groups on anhydroglucose units of cellulose. Hence, the most widely used are methyl cellulose, carboxymethyl cellulose, hydroxypropyl cellulose, hydroxypropyl methyl cellulose (HPMC), hydroxyethyl cellulose, and ethylhydroxyethyl cellulose. Bacterial cellulose (BC), originally reported by Brown (Brown 1886), has attracted considerable attention in both drug delivery and biomedical fields due to its unique fibrillar nanostructure, high water holding capacity, high degree of polymerization, high mechanical strength, and degree of crystallinity, as well as its availability for being effectively produced in high purity by

Acetobacterxylinum (Esa et al. 2014). Cellulose and its derivatives have been widely used in the pharmaceutical industry due to their ability to swell in contact with water and their high compatibility which makes them suitable as a binder/diluent and also as an disintegrant agent in oral tablets and capsules, depending on the substitution degree (SD). Cellulose derivatives are able to form hydrogels and therefore, are appropriate as suspending or viscosity-increasing agents for oral suspensions. Other kind of applications such as wound dressing, transdermal patches, and ophthalmic preparations have also been reported for some of these derivatives; these traditional applications have been extensively discussed in literature (Shokri and Adibkia 2013; Kamel et al. 2008; Rowe et al. 2009).

In native cellulose, the adjacent chains of the polymer fit closely together in an ordered crystalline region, resulting in a product with high strength. Different degrees of crystallinity can be found according to the source and degree of processing of the raw material which, in turn, varies the mechanical properties of the final product. Young's Modulus, for example, can vary from 20.8 to 60.1 GPa in cellulose obtained from wood fibers (Wang 2010). As mentioned before, cellulose derivatives are able to form gels and a wide range of mechanical properties can be obtained depending on the SD, nature of the solvent, and concentration (Jain et al. 2013). Bacterial cellulose exists as a basic fibrillar structure 100 times smaller than plant cellulose and highly crystalline (Esa et al. 2014). Its reported elastic modulus was approximately 10 GPa (Iguchi et al. 2000; Svensson et al. 2005), which is comparable to that of the articular cartilage, and this is extraordinary large for an organic material with a two dimensional structure. Therefore, bacterial cellulose is a suitable candidate to be applied in tissue engineering and also to develop membranes for controlled release for drugs.

Cellulose and its ethers commonly used in the pharmaceutical industry induce negligible foreign body and inflammatory responses, being generally regarded as a non-toxic and non-irritant material. However, oral consumption of large amounts of them may have a laxative effect. *In vivo* biocompatibility of BC implanted subcutaneously in rats for up to 12 weeks has been studied, proving good integration into the host tissue, and no signs of inflammation or foreign body response (Helenius et al. 2006). Regarding their degradation, these materials are considered non- or slowly biodegradable *in vivo*, due to the lack of cellulase enzymes in animals (Dugan et al. 2013).

Bacterial cellulose and its ethers can be used to create "smart" materials, which present differential behaviors under environmental stimulus. This fact constitutes a very versatile feature for drug delivery systems. Hydrogels, membranes, self-assembled systems, and nanocomposites are among the most widely investigated alternatives (Edgar 2007). In the particular case of BC, sources directly influence structure because its properties vary with bacterial strain and culture media; therefore, its knowledge can be used to tailor the material for different drug delivery purposes.

A cellulose nanofibers–titania composite is currently under development for drug delivery of anesthetics, analgesics, and antibiotics (Galkina et al. 2015). This material is presented as an interesting alternative for wound-dressing with transdermal drug delivery properties. Sodium diclofenac, D-penicillamine, and phosphomycin were used as model drugs, showing uniform distribution within the nanofiber film and long-term drug release with different profiles: the quickest release was observed for the painkiller, a slower one for the anti-inflammatory agent, and the longest release took place for the strongly chemisorbed antibiotic agent.

Polymer-nanoparticle (PNP) hydrogels were recently developed by mixing HPMC and carboxy-functionalized polystyrene nanoparticles (PSNPs) by Appel et al. (2015). Interestingly, these self-assembled hydrogels are able to flow under applied shear stress, followed by rapid self-healing when the stress is relaxed, allowing its safe subcutaneous injection. Moreover, owing to the hierarchical structure of the gel, molecular delivery was controlled allowing differential release of multiple compounds (tested with hydrophobic and hydrophilic therapeutic models, in both *in vitro* and *in vivo* systems). BC membranes produced from *Gluconacetobactersacchari* have been developed as systems for topical and transdermal drug delivery; using lidocaine hydrochloride and ibuprofen as models for hydrophilic and hydrophobic drugs, respectively. Trovatti et al. (Trovatti et al. 2012) proved that permeation rate is higher for the hydrophobic drug than for the hydrophilic one, demonstrating that these delivery systems can be tuned to modulate the bioavailability of drugs for percutaneous administration, having the advantage of using a membrane that is also able to absorb exudates and to adhere to irregular skin surfaces. Recently, Amin et al. (2012) combined BC obtained from cream of coconut (also known as nata de coco) and different proportions of acrylic acid to fabricate thermally stable hydrogels with moldable pore sizes. Therefore, *in vitro* drug release studies with bovine serum albumin showed a thermo- and pH-responsive behavior of the hydrogels suggesting them as a suitable system for temperature-controlled delivery of protein-based drugs.

Guar gum

Guar gum is a hydrocolloidal galactomannan that structurally comprises long and straight chains of (1→4)-α-D-mannopyranosyl units linked together by (1→4)-β-D-galactopyranosyl units by (1→6) linkages. The ratio of D-mannose to D-galactose of guar gum has been known to be approximately 2:1 and 1.4:1. A single molecular weight is estimated to be in the range of 200 kDa to 300 kDa (Schierbaum 1971). Guar gum is obtained by grinding the endosperm portion of a leguminous plant called *Cyamoposistetragonolobus* (L.) *Taub*. that is grown mainly in India, Pakistan, and United States to produce seeds used for human and animal food (Rowe et al. 2009). Additionally, guar gum exhibits potential applications in various fields such as drugs, cosmetic, food, and textile industries. Different guar gum composites have been studied to improve the properties of conventional food technologies such as thermoplastic polymers and fillers (Funami et al. 2005). Generally, this hydrocolloidal agent is used as an additive in the food industry to facilitate gelling, thickening, firming, and emulsification of food products but a high viscosity (2,000 to 3,000 mPa.s) is reached when its concentration is above 1% w/v and this is a limiting factor for its use in food products (McCleary 1979), resulting in liquid products which are highly viscous. In order to reduce its viscosity, it may be processed into partially hydrolysed guar gum (PHGG), which is obtained by controlled partial enzymatic hydrolysis of guar gum seeds (Flammang et al. 2006). PHGG has the same chemical structure as the original guar gum, but with a significantly reduced molecular weight of around 20 kDa and one-tenth of the original chain length (Yoon et al. 2008). Guar gum produces a pseudoplastic viscous solution when hydrated in cold water and it also has a low-shear viscosity greater than other hydrocolloids (Brosio et al. 1994).

Mechanical properties studies of low concentrated and almost monodisperse guar gums suspensions have shown that there is a plateau in the storage modulus at a frequency of $\omega = 10^{-3}$. It was demonstrated that guar gum enhance rheological and large deformation properties of soybean β-conglycinin gel. Moreover, due to increasing concentrations of guar gum the elastic modulus of the composite is also increased (Zhu et al. 2009). Guar gum has many desirable properties for drug delivery applications and is generally used as a sustained release excipient owing to its high viscosity, low cost, and commercial availability. This compound forms a hydrophilic matrix that could be used as oral carrier for controlled delivery of drugs with varying solubility; therefore, its gelling property retards the release of drugs from the dosage form and it is susceptible to degradation in the colonic environment (Jain et al. 1992; Bhalla and Shah 1991; Krishnaiah et al. 1998). In order to improve its applications as drug delivery carrier, several chemical modifications have been made on guar gum such as cross-linking with borax, glutaraldehyde, and trisodiumtrimeta phosphate. These cross-linked formations reduce its enormous swelling. Furthermore, for the preparation of different guar gum-based systems, combinations with other natural or synthetic polymers such as polyacrylamide, polyvinylpyrrolidone, ethyl cellulose, hydroxypropyl methyl cellulose, polyvinyl alcohol, polyacrylic acid, sodium carboxymethyl cellulose, sodium alginate, xanthan gum, chitosan, carrageenan, hydroxypropyl cellulose, and carboxymethyl cellulose could be considered.

In recent years, stimuli-responsive micro and nanogels have been designed, which respond to external stimuli such as pH, ionic strength, temperature, and electric current in order to deliver a specific drug dosage in a specific site (Prabaharan 2011). George et al. (George and Abraham 2007) have designed a pH sensitive system made of alginate-guar gum hydrogel cross-linked with glutaraldehyde for controlled delivery of proteins. These authors found that the presence of this modified guar gum increases the entrapment efficiency and prevents the rapid dissolution of alginate in a basic pH as the pH found in the intestine, ensuring a controlled release of the entrapped drug. Furthermore, guar gum has been used to develop sustained-release devices of water soluble antihypertensive drugs such as nifedipine, diltiazem hydrochloride, and other such as ketoprofen. Recent studies carried out by Das et al. (Das and Subuddhi 2015) have shown very encouraging results using pH-responsive hydrogel systems based on guar gum, poly(acrylic acid), and cross-linked cyclodextrin with tetraethyl orthosilicate for intestinal delivery of dexamethasone. They found that as the guar gum content increases, the rate of drug release decreases considerably and the drug release is prolonged. On the other hand, considering that guar gum and its derivatives have good film forming and controlled drug release abilities, they have the potential to be used as transdermal drug delivery devices (Altaf et al. 1998).

The physiological effects of guar gum have been extensively studied, first on animals and then on humans. Studies revealed that guar gum is non-toxic; additionally, it does not have carcinogenic or teratogenic effects (Melnick et al. 1983). In addition, due to its high biocompatibility and biodegradability it is extensively used as a biomaterial. Guar gum cannot be degraded in the small intestine; however, in the large intestine, the glycosidic linkage present in guar gum is degraded due to the microbial enzyme present there (Tomlin et al. 1986). One of the bacteria responsible for guar gum degradation is *Clostridium butyricum* (Mudgil et al. 2014).

Carrageenan

Carrageenans are a family of high molecular weight sulfated polysaccharides obtained by extraction from some members of the algae class Rhodophyceae (red seaweed). They are composed of galactose and anhydrogalactose units, linked by glycosidic unions. Depending on the method and the algae from which carrageenan is extracted, three main types of carrageenans can be obtained: kappa (κ), iota (ι), and lambda (λ) (Sankalia et al. 2006). The primary differences which influence the properties of carrageenan type are the number and position of sulfate ester groups as well as the content of 3,6-anhydrogalactose. Typically, commercial λ-carrageenan contains approximately 35% sulfate ester by weight and little or no 3,6-anhydrogalactose, ι-carrageenan contains about 32% sulfate ester by weight and approximately 30% 3,6-anhydrogalactose, and κ-carrageenan contains 25% sulfate ester by weight and approximately 34% 3,6-anhydrogalactose (Jana et al. 2011). Even though these three types of carrageenans have similar characteristics in their chemical structure, it was reported that higher levels of sulfate ester resulted in lower solubility temperature and lower gel strength (Necas and Bartosikova 2013). Moreover, given the ionic nature of the polymer, its gelation is strongly influenced by the presence of electrolytes and, among these three types, only κ- and ι-carrageenans evidence gel-forming ability; the κ-carrageenan gels are firmer than those obtained with ι-carrageenan, which are more elastic and soft (Bixler 1994).

Carrageenan is widely used in the food industry due to its excellent gelling, thickening, emulsifying, and stabilizing abilities. Furthermore, it is also applied in other commercial products such as cosmetics, air freshener gels, and fire fighting foam (Necas and Bartosikova 2013), and recently, it is increasingly being used in pharmaceutical formulations as well (Li et al. 2014).

Mechanical and rheological properties of carrageenan gels have been widely studied in the presence of ions. Carrageenans exist as a random coil at high temperature; and temperature reduction induces the formation of double helices. This leads to the formation of small independent domains involving a limited number of chains via intermolecular association. However, when cations are incorporated into carrageenan suspensions, helices of different domains aggregate to enable long range cross-linking which forms a cohesive network and this quaternary structure contributes to the final properties of the resultant gels (Morris et al. 1980). However, Thrimawithana et al. have demonstrated that increasing ion concentrations beyond a threshold also had a negative impact on some mechanical properties of carrageenan gels (Thrimawithana et al. 2010).

Different carrageenan drug delivery systems have been developed, and they are mainly used as a polymer matrix in oral extended-release tablets (Hariharan et al. 1997), as a novel extrusion aid for the production of pellets (Thommes and Kleinebudde), and as a carrier in micro and nanoparticles systems (Cheng et al. 2015). In addition, based on their strong negative charge, carrageenans have been used as gelling and viscosity enhancing agents for the design of drug controlled-release systems which could be used, for example, as prolonged retention systems. It can be found combined with locust bean gum and gellan gum, in chitosan/carrageenan nanoparticles, agarose/carrageenan hydrogels, and carrageenan/gelatin mucoadhesive systems, among others (Jana et al. 2011). In particular, κ-carrageenan is widely used due to their hydrogen bond-forming capability in several sites which impart bioadhesive properties to the final formulation. Moreover, its mucoadhesive property could be further enhanced by the negative charge of the sulfate group in the carrageenan structure; as a consequence, ionic bonds are formed with the positively charged mucin present on the buccal mucosa (Kianfar et al. 2011).

Carrageenans have shown several potential pharmaceutical properties including anticoagulant, anticancer, antihyperlipidemic, and immunomodulatory activities (Wijesekara et al. 2011; Campo et al. 2009). Comparison of a variety of compounds reveals that carrageenan is an extremely potent infection inhibitor for a broad range of sexually transmitted human papillomavirus (Buck et al. 2006); in fact, it was reported that carrageenans-based gels used in sexual lubricant may offer protection against human papillomavirus transmission (Campo et al. 2009; Roberts et al. 2007). Additionally, Rocha de Souza et al. (Rocha de Souza et al. 2007) found a positive correlation between sulfate content and antioxidant activity of carrageenan. In contrast, it is known that carrageenans induce inflammatory responses in laboratory animals (Tobacman 2001; van der Kam et al. 2008; Sadeghi et al. 2011); and some studies showed that long-term administration of carrageenans in animal models caused ulcerative colitis or intestine mucous membrane damage. It was also reported that these compounds promote tumor growth (Tobacman 2001). Finally, specialists concluded that it is necessary to perform more epidemiological and essential studies to evaluate the safety of carrageenan (Li et al. 2014).

Hyaluronan

Hyaluronan (HA), also known as hyaluronic acid or hyaluronate, is a negatively charged, linear and unbranched polysaccharide with a simple chemical structure consisting of alternating units of D-glucuronic acid and N-acetyl-D-glucosamine. It is considered the largest glycosaminoglycan, with a molecular weight ranged from 103 to 104 kDa (Rowe et al. 2009). HA was first isolated from bovine vitreous humor in 1934 by Meyer and Palmer (Meyer and Palmer 1934). It is currently extracted from animal waste (e.g., rooster comb) and it has been obtained by different biotechnological methods such as microbial (Widner et al. 2005) and enzymatic production (Kooy et al. 2009). HA has been widely studied because of its unique properties, such as aqueous solubility, and its viscoelastic properties that allow it to form highly viscous solutions and three dimensional structures. It has been reported that HA plays an important role in the structure and viscoelastic properties of different tissues such as skin and articular cartilage (Nair and Laurencin 2007).

Regarding its mechanical properties, a single HA molecule is very flexible and its viscoelasticity is affected by the pH and ionic strength of its environment (Kobayashi et al. 1994). Furthermore, HA has a pKa value of about 3.0 and therefore, a change in pH will affect the extent of ionization of the HA chains (Mi et al. 1996). To improve its mechanical properties HA can be chemically modified or cross-linked. Generally carboxylic acid and alcohol groups have been modified by esterification and by crosslinkers such as dihydrazide, dialdehyde, divinylsulfone, diglycidyl ethers, or disulfide (Jeon et al. 2007). Several investigations have shown that parameters such as elastic modulus, shear modulus, viscosity, and viscoelasticity depend on HA concentration and cross-linked degree of hydrogels (Balazs and Denlinger 1993; Altman and Moskowitz 1998; Nijenhuis et al. 2008). Mainly, it is possible to increase the hydrogel's storage modulus by increasing the gel precursor solution's HA concentration, with stiffness ranging from 100 Pa to 1000 Pa (Lam et al. 2014). Although, a research have shown that the elastic modulus rises while HA concentration keeps below 20%, however above this value the elastic modulus decreases due to a significant growth of swelling of the hydrogel (Jeon et al. 2007).

HA has a great potential to be used as a specific-target carrier and long-acting delivery systems of various molecules including proteins, peptides, and nucleotides. In encapsulation of proteins, HA provides a well-hydrated environment, helping them to retain their biological activity and to limit denaturation (Hoffman 2002). Recently, HA has been investigated as a drug delivery agent for various routes of administration, including dermal, ophthalmic, nasal, pulmonary, parenteral, and topical. Regarding dermal applications, Solaraze®, a HA gel with a commercial drug (diclofenac), was developed for the topical treatment of actinic keratosis. In this formulation, HA enhances significantly the partitioning of diclofenac into human skin and its retention and localization in the epidermis (Del Rosso 2003). Due to its mucoadhesive capacity, microspheres delivery systems made of HA have been used as a vehicle for topical ophthalmic drugs (Lim et al. 2000). Microspheres have also been used experimentally as delivery devices for nerve growth factors (Mohammad et al. 2000), and as a nasal delivery system for insulin (Illum et al. 1994). Moreover, paclitaxel and doxorubicin, both anticancer drugs, have been chemically linked to HA systems and it was found to selectively target human cancer cells because HA is the main ligand for CD44 and RHAMM receptors, which are over-expressed in a variety of tumor cell surfaces (Culty et al. 1994) including colon cancer (Tanabe et al. 1993), human breast epithelial cells (Bourguignon et al. 2009), lung cancer (Matsubara et al. 2000), and acute leukemia cells (Yokota et al. 1999).

HA biocompatibility, non-toxic properties and lack of immunogenicity, make it an ideal scaffold for tissue engineering. In terms of biodegradation in human tissues, HA has a half-life from less than 1 to several days. Once it reaches the blood stream, about 85–95% is eliminated by the liver; while kidneys extract 10% but excrete about 1–2% in urine (Fraser et al. 1997). On the other hand, it was shown that HA is related to different kinds of diseases. Elevated proportions of HA, HA synthase, and hyaluronidase are involved in cell migration and metastasis at various stages of cancer progression (Lokeshwar et al. 1997). Moreover, HA oligomers formed by hyaluronidase degradation are pro-angiogenic (Liu et al. 1996) and have inflammatory and immuno-stimulatory properties (Xu et al. 2002).

Alginates

Alginates are mainly obtained from cell walls of different species of brown algae belonging to Phaeophyceae class. Since that these algae are harvested from nature, there is a variety of types of alginates depending on the selected species, the time of collection and the region where each species is found. In this context, alginate allows significant variation of material properties solely based on polysaccharide composition (Grasdalen et al. 1981) and these properties allow tailoring of a variety of biomaterials suitable for tissue engineering.

Alginates are water soluble and anionic linear hetero-polysaccharide composed of two different monomers $(1{\rightarrow}4)$-β-linked: the β-D-mannuronic acid (M) (pKa = 3.38) and the α-L-guluronic acid (G) (pKa = 3.65). Therefore, if the pH of the alginate-containing solution is lowered below the pKa of the constituting acids, phase separation or hydrogel formation occurs. Generally, they are composed of three different forms of polymer segments: consecutive G residues, consecutive M residues, and alternating MG residues. The resulting variability of alginate composition significantly affects its physical properties, for example: G rich domains with more than 6–10 residues bind divalent ions (Ca2+, Ba2+, etc.) forming cross-links between different chains in a so-called 'egg-box arrangement' (Grant et al. 1973). These polysaccharides are insoluble in aqueous-alcoholic solutions and also in organic solvents. Their use has been widely diffused in different industries such as pharmaceutical ones. Here, they are part of tablets and ophthalmic preparations, among others; however, nowadays the most important field of interest is the production of hydrogels. Alginates can be found forming salts with different cations: ammonium, potassium, sodium, and propylene glycol. Typically, alginate salts are prepared at 1% w/v in aqueous solution, and at 20°C they have a viscosity of 20–400 mPa x s. The viscosity of these gels may vary depending upon concentration, pH, temperature, or the presence of metal ions, for instance, above pH 10, their viscosity decreases (Rowe et al. 2009).

The design of drug delivery systems based on alginates can be performed due to the sol-gel transition behavior of the alginate in the presence of divalent cations such as Ca2+, Sr2+, and Ba2+. After this reaction, the water solubility of the monovalent alginate decreases converting it into a water insoluble salt. Furthermore, GG blocks have shown to be more rigid than MM blocks because of axial–axial or diequatorial linkage (Rinaudo 2008). Therefore, gels formed from alginate with a high M content are typically softer and less porous than high G alginate gels, showing a higher degree of swelling and shrinking. Consequently, a high G alginate is advantageous in terms of maintenance of form and integrity over extended time (Simpson et al. 2004; De Vos et al. 1996).

In drug delivery systems' design, alginates are used as a stabilizing agent, suspending agent, tablet and capsule disintegrant, tablet binder, and viscosity increasing agent (Rowe et al. 2009). Moreover, different systems with applications in regenerative medicine, such as microspheres, microcapsules, sponges, foams, and fibers, have been developed. Alginates may be used to develop delivery systems for cationic polyelectrolytes and proteoglycans through simple electrostatic interactions due to its pH dependent anionic nature (Yu et al. 2009). Recently several different formulations were developed where this polymer was included; however, only two of them will be highlighted in this section: the development of nanoparticles and the production of hydrogels. The most important feature of these hydrogels is their adhesion to different tissues. The adhesive devices can be formulated for drug release into different mucosal tissues such as oral and vaginal ones, and can be developed as *in situ*-formed gels to be applied in buccal and ophthalmic mucosa to controllably release the API. The esophageal bio-adhesion of alginate suspensions may provide a barrier against gastric reflux or site-specific delivery of therapeutic agents (Richardson et al. 2005). Furthermore, nasal delivery systems based on mucoadhesive microspheres (Gavini et al. 2005), and a freeze-dried device intended for the delivery of bone-growth factors have been reported. One of the most important applications of the alginates is the development of hydrogel systems for delivery of sensitive drugs such as proteins and peptides (Gombotz and Pettit 1995). In these groups of drugs are included several proteins such as immunoglobulin, fibrinogen, insulin, melatonin, heparin, and hemoglobin. Related to peptides delivery, this polymer was blended with another natural polysaccharide, guar gum (George and Abraham 2007), to overcome the rapid dissolution of the alginate at high pH, a major limitation during delivery of peptide drugs (Yu et al. 2009; Li et al. 2006). In addition, sodium alginate microspheres have been used in the preparation of a DNA vaccine for the foot-mouth disease (Liu et al. 2004), and therefore, the incorporation of functional small interfering siRNAs proves the significance of this polyanionic polysaccharide. Moreover, the use of alginate-based delivery systems for distribution of cell induction ligands and also for bioactive molecules for signaling was reported (Kulkarni et al. 2012).

Alginates are generally regarded as non-toxic and non-irritant materials. However, biocompatibilities of alginates were significantly affected by their composition and their molecular weight. In this context, it was suggested that unbound alginate oligosaccharides may be responsible for the induction of inflammatory reactions, and the purification of the alginate reduces the low molecular weight fraction which may lead to improved biocompatibility. In this context, their biodegradability strongly depends on the characteristics of each polymer and hence, the biodegradability of high molecular weight alginates is hampered when they are parenterally administered as they may exceed the threshold of renal clearance. Due to that fact, to improve the biodegradability of alginates, low molecular weight polymers are cross-linked with biodegradable molecules to obtain high molecular weight alginates with enhanced renal clearance. Nevertheless, this strategy has a disadvantage related with the high purification process required to use these assembled polymers (Germershaus et al. 2015).

Proteins

Essentially, proteins are a polymeric arrangement of amino acids in a three-dimensional folded structure forming the major structural components of many human tissues; they also are one of the most important classes of identified biomolecules. There are at least two fundamental factors in the characterization of proteins. The first one is related to their morphology, which affects their solubility and the other is related to their biological function, that is, if a protein is a structural protein or a transport protein. Morphologically, proteins are divided into fibrous and globular proteins. The main difference between these two kinds of proteins is that fibrous proteins generally have only primary and secondary structures; whereas globular proteins have also tertiary and sometimes quaternary structures. In contrast to globular proteins, fibrous proteins provide mechanical and structural support in the body whereas globular proteins are related to transport function (Nelson et al. 2008). Fibrous proteins form the extra cellular matrix and/or basal lamina of the cells in different tissues such as ligament, bone, and skin.

As mentioned above, proteins are the major component of natural tissues; therefore, this is one of the reasons why proteins and other amino acid-derived polymers have been a preferred biomaterial for medical uses such as haemostatic agents, scaffolds for tissue engineering, and drug delivery vehicles (Meinel et al. 2005). The use of biodegradable hydrogels based on proteins as drug delivery systems has a particular interest due to their biocompatibility and their relative inertness. For this reason, in this section we will show examples related to proteins forming hydrogels. Finally, it is important to remark that protein-based biomaterials are known to undergo naturally-controlled degradation processes.

Collagen I

Collagen is the main structural protein in vertebrates, and it represents approximately 30% of all body proteins. Collagen's family is characterized by a unique triple-helix configuration of three polypeptide subunits known as a α-chain. Due to differences in the helix's lengths and in the nature of the non-helical portions have been separated, at least, 13 types of collagens. The basic collagen molecule is formed by more than 1000 amino acids which develop a unique triple-helix sequence, which in turn is composed by α-chains. A right-handed helix is formed by 3 α-chains (Friess 1998) and it is stabilized by hydrogen bonds, intra-molecular van de Waals interactions (Brinckmann et al. 2005), and some covalent bonds (Harkness 1965). The helix has an average molecular weight of 300 kDa, a length of 300 nm, and a diameter of 1.5 nm (Friess 1998). Moreover the helices are associated into right handed microfibrils (40 nm in diameter) which are assembled into fibrils (100–200 nm in diameter). Finally, a group of fibrils form collagen fibers (He, Mu et al. 2011). In addition, a distinctive collagen marker is the presence of 4-hydroxyproline in the triple-helix (Cen et al. 2008).

The unique physiological characteristics of collagen and its capability to develop biomaterials derive from the structural complexity of the collagen molecule (Friess 1998). Reconstituted collagen fibrils have mechanical properties sensitive to their hydration state (van der Rijt et al. 2006) and are able to be manipulated by controlling their aqueous environment (Grant et al. 2009). Although it has been reported that a tendon's collagen fibrils form a rope-like structure, mechanical properties at a sub-fibrillar level are not fully understood (Bozec et al. 2007). The self-assembly mechanism generates a homogeneous single fibril of collagen (Yang et al. 2008). However, the alignment of collagen molecules along the longitudinal fibril direction could cause a mechanical anisotropy. Tensile test has been performed on single collagen type I fibrils. For example, a Young's modulus value of 5 ± 2 GPa was found for dry fibrils of type I collagen and when these fibrils were immersed in phosphate-buffered saline, its elasticity decreased to 0.2 to 0.5 GPa. These results support the hypothesis that the anisotropy of collagen arises from the alignment of sub fibrils along the fibril axis (Yang et al. 2008). Atomic Force Microscopy has been used to infer the elasticity of these structures and thus, the modulus of several collagen fibrils in air and aqueous fluid were compared. Therefore, this study (Atomic force microscopy) was carried out to describe the effect of hydration on the mechanical response (Grant et al. 2009).

This behavior is due to that the cross-linking process increases the stiffness of the material and also sterilization with glutaraldehyde. On the other hand, thermal sterilization can decrease its stiffness (Lesiak-Cyganowska et al. 2000; Angele et al. 2004; Friess 2000). Different kinds of collagen such as powders, liquids, solid compressed masses, membranes, or sponges have been reported. The obtained behavior, which is result of a study of different drug delivery systems, must be in concordance or should explain the properties of these systems (Ruszczak and Friess 2003). Nowadays, different efforts to attach drugs or polymers structures to collagen have been described in literature. Controlling drug conjugates would allow the immobilization of therapeutic enzymes or drug delivery; in this regard, kanamycin and pilocarpine have been investigated as conjugate options (Friess 1998).

Sheets, tubes, sponges, powders, fleeces, injectable solutions and dispersions are some of the forms in which collagen can be processed (Chvapil et al. 1973; Byrom 1991; Fu Lu and Thies 1991). Inserts and shields are among the most studied drug carrier applications of collagen. They are used for drug delivery above the corneal surface or for forming the cornea itself (Friess 1998). Inserts are cut from films or fabricated as molded rods prepared out of mixtures of drug and collagen by air-drying (Rubin et al. 1973).

There are different kinds of injectable systems carried out as gels. One of them is initially liquid, which when is injected inside the eye, coagulate in it, turning into a gel. These gels are able to remain longer than liquid formulations and could achieve a sustained delivery of non-steroidal anti-inflammatory drugs or antibiotics (Friess 1998).

A formulation of collagen with epinephrine for local vasoconstriction was tested aiming to enhance local drug retention, minimization of systemic side effects, and reduction of the required dose (Friess 1998).

In order to deal with a key complication in surgery, which is the local treatment of soft tissue infections, combinations with antibiotics are being developed (Taylor 1997). Collagen products are appropriate for medical uses because of their low antigenicity, excellent biocompatibility, low immunoreactions, clear association with other biological species and polyelectrolyte behaviour. In addition, final products such as threads, sponges, films, and drug delivery systems are important considering the reconstitution of collagen into native fibres starting from collagen solutions (Chirita 2008). Since there are similarities between amino acids of collagen of different animal species and the low content of aromatic residues, generally, collagen fibres behave as a non-antigenic protein. However, there are massive concerns about massive immune responses or autoimmune diseases triggered by antibodies which may produce cross-reactions by collagen derived from animal tissues (Friess 1998). Despite their ability to interact with antibodies, collagens are weakly immunogenic in comparison to other proteins (Byrom 1991). Antigenic determinants of collagen can be classified into three following categories: 1) tridimensional conformation recognition by antibodies; 2) recognition of amino acid sequence located within the triple helical portion (Lynn et al. 2004); 3) recognition of terminal and non-helical regions (Lee et al. 2001; Chevallay and Herbage 2000; Hsu et al. 1999; Kikuchi et al. 2004).

During the *in vivo* process, collagen is infiltrated by inflammatory cells such as fibroblasts, macrophages, or neutrophils, which secrete enzymes, activators, inhibitors, and regulatory molecules (Byrom 1991). Water, enzymes, and the digestion of linkages are required for collagen degradation. After a process of swelling by exposure to water, collagen is only completely digested by specific collagenases and cleaving enzymes (Harrington 1996). Collagen is degraded by endopeptidases and some non-enzymatic degradation mechanisms like hydrolysis (Okada et al. 1992). The connective tissue is digested by proteases, whereas metalloproteinases (MMPs) carry out the extracellular matrix degradation. Cysteine and aspartic proteases (cathepsins) degraded connective tissue intracellularly, while serine and MMP matrix degrade it extracellularly (Shingleton et al. 1996).

Gelatin

Gelatines are proteins derived from collagen, soluble in warm water, and with molecular weights ranging from ~ 20 to 250 kDa; and like in collagen, glycine (~ 24%), proline (~ 17%), alanine (~ 14%), and hydroxyproline (~ 10%) are the four most abundant amino acids. The essential amino acid, tryptophan, is not found in gelatin. The helical conformation can reach 70% and may be found in the gel form of gelatin. These regions have many inter and intramolecular associations and the α-chain of gelatin, which has a highly ordered sequence of amino acids, behaves like a random-coil polymer in the solution. The gel structure is a combination of fine and coarse interchain networks, and the ratio is defined as a proportional relation between fine chains and coarse depends on the gel formation temperature. In addition, the rigidity of the gel is approximately proportional to the square of the gelatin concentration (Gurr and Mülhaupt 2012). The gelatines are known as type A and type B depending on the production process; thus, if it is treated with acid, it is called type A, and if it is alkali treated, it is type B. These treatments cause de-amidation of asparagine and glutamine resulting in an increase in the number of acids, aspartic and glutamic (Eysturskarð et al. 2009).

Physical-chemical and rheological properties depend on their amino acid content. Rheological properties are important considerations in process design, evaluation, as well as in modelling. Hence, these are properties that indicate the quality of the product. Dynamic viscoelastic properties and flow properties provide information about their molecular arrangements. Hence, it is important to assess the rheological properties of gelatin along with its physical-chemical properties (Chandra and Shamasundar 2015). Mechanical properties such as the dynamic storage modulus and bloom value for gelatines are dependent on the average molecular weight and its distribution, whereas the content of the amino acids affects their physical properties. Low molecular weight fractions of gelatin block the helix assembly, perturbing the formation of the network. Both proline and hydroxyproline have stabilizing effects on the helices due to their ring conformation, and they also influence the flexibility of the chains. Consequently, the lower content of these amino acids increases the flexibility and, as a result, facilitates the reorganization of the network (Eysturskarð et al. 2009).

Gelatin may be loaded with charged biomolecules due to its intrinsic features, and it can be used as a drug delivery carrier. The drug loading efficiency depends on the treatment that collagen received to produce the gelatin, that is, alkaline or acidic, and also the nature of the guest drug. The cross-linking and the gelatin molecular weight can be tuned to control the release kinetics of gelatin. This polymer gives the possibility to control both aspects, that is, drug loading and release kinetics (Santoro et al. 2014). Oral administration is the main use for gelatin capsules. Solid, semisolid, and liquid fillings can be carried in hard capsules, whereas soft capsules are mainly for semisolids or liquids. Active ingredients can be incorporated differently depending on the capsule: as a filling in the hard ones; whereas the soft ones are able to carry the drug within their soft shell as well as in the filling. In addition, they can release the content rapidly thanks to a fast swelling and dissolving. Gelatines can contain coloring and antimicrobial agents, and they can also be used for the microencapsulation of drugs where the API is sealed inside a microsized capsule or beadlet. Other examples of gelatin uses are ibuprofen-gelatin micropellets, pastes, pastilles, pessaries, and suppositories. It is also used as tablet binder, coating agent, and viscosity increasing agent (Rowe et al. 2009). In more specific examples, studies of releasing lysozyme from hydrogels are being conducted in order to deliver antibacterial proteins into prosthesis of heart valves to prevent valve endocarditis. There has been a recent development in long-circulating gelatine controlled release systems which improve the applications in chemotherapy because they can gradually be accumulated at the tumor site thanks to the leaky vasculature and lack of lymph vessels around tumors (Young et al. 2005). Releasing tetracycline and bisphosphonate from Gelfoam® pellets to reduce periodontal bone loss and controlled-release vehicles for chemo-therapeutic agents are other examples of current researches (Yaffe et al. 2003).

As a collagen derivative, gelatin is a non-toxic, biodegradable, inexpensive, non-immunogenic material; therefore, it has a high potential to be used in a variety of medicinal agents. In addition, its water solubility and lesser cost are advantageous over its precursor (Varghese et al. 2014). As it was mentioned before, gelatin is highly biocompatible and biodegradable in a physiological environment. The digestive process confers to gelatin a very low antigenicity, with the formation of harmless metabolic products upon degradation. The presence of amino acidic sequences such as Arg-Gly-Asp (RGD) in the structure, improves the final biological performance of gelatin over synthetic polymers that lack these cell-recognition motifs (Santoro et al. 2014).

Human Serum Albumin

Human Serum Albumin (HSA) is the main protein of the blood plasma, accounting for over 50% of its total protein content, and its concentration range is from 3.5 to 5 g/dl. HSA is a small globular protein with a molecular weight of 66.5 kDa comprised of a single polypeptide chain of 585 amino acids; it is also the only major plasma protein that does not contain carbohydrate constituents (Rowe et al. 2009). Regarding its biological properties, albumin is responsible for 75–80% of the colloid osmotic pressure of plasma (Scatchard et al. 1944); it is also involved in transport and metabolism of several endogenous and exogenous compounds, such as hormones, bile acids, amino acids, fatty acids, toxic metabolites, metals, and drugs (Kratz 2008). The protein contains a single thiol group from a cysteine residue at position 34 (Cys34) that acts both as a binding site for many biologically active molecules and also providing antioxidant activity, and constituting the largest fraction of free thiol groups in the blood (Stewart et al. 2005). Due to the presence of undissociated acid content within the polypeptide, HSA participates in the regulation of acid-base balance (Bruegger et al. 2005).

Albumin and other small macromolecules accumulate in the tumor area due to extensive angiogenesis, increased permeability, and lack of lymphatic drainage in a phenomenon that is universal in solid tumors and it is called enhanced permeability and retention (EPR) effect (Maeda et al. 1985), providing an attractive strategy for passive targeting of drugs into the tumoral tissue. Furthermore, albumin-binding proteins such as membrane associated gp60 and osteonectin (SPARC), which promote the accumulation of albumin within the tumor interstitium, can also be used in the targeting of tumors by the simple formation of the drug-albumin conjugation (Kratz 2008).

Since Albumin is a naturally-occurring protein found in the body, it is not surprising that the protein is cataloged as a non-toxic material (Rowe et al. 2009). HSA has an average half-life of 19 days, which provides an attractive approach for improving the pharmacokinetic profiles of peptides and cytokines. Therefore, biodegradability has to be considered for each particular albumin-based drug delivery system because it has proven its strong dependence on the degree of cross-linking (Langer et al. 2008), pH, and temperature of preparation (Rohanizadeh and Kokabi 2009).

Nowadays, albumin is used as a versatile protein carrier for drug targeting and for improving the pharmacokinetic profile of peptide or protein-based drugs. There are mainly three drug delivery technologies: coupling of low-molecular weight drugs to exogenous or endogenous albumin, conjugation with bioactive proteins, and encapsulation of drugs into albumin particulate systems such as nanoparticles or micelar structures. Several examples of these systems are presented below. The first drug-albumin conjugates were obtained by direct binding peptides or prodrugs to the Cys34 position of exogenous and endogenous albumin. Commercially available albumin can be successfully conjugated with doxorubicin maleimide derivatives (an antibiotic with antineoplastic activity), as reported by Drevs et al. (2000), to obtain the A-DOXO-HYD conjugate, which has proved to have a superior effect against murine renal carcinoma compared to free doxorubicin at the equitoxic dose. Endogenous albumin can also be used as a drug carrier as in the case of AldoxorubicinTM (CytRx Corporation, Los Angeles, CA, USA), a prodrug of doxorubicin that, following intravenous administration, is able to bind rapidly and selectively to the Cys34 position of albumin, leading to passive accumulation within the tumor; currently this prodrug is being tested in phase 3 clinical trials in patients with soft tissue sarcomas whose tumors have progressed after treatment with chemotherapy.

Bioactive peptides, such as Insulin were successfully conjugated with albumin in the so called PC-DAC™:Insulin by ConjuChem, Inc. (Los Angeles, CA, USA), demonstrating more efficiency than insulin Glargine in diabetic rats and a prolonged duration of activity in preclinical pharmacodynamics studies. Albinterferon-α-2bTM, a fusion protein of recombinant HSA and interferon α-2b, was developed as a long-acting interferon for the treatment of chronic hepatitis C by Human Genome Sciences in collaboration with Novartis. In this system, albumin was used to increase circulation half-life of interferon-α leading to a significant reduction of the dosing interval, granting a successful phase 3 clinical trial approval; however, Food and Drug Administration's concerns regarding reduced performance led to the cancellation of the program in 2010. Albumin can also be used for encapsulating lipophilic drugs into nanoparticles using a quite elegant technology (nab or NP albumin bound) in which the drug is mixed with aqueous HSA and passed under high pressure through a jet to yield nanoparticles with sizes of 100–200 nm. An example of this is the commercially available nab-paclitaxel, also known as AbraxaneTM, a variation of paclitaxel in which the taxane is bond to albumin forming nanoparticles of an approximate diameter of 130 nm, that was approved in 2005 for the treatment of metastatic breast cancer. The enhanced uptake of these albumin-based drug delivery systems in solid tumors can be ascribed to the EPR effect as well as to transcytosis initiated by binding of albumin with gp-60 and SPARC (Desai et al. 2006).

Miscellaneous

Polyethylene glycols

Polyethylene glycol polymers (PEGs) are polyalcohols that have been described as an addition of polymers of ethylene oxide and water. These polymers are commonly named macrogols followed by a number indicating their molecular weight, which varies depending on the polymerization degree. Hence, polyethylene glycol grades from 200 to 600 (or macrogols 200 to 600) are liquids and grades up to 1000 are solids at 25°C. The empirical formula can be written as: $HOCH_2(CH_2OCH_2)mCH_2OH$ where m represents the average number of oxyethylene groups that ranges from 200 to 8000, and their molecular weights ranges are from 190 to 9000. However, there are grades of PEGs near to 35000. The number can be used to indicate the approximate molecular weight of a macrogol. All grades of polyethylene glycol are soluble in water and miscible in all proportions with other polyethylene glycols. Aqueous solutions of high molecular weight glycols (or high grades), may form gels with different viscosity (Rowe et al. 2009).

PEGs are widely used in the manufacture of surfactants, pharmaceuticals, cosmetics, polyurethanes, as well as in a variety of different fields. Regarding pharmaceutical formulations they are used as excipient, being included in parenteral, topical, ophthalmic, oral, rectal preparations; and also have been used experimentally in biodegradable polymeric matrices and in controlled-release systems. Functionally, the pharmaceutical industry uses these compounds as an ointment base, plasticizer, solvent, suppository base, tablet, and capsule lubricant. PEGs are stable and aqueous polyethylene glycol solutions can be used either as suspending agents or to adjust the viscosity and consistency of other suspending vehicles. These compounds can also be used as a co-solvent in order to enhance the aqueous solubility or dissolution characteristics of poorly soluble compounds by making solid dispersions with an appropriate polyethylene glycol. In this context, PEGs enhance the stability of aspartame solutions (Yalwsky et al. 1993); they can be used in diazepam solutions for parenteral administration (Shah et al. 1991) and can also improve bentonite dispersions. First Ambrosi et al. (2004) and later Benedini et al. (2012) have used PEG400 to modify the transition temperature of coagels of ascorbylpalmitate and shift the existence limits of liquid crystals of ascorbylpalmitate.

PEGs are essentially non-irritant to the skin and biocompatible, however they are not easily degradable polymers. PEGs with molecular weight lower than 4000 can be degraded by many bacteria species whereas those with higher molecular weights are significantly more resistant (Marchal et al. 2008). The oxidation of the terminal hydroxyl group and sequential shortening by a single oxyethylene unit is considered, by many authors, as a predominant pathway (Zgoła-Grześkowiak et al. 2006).

Polyacrylic acid

Polyacrylic acids, also known as carbomers, belong to the polyacids family. They are synthetic high molecular-weight polymers of acrylic acid repeated units. These polymers can be classified by grades, each one representing a variation in the chemical structure, degree of cross-linking, and residual components of the polymers. These differences account for the specific rheological behavior, handling, and the particular use of each grade. Their molecular weight is theoretically estimated at 700 to 4 x 106 kDa. Generally, carbomer polymers show lower viscosity and rigidity when most of the molecule is found without cross-links. Conversely, carbomer polymers with more cross-linked areas will have high-viscosity and rigidity. Carbomers swell, but do not dissolve in water and glycerin when they are neutralized. One gram of carbomer is neutralized by approximately 0.4 g of sodium hydroxide. Neutralized aqueous gels are more viscous at pH 6–11. These compounds can be used to perform liquid or semisolid pharmaceutical formulations, and their selection depends on their intrinsic rheological properties. Their viscosity is considerably reduced at pH values less than 3, greater than 12, or in the presence of strong electrolytes (Neau et al. 1996). During the exposure to ultraviolet light, gels rapidly lose their viscosity; however, this effect can be minimized by addition of a suitable antioxidant. Furthermore, carbomer polymers are incompatible with strong acids, cationic polymers, and high levels of electrolytes (Rowe et al. 2009) which accelerate drug release rates and reduce its bioadhesive properties.

Carbomers designated with the letter 'P', e.g., Carbopol 971P, are the pharmaceutical grade polymers for oral or mucosal contact products; however, during handling, it must be considered that carbomer dust is irritating to the eyes, mucous membranes, and respiratory tract.

Due to its bioadhesive capability, it has been widely used in ophthalmology improving the drug eye residence and its bioavailability (Edsman et al. 1996; von der Ohe et al. 1996) in cervix (Woolfson et al. 1995), and oral paths (Singla et al. 2000). They have also been used as controlled-release agent in other kinds of formulations; thus, it must be considered that lightly cross-linked carbomers (lower viscosity) are generally more efficient in controlling drug release than highly cross-linked ones (higher viscosity). These polymers are also used as emulsifying agents and emulsion stabilizers when oil-in-water emulsions for external administration are performed. Finally, carbomers are also used as rheology modifiers, stabilizing agents, and suspending agents in other kinds of formulations; furthermore, their role as a tablet binder was also reported.

Polyhydroxyalkanoates and derivatives

Polyhydroxyalkanoates (PHAs) are polyesters that belong to a class of intracellular biopolymers synthesized by many bacteria and/or plants. The main biopolymer of the PHA family is the polyhyroxybutyrate (PHB). PHBs are biodegradable polymers with thermoplastics properties synthesized by PHB synthases (PhaC) using (R)-3-hydroxybutyryl coenzyme A as a substrate. These polymers were discovered in 1920 as bacteria Bacillus megaterium's products. Under starvation conditions, many bacteria generate these polymers when an appropriate carbon source is available (Anderson and Dawes 1990). Furthermore, PHB serves as an energy source and as carbon storage product; that capacity can also be compared with glycogen in mammalian systems and starch in plants (Dawes 1973). PHB is a semi-crystalline isotactic polymer that undergoes surface erosion by hydrolytic cleavage of the ester bonds and has a melting temperature in the range of 160–180°C (Zinn et al. 2001). To improve its features PHB can be polymerized with 3 hydroxyvalerate (HV) obtaining P(HB-HV) which has similar semi-crystalline properties as PHB and lower melting temperature depending on the HV content. Both PHB and P(HB-HV) have been found to be soluble in a wide range of solvents and can be processed into different shapes and structures. The homopolymer PHB is tough and brittle, however, the co-polymer is less brittle and tougher, therefore, it has more potential as biomaterial (Nair and Laurencin 2007). In this context, biocompatibility and biodegradability by simple hydrolysis of ester bonds in aerobic conditions as well as piezoelectric properties make them suitable for drug delivery, tissue engineering, and orthopedic applications (Ueda and Tabata 2003). PHAs have emerged as a vast family of potential candidates of biodegradable polymers for drug delivery systems. PHA-based drug delivery systems form mainly subcutaneous implant covers, as well as compressed tablets for oral administration and micro particulate carriers for subcutaneous and intravenous use (Nigmatullin et al. 2015). Moreover, PHA rods can be loaded with different antibiotics that include sulbactam-cefoperazone and sulbactam-ampicillin combinations, and gentamicin alone. These formulations were prepared as a polymer matrix by casting drug/polymer pastes (Nigmatullin et al. 2015).

PHAs are biocompatible and degrade within desirable time frames under physiological conditions. These PHA materials provide a wider range of degradation rates than those currently available (Martin et al. 2003). Methods for manufacturing devices, which increase porosity or exposed surface area can be used to alter their degradability. For example, porous PHA can be made using methods that creates pores, voids, or interstitial spacing, such as an emulsion or spray drying technique, or those methods which incorporate leachable or lyophilizable particles within the polymer (Chen and Wu 2005). It has been reported that the deprivation of PHB *in vivo* is faster than *in vitro* hydrolysis at body temperature, indicating that enzymes existing *in vivo* catalyze the degradation (Piskin 1995). Other authors (Lo et al. 1999) detected lipase activities in the rat gastrointestinal tract near the PHA implant, suggesting the involvement of lipases in the metabolism of PHA *in vivo*. Hence, degradation of PHA matrices in the tissues of the host organism offers the possibility of coupling this phenomenon with release of bioactive compounds, such as the antibiotic or antitumor drug. If a PHA insert is impregnated with a compound, the degradation over time will release the compound, acting as an automatic dosing agent (Shrivastav et al. 2013). Various tests with members of the PHA family were conducted on animal models, showing good compatibility with a variety of tissues. Surface properties of PHA films have been shown to be favorable for proliferation and attachment of tissue cells (Misra et al. 2006; Wu et al. 2009). *In vivo* and *in vitro* biocompatibility of PHB and P(HBV) copolymers have been studied on the growth of Chinese hamster ovary cells, showing favorable results (Pouton and Akhtar 1996). In another study, P(HBHV) polymers generally showed good *in vitro* and *in vivo* biocompatibility despite the initial acute inflammation observed *in vivo* with P(HB-HV), which was probably in response to the trauma of implantation or injection (Pouton et al. 1988).

Acknowledgments

The authors acknowledge Universidad Nacional del Sur (PGI 24/Q064), Concejo Nacional de Investigaciones Científicas de la República Argentina (CONICET, PIP 11220130100100CO). JS, NLD, and ANG have doctoral fellowships at CONICET; LAB is an assistant researcher at CONICET.

References

Altaf, S. A., K. Yu, J. Parasrampuria and D. R. Friend. 1998. Guar gum-based sustained release diltiazem. Pharm. Res. 15: 1196–1201.

Altman, R. D. and R. Moskowitz. 1998. Intraarticular sodium hyaluronate (Hyalgan) in the treatment of patients with osteoarthritis of the knee: a randomized clinical trial. Hyalgan Study Group. J. Rheumatol. 25: 2203–2212.

Amann, M. and G. Dressnandt. 1993. Solving problems with cyclodextrins in cosmetics. Cosmet. Toiletries. 108: 90–95.

Ambrosi, M., P. L. Nostro, L. Fratoni, L. Dei, B. W. Ninham, S. Palma et al. 2004. Water of hydration in coagels. Phys. Chem. Chem. Phys. 6: 1401–1407.

Amin, M. C. I. M., N. Ahmad, N. Halib and I. Ahmad. 2012. Synthesis and characterization of thermo- and pH-responsive bacterial cellulose/acrylic acid hydrogels for drug delivery. Carbohydr. Polym. 88: 465–473.

Anderson, A. J. and E. A. Dawes. 1990. Occurrence, metabolism, metabolic role, and industrial uses of bacterial polyhydroxyalkanoates. Microbiol. Rev. 54: 450–472.

Angele, P., J. Abke, R. Kujat, H. Faltermeier, D. Schumann, M. Nerlich et al. 2004. Influence of different collagen species on physico-chemical properties of cross-linked collagen matrices. Biomaterials 25: 2831–2841.

Appel, E. A., M. W. Tibbitt, M. J. Webber, B. A. Mattix, O. Veiseh and R. Langer. 2015. Self-assembled hydrogels utilizing polymer–nanoparticle interactions. Nat. Commun. 6: 1–9.

Balazs, E. A. and J. L. Denlinger. 1993. Viscosupplementation: a new concept in the treatment of osteoarthritis. J. Rheumatol. Suppl. 39: 3–9.

Benedini, L., P. V. Messina, S. D. Palma, D. A. Allemandi and P. C. Schulz. 2012. The ascorbyl palmitate– polyethyleneglycol 400–water system phase behavior. Colloids Surf. B Biointerfaces 89: 265–270.

Bhalla, H. L. and A. A. Shah. 1991. Controlled release matrices for ketoprofen. Indian Drugs 28: 420–422.

Bixler, H. 1994. The carrageenan connection IV. British Food J. 96: 12–17.

Bourguignon, L. Y., C. C. Spevak, G. Wong, W. Xia and E. Gilad. 2009. Hyaluronan-CD44 interaction with protein kinase C(epsilon) promotes oncogenic signaling by the stem cell marker Nanog and the Production of microRNA-21, leading to down-regulation of the tumor suppressor protein PDCD4, anti-apoptosis, and chemotherapy resistance in breast tumor cells. J. Biol. Chem. 284: 26533–26546.

Bozec, L., G. van der Heijden and M. Horton. 2007. Collagen fibrils: nanoscale ropes. Biophys. J. 92: 70–75.

Brosio, E., A. D'Ubaldo and B. Verzegnassi. 1994. Pulsed field gradient spin-echo NMR measurement of water diffusion coefficient in thickening and gelling agents: guar galactomannan solutions and pectin gels. Cell Mol. Biol. 40: 569–573.

Brown, A. J. 1886. On an acetic ferment which forms cellulose. J. Chem. Soc. Trans. 49: 432–439.

Bruegger, D., M. Jacob, S. Scheingraber, P. Conzen, B. F. Becker, U. Finsterer et al. 2005. Changes in acid-base balance following bolus infusion of 20% albumin solution in humans. Intensive Care Med. 31: 1123–1127.

Buck, C. B., C. D. Thompson, J. N. Roberts, M. Müller, D. R. Lowy and J. T. Schiller. 2006. Carrageenan is a potent inhibitor of papillomavirus infection. PLoS Pathog. 2: e69.

Buschmann, H. J. and E. Schollmeyer. 2002. Applications of cyclodextrins in cosmetic products: a review. J. Cosmet. Sci. 53: 185–192.

Byrom, D. 1991. Biomaterials: Novel Materials from Biological Sources. Macmillan, New York.

Campo, V. L., D. F. Kawano, D. B. D. Silva, Jr. and I. Carvalho. 2009. Carrageenans: biological properties, chemical modifications and structural analysis—A review. Carbohydr. Polym. 77: 167–180.

Culty, M., M. Shizari, E. W. Thompson and C. B. Underhill. 1994. Binding and degradation of hyaluronan by human breast cancer cell lines expressing different forms of CD44: correlation with invasive potential. J. Cell. Physiol. 160: 275–286.

Challa, R., A. Ahuja, J. Ali and R. Khar. 2005. Cyclodextrins in drug delivery: an updated review. AAPS PharmSciTech. 6: E329–E357.

Chandra, M. and B. Shamasundar. 2015. Rheological properties of gelatin prepared from the swim bladders of freshwater fish Catlacatla. Food Hydrocolloid. 48: 47–54.

Chen, G. Q. and Q. Wu. 2005. The application of polyhydroxyalkanoates as tissue engineering materials. Biomaterials 26: 6565–6578.

Cheng, L., C. Bulmer and A. Margaritis. 2015. Characterization of novel composite alginate chitosan-carrageenan nanoparticles for encapsulation of BSA as a model drug delivery system. Curr. Drug. Deliv. 14: 14.

Chevallay, B. and D. Herbage. 2000. Collagen-based biomaterials as 3D scaffold for cell cultures: applications for tissue engineering and gene therapy. Med. Biol. Eng. Comput. 38: 211–218.

Chirita, M. 2008. Mechanical properties of collagen biomimetic films formed in the presence of calcium, silica and chitosan. J. Bionic. Eng. 5: 149–158.

Chvapil, M., R. L. Kronenthal and W. van Winkle. 1973. Medical and surgical applications of collagen. Int. Rev. Connect. Tissue Res. 6: 1–61.

Das, S. and U. Subuddhi. 2015. pH-responsive guar gum hydrogels for controlled delivery of dexamethasone to the intestine. Int. J. Biol. Macromolec. 79: 856–863.

Dawes, E. S. and P. J. Senior. 1973. The role and regulation of energy reserve polymers in microorganisms polyhydroxybutyrate. Adv. Microbiol. Physiol. 10: 135–266.

De Vos, P., B. De Haan, G. H. Wolters and R. Van Schilfgaarde. 1996. Factors influencing the adequacy of microencapsulation of rat pancreatic islets 1. Transplantation 62: 888–893.

Del Rosso, J. Q. 2003. New and emerging topical approaches for actinic keratoses. Cutis 72: 273–276, 279.

Desai, N., V. Trieu, Z. Yao, L. Louie, S. Ci, A. Yang et al. 2006. Increased antitumor activity, intratumor paclitaxel concentrations, and endothelial cell transport of cremophor-free, albumin-bound paclitaxel, ABI-007, compared with cremophor-based paclitaxel. Clin. Cancer. Res. 12: 1317–1324.

Drevs, J., N. Esser, H. Richly, M. Skorzec, M. Scheulen, C. Unger et al. 2000. *In vivo* activity and pharmacokinetic study of an acid-sensitive doxorubicin albumin conjugate in murine renal cell carcinoma in comparison to free doxorubicin. Clin. Cancer. Res. 6: a120.

Dugan, J. M., J. E. Gough and S. J. Eichhorn. 2013. Bacterial cellulose scaffolds and cellulose nanowhiskers for tissue engineering. Nanomedicine 8: 287–298.

Edgar, K. J. 2007. Cellulose esters in drug delivery. Cellulose 14: 49–64.

Edsman, K., J. Carlfors and K. Harju. 1996. Rheological evaluation and ocular contact time of some carbomer gels for ophthalmic use. Int. J. Pharm. 137: 233–241.

Endo, T., H. Nagase, H. Ueda, S. Kobayashi and T. Nagai. 1997. Isolation, purification, and characterization of cyclomaltodecaose (epsilon-cyclodextrin), cyclomaltoundecaose (zeta-cyclodextrin) and cyclomaltotridecaose (theta-cyclodextrin). Chem. Pharm. Bull. 45: 532–536.

Esa, F., S. M. Tasirin and N. A. Rahman. 2014. Overview of bacterial cellulose production and application. Agric. Agric. Sci. Procedia. 2: 113–119.

Eysturskarð, J., I. J. Haug, A. S. Ulset and K. I. Draget. 2009. Mechanical properties of mammalian and fish gelatins based on their weight average molecular weight and molecular weight distribution. Food Hydrocoll. 23: 2315–2321.

Flammang, A. M., D. M. Kendall, C. J. Baumgartner, T. D. Slagle and Y. S. Choe. 2006. Effect of a viscous fiber bar on postprandial glycemia in subjects with type 2 diabetes. J. Am. Coll. Nutr. 25: 409–414.

Fraser, J. R., T. C. Laurent and U. B. Laurent. 1997. Hyaluronan: its nature, distribution, functions and turnover. J. Intern. Med. 242: 27–33.

Friess, W. 1998. Collagen–biomaterial for drug delivery. Eur. J. Pharm. Biopharm. 45: 113–136.

Friess, W. 2000. Drug Delivery Systems Based on Collagen. Berichteaus der Pharmazie, Shaker Verlag, Aachen.

Fu Lu, M. and C. Thies. 1991. Collagen-based drug delivery devices. pp. 149–161. *In*: Tarche, P. (ed.). Polymers for Controlled Drug Delivery. CRC Press, Boca Raton, FL.

Funami, T., Y. Kataoka, T. Omoto, Y. Goto, I. Asai and K. Nishinari. 2005. Effects of non-ionic polysaccharides on the gelatinization and retrogradation behavior of wheat starch. Food Hydrocolloid 19: 1–13.

Galkina, O.L., V. Ivanov, A.V. Agafonov, G.A. Seisenbaeva and V.G. Kessler. 2015. Cellulose nanofiber–titania nanocomposites as potential drug delivery systems for dermal applications. J. Mater. Chem. B 3: 1688–1698.

Gavini, E., G. Rassu, V. Sanna, M. Cossu and P. Giunchedi. 2005. Mucoadhesive microspheres for nasal administration of an antiemetic drug, metoclopramide: *in-vitro/ex-vivo* studies. J. Pharm. Pharmacol. 57: 287–294.

George, M. and T. E. Abraham. 2007. pH sensitive alginate-guar gum hydrogel for the controlled delivery of protein drugs. Int. J. Pharm. 335: 123–129.

Germershaus, O., T. Lühmann, J. C. Rybak, J. Ritzer and L. Meinel. 2015. Application of natural and semi-synthetic polymers for the delivery of sensitive drugs. Int. Mater. Rev. 60: 101–131.

Gombotz, W. R. and D. K. Pettit. 1995. Biodegradable polymers for protein and peptide drug delivery. Bioconjug. Chem. 6: 332–351.

Grant, C. A., D. J. Brockwell, S. E. Radford and N. H. Thomson. 2009. Tuning the elastic modulus of hydrated collagen fibrils. Biophys. J. 97: 2985–2992.

Grant, G. T., E. R. Morris, D. A. Rees, P. J. Smith and D. Thom. 1973. Biological interactions between polysaccharides and divalent cations: the egg-box model. FEBS Lett. 32: 195–198.

Grasdalen, H., B. Larsen and O. Smisrod. 1981. 13C NMR studies of monomeric composition and sequence in alginate. Carbohydr. Res. 89: 179–191.

Gurr, M. and R. Mülhaupt. 2012. Rapid prototyping. pp. 77–99. *In*: Matyjaszewski, K. and M. Möller (eds.). Polymer Science: A Comprehensive Reference. Elsevier, Amsterdam.

Hariharan, M., T. A. Wheatley and J. C. Price. 1997. Controlled-release tablet matrices from carrageenans: compression and dissolution studies. Pharm. Dev. Technol. 2: 383–393.

Harkness, R. 1965. Collagen. Sci. Prog. 54: 257–274.

Harrington, D. J. 1996. Bacterial collagenases and collagen-degrading enzymes and their potential role in human disease. Infect. Immun. 64: 1885.

He, L., C. Mu, J. Ski, Q. Zhang, B. Shi and Q. Lin. 2011. Modification of collagen with a natural cross-linker, procyanidin. Int. J. Biol. Macr. 48: 354–359.

Helenius, G., H. Bäckdahl, A. Bodin, U. Nannmark, P. Gatenholm and B. Risberg. 2006. *In vivo* biocompatibility of bacterial cellulose. J. Biomed. Mater. Res. A 76: 431–438.

Hinterstoisser, B. and L. Salmén. 2000. Application of dynamic 2D FTIR to cellulose. Vib. Spectr. 22: 111–118.

Hoffman, A. S. 2002. Hydrogels for biomedical applications. Adv. Drug Delivery Rev. 54: 3–12.

Hsu, F. Y., S. C. Chueh and Y. J. Wang. 1999. Microspheres of hydroxyapatite/reconstituted collagen as supports for osteoblast cell growth. Biomaterials 20: 1931–1936.

Iguchi, M., S. Yamanaka and A. Budhiono. 2000. Bacterial cellulose—a masterpiece of nature's arts. J. Mate. Sci. 3: 261–270.

Illum, L., N. F. Farraj, A. N. Fisher, I. Gill, M. Miglietta and L. M. Benedetti. 1994. Hyaluronic acid ester microspheres as a nasal delivery system for insulin. J. Control. Rel. 29: 133–141.

Irie, T. and K. Uekama. 1997. Pharmaceutical applications of cyclodextrins. III. Toxicological issues and safety evaluation. J. Pharm. Sci. 86: 147–162.

Jain, N. K., K. Kulkarni and N. Talwar. 1992. Controlled-release tablet formulation of isoniazid. Pharmazie 47: 277–278.

Jain, S., P. S. Sandhu, R. Malvi and B. Gupta. 2013. Cellulose derivatives as thermoresponsive polymer: an overview. J. Appl. Pharm. Sci. 3: 139–144.

Jana, S., A. Gandhi, K. Sen and S. Basu. 2011. Natural polymers and their application in drug delivery and biomedical field. J. Pharma. SciTech. 1: 16–27.

Jeon, O., S. J. Song, K.-J. Lee, M. H. Park, S.-H. Lee, S. K. Hahn et al. 2007. Mechanical properties and degradation behaviors of hyaluronic acid hydrogels cross-linked at various cross-linking densities. Carb. Polym. 70: 251–257.

Kamel, S., N. Ali, K. Jahangir, S. Shah and A. El-Gendy. 2008. Pharmaceutical significance of cellulose: a review. Express Polym. Lett. 2: 758–778.

Kianfar, F., M. Antonijevic, B. Chowdhry and J. Boateng. 2011. Formulation development of a carrageenan based delivery system for buccal drug delivery using ibuprofen as a model drug. J. Biomat. Nanobiotec. 2: 582–595.

Kikuchi, M., H. N. Matsumoto, T. Yamada, Y. Koyama, K. Takakuda and J. Tanaka. 2004. Glutaraldehyde cross-linked hydroxyapatite/collagen self-organized nanocomposites. Biomaterials 25: 63–69.

Kobayashi, Y., A. Okamoto and K. Nishinari. 1994. Viscoelasticity of hyaluronic acid with different molecular weights. Biorheology 31: 235–244.

Kooy, F. K., M. Ma, H. H. Beeftink, G. Eggink, J. Tramper and C. G. Boeriu. 2009. Quantification and characterization of enzymatically produced hyaluronan with fluorophore-assisted carbohydrate electrophoresis. Anal. Biochem. 384: 329–336.

Kratz, F. 2008. Albumin as a drug carrier: design of prodrugs, drug conjugates and nanoparticles. J. Control. Rel. 132: 171–183.

Krishnaiah, Y. S., S. Satyanarayana, Y. V. Rama Prasad and S. Narasimha Rao. 1998. Gamma scintigraphic studies on guar gum matrix tablets for colonic drug delivery in healthy human volunteers. J. Control. Rel. 55: 245–252.

Kulkarni, R. V., R. Boppana, G. K. Mohan, S. Mutalik and N. V. Kalyane. 2012. pH-responsive interpenetrating network hydrogel beads of poly (acrylamide)-g-carrageenan and sodium alginate for intestinal targeted drug delivery: Synthesis, *in vitro* and *in vivo* evaluation. J. Col. Int. Sci. 367: 509–517.

Lai, W.-F. 2014. Cyclodextrins in non-viral gene delivery. Biomaterials 35: 401–411.

Lam, J., N. F. Truong and T. Segura. 2014. Design of cell-matrix interactions in hyaluronic acid hydrogel scaffolds. ActaBiomater. 10: 1571–1580.

Langer, K., M. Anhorn, I. Steinhauser, S. Dreis, D. Celebi, N. Schrickel et al. 2008. Human serum albumin (HSA) nanoparticles: reproducibility of preparation process and kinetics of enzymatic degradation. Int. J. Pharm. 347: 109–117.

Lee, C. H., A. Singla and Y. Lee. 2001. Biomedical applications of collagen. Int. J. Pharm. 221: 1–22.

Lesiak-Cyganowska, E., D. Sladowski and J. Komender. 2000. Modification of collagen film by certain chemical agents. Archi. Immunol. Ther. Experim. 49: 247–251.

Li, L., R. Ni, Y. Shao and S. Mao. 2014. Carrageenan and its applications in drug delivery. Carbohydr. Polym. 103: 1–11.

Li, X., W. Wu, J. Wang and Y. Duan. 2006. The swelling behavior and network parameters of guar gum/poly (acrylic acid) semi-interpenetrating polymer network hydrogels. Carbohydr. Polym. 66: 473–479.

Lim, S. T., G. P. Martin, D. J. Berry and M. B. Brown. 2000. Preparation and evaluation of the *in vitro* drug release properties and mucoadhesion of novel microspheres of hyaluronic acid and chitosan. J. Control. Release 66: 281–292.

Liu, D., E. Pearlman, E. Diaconu, K. Guo, H. Mori, T. Haqqi et al. 1996. Expression of hyaluronidase by tumor cells induces angiogenesis *in vivo*. Proc. Natl. Acad. Sci. 93: 7832–7837.

Liu, S.-K., Y.-Q. Zhong and F. Wang. 2004. Preparation and *in vitro* release of foot-mouth-disease DNA vaccine-loaded sodium alginate microspheres. Pharm. Care. Resch. 4: 107–110.

Lo, M., M. Sass, P. Michel, U. Hopt, C. Kunze and K.-P. Schmitz. 1999. Differential gene expression after implantation of biomaterials into rat gastrointestine. J. Mat. Sci.: Mat. Med. 10: 797–799.

Loftsson, T. and E. Stefánsson. 2002. Cyclodextrins in eye drop formulations: enhanced topical delivery of corticosteroids to the eye. Acta Ophthal. 80: 144–150.

Lokeshwar, V. B., C. Obek, M. S. Soloway and N. L. Block. 1997. Tumor-associated hyaluronic acid: a new sensitive and specific urine marker for bladder cancer. Cancer Res. 57: 773–777.

Lynn, A., I. Yannas and W. Bonfield. 2004. Antigenicity and immunogenicity of collagen. J. Biomed. Mat. Res. B: Appl. Biomat. 71: 343–354.

Maeda, H., M. Ueda, T. Morinaga and T. Matsumoto. 1985. Conjugation of poly (styrene-co-maleic acid) derivatives to the antitumor protein neocarzinostatin: pronounced improvements in pharmacological properties. J. Med. Chem. 28: 455–461.

Marchal, R., E. Nicolau, J.-P. Ballaguet and F. Bertoncini. 2008. Biodegradability of polyethylene glycol 400 by complex microfloras. Internat. Biodeterior. Biodegrad. 62: 384–390.

Martin, D. P., F. Skraly and S. F. Williams. 2003. Polyhydroxyalkanoate compositions having controlled degradation rates: #US 6610764 B1.

Matsubara, Y., S. Katoh, H. Taniguchii, M. Oka, J. Kadota and S. Kohno. 2000. Expression of CD44 variants in lung cancer and its relationship to hyaluronan binding. J. Int. Med. Res. 28: 78–90.

McCleary, B. B. 1979. Enzymic hydrolysis, fine structure, and gelling interaction of legume-seed D-galacto-D-mannans. Carbohydr. Res. 71: 205–230.

Meinel, L., S. Hofmann, V. Karageorgiou, C. Kirker-Head, J. McCool, G. Gronowicz et al. 2005. The inflammatory responses to silk films *in vitro* and *in vivo*. Biomaterials 26: 147–155.

Melnick, R. L., J. Huff, J. K. Haseman, M. P. Dieter, C. K. Grieshaber, D. S. Wyand et al. 1983. Chronic effects of agar, guar gum, gum arabic, locust-bean gum, or tara gum in F344 rats and B6C3F1 mice. Food Chem. Toxicol. 21: 305–311.

Meyer, K. and J. W. Palmer. 1934. The polysaccharide of the vitreous humor. J. Biolog. Chem. 107: 629–634.

Misra, S. K., S. P. Valappil, I. Roy and A. R. Boccaccini. 2006. Polyhydroxyalkanoate (PHA)/inorganic phase composites for tissue engineering applications. Biomacromolecules 7: 2249–2258.

Mo, Y., T. Takaya and K. Nishinari. 1996. Effects of sodium chloride, guanidine hydrochloride and sucrose on the rheological properties of hyaluronic acid solutions. Biorheology 33: 79.

Mohammad, J. A., P. H. Warnke, Y. C. Pan and S. Shenaq. 2000. Increased axonal regeneration through a biodegradable amnionic tube nerve conduit: effect of local delivery and incorporation of nerve growth factor/hyaluronic acid media. Ann. Plast. Surg. 44: 59–64.

Morris, E. R., D. A. Rees and G. Robinson. 1980. Cation-specific aggregation of carrageenan helices: domain model of polymer gel structure. J. Mol. Biol. 138: 349–362.

Mudgil, D., S. Barak and B. S. Khatkar. 2014. Guar gum: processing, properties and food applications: a review. J. Food Sci. Technol. 51: 409–18.

Mura, P., E. Adragna, A. Rabasco, J. Moyano, J. Perez-Martinez, M. Arias et al. 1999. Effects of the host cavity size and the preparation method on the physicochemical properties of ibuproxam-cyclodextrin systems. Drug Development Ind. Pharm. 25: 279–287.

Nagase, Y., M. Hirata, K. Wada, H. Arima, F. Hirayama, T. Irie et al. 2001. Improvement of some pharmaceutical properties of DY-9760e by sulfobutyl ether β-cyclodextrin. Int. J. Pharm. 229: 163–172.

Nair, L. S. and C. T. Laurencin. 2007. Biodegradable polymers as biomaterials. Prog. Polym. Sci. 32: 762–798.

Neau, S. H., M. Y. Chow and M. J. Durrani. 1996. Fabrication and characterization of extruded and spheronized beads containing Carbopol® 974P, NF resin. Int. J. Pharm. 13: 47–55.

Necas, J. and L. Bartosikova. 2013. Carrageenan: a review. Vet. Med. 58: 187–205.

Nelson, D. L., A. L. Lehninger and M. M. Cox. 2008. Lehninger Principles of Biochemistry. Macmillan, London.

Nigmatullin, R., P. Thomas, B. Lukasiewicz, H. Puthussery and I. Roy. 2015. Polyhydroxyalkanoates, a family of natural polymers, and their applications in drug delivery. J. Chem. Technol. Biotechnol. 90: 1209–1221.

Nijenhuis, N., D. Mizuno, C. F. Schmidt, H. Vink and J. A. Spaan. 2008. Microrheology of hyaluronan solutions: implications for the endothelial glycocalyx. Biomacromolecules 9: 2390–2398.

O'Neill, M. J., A. M. O'Mahony, C. Byrne, R. Darcy and C. M. O'Driscoll. 2013. Gastrointestinal gene delivery by cyclodextrins–*In vitro* quantification of extracellular barriers. Int. J. Pharm. 456: 390–399.

Okada, T., T. Hayashi and Y. Ikada. 1992. Degradation of collagen suture *in vitro* and *in vivo*. Biomaterials 13: 448–454.

Palmieri, G. F., P. Wehrlé and A. Stamm. 1993. Inclusion of vitamin D2 in β-cyclodextrin. Evaluation of different complexation methods. Drug DevelIndust. Pharm. 19: 875–885.

Piskin, E. 1995. Biodegradable polymers as biomaterials. J. Biomater. Sci. Polym. Ed. 6: 775–795.

Pouton, C. W., J. E. Kennedy, L. J. Notarianni and P. L. Gould. 1988. Biocompatibility of polyhydroxybutyrate and related copolymers. In. Proc. Int., Symp. Controlled Release Bioact. Mater. 15: 179–180.

Pouton, C. W. and S. Akhtar. 1996. Biosynthetic polyhydroxyalkanoates and their potential in drug delivery. Adv. Drug Deliv. Rev. 18: 133–162.

Prabaharan, M. 2011. Prospective of guar gum and its derivatives as controlled drug delivery systems. Int. J. Biol. Macromol. 49: 117–124.

Prankerd, R. J., H. W. Stone, K. B. Sloan and J. H. Perrin. 1992. Degradation of aspartame in acidic aqueous media and its stabilization by complexation with cyclodextrins or modified cyclodextrins. Int. J. Pharm. 88: 189–199.

Redenti, E., C. Pietra, A. Gerloczy and L. Szente. 2001. Cyclodextrins in oligonucleotide delivery. Adv. Drug Deliv. Rev. 53: 235–244.

Richardson, J. C., P. W. Dettmar, F. C. Hampson and C. D. Melia. 2005. Oesophageal bioadhesion of sodium alginate suspensions: 2. Suspension behaviour on oesophageal mucosa. Eur. J. Pharm. Sci. 24: 107–114.

Rinaudo, M. 2008. Main properties and current applications of some polysaccharides as biomaterials. Polym. Int. 57: 397–430.

Roberts, J. N., C. B. Buck, C. D. Thompson, R. Kines, M. Bernardo, P. L. Choyke et al. 2007. Genital transmission of HPV in a mouse model is potentiated by nonoxynol-9 and inhibited by carrageenan. Nat. Med. 13: 857–861.

Rocha de Souza, M. C., C. T. Marques, C. M. Guerra Dore, F. R. Ferreira da Silva, H. A. Oliveira Rocha and E. L. Leite. 2007. Antioxidant activities of sulfated polysaccharides from brown and red seaweeds. J. Appl. Phycol. 19: 153–60.

Rohanizadeh, R. and N. Kokabi. 2009. Heat denatured/aggregated albumin-based biomaterial: effects of preparation parameters on biodegradability and mechanical properties. J. Mater. Sci. Mater. Med. 20: 2413–2418.

Rowe, R. C., P. J. Sheskey, M. E. and A. P. Quinn. 2009. Handbook of Pharmaceutical Excipients. Vol. 6. Pharmaceutical Press, London.

Rubin, A. L., K. H. Stenzel, T. Miyata, M. J. White and M. Dunn. 1973. Collagen as a vehicle for drug delivery. J. Clin. Pharmacol. New Drugs. 13: 309–312.

Ruszczak, Z. and W. Friess. 2003. Collagen as a carrier for on-site delivery of antibacterial drugs. Adv. Drug Deliv. Rev. 55: 1679–1698.

Sadeghi, H., V. Hajhashemi, M. Minaiyan, A. Movahedian and A. Talebi. 2011. A study on the mechanisms involving the anti-inflammatory effect of amitriptyline in carrageenan-induced paw edema in rats. Eur. J. Phycol. 667: 396–401.

Sankalia, M. G., R. C. Mashru, J. M. Sankalia and V. B. Sutariya. 2006. Stability improvement of alpha-amylase entrapped in kappa-carrageenan beads: physicochemical characterization and optimization using composite index. Int. J. Pharm. 312: 1–14.

Santoro, M., A. M. Tatara and A. G. Mikos. 2014. Gelatin carriers for drug and cell delivery in tissue engineering. J. Controlled Release. 190: 210–218.

Scatchard, G., A. Batchelder and A. Brown. 1944. Chemical, clinical, and immunological studies on the products of human plasma fractionation. VI. The osmotic pressure of plasma and of serum albumin. J. Clin. Invest. 23: 458.

Schardinger, F. 1903. Über Thermophile Bakterien aus verschiedenen Speisen und Milch, sowie über einige Umsetzungsprodukte derselben in kohlenhydrathaltigen Nährlösungen, darunter krystallisierte Polysaccharide (Dextrine) aus Stärke. Z. Untersuch. Nahr. u. Genussm. 6: 865–880.

Schierbaum, F. 1971. Glicksman, M.: Gum Technology in the Food Industry. Academic Press, New York and London, 1969. XIII, 590 S., 8°, mit zahlreichen Abb. und Tab., Ganzleinen. Starch – Stärke. 23: 372–373.

Shah, A. K., K. J. Simons and C. J. Briggs. 1991. Physical, chemical, and bioavailability studies of parenteral diazepam formulations containing propylene glycol and polyethylene glycol 400. Drug dev. Ind. Pharm. 17: 1635–1654.

Shingleton, W., T. Cawston, D. Hodges and P. Brick. 1996. Collagenase: a key enzyme in collagen turnover. Biochem. Cell Biol. 74: 759–775.

Shokri, J. and K. Adibkia. 2013. Application of Cellulose and Cellulose Derivatives in Pharmaceutical Industries: Cellulose-Medical, Pharmaceutical and Electronic Applications, InTech, Open access.

Shrivastav, A., H. Y. Kim and Y. R. Kim. 2013. Advances in the applications of polyhydroxyalkanoate nanoparticles for novel drug delivery system. BioMed. Res. Int., Article ID: 581684.

Simpson, N. E., C. L. Stabler, C. P. Simpson, A. Sambanis and I. Constantinidis. 2004. The role of the $CaCl_2$–gulronic acid interaction on alginate encapsulated βTC3 cells. Biomaterials 25: 2603–2610.

Singla, A. K., M. Chawla and A. Singh. 2000. Potential applications of carbomer in oral mucoadhesive controlled drug delivery system: a review. Drug Dev. Ind. Pharm. 26: 913–924.

Stewart, A. J., C. A. Blindauer, S. Berezenko, D. Sleep, D. Tooth and P. J. Sadler. 2005. Role of Tyr84 in controlling the reactivity of Cys34 of human albumin. Febs J. 272: 353–362.

Svensson, A., E. Nicklasson, T. Harrah, B. Panilaitis, D. Kaplan, M. Brittberg et al. 2005. Bacterial cellulose as a potential scaffold for tissue engineering of cartilage. Biomaterials 26: 419–431.

Szejtli, J. 1998. Introduction and general overview of cyclodextrin chemistry. Chem. Rev. 98: 1743–1754.

Szente, L., I. Apostol and J. Szejtli. 1984. Suppositories containing beta-cyclodextrin complexes. Part 1: Stability studies. Pharmazie. 39: 697–699.

Szente, L., I. Apostol, A. Gerloczy and J. Szejtli. 1985. Suppositories containing cyclodextrin complexes. Part 2: Dissolution and absorption studies. Pharmazie. 40: 406–407.

Tan, H., F. Qin, D. Chen, S. Han, W. Lu and X. Yao. 2013. Study of glycol chitosan-carboxymethyl β-cyclodextrins as anticancer drugs carrier. Carbohyd. Polym. 93: 679–685.

Tanabe, K. K., L. M. Ellis and H. Saya. 1993. Expression of CD44R1 adhesion molecule in colon carcinomas and metastases. Lancet. 341: 725–726.

Tasić, L. M., M. Jovanović and Z. Djurić. 1992. The influence of β-cyclodextrin on the solubility and dissolution rate of paracetamol solid dispersions. J. Pharm. Pharmacol. 44: 52–55.

Taylor, E. 1997. Surgical infection: current concerns. Eur. J. Surg. Suppl./Acta chirurgica. Supplement. 578: 5.

Thommes, M. and P. Kleinebudde. 2007. Properties of pellets manufactured by wet extrusion/spheronization process using κ-carrageenan: effect of process parameters. AAPS Pharm. Sci. Tech. 8: 101–108.

Thrimawithana, T. R., S. Young, D. E. Dunstan and R. G. Alany. 2010. Texture and rheological characterization of kappa and iota carrageenan in the presence of counter ions. Carbohyd. Polym. 82: 69–77.

Tobacman, J. K. 2001. Review of harmful gastrointestinal effects of carrageenan in animal experiments. Environ. Health. Perspect. 109: 983–994.

Tomlin, J., N. W. Read, C. A. Edwards and B. I. Duerden. 1986. The degradation of guar gum by a faecal incubation system. Br. J. Nutr. 55: 481–486.

Trovatti, E., C. S. Freire, P. C. Pinto, I. F. Almeida, P. Costa, A. J. Silvestre et al. 2012. Bacterial cellulose membranes applied in topical and transdermal delivery of lidocaine hydrochloride and ibuprofen: *in vitro* diffusion studies. Int. J. Pharm. 435: 83–87.

Ueda, H. and Y. Tabata. 2003. Polyhydroxyalkanonate derivatives in current clinical applications and trials. Adv. Drug Deliv. Rev. 55: 501–518.

van der Kam, E. L., J. D. Vry, K. Schiene and T. M. Tzschentke. 2008. Differential effects of morphine on the affective and the sensory component of carrageenan-induced nociception in the rat. Pain 136: 373–379.

van der Rijt, J. A., K. O. van der Werf, M. L. Bennink, P. J. Dijkstra and J. Feijen. 2006. Micromechanical testing of individual collagen fibrils. Macromol. Biosci. 6: 697–702.

Varghese, J. S., N. Chellappa and N. N. Fathima. 2014. Gelatin–carrageenan hydrogels: role of pore size distribution on drug delivery process. Colloids Surf. B. Biointerfaces 113: 346–351.

Villiers, A. 1891. Sur la fermentation de la fécule par láction du ferment butyrique. Compt. Rend. Acad. Sci. 112: 536–538.

von der Ohe, N., M. Stark, H. Mayer and H. Brewitt. 1996. How can the bioavailability of timolol be enhanced? A pharmacokinetic pilot study of novel hydrogels. Ger. J. Ophthalmol. 234: 452–456.

Wang, S., S. H. Lee and Q. Cheng. 2010. Mechanical properties of cellulosic materials at micro- and nanoscale levels, cellulose: structure and properties. pp. 459–500. *In*: Lejeune, A. and D. Thibaut (eds.). Cellulose: Structure and Properties, Derivatives and Industrial Uses. Nova Publishers, USA.

Widner, B., R. Behr, S. Von Dollen, M. Tang, T. Heu, A. Sloma et al. 2005. Hyaluronic acid production in Bacillus subtilis. Appl. Environ. Microbiol. 71: 3747–3752.

Wijesekara, I., R. Pangestuti and S. K. Kim. 2011. Biological activities and potential health benefits of sulfated polysaccharides derived from marine algae. Carbohyd. Polym. 84: 14–21.

Woolfson, A., D. McCafferty, P. McCarron and J. Price. 1995. A bioadhesive patch cervical drug delivery system for the administration of 5-fluorouracil to cervical tissue. J. Control. Release 35: 49–58.

Wu, Q., Y. Wang and G. Q. Chen. 2009. Medical application of microbial biopolyesters polyhydroxyalkanoates. Artif. Cells Blood Substit. Immobil. Biotechnol. 37: 1–12.

Xu, H., T. Ito, A. Tawada, H. Maeda, H. Yamanokuchi, K. Isahara et al. 2002. Effect of hyaluronan oligosaccharides on the expression of heat shock protein 72. J. Biol. Chem. 277: 17308–17314.

Yaffe, A., A. Herman, H. Bahar and I. Binderman. 2003. Combined local application of tetracycline and bisphosphonate reduces alveolar bone resorption in rats. J. Periodontol. 74: 1038–1042.

Yalwsky, S. H., E. Davis and T. Clark. 1993. Stabilization of aspartame by polyethylene glycol 400. J. Pharm. Sci. 82: 978–978.

Yang, L., K. O. Van der Werf, C. F. Fitié, M. L. Bennink, P. J. Dijkstra and J. Feijen. 2008. Mechanical properties of native and cross-linked type I collagen fibrils. Biophys. J. 94: 2204–2211.

Yokota, A., G. Ishii, Y. Sugaya, M. Nishimura, Y. Saito and K. Harigaya. 1999. Potential use of serum CD44 as an indicator of tumour progression in acute leukemia. Hematol. Oncol. 17: 161–168.

Yoon, S. J., D. C. Chu and L. Raj Juneja. 2008. Chemical and physical properties, safety and application of partially hydrolized guar gum as dietary fiber. J. Clin. Biochem. Nutr. 42: 1–7.

Young, S., M. Wong, Y. Tabata and A. G. Mikos. 2005. Gelatin as a delivery vehicle for the controlled release of bioactive molecules. J. Control. Release 109: 256–274.

Yu, C. Y., B. C. Yin, W. Zhang, S. X. Cheng, X. Z. Zhang and R. X. Zhuo. 2009. Composite microparticle drug delivery systems based on chitosan, alginate and pectin with improved pH-sensitive drug release property. Colloids Surf B Biointerfaces 68: 245–249.

Zgoła-Grześkowiak, A., T. Grześkowiak, J. Zembrzuska and Z. Łukaszewski. 2006. Comparison of biodegradation of poly(ethyleneglycol)s and poly(propyleneglycol)s. Chemosphere. 64: 803–809.

Zhu, J. H., X. Q. Yang, I. Ahmad, Y. Jiang, X. Y. Wang and L. Y. Wu. 2009. Effect of guar gum on the rheological, thermal and textural properties of soybean β-conglycinin gel. Int. J. Food Sci. Technol. 44: 1314–1322.

Zinn, M., B. Witholt and T. Egli. 2001. Occurrence, synthesis and medical application of bacterial polyhydroxyalkanoate. Adv. Drug Deliv. Rev. 53: 5–21.

3

Polysaccharide Based Biomaterials

*Narendra Reddy** and *Divya Natraj*

Introduction

There is an increasing interest in using biopolymeric materials for medical applications due to their biocompatibility, ability to support attachment and growth of cells, deliver drugs to targeted organs, and easy degradability. Unlike metals or synthetic polymers, biopolymeric materials have limited risk of immunogenic response and accumulation in the body. Also, biopolymers are readily available and easily modifiable for specific applications. Proteins and polysaccharides are the two most common biopolymers. Although proteins are preferred over polysaccharides, proteins have several limitations. Despite limitations, polysaccharides have unique properties and several advantages that make them useful for medical applications. Compared to proteins, polysaccharides are more stable and provide biomaterials with required mechanical properties and aqueous stability. In addition, polysaccharides are more readily available than proteins and can better withstand processing conditions and can be more easily made into various shapes and sizes.

Starch, cellulose, chitosan, and alginate are the most common polysaccharides. Bacterial cellulose is another polysaccharide that has been extensively studied and used for medical applications. In addition to these, hyaluronic acid, pullalan, and

Center for Emerging Technologies, Jain University, Jain Global Campus, Jakkasandra Post, Ramanagar District, Bengaluru 562112, India.
* Corresponding author: narendra.reddy@jainuniversity.ac.in

cyclodextrin are lesser known polysaccharides that have been considered for medical applications. Cotton, one of the most widely available polysaccharide, has been used as wound dressings (gauze) and in other forms for medical applications since ancient times. Many literatures cite the advantages of using cotton for *in vitro* and *in vivo* use. However, polysaccharides including cellulose have several limitations that restricts their widespread use. For example, the human body does not generate enzymes that degrade cellulose thereby making cellulosic materials undesirable for *in vivo* medical applications. Similarly, polysaccharides have limited free functional groups available for chemical modifications or for attaching drugs and pharmaceuticals. Developing biomaterials from polysaccharides such as cellulose is also a challenge since polysaccharides do not dissolve in common solvents. Although starch and chitosan dissolve in common solvents, the properties of the products obtained using these materials may not meet the requirements.

Despite these limitations, starch, cellulose, chitosan, and alginate have all been made into films, fibers (micro and nano), hydrogels, 3D scaffolds, micro and nanoparticles, vascular grafts, artificial red blood cells, etc., for medical use. Since a single polysaccharide cannot provide the desired properties and functionalities, most often a blend of the polymers have been used to develop the biomaterials. In addition, synthetic polymers such as polycaprolactone and polyethylene glycol have also been blended with polysaccharides to improve performance properties or biocompatibility. Similarly, chemical modifications such as grafting have also been done to make polysaccharides suitable for medical applications.

Since there is a vast amount of literature available on polysaccharides for medical applications, we have been compelled to restrict our discussions. In this chapter, we will provide an overview of biomaterials developed from alginate, starch, and cellulose (including bacterial cellulose) for various medical applications. We have excluded chitosan from this review due to the large number of papers available on the use of chitosan for medical applications. Condensing the available literature on chitosan into part of this chapter would exclude many important papers. Also, instead of discussing a particular polymer or a specific biomaterial (film, hydrogel, etc.) in detail, we have attempted to provide a glimpse of the various possibilities of using polysaccharides for medical applications. Efforts have been made to cover recent literature and trends but this review is by no means exhaustive.

Alginate

Alginate is one of the most common biopolymers used for medical applications. Alginate is available in many sea weeds and usually extracted from brown algae. Several species of brown algae are used to extract alginate. Extraction of algae from sea weed is simple and achieved by treating it with sodium hydroxide. Alginates are commercially produced and sold in various forms (http://www.fao.org/docrep/006/y4765e/y4765e08.htm; http://www.fmcbiopolymer.com/portals/pharm/content/docs/alginates.pdf). A simplified process of producing various types of alginates is shown in Fig. 1.

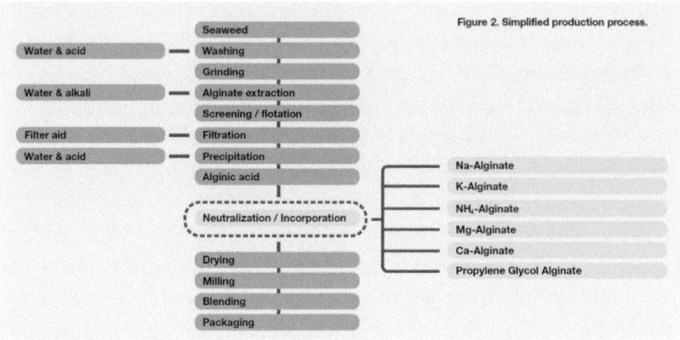

Fig. 1: Simplified depiction of the process of producing various types of alginates (http://www. fmcbiopolymer.com/portals/pharm/content/docs/alginates.pdf).

Alginate based hydrogels

Hydrogels are one of the most common forms of biomaterials used for medical applications. In addition to making hydrogels from individual polysaccharides, blends of polymers have also been made into hydrogels. Chitosan and alginate were blended together to form semi interpenetrating polymer network (IPN) hydrogels. IPNs are network of polymers where one of the polymer is crosslinked due to which an non-covalent interaction occurs with the other polymer (Treenate et al. 2014). Hydrogels could swell up to 600% depending on the ratio of chitosan to alginate. Increasing the amount of calcium chloride increased the crosslinking density and uniformity in distribution of the crosslinking ions (Fig. 2). Increasing the alginate to chitosan ratio decreased the ion content (b, d). MTT assay did not show any cytotoxicity and the hydrogels were considered to be suitable for medical applications (Treenate et al. 2014). IPNs could also be obtained when calcium alginate was combined with methacrylted dextran and photocrosslinked *in situ* (Matricardi et al. 2008). Rheological properties of the combined hydrogel was considerable different than the hydrogels made from calcium alginate. The gels could be easily injected using a hypodermic needle. Various model drugs were added into the alginate solution and made into gels and the release profile was studied. Mechanical properties, ability to degrade completely in the body, and sustained release of drugs from the IPN hydrogels were studied and found to be suitable for medical applications (Matricardi et al. 2008; Pescosolido et al. 2011). In another study, alginate was methacrylated and the modified gel was photocrosslinked for potential use as scaffold for regeneration of the intervertebral disc. Hydrogels with tunable degradation and Young's modulus of 0.6 to 8.8 MPa were obtained (Chou et al. 2007). Hydrogels made from methacrylated alginate and photo crosslinked by exposure to UV light were used as substrates for regeneration of nucleus pulposus (NP) damaged during intervertebral disc degeneration (Chou et al. 2009). NP cells were encapsulated into the alginate, injected into the intervertebral disc, and the ability of the hydrogels to promote the regeneration of the extracellular matrix and repair disc damage was studied. It was observed that photocrosslinked hydrogels had higher viability of cells after four weeks of culture and with the hydrogels being intact without any physical damage (Fig. 3) compared to the ionically crosslinked hydrogels that had disintegrated by four weeks. Also, photocrosslinked hydrogels had higher amount of extracellular matrix (ECM), type II collagen, and chondrotin sulfate proteoglycan implying that the gels were well suited for tissue regeneration (Chou et al. 2009).

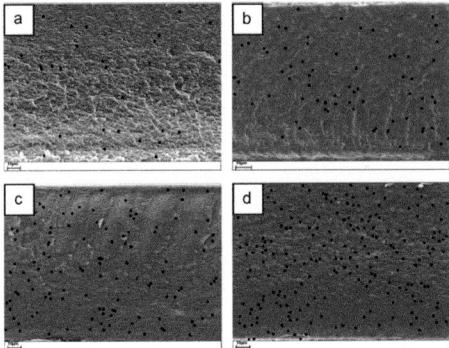

Fig. 2: Distribution of Ca2+ ions in the two dimensional hydrogels films containing different ratios of sodium alginate (SA), chitosan (HC) and calcium ions (Ca) (Treenate et al. 2014). HC75SA25Ca0.05 (a), HC75SA25Ca0.25 (b), HC50SA50Ca0.25 (c); HC25SA75Ca0.25 (d). Reproduced with permission from Springer.

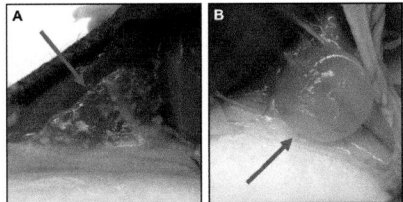

Fig. 3: Digital images of the ionically (left) and photocrosslinked (right) methacryalted alginate hydrogels after four weeks of implantation. The ionically crosslinked hydrogels show substantial degradation whereas the photocrosslinked hydrogels maintain their shape and promote the formation of ECM (Chou et al. 2009). Reproduced with permission from Elseiver.

Alginates have also been made into 2D hydrogels and 3D tubes for tissue engineering applications. The gels and tubes were crosslinked using calcium chloride and later seeded with rBMC cells. The cells were able to proliferate to a considerably large extent on the 3D tubes compared to the hydrogels. Substantial differentiation of cells was also observed on the scaffolds (Lee et al. 2013).

To avoid the use of chemcial crosslinkers, alginate hydrogels were crosslinked by conjugation with a natural crosslinker (3,4-dihydroxy-L-phenylalanine (L-DOPA) found in mussel bysuss. This natural crosslinker is reported to oxidatively crosslink proteins (Lee 2013). The oxidative crosslinking leads to the formation of catechol-catechol adducts that not only provide physical stability but are also non-toxic. Alginate-catechol conjugates were dissolved in cell culture media (Dulbecco's Phosphate Buffered Saling (DPBS)) and mixed with a gelation solution.

Hydrogels were also formed by crosslinking using calcium chloride for comparison with the catechol crosslinked gels. Alginate hydrogels had a pore size of 37 μm and were highly porous that would facilitate cell adhesion, proliferation, and migration (Lee et al. 2013). Catechol crosslinking showed considerably higher stability in aqueous conditions due to the higher resistance to ion exchange. In terms of mechanical properties, the alginate-catechol hydrogels were considered to be "soft hydrogels" with a modulus of 6 kPa. *In vitro* studies showed that the alginate-catechol hydrogels had good viability to Huh-7 and Neuro-2a cells and were also able to provide better (99–100% viability) support for primary and stem cells compared to calcium crosslinked alginate hydrogels (86% viability). Further, the hydrogels were able to provide a sustained release of growth factors and therefore considered to be suitable for medical applications (Lee et al. 2013). More importantly, the catechol crosslinking enabled controlling the physical and mechanical properties of the hydrogel and promote cell attachment and proliferation.

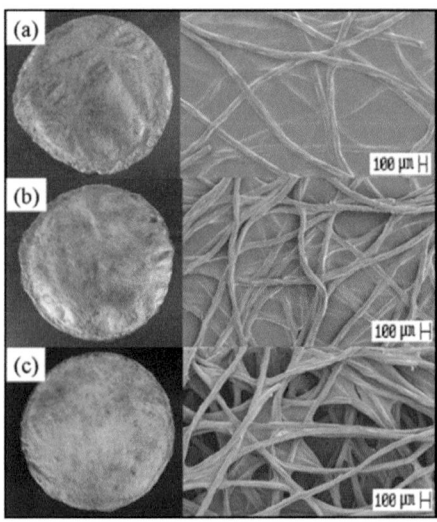

Fig. 4: Digital and SEM images of alginate and silk fiber composites at various levels of alginate fibers (Moraes and Beppu 2013). Part (a) has 20%, (b) has 40%, and (c) has 60% by weight of silk fibroin fibers. Reproduced with permission from John Wiley and Sons.

To prepare hydrogels for cartilage regeneration and enable complete degradation of the alginate, the alginate was oxidized using sodium periodate and later combined with hyaluronate and ionically crosslinked. Developed hydrogels were injected into the mice and the ability of the hydrogels to support cartilage regeneration was investigated (Park and Lee 2014). Oxidation of the alginate hydrogels increased the resistance to degradation in PBS and the extent of degradation was proportional to the level of oxidation. Hydrogels made from the alginate/hyaluronate blends were transplanted with primary chondrocytes and implanted in mice for cartilage regeneration. Implanted hydrogels were able to support the regeneration of cartilage (Park and Lee 2014). Rate of gelation, mechanical properties, and hydrogels with required dimensions could be achieved by varying the calcium source and extent of crosslinking (Kuo and Ma 2001). In a different approach towards preparing hydrogels, sodium alginate (low and high viscosity) was dissolved in water using calcium sulfate or calcium carbonate and D-glucono-δ-lactone as the gelling agent. Gels obtained with calcium sulfate and water solution were non-uniform whereas the calcium carbonate and D-glucono-δ-lactone gels were stable, uniform in size, and transparent (Fig. 6). Hydrogels could be tailored to have the required degradation rate, dimensions, and biocompatibility and therefore considered to be suitable for medical applications.

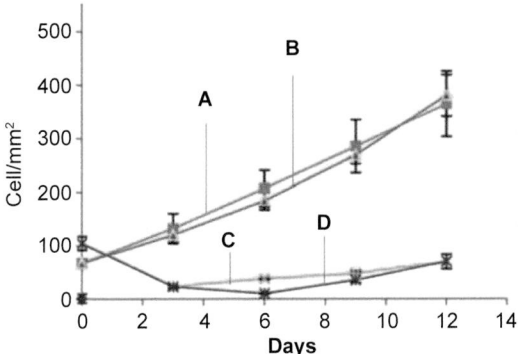

Fig. 5: Proliferation of the rBMC cells on the alginate hydrogels (discs) and 3D tubes (Barallet et al. 2005). Reproduced with permission from Springer. A is 8% alginate tubes, B is 8% alginate + tricalcium phosphate tubes, C is 8% alginate + TCP + cell disc and D is 8% alginate disc.

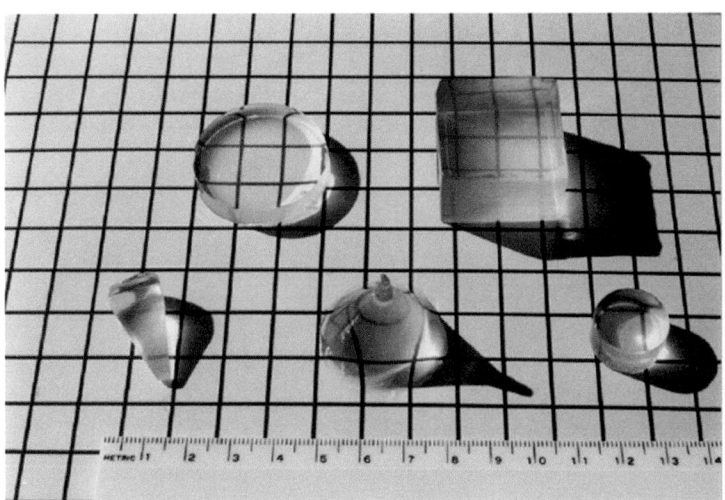

Fig. 6: Alginate gels of various shapes and sized made from an alginate solution using calcium carbonate and D-glucono-δ-lactone (Kuo and Ma 2001). Reproduced with permission from Elsevier.

Biocomposites

Since a single polymer most often is unable to provide the desired properties, a blend of polymers (typically synthetic polymers) have been used to develop biomaterials. Instead of combining alginate with synthetic polymers such as PEO, alginate was blended with silk fibroin and made into biocomposite films by casting. Silk fibers of about 50 µm in diameter were cut into length of 1 cm and dispersed in a sodium alginate solution (Moraes and Beppu 2013). Digital and SEM images of the composites containing various levels of silk fibers showed that increasing the concentration of feathers in the alginate matrix increased the density of the films and therefore the tensile properties. Unreinforced alginate films had a tensile strength of 73 N compared to 180 N for the composites containing 60% silk fibers which is expected due to the inherently higher strength of the silk fibers (Moraes and Beppu 2013). Silk fibers also increased the thermal stability of the alginate. Also, the composites had similar attachment and proliferation of CHO cells compared to pure alginate suggesting that the addition of silk fibers did not decrease the biocompatibility (Moraes and Beppu 2013). In another study, incorporating ferric ions instead of calcium ions was found to promote the attachment and proliferation of human fibroblasts (Machida-Sano et al. 2009). Fe-alginate was found to absorb more proteins and also had higher surface hydrophobicity which resulted in higher level of cell growth.

A ternary mixture of alginate, N-succinylchitosan and calcium sulfate were used to form composites for bone regeneration (Gomez d'Ayala et al. 2007). Composites obtained had varying strength and modulus depending on the ratio of the three polymers (Table 1). Addition of calcium sulfate improved adhesion and interaction between the alginate and chitosan without affecting the biocompatibility of the scaffolds (Gomez d'Ayala et al. 2007). Similarly, sodium alginate, gelatin and hyaluronic acid were blended and made into hydrogels using 1-ethyl-3-(3-dimethyl aminopropyl)

Table 1: Comparison of the strength and modulus of composites made using various ratios of alginate (Alg), chitosan (sCH), and 50% calcium sulfate (CHS) (Gomez d'Ayala et al. 2007).

Sample	Strength, MPa	Modulus, MPa
CHS/Alg (50/50)	0.03 ± 0.01	20.2 ± 3.5
CHS/sCh (50/50)	0.80 ± 0.21	14.7 ± 4.3
CHS/Alg/sCh (50/10/40)	4.58 ± 1.63	427.4 ± 79.8
CHS/Alg/sCh (50/20/30)	13.62 ± 0.41	873.9 ± 145.8
CHS/Alg/sCh (50/25/25)	8.20 ± 0.15	370.8 ± 73.7
CHS/Alg/sCh (50/30/20)	9.02 ± 2.62	437.9 ± 83.5
CHS/Alg/sCh (50/40/10)	3.22 ± 0.59	444.2 ± 74.7
CHS/Alg/Ch (50/30/20)	0.04 ± 0.01	9.9 ± 0.6

carbodiimide (EDC) as the crosslinking agent (Zhou et al. 2014). Gels made with different proportions of the blends had uniform and interconnected pores. The addition of sodium alginate increased the water absorption of the hydrogels due to the high hydrophilicity of sodium alginate (Zhou et al. 2014).

Electrospun fibers from alginate

To exploit the advantages of electrospun nano and microfibers for medical applications, alginate has been electrospun into fibers. Since typical electrospinning is slow and not suitable for mass production, a multi-nozzle set-up was used to produce nanofibers from the alginate. Sodium alginate with molecular weight of 9,000,000 was dissolved in water. Poly(ethylene oxide) was blended with the alginate and a surfactant lecithin was included to improve electrospinnability and the properties of the fibers (Kim and Park 2009). A 50/50 ratio of alginate and PEO produced nanofibers without any beads. Most of the fibers had diameters in the range of 200 to 300 nm with the lowest diameter being about 75 nm. Using auxiliary electrodes during electrospinning further reduced the diameters to 100 from 200 nm (Kim and Park 2009). Cells cultured on the blend electrospun fibers showed limited attachment but were able to spread and proliferate indicating biocompatibility (Kim and Park 2009). In a similar approach, alginate fibers were combined with poly(vinyl alcohol) (PVA) in various ratios and electrospun into fibers (Shen and Hsieh 2014). Two types of alginate (low and medium viscosity) were used for fiber production. Electrospinning conditions, particularly, viscosity played a critical role in determining spinnability and fiber diameters. A ratio of 3:7 of low viscosity alginate and PVA produced the most uniform fibers without beads. However, alginate/PVA blend fibers were unstable in water. To improve the stability, fibers were treated with ethanol followed by ethanol/$CaCl_2$ solution. After crosslinking, the fibers were immersed in water for two hours to determine the increase in stability. Treating the fibers in 5% $CaCl_2$ in 75% ethanol for 30 minutes made the fibers remain stable in aqueous conditions. Simultaneous crosslinking and treating with ethanol induced crystallization. Although stable electrospun fibers were produced, the size of the fibers and the ability of the fibers to be used for various applications was not studied (Shen and Hsieh 2014).

Although electrospinning produces nano and micro level fibers, the production rate is quite low and it is also difficult to obtain uniform and consistent fibers. To overcome this limitation, solid and hollow alginate tubes were prepared using a molding technique (Fig. 7) (Yoo and Ghosh 2014). Fibers formed were *in situ* crosslinked with calcium ions. To understand the potential of the alginate fibers for medical applications, human umbilical vein endothelial cells were added into the sodium alginate solution and made into tubes (Yoo and Ghosh 2014). Concentrations of alginate, the crosslinking agent and the production conditions resulted in fibers with various dimensions. Hollow fibers had tensile strength of up to 70 kN/m^2. Cells seeded on the tubes were uniformly distributed inside (Fig. 8) and the cells showed good prolifertion suggesting that the tubes are suitable for medical applications (Yoo and Ghosh 2014). However, it was cautioned that the molding method had restrictions and it was not possible to obtain long fibers.

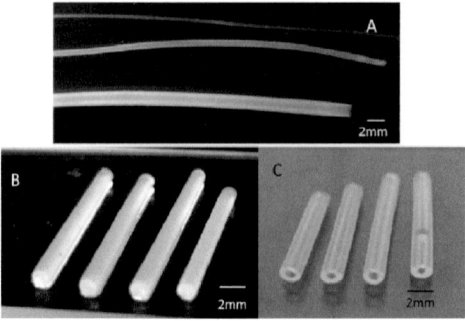

Fig. 7: Digital images of solid and hollow alginate fibers (Yoo and Ghosh 2014). Reproduced with permission from Elsevier.

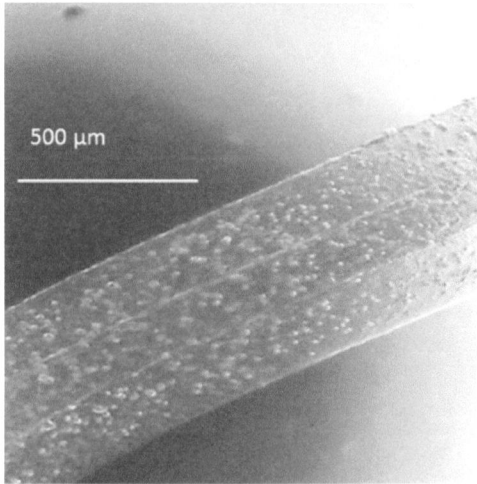

Fig. 8: Light microscopy image of hollow alginate fibers containing embedded HUVEC, one day after incubation (Yoo and Ghosh 2014). Reproduced with permission from Elsevier.

Micro and nanoparticles

In addition to fibers, films and hydrogels, alginates have also been made into beads (400 μm) and nanoparticles. Calcium alginate beads were prepared by adding sodium alginate solution into calcium solution and crosslinking. Iron oxide nanoparticles were grown in pre-formed calcium alginate beads or preformed particles were encapsulated within the beads (Morales et al. 2008). Ability to load the nanoparticles into biocompatible gels was considered to be useful for controlled delivery applications (Morales et al. 2008). Alginate beads were also mineralized using calcium phosphate or using phosphate ions released by the enzyme alkaline phosphatase (Olderoy et al. 2012). Enzymatically crosslinked beads had higher stiffness and mechanical properties similar to that of alginate hydrogels previously reported. Alginate (low and high molecular weight) microspheres were grafted with RGD peptides and used to encapsulate human mesenchymal stem cells and studied for the potential for osteogenic differentiation (Bidarra et al. 2010). The microspheres had excellent ability to attach and proliferate the cells and after 21 days, extensive formation of the cytoskeleton inside the alginate microspheres (Fig. 9) was observed. In fact, tube like structures were formed due to stimulation of neighbouring endothelial cells by the encapsulated cells. Alginate microspheres were considered to be suitable for bone regeneration (Bidarra et al. 2010).

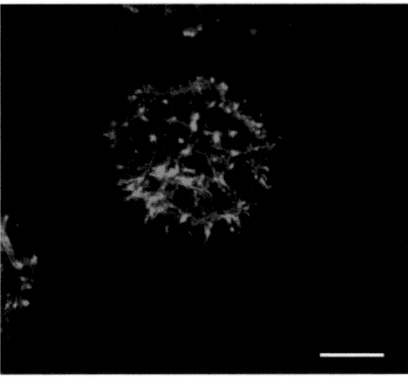

Fig. 9: Picture shows the development of cytoskeleton by the mesenchymal stem cells inside the alginate microspheres (Bidarra et al. 2010). Reproduced with permission from the American Chemical Society.

Miscellaneous structures

In addition to the conventional films, hydrogels and micro and nanoparticles, attempts have been made to develop unique structures for medical applications. In one such attempt, a unique foaming and freeze-drying approach was used to manufacture highly porous scaffolds from various polysaccharides (Barbetta et al. 2010). In this gas-in-liquid templating approach, solutions of the polysaccharides were made into foams stabilized using a surfactant and instantly freeze dried. Scaffolds were later crosslinked with N-ethyl-N'-(3-dimethylaminopropyl)carbodiimide hydrochloride (EDC) and characterized for their structure. Alginate scaffolds made using this approach had pores with diameters in the range of 5 to 10 μm and the distribution of voids was between 100 to 350 μm with extensive interconnections (Fig. 10) (Barbetta et al. 2010). The scaffolds developed were considered to have the ideal porosity for cell infiltration and the biocompatibility and stability required for medical applications (Barbetta et al. 2010).

A thermally induced phase separation approach was used to manufacture nanofibrous scaffolds from a mixture of alginate and silk fibroin. Alginate and silk fibroin solution were mixed together and freeze dried to form a gel (Zhang et al. 2015). The gel was thawed and again washed with ethanol at –20°C and later re-washed with water to remove the solvents and form a solid scaffold. Addition of alginate into silk fibroin facilitated the formation of nanofibers (50–500 nm) and increase in porosity. Scaffolds with porosity as high as 92% were obtained using a 5:1 ratio of silk fibroin

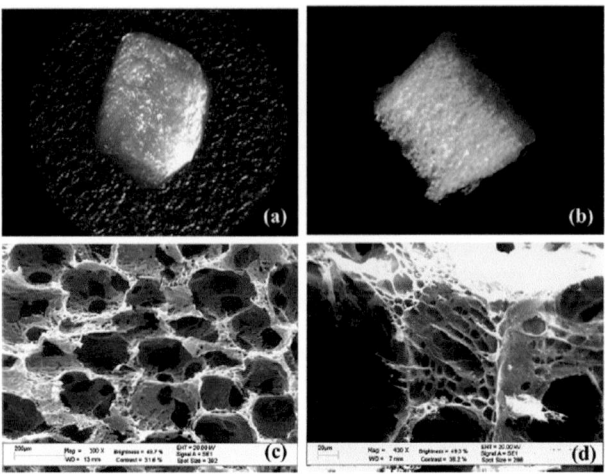

Fig. 10: Images of the EDC crosslinked alginate scaffold. Swollen state (a), freeze-dried state (b), and SEM images revealing the highly porous nature of the scaffold (Barbetta et al. 2010). Reproduced with permission from the Royal Society of Chemistry.

and alginate. Osteoblasts cultured on the scaffolds showed good proliferation indicating the suitability of the scaffolds for tissue engineering (Zhang et al. 2015).

Cellulose

Hydrogels

Hydrogels have been made from cellulose nanofibrils obtained from wood pulp. To form the hydrogels, various monovalent and multivalent metal ions were added into the cellulose solution (1.27%). The binding affinity of the metal cations with carboxylate groups leads to the formation of the gels and the addition of divalent cations or transistion metal ions led to rapid gelation. Gels of various colors were obtained depending on the type of cation added (Fig. 11) (Dong et al. 2013). When the dried gels were observed under FESEM, a three dimensional extensively interconnected structure was observed. Fibrils in the gels had diameters in the range of 4–7 nm and the structure and size of the fibrils in the gels also varied with the type of metal ion present. Mechanical properties of the hydrogels also depended on the type of metal ion present. For instance, gels made from Cu^{2+} salt solutions had modulus of 11.8 kPa, substantially lower than that of gels made from Al^{3+} and Fe^{3+}. Formation of hydrogels directly from a cellulose obtained from biomass and the biocompatibility and ability to control the modulus of the gels by varying the metal salts were considered to be very unique. It was suggested that such hydrogels were ideal for drug delivery and other medical applications (Dong et al. 2013).

In a similar approach, carboxymethyl cellulose (CMC) hydrogels with antibacterial properties were manufactured by *in situ* oxidation of Cu^{2+} ions in the hydrogel (Yadollahi et al. 2015a). For preparation of the hydrogels, CMC was dissolved in

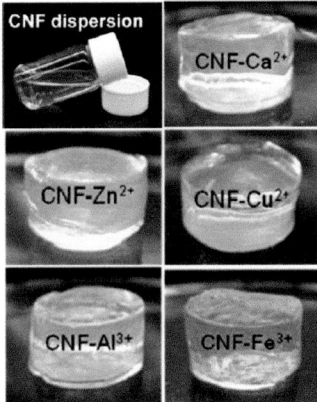

Fig. 11: Gels obtained from cellulose nanofibrils after addition of various metal salts (Dong et al. 2013). Reproduced with permission from the American Chemical Society.

NaOH and the crosslinker epichlorohydrin was added. Solution was heated to 80°C for 2 hours and the crosslinked solution formed an hydrogel which was washed to remove excess NaOH and epichlorohydrin. Hydrogels obtained were later immersed in various concentrations of copper chloride and then oxidized resulting in the *in situ* formation of CuO nanoparticles. Native CMC hydrogels were clear but the addition of the Cu^{2+} turned the hydrogel blue and later green after oxidation (Fig. 12). The hydrogels were also pH responsive in the sense that the swelling varied considerably with change in pH. Swelling of the gels increased with increasing pH from 2 to 7 but decreased when the pH was above 7. Gels containing CuO nanoparticles had higher swelling due to the increase in the penetration and pores size in the hydrogels (Yadollahi et al. 2015a). Antibacterial activity increased linearly with increasing concentration of the Cu^{2+} ions. The zone of inhibition for the hydrogels containing 0.030 M of $CaCl_2$ was 14 mm for *E. coli* and 19 mm for *S. aureus* whereas the pure hydrogels did not show any inhibition suggesting that the nanocomposite hydrogels are suitable for medical applications. Using a similar approach, zinc nanoparticles (10–20 nm) were used instead of Cu^{2+} ions to obtain antimicrobial hydrogels. Higher level (zone of inhibition of up to 28 mm) of antimicrobial activity were obtained for the ZnO hydrogels compared to the CuO containing hydrogels (Yadollahi et al. 2015b).

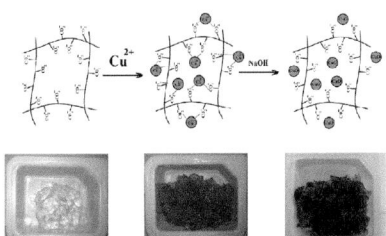

Fig. 12: Mechanism of formation of the CMC hydrogel (Top) and changes in the color and appearance after addition of Cu^{2+} ions and oxidation (Yadollahi et al. 2015a). Reproduced with permission from Elsevier.

Films/membranes

Membranes and hollow tubes for use as coronary artery were prepared using a blend of chitosan and cellulose. Cellulose was converted to methylol cellulose to make it soluble in DMSO. Chitosan was dissolved in HCl and the two solutions were combined in various ratios to form the membranes and hollow tubes (Azevedo et al. 2013). Tensile strength of the membranes decreased whereas modulus increased with the addition of chitosan into cellulose. Among the various ratios of cellulose and chitosan studied, a ratio of 5:5 provided optimal tensile properties and this blend was further made into hollow tubes with diameters of 2 to 4 mm and thickness ranging from 0.3 to 1.2 mm. Since the tubes were intended for use as arteries, the change in the diameter of the tubes with increasing pressure (up to 300 mm Hg), termed as compliance was measured. Compliance (Table 2) of the 5:5 chitosan:cellulose tubes was considerably higher than dacron, PTFE, and similar to that of human artery. Morphologically, the tubes had a dense membrane on the outside but were porous

Table 2: Comparison of the compliance of the cellulose-chitosan tubes of various diameter and thickness with commercially used tubes and human artery and veins (Azevedo et al. 2013).

Sample	Compliance (% per mm Hg x 10^{-2})
Cellulose:Chitosan (D = 4 mm, t = 1.2 mm)	2.91 (1.88)
Cellulose:Chitosan (D = 2 mm, t = 1.2 mm)	4.39 (2.09)
Cellulose:Chitosan (D = 4 mm, t = 0.3 mm)	9.34 (2.65)
Human coronary artery	5.9–8.0
Human saphenous vein	4.4–5.0
Dacron	1.9
ePTFE	1.2–1.6

in their cross-section. When myofibroblasts were seeded on the tubes, there was no cell attachment on the pure cellulose tubes whereas considerable attachment and proliferation was observed on the blend tubes. Although this study showed promising results on the potential of using cellulose:chitosan blend tubes as coronary grafts, the *in vivo* compatibility and performance of the tubes under physiological conditions has to be known before adapting the tubes for practical applications (Azevedo et al. 2013).

Bacterial cellulose is considered to be a promising candidate for biomedical applications. However, bacterial cellulose has relatively poor adhesion for cells. To improve adhesion and proliferation, bacterial cellulose membrane were attached to a peptide IKVAV which was fused to a carbohydrate binding module (CBM3) for promotion of neuronal and mesenchymal stem cells adhesion (Pertile et al. 2012). Cell activity assays showed that adhesion of the cells was higher by more than 100% on the treated bacterial cellulose membranes. Further, the membranes were able to release growth factors suggesting that the modified bacterial cellulose was suitable for tissue engineering applications (Pertile et al. 2012). In addition to using native bacterial cellulose, nanocomposites films have been made using regenerated bacterial cellulose with the addition of zinc oxide nanoparticles (Ul-Islam 2014). Bacterial cellulose was dissolved in the NMMO solution and heated at 80°C for 12 hours and freeze dried to form films. Similarly, nanocomposites were formed with the addition of 1 to 2% of ZnO nanoparticles into the cellulose solution and freeze drying. Compared to using native bacterial cellulose, films obtained using the regenerated cellulose had a more compact fibril arrangement and with uniform attachment of the nanoparticles throughout the surface (Ul-Islam et al. 2014). Tensile properties of the nanocomposites were higher than that of the films made from pure regenerated cellulose. Although bacterial cellulose did not show any antibacterial inhibition, addition of 1 and 2% of ZnO showed large zones of inhibitions but there was no negative effect of ZnO on the cell attachment or proliferation indicating that the scaffolds are suitable for tissue engineering and other medical applications.

Since cellulose has limited solubility, chemical modifications have been done to improve the biomedical applications of cellulose. Cellulose acetate phthalate (CAP) and hydroxypropyl cellulose (HPC) were blended and their properties and potential applications were studied (Onofrei et al. 2015). The two cellulose blends were dissolved in N,N-dimethylacetamide and cast into films. Compatibility of the cellulose membranes to various blood components was investigated. Interaction (Fig. 13) of the blood components with the blend membranes was determined by the hydrophilic/hydrophobic character based on the amount of each polymer in the blend. HPC showed higher affinity for the proteins than CAP. However, CAP had higher inhibition against both *S. aureus* and *E. coli* than HPC.

Although bacterial cellulose is widely considered to be suitable for medical applications, the poor degradability of cellulose is a concern. To overcome this limitation, bacterial cellulose was engineered to have lower crystallinity and higher N-acetylglucosamine residues which increases their degradability (Yadav et al. 2010). The degree of crystallinity of the modified cellulose was lower by about 50% compared to the normal bacterial cellulose. When implanted into mice, the modified bacterial cellulose scaffolds were completely degraded after 10 days but showed slight inflammation whereas the regular bacterial scaffolds only partially degraded.

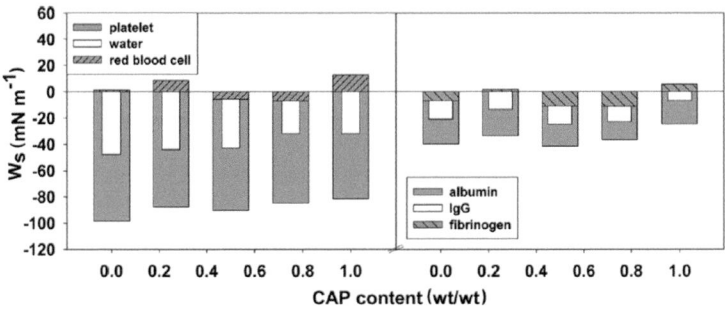

Fig. 13: Interaction of the CAP/HPC blend films with various blood components (Onofrei et al. 2015). Reproduced with permission from John Wiley and Sons.

After 20 days of implantation, there was no inflammation and both the scaffolds had assimilated into the tissue.

Biocomposites

Bacterial cellulose nanocomposites were made by adding carboxyl methyl cellulose (CMC) into the bacterial culture and later combining with hydroxyapatite (Grande et al. 2009). Gels of pure bacterial cellulose, bacterial cellulose with CMC, and bacterial cellulose with CMC and hydroxyapatite nanoparticles were made. The gels were also dried and made into films for analysis and cell culture. Addition of bacterial cellulose resulted in fibers with diameters of 60 nm compared to fibers with diameters of 118 nm when CMC was not added. Chemical interaction between hydroxyapatite and bacterial cellulose was observed and the nanocomposites had lower % crystallinity compared to the pure hydroxyapatite (Grande et al. 2009). Nanocomposites containing the hydroxyapatite and CMC showed considerably higher viability for HEK cells indicating the suitability of the films for biomedical applications. In another approach, bacterial cellulose nanocomposites were formed with hydroxyapatite using a biological route. Bacterial cellulose was phosphorylated and then treated with $CaCl_2$. For biomineralization, the treated bacterial cellulose was immersed in simulated body fluid at 37°C for 7 to 14 days. Mineralization increased the % crystallinity and crystal size and SEM observations revealed that the bacterial cellulose has a 3D network with interconnected pores. Needle shaped hydroxyapatite crystals were formed on the surface of the bacterial cellulose network. Phosphorylated samples had uniform distribution of the crystals on the surface and also within the network (Fig. 14). It was suggested that biomineralization by phosphorylation of bacterial cellulose would be a viable and effective method to develop scaffolds for tissue engineering (Wan et al. 2007).

Microfibrillated cellulose was combined with calcium peroxide to form nanocomposites with ability to modulate the release of hydrogen peroxide or oxygen (Chang and Wang 2013). Catalase was added into the nanocomposites to convert peroxide into oxygen and the ability of the composites to support the attachment and

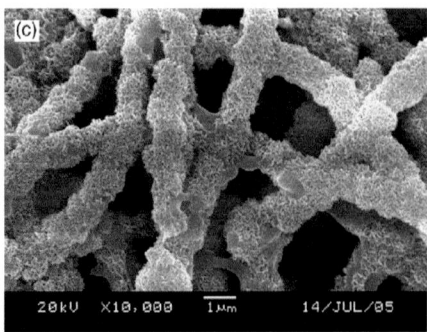

Fig. 14: SEM image of the surface of bacterial cellulose fibers coated with nano-scale hydroxyapatite crystals that were phosphorylated and immersed in simulated body fluid for biomineralization (Wan et al. 2007). Reproduced with permission from Elsevier.

proliferation of L-929 fibroblasts was studied. Morphologically, the microfibrillated cellulose was highly porous which faciliated the movement of gases and the porous structure was maintained even after the addition of calcium peroxide and catalase. After five days of culture, fibroblasts showed higher cell density on the pristine cellulose than culture plates due to the porous morphology of the fibers. However, significant toxicity and apotposis was observed on the cellulose-peroxide composites due to the release of hydrogen peroxide and hydroxyl radicals. Contrarily, cell proliferation was considerably higher on the catalase containing composite with cell densities up to 32400 cells/cm^2 since the peroxide was converted into oxygen. Cell morphologies (Fig. 15) clearly show the differences in the density and proliferation of microfibrillated cellulose, hydrogen peroxide, and catalase containing nanocomposites. Generation of oxygen by the catalase served as support for the cells and eliminated the need for serum in the cell culture media. The nanocomposites with peroxide were considered particularly suitable for wound dressing, tooth bleaching, and antimicrobial applications and those containing the catalase were suitable for tissue engineering (Chang and Wang 2013).

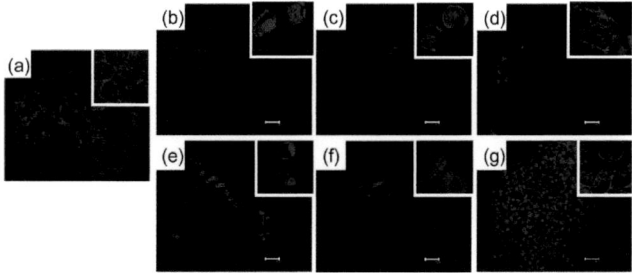

Fig. 15: Morphologies of fibroblasts on the microfibrillated cellulose (a), cellulose-peroxide (5,10,15%-b,c,d), and cellulose-catalase and peroxide (5,10,15%-e,f,g) concentrations (Chang and Wang 2013). Reproduced with permission from the American Chemical Society.

Bionanocomposites that become stiff when dry and soft when wet were developed using poly(vinylalcohol) and cellulose nanocrystals (CNCs) (Jorfi et al. 2013). Cellulose nanocrystals in the form of powder were prepared from two sources, tunicates (t-CNC) and cotton (c-CNC). Nanocrystals obtained from the tunicates had a average length and width of 2500 nm and 30 nm, respectively compared to 200 and 22 nm for the cellulose nanocrystals, respectively. Nanocrystals and PVOH dissolved in water were mixed together and made into a film by solvent casting. The films were further compression molded to form the composites. Mechanical properties of the films containing various amounts of nanocrystals in dry state and after immersion in artificial cerebrospinal fluid (ACSF) are seen in Table 3. Modulus of the films varies by as much as four times in the dry condition when measured between 25 and 100°C. Films made from c-CNC had lower modulus than the t-CNC due to lower aspect ratio and stiffness (Jorfi et al. 2013). Under the swollen state, the films had considerably lower modulus (up to 900 times lower) and the films were therefore considered to be responsive to thermal treatment and useful as a neural prosthetic device.

Table 3: Modulus of the cellulose nanocrystal-PVOH films in dry and swollen condition when measured at different temperatures and various levels of CNC content (Jorfi et al. 2013).

Sample	%CNC	Dry Nanocomposites, GPa		Swollen Nanocomposites, MPa	
		25°C	100°C	1 week	1 month
Neat PVOH		7.3	0.84	11.1	6.9
PVOH/t-CNC	4	10.5	2.1	45.4	46.8
	8	11.1	3.7	78.3	85.2
	12	11.7	4.7	124	108
	16	13.7	5.4	164	173
	16	12.3	3.0	60	-
Neat PVOH		7.0	0.7	1.4	-
PVOH/c-CNC	4	6.8	0.5	1.5	-
	8	7.7	0.8	3.6	-
	12	8.3	1.0	1.6	-
	16	9.0	1.4	1.9	-
	16	8.4	2.1	13	-

Fibers

Fibers, particularly in nanoscale, are structures that more closely mimic the extracellular matrix and therefore attempts have been made to develop micro and nanofibers for tissue engineering and other medical applications. A nanofibrillar composite of bacterial cellulose and chitosan (75/25) was prepared by immersing bacterial cellulose pellicles into 1% chitosan solution for six hours. Bacterial cellulose nanofibrils (40 nm) were extensively coated with chitosan and the chitosan was able to penetrate into the inner porous surface of the cellulose (Fig. 16) (Kim et al. 2011). Inclusion of chitosan into bacterial cellulose decreased the % crystallinity but thermal resistance and mechanical properties showed marginal improvements (Kim et al. 2011).

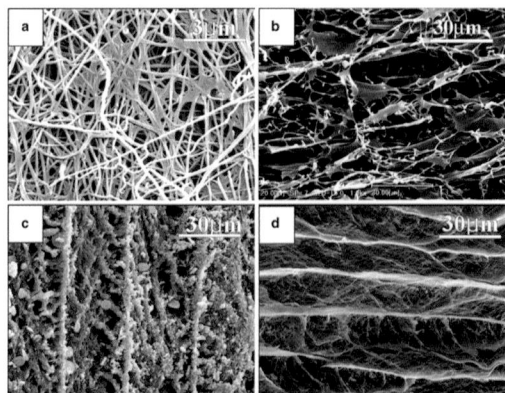

Fig. 16: SEM image of the surface (a) and cross-section (c) of pure bacterial cellulose and the cellulose-chitosan composite (b, d) (Kim et al. 2011). Reproduced with permission from Springer.

Compared to pure bacterial cellulose, the cellulose-chitosan composite showed higher attachment, proliferation, and spreading of fibroblasts suggesting that the scaffolds would be suitable for tissue engineering.

In another novel approach, bacterial cellulose was modified by adding cell binding peptides (RGD and GRGDY) by fusing them using a cell binding module (CBM). Proteins containing the cell binding peptides were recombinantly produced using *E. coli* and the proteins obtained were coated (absorbed) onto bacterial cellulose fibers (Andrade et al. 2010). Fibroblasts showed considerably higher adhesion and proliferation on the RGD containing cellulose fibers.

Cellulose nanowhiskers have excellent structural diversity and are porous and permeable, which is well suited for neo-tissue development for bone and cartilage regeneration, wound healing, etc. To exploit the advantages of cellulose nanowhiskers, a biocomposite comprised of the nanowhiskers (10–50 nm in diameter and 1–2 µm in length) as reinforcement (0.2 to 9%) and cellulose acetate propionate as matrix was developed (Pooyan et al. 2012a). A porous 3D scaffold with the ability to allow percolation of cells (Fig. 17) was obtained by controlling the dispersion of the nanowhiskers. Average size of the pores in the scaffolds was about 3 µm and void fraction was about 15% (Pooyan et al. 2013). Nanowhiskers could be aligned in the composite by using magnetic fields which led to an increase in more than twice the strength of the matrix even at a concentration of 0.2 wt%. However, no studies were conducted to understand the ability of the scaffolds to support cell attachment and growth or the *in vitro/in vivo* degradation of the scaffolds (Pooyan et al. 2012). Scaffolds were considered to be suitable for development of artificial conduits and blood vessels (Pooyan et al. 2013).

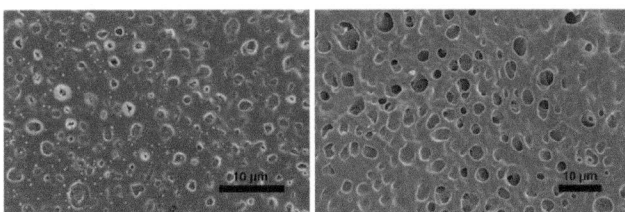

Fig. 17: SEM images showing the porous nature of the cellulose nanowhisker reinforced scaffold with 0.2% (left) and 9% whisker content (right) (Pooyan et al. 2012). Reproduced with permission from Elsevier.

Cellulose based fibrous meshes as tissue engineering scaffolds were obtained through a series of chemical modifications. In this approach, cellulose acetate was electrospun into a fibrous mesh and later treated to form regenerated cellulose. The regenerated cellulose mesh (Fig. 18) was further oxidized and sulfated and also thermally processed to obtain a mechanically and water stable mesh (Filion et al. 2011). Thermal and chemical treatments lead to considerable increase in strength and stability. Sulfated fibrous meshes have higher retention ability for growth factors and considerably higher attachment and differentiation of mesenchymal stem cells and therefore considered to have great potential for bone regeneration (Filion et al. 2011).

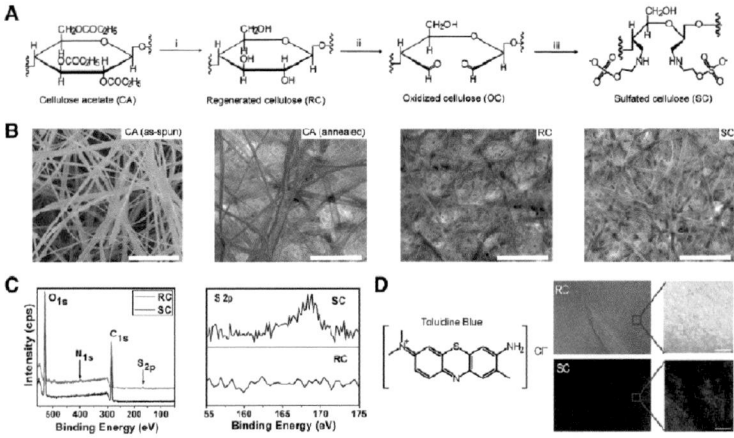

Fig. 18: Depiction of the process used to chemically modify the cellulose meshes and the corresponding changes in the morphology of the meshes (Filion et al. 2011). Reproduced with permission from Elsevier.

Micro and nanoparticles

Cellulose microparticles as substrates for controlled drug delivery were prepared using microfibrillated cellulose as the matrix. To prepare the particles, nanofibrillated cellulose in solution form was obtained and combined with various drugs. The mixture was later spray dried to form particles using a spray dryer (Kolakovic et al. 2012). Particles were spherical with diameters of about 5 μm and had a fibrous morphology when observed at higher magnifications (Fig. 19). Drugs attached onto the microparticles could also be seen. Up to 15% drug loading could be achieved depending on the drug used. Although there was an initial burst release, a sustained release of up to two months was seen for all the drugs (Fig. 20) (Kolakovic et al. 2012).

Hollow cellulose capsules with capacity to hold up to 10 μl were prepared using a unique three-step approach (Carrick et al. 2013). Cellulose with a degree

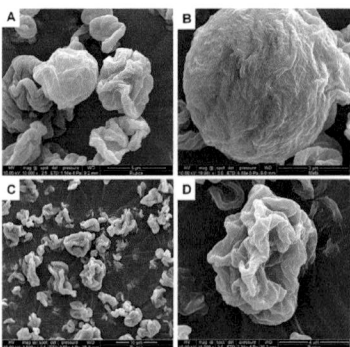

Fig. 19: SEM image of the cellulose microparticles containing 20% metoprolol (a, b) and 20% verapamil (c, d) reveals the fibrous nature of the particles (Kolakovic et al. 2012). Reproduced with permission from Elsevier.

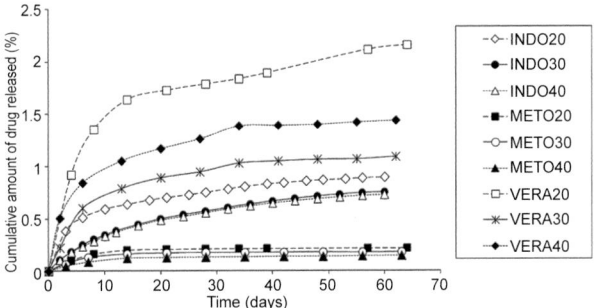

Fig. 20: Ability of the cellulose microparticles to release various drugs (Kolakovic et al. 2012). Reproduced with permission from Elsevier.

of polymerization (DP) of about 780 was dissolved using lithium chloride–N,N-dimethylacetamide (LiCl–DMAc). Dissolved cellulose solution was saturated with CO_2 and the gas saturated solution was added into water to instantly form capsules. Schematic of the three-step process used to form the capsules is shown in Fig. 21. Capsules with various wall thickness and volume were obtained by varying the concentration of the cellulose in the solution or treatment time with CO_2, type of gas, and pressure of gas. Pore diameter of the capsules varied from 14.7 to 24.1 nm when the cellulose concentration was increased from 1 to 2%. Increasing concentration from 1 to 2% also resulted in increase in modulus of the capsules from 1.8 to 7.3 MPa (Carrick et al. 2013). Although cellulose nanocapsules were obtained, the ability of the capsules to load drugs and their *in vitro* or *in vivo* behavior was not reported. In a different study, cellulose nanocrystals obtained by dissolving microcrystalline cellulose in sulfuric acid were used as carriers for hydroquinone. Nanocrystals (301 nm) were able to load up to 79% of hydroquinone and had a sustained release with about 80% of bound drug released in about four hours (Taheri and Mohammadi 2015). These cellulose nanocrystals were considered suitable to deliver drugs to the skin for treatment of hyperpigmentation and other disorders.

Porous cellulose scaffolds that had excellent biocompatibility and potential for tissue engineering were prepared using a salt leaching approach (Shin et al. 2014). In

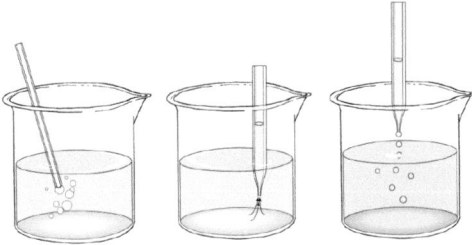

Fig. 21: Three-step approach used to form cellulose nanocapsules. Cellulose solution is saturated with gas (left), collection of cellulose saturated with gas (center), and addition of the cellulose solution into water (right) resulting in formation of the cellulose nanocrystals (Carrick et al. 2013). Reproduced with permission from the Royal Society of Chemistry.

this method, cellulose linters were dissolved in AmimCl in 2, 4 or 6% concentrations by heating at 90°C. Sodium chloride having particle size of 210–270 µm was added into the cellulose solution which was allowed to gel at –10°C. Obtained gels were throughly washed to remove the solvent and NaCl particles. Scaffolds with a highly porous structure were obtained at all three concentrations of cellulose (Fig. 22). However, the pore size was dependent on the concentration of cellulose in the solution. For example, gels made with 2% cellulose had pore diameter of 200 µm but the pore diameters increase to 300 and 500 µm when the concentration is increased to 4 and 6%, respectively. Porosity of the scaffolds varied from 92–97% for the different scaffolds. Tensile stress (5 MPa) was highest for the scaffold made using 4% cellulose and modulus was highest for 2% cellulose containing scaffold. Up to 2500% water uptake was observed but only 10% of the hydrogel was degraded *in vitro* after 90 days of degradation which could be considerably slow for several applications. *In vitro* studies showed high attachment and proliferation and when implanted in mice, the scaffolds were non-immunogenic and supported growth of tissue (Shin et al. 2014).

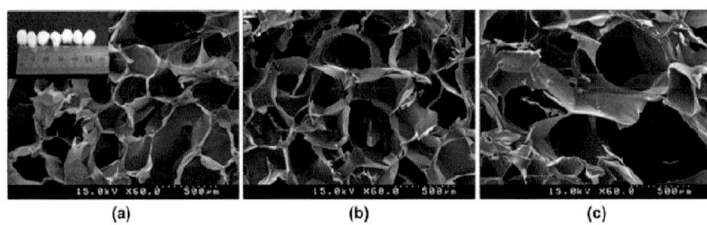

Fig. 22: Cellulose scaffolds had a porous structure with the pore sizes increasing with increasing cellulose concentration. The three images represent scaffolds made from 2% (a), 4% (b), and 6% (c) cellulose (Shin et al. 2014). Reproduced with permission from Springer.

Starch

Films

Starch based biomaterials have been developed for wound dressing, regeneration of skin, drug and hormone carriers, and for cartilage and vascular regeneration. In most applications, thermoplastic starch, chemically modified starch or blends of starch have been made into various forms for medical applications. Native starch obtained from various Andean crops was dissolved in water, hydrolyzed using hydrochloric acid and made into films (Fig. 23) with the addition of glycerol (Torres et al. 2011). Films were seeded with 3T3 fibroblast cells and their attachment and proliferation was studied. Considerable variations in confluence of cells on the different films was observed. However, authors claimed that the starch films offered poor adhesion to cells and surface modification of the films was necessary to improve adhesion (Torres et al. 2011). A blend of sago starch and silver nanoparticles (8 to 20 nm) containing chitosan was made into films. An antibacterial drug gentamycin was also included when the films were implanted into mice (Arockianathan 2015). Films had a porous and rough surface which was suggested to help in absorption of wound exudates and

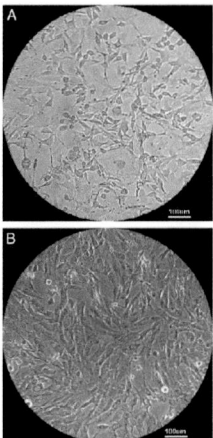

Fig. 23: Proliferation of 3T3 fibroblast cells on the cell culture plate and on muro-huayro potato starch films after 3 days of culture (Torres et al. 2011). Reproduced with permission from Elsevier.

for oxygen exchange. Addition of the nanoparticles resulted in lower elongation at break but considerably higher tensile strength. The films were implanted into mice at a wound site and ability of the films to support the healing of the wound was studied. It was observed that the wounds healed faster in the presence of the nanocomposites compared to pure starch films. Complete closure of wound occurred after 16 days for the nanocomposite film but it took 24 days for the wound to heal without the films (Fig. 24). Based on these results it was concluded that the starch nanocomposite films were suitable for wound healing (Arockianathan 2015).

Starch functionalized graphene nanosheets were prepared by reduction of exfoliated graphene oxides for potential use as drug carriers (Liu et al. 2015). Graphene oxide was exfoliated in water to form graphene oxide nanosheets which were chemically reduced to form graphene nanosheets using soluble starch. The

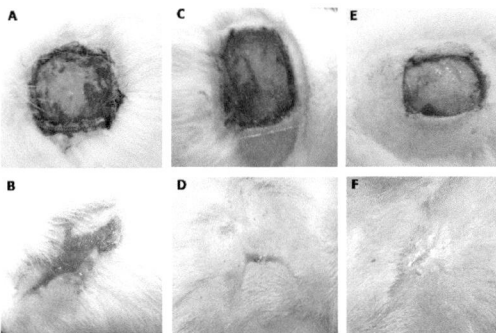

Fig. 24: Images of wounds on mice without (a), with the starch nanocomposite films (b) and with the nanocomposite film containing gentamycin (c) on the day of wound formation. B, D and F are corresponding wounds after 16 days show that the nanocomposite films were able to accelerate wound healing (Arockianathan 2012). Reproduced with permission from Elsevier.

starch graphene sheet had a thickness of about 4 nm, considerably higher compared to 0.8 nm for the exfoliated graphene sheet. Rhodamine 6G was selected as a model drug to understand the loading and release potential of the graphene sheets. Highest amount of drug that could be loaded was 8 µg per 140 µg of starch-graphene sheet which was considerably higher than other common materials used for drug loading. Release of the drug from the sheets was heavily dependent on the pH of the solution. Acidic pH resulted in higher release (up to 15%) compared to release at pH 7.4. Higher release under acidic conditions was suggested to be due to the dissociation of the hydrogen bonding interaction between the drug and the nanosheets. Ability of the nanosheets to attach and release an anticancer drug hydroxycampthothecin (HCPT) was also studied. Up to 12 µg of HCPT could be absorbed on the sheets. Viability studies of SW-620 cancer cells showed that the cellulose-graphene sheets had no cytotoxicity whereas the free HCPT was cytotoxic with considerable decrease in viable cells with increasing incubation time (Fig. 24) (Liu et al. 2015). However, HCPT embedded into the starch-graphene sheets had low cytotoxicity since the HCPT was encapsulated and had a slow release.

Biocomposites

Starch based biocomposites for tissue engineering were developed by blending starch with ethylene vinyl alcohol (SEVA-C), cellulose acetate (SCA), polycaprolactone (SPCL), and hydroxyapatite (HA) and the biocompatibility of these composites was studied by implanting the scaffolds into mice (Marques et al. 2005). Composites were made by injection molding and samples suitable for *in vivo* implantation were prepared. None of the starch based biomaterials invoked strong inflammatory reaction and no cellular exudate was formed suggesting the suitability of the materials for *in vivo* applications. However, SPCL and SCA composites had a stronger immune response compared to the other starch based scaffolds (Marques et al. 2005). Composites developed were considered suitable for biomedical applications but the degradability of the scaffolds under *in vivo* conditions was not studied. In a similar study, scaffolds were made from a blend of starch/ethylene vinyl alcohol and the ability of the scaffold to support generation of collagen and support mineralization of bone was studied (Salgado et al. 2004). Scaffolds had a porosity of 60% with pore sizes between 200 to 900 µm. Compressive strength and modulus of the scaffolds was 20.8 and 118 MPa, respectively. The scaffolds did not show any cytotoxicity and were able to support the growth of cells for four weeks. Deposition of collagen and expression of osteopontin was detected in the scaffolds suggesting that the scaffolds are suitable for bone tissue engineering (Salgado et al. 2004).

Scaffolds made from SEVA-C, SEVA-C coated with calcium phosphate, and 50/50 blend of corn starch and cellulose acetate when implanted in mice showed the ability to support connective tissue and bone formation (Salgado et al. 2007). Influence of crystalline structure and plasticizer content on the mechanical properties and *in vitro* and *in vivo* viability of two varieties (potato and amylomaize) of botanical starch was studied (Velasquez et al. 2015). Starch with and without glycerol were extruded, compression molded, and cut into samples of 1 cm^2 dimension and thickness of 1.5 mm. These samples were immersed in PBS and their swelling was studied for

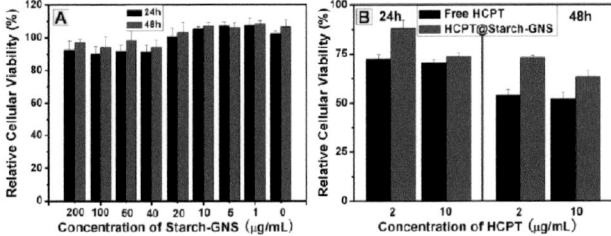

Fig. 25: Viability of SW-620 cells containing starch-graphene sheets, free HCPT and HCPT embedded into the starch-graphene sheets when incubated for 24 and 48 hours (Liu et al. 2015). Reproduced with permission from Elsevier.

up to 30 days. Starch scaffolds were cultured with cells and also implanted in mice. The addition of glycerol decreased the modulus and glass transistion temperature but increased moisture content (Table 4). The scaffolds made from potato starch had lower strength than the amylomaize starch. Both *in vitro* and *in vivo* studies did not show any cytotoxicity of the scaffolds to the cells. Potato starch materials were found integrated with the tissue better than that of amylomaize starch due to the differences in the composition of the two starches.

Table 4: Properties of scaffolds developed from potato and amylomaize starch with three levels (0, 10, and 20%) of glycerol content (Velasquez et al. 2015).

Sample	Moisture Content, %	Tg, °C	Initial Elastic Modulus, MPa
Potato starch, 0%	10.5	87	105 ± 4
Potato starch, 10%	10.4	40	89.9 ± 1.3
Potato starch, 20%	12.6	16	64.8 ± 0.6
Amylomaize, 0%	11.9	77	114 ± 16
Amylomaize, 10%	10.7	32	107 ± 16
Amylomaize, 20%	15	17	83 ± 4

Hydrogels

Similar to other polysaccharides, starch has been widely used to develop hydrogels using both chemical and physical approaches. Crosslinking, blending with other polymers, grafting of vinyl monomers, and esterification are some of the common approaches used to obtain stable starch hydrogels (Xiao 2013; Zhang et al. 2005). Cassava starch was methylated and combined with chitosan (1%) dissolved in acetic acid and the individual polymers and blend of starch-chitosan were made into hydrogels. The chitosan used was also crosslinked using glutaraldehyde and made into hydrogel for comparison (Sivoli et al. 2013). Composite hydrogels had a stable porous structure whereas the porous structure in chitosan hydrogels was unstable. Hydrogels were seeded with human dermal fibroblasts and the ability of the hydrogels to support attachment and proliferation was studied. Starch based hydrogels had similar cell adhesion and proliferation compared to the crosslinked chitosan hydrogels and therefore considered to be suitable for medical applications. Starch was also made into hydrogels after grafting with poly(acrylamide-co-acrylic acid) and irradiating with γ-rays (Erizal et al. 2014). Gels were able to swell instantly and absorb up to 300% of water within 15 seconds of immersion. Further immersion (3 minutes) led to an absorption of up to 400%. However, the swelling of the hydrogels was lower (up to 175%) in saline solutions.

To reduce protein absorption (biofouling), ionic solvation hydration groups were introduced onto starch hydrogels by preparing anionic (a), cationic (c), and zwitterionic (z) starches through etherification and crosslinking with poly(ethylene glycol) diglycidyl ether (PEGDE). Chemical modifications led to the formation of hydrogels with different surface charges. While native starch was neutral, anionic starch had considerably high negative zeta potential and c-starch had positive zeta potential (Wang et al. 2015a). Modified starch hydrogels also had higher capacity to absorb water due to higher hydrogen bonding and ionic solvation (Fig. 26). With respect to protein adsorption, C-starch had low protein resistance whereas A and Z starches had considerably high resistance due to better hydrogen bonding and ionic solvation (Fig. 27). The Z and A starch hydrogels had good biocompatibility and resisted cell adhesion. Among the three types of hydrogels, the Z-starch hydrogels were considered to show higher promise for non-fouling applications. Further studies showed that the cytotoxicity and protein resistance of the Z-starch hydrogels was a function of the degree of substitution of the zwitter ions (Wang et al. 2015b). A substition of 0.26 promoted cell adhesion but increased level of substitution and decreased protein absorption. Carboxymethylation and addition of dextran sulfate to starch produced hydrogels that could encapsulate 5-,10-,15-,20-tetrakis(meso-hydroxyphenyl) porphyrin (mTHPP) and therefore considered to treat cancer through photodynamic therapy (Saboktakin et al. 2012). The hydrogels had relatively low level of swelling

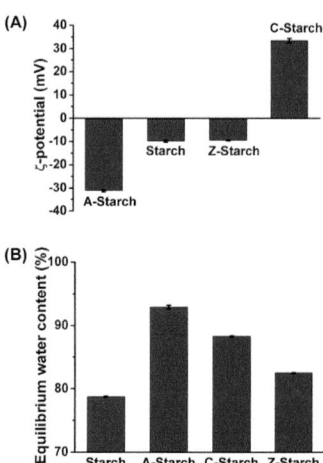

Fig. 26: Zeta potential and water content in the three types of modified starches compared to native starch (Wang et al. 2015). Reproduced with permission from John Wiley and Sons.

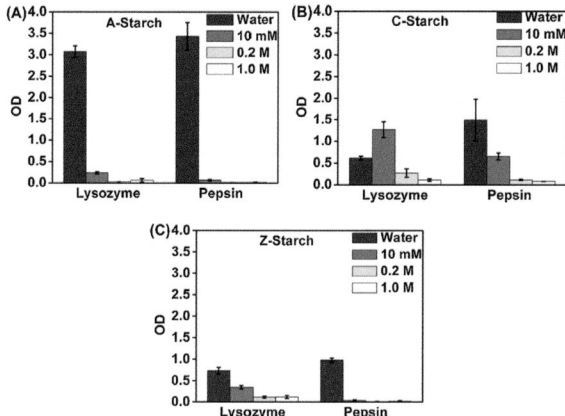

Fig. 27: Protein absorption of the modified starches in water and at different levels of ionic strengths (Wang et al. 2015). Reproduced with permission from John Wiley and Sons.

but high encapsulation efficiency (Table 5). Up to 100% of the encapsulated drug was released within 10 hours in pH 7.4 solution at 37°C. However, no *in vivo* release and targeted delivery studies were done.

A superabsorbent hydrogel with network structure resembling that of the brain was developed by UV induced copolymerization crosslinking of vinyl modified starch with acrylic acid and N,N-dimethylacrylamide and Fe_3O_4 particles (Guilherme et al. 2012). In this research, starch was first chemically modified using glycidyl methacrylate. Later, the modified starch was combined with dimethylacrylamide and Fe_3O_4 particles and made into an hydrogel. Albumin was also included into the hydrogel as a model drug for release studies. FTIR, X-ray, and EDS studies suggested some interaction between the mineral and the hydrogel. Digital images of the hydrogel taken after addition of iodine revealed the phenomenol network structure of the hydrogel (Fig. 28). A 3D

Table 5: Properties of the mTHPP loaded CMS-DS hydrogels (Saboktakin et al. 2012).

Parameter	Values	Degree of swelling, %	Average Particle Size, nm	Encapsulation efficiency, %
mTHPP	0	1.64 ± 0.10	1.76 ± 0.12	–
	5	1.34 ± 0.03	2.00 ± 0.10	73.41 ± 0.12
	10	0.86 ± 0.12	2.45 ± 0.04	80.10 ± 0.10
	15	0.68 ± 0.05	2.43 ± 0.80	83.64 ± 0.05
	20	0.49 ± 0.08	3.00 ± 0.06	92.18 ± 0.08
Time (min)	10	0.45 ± 0.34	1.74 ± 0.13	65.56 ± 0.24
	20	0.67 ± 0.12	1.62 ± 0.10	87.12 ± 0.10
	40	0.87 ± 0.03	1.43 ± 0.04	75.49 ± 0.02
Drying	Lyophilization	0.75 ± 0.06	1.15 ± 0.16	68.10 ± 0.03
	45°C	0.61 ± 0.10	1.24 ± 0.04	57.12 ± 0.12

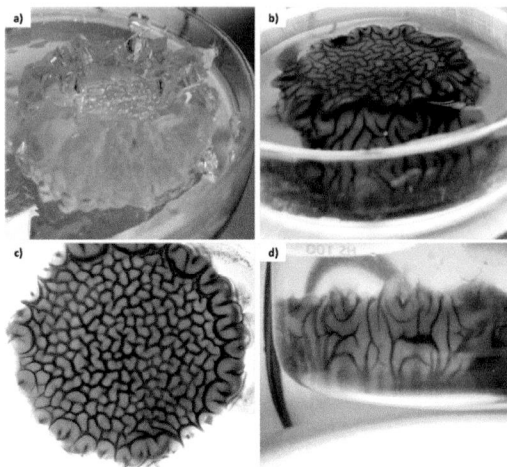

Fig. 28: Digital images of the modified starch hydrogels before and after swelling. A 3D network is seen when the gels are stained with iodine (Guilherme et al. 2012). Reproduced with permission from the Royal Society of Chemistry.

network with interconnected lines were observed when the gel was swollen in water. Hydrogel without the Fe_3O_4 particles were able to swell up to 150 times whereas the swelling was limited to about 70 times when the particles were present. Release of albumin from the hydrogel could be controlled by varying the Fe_3O_4 particle content and by applying a magnetic field. The unique hydrogels developed in this research were considered to be particularly suitable for oral delivery of acid responsive drugs (Guilherme et al. 2012).

The ability of boiled starch and soluble starch to form phase separated hydrogels with gelatin in comparison to normal commercial starch-gelatin mixture was studied (Mallick et al. 2014). Microscopical examination revealed that the starch in the form of dark globules were dispersed in a continous gelatin matrix indicating phase separation. Addition of starch decreased the melting temperature and the blend hydrogels also had lower strength when compared to pure gelatin hydrogel. Among the different starches, soluble starch produced stronger hydrogels than the boiled and commercial starches. When used for drug release, the gelatin hydrogels had a quick release of 98% of the drug. Increasing starch concentration decreased the drug release. Due to the quick release, gelatin hydrogels also showed higher inhibition against gram positive and gram negative bacteria than the starch hydrogels. *In situ* formed hydrogels were obtained by combining cholestrol modified oxidized starch in nanoparticle form with O-carboxymethyl chitosan in various ratios (Li et al. 2015). Chitosan in the gel was in fibrous form and the starch in particle form making it an unique hydrogel with highly porous structures. Gels could swell up to 68% in distilled water but only to about 23% under acidic conditions. Release of drug from the hydrogel was dependent on the pH and about 75% of the drug was released in 400 hours and no cytotoxicity was observed (Li et al. 2015).

Micro and nanoparticles

Starch has been traditionally used for pharmaceutical applications in the form of binder, diluent, and disintegrant. To improve the applicability of starch for medical applications, particularly drug delivery, micro and nanoparticles have been developed from starch and starch derivatives (Rodrigues 2012). For example, starch-polycaprolactone (SPCL) was made into microparticles as potential carrier for bioactive agents (Balmayor et al. 2009). Particles with size ranging from 5.7 to 913 μm were obtained depending on the conditions used during preparation (Fig. 29). Up to 94% of the drug dexamethasone could be loaded onto the particles. A sustained release profile was observed for the particles with 60% of the drug being released in about 600 hours. In another study, starch was combined with the drug diclofenac and heated to form a gel. The gel was spray dried to form microparticles with particle size between 10.3 to 13.1 μm (Table 6). A high level (95 to 98%) of drug encapsulation was achieved and a sustained release (100%) was obtained for up to six hours (Liu et al. 2007).

Unique multicompartmental and thermoresponsive microcapsules were prepared from starch. The microspheres were also able to bind drugs thermostatically. To prepare such unique microparticles, starch was crosslinked with epichlorohydrin

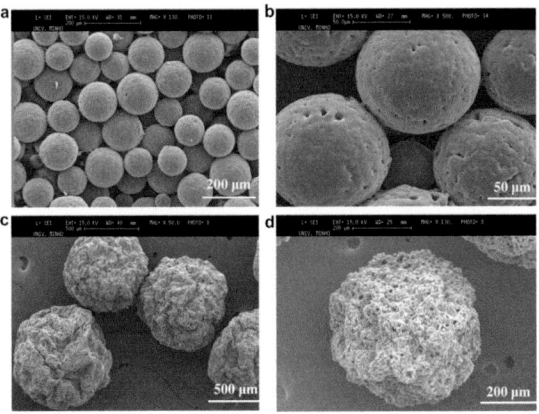

Fig. 29: Morphologies of starch polycaprolactone microparticles obtained under different experimental conditions. a and b are particles obtained using 5% SPCL and c and d are particles obtained using 10% SPCL (Balmayor et al. 2009). Reproduced with permission from Elsevier.

Table 6: Properties of starch polycaprolactone microparticles obtained at different concentrations of starch and their corresponding particle size and encapsulation efficiency (Liu et al. 2007).

SPS, % w/v	Drug loading, %	Mean particle size, μm	Encapsulation efficiency, %	Yield, %
2	1	10.3 ± 2.1	95.1 ± 1.8	65.2
3	1	11.2 ± 1.5	97.4 ± 2.2	68.3
4	1	13.1 ± 1.1	98.2 ± 1.2	70.1
2	2	10.8 ± 1.2	96.3 ± 2.3	69.6

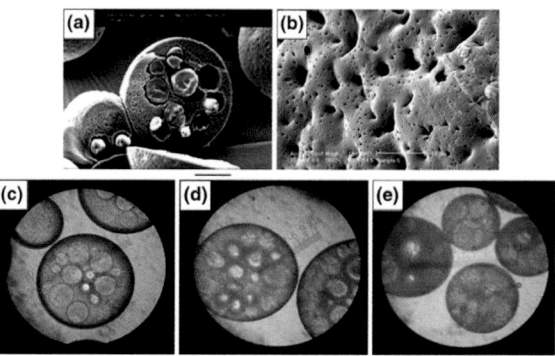

Fig. 30: Scanning electron images of the cross-section (a) and surface of cellulose acetate butyrate microcapsules containing the starch microspheres. c to e are digital images showing the formation of the microcapsules after 10, 30, and 60 minutes (Fundueanu et al. 2010). Reproduced with permission from Springer.

and the particles obtained were later grafted with poly(NIPAAm-co-DMAAm) to impart thermosensitivity through the addtion of SO_3H groups. Later, the grafted starch microparticles were complexed with metoclopramide as the model drug. The thermosensitive starch microparticles containing the model drug was encapsulated into cellulose acetate butyrate microcapsules to form the multicompartmental microcapsules (Fig. 29) (Fundueanu et al. 2010). Due to the differences in the volume phase transisition temperature of the microspheres, the multicompartmental system could behave as a smart drug delivery system. For instance, the capsules swell extensively in body fluids at below normal body temperature and hence bioactive compounds that can maintain body activity can be released. However, at normal body conditions, the microspheres exhibit marginal swelling and have a long and sustained release (Fundueanu et al. 2010). The amount of drug release and the transisition temperature could be controlled leading to the ability to develop materials for specific applications.

Sago starch was capped with silver nanoparticles which were added into gelatin and formed into a scaffold for potential medical applications (Mandal et al. 2014). Silver nanoparticles with sizes ranging from 15 to 90 nm were obtained by varying the concentration of starch used as the capping agent. Zeta potential studies showed that the capped nanoparticles were stable due to steric repulsion since starch stabilizes the nanoparticles and restrictes the mobility of the ions. Increasing the concentration of starch resulted in increase in pore size that leads to higher water storage. Increase in collagen/gelatin content and subsequently the amine and carboxlic groups reduces hydrophilicity and therefore swelling. In terms of mechanical properties, the collagen-nanoparticle scaffold had highest strength and elongation but lower modulus (Table 7). Addition of starch into the collagen-nanoparticle scaffold decreased the elongation and strength but increased modulus.

Nanoparticles prepared from propyl starch derivatives with two degrees of substitution (DS) (1.05 and 1.45) were studied for their potential for transdermal drug delivery (Santander-Ortega et al. 2010). Particles were prepared using a emulsion diffusion method and characterized for their structure and properties. Nanoparticles

Table 7: Mechanical properties of scaffolds made from sago starch, gelatin containing uncapped silver nanoparticles (FSC-AgNPs), and the gelation starch capped nanoparticles at three different levels of starch (Mandal et al. 2014).

Scaffold	Strength, MPa	Elongation, %	Modulus, MPa
Sago starch	10.1 ± 0.7	8.3 ± 0.7	490 ± 17
Collagen-uncapped Nanoparticles	24.3 ± 1.3	32.8 ± 2.4	116 ± 22
Collagen capped (1 µM) nanoparticles	19.5 ± 0.9	7.9 ± 0.5	598 ± 13
Collagen capped (2 µM) nanoparticles	15.5 ± 0.6	6.8 ± 0.3	953 ± 18
Collagen capped (3 µM) nanoparticles	13.4 ± 0.7	5.1 ± 0.4	649 ± 15

had average diameters of 150 and 183 nm for the starches made from DS of 1.05 and 1.45, respectively. No cytotoxicity was observed when the nanoparticles were added into a CaCO-2 test model. Encapsulation efficiency of drugs varied from 80 to 95% depending on the type of drug. A linear release profile without any burst release was observed for the three drugs loaded onto the nanoparticles and rate of release was governed by the hydrophobic and ionic interactions between the particles and the drugs. However, flufenamic acid loaded onto nanoparticles had a 10 times higher permeability across the skin but caffein and testestorone did not have an increased permeation. It was suggested that the modified starch nanoparticles could be used for transdermal delivery of certain drugs (Santander-Ortega et al. 2010). Similarly, anionic starch nanoparticles (113–154 nm) modified by oxidation were also found suitable for delivery of drugs by controlling the pH (Thiele et al. 2011).

Fluorescent starch nanoparticles for imaging applications have been developed by hydrothermal treatment of starch with polyethyleneimine (Liu et al. 2015). Such fluorescent organic nanoparticles were obtained by mixing solutions of starch and polyethyleneimine and heating the mixture at 100°C for 2 hours. Nanoparticles had a average diameter of about 195 nm and the fluorescene quantum yield was 9.8%. When incubated with cells, the nanoparticles did not show any cytotoxicity. However, the nanoparticles were able to enter cells but not the nucleus. Depending on the wave length, the cells containing the nanoparticles could emit blue and green fluorescene suggesting that the nanoparticles could be used for biological imaging (Liu et al. 2015).

Artificial red blood cells

Unlike other polysaccharides, starch has the distinction of being used to develop artificial red blood cells by encapsulating hemoglobin (Xu et al. 2015). To achieve this, starch was first grafted with oleic acid and the grafted starch was mixed with hemoglobin in different proportions and freeze dried to form nanoparticles with an average diameter of about 250 nm. An encapsulation efficiency of up to 98% of hemoglobin was achieved by varying the parameters. Nanoparticles also had similar oxygen carrying capacity compared to that of native hemoglobin. Further, the circulation half time of the grafted starch encapsulated hemoglobin samples was about 11.5 hours. Nanoparticles were injected into mice which were subject to hemorrhagic shock. Tissue sections collected from normal mice and mice injected with the nanoparticles did not show any obvious histological difference suggesting that the mice were able to recover from the shock and the hemoglobin in the starch nanoparticles was active (Fig. 31). The grafted starch nanoparticles developed were considered to be suitable to develop artificial red blood cells with the biocompatibility and oxygen carrying capacity required for medical applications (Xu et al. 2015).

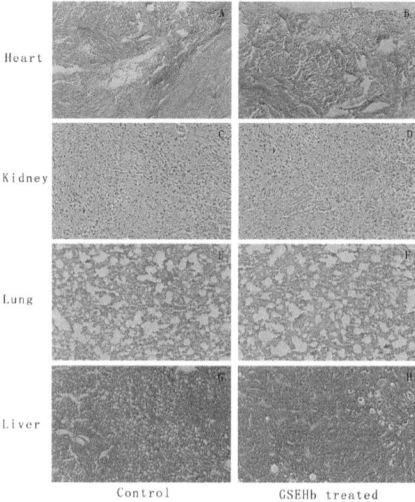

Fig. 31: Histological sections of the various organs in mice with and without the grafted starch nanoparticles containing hemoglobin after hemorrhagic shock show no obvious differences suggesting that the nanocapsules and hemoglobin induced are biocompatible (Xu et al. 2015). Reproduced with permission from the Royal Society of Chemistry.

Fibers

Fibrous structures particularly nanofibers more closely mimic the extracellular matrix and therefore attempts have been made to develop fibrous structures from starch for medical applications. In one such attempt, hierarchial fibrous structure was built using starch-polycaprolactone micro and nano motifs (Martins et al. 2009). To develop such as structure, a 30/70 blend of starch/polycaprolactone was extruded into fiber mesh form using a 3D printer. Layers of nanofibers formed earlier were placed between each layer of the 3D printed structure to form the hierarchial scaffold (Fig. 32). Fibers obtained by 3D printing had diameters of 300 μm and the electrospun fibers had diameters of 1.4 μm to 400 nm with a porosity of about 68% (Martins et al. 2009). Cells seeded on the scaffold showed uniform distribution but preferentially attached to the nanofiber mats. Higher proliferation of osteoblast cells was observed on the hierarchial fibrous structure suggesting suitability of the scaffolds for bone tissue engineering.

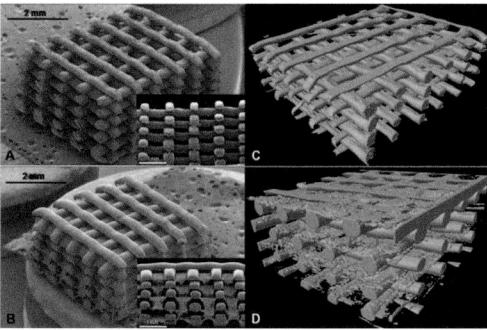

Fig. 32: SEM and μ-ct images of the starch polycaprolactone 3D printed structure (a, c) and the hierarchial structure comprising the 3D printed fibers and electrospun fiber meshes (Martins et al. 2009). Reproduced with permission from John Wiley and Sons.

Conclusions

There is incredible information on the development and use of polysaccharides for medical applications. Although traditional applications of polysaccharides for medical applications continues, several new polymers, polymeric blends and applications have been developed albeit most of them are still in laboratory stage. Abundant availability, excellent mechanical properties, and processability into various forms make polysaccharides preferable for medical applications. In addition to the conventional approaches, it is necessay to adopt latest techniques to develop biomaterials for medical applications. Increasing the stability, biocompatibility and ability to tailor the polysaccharide based biomaterials for specific applications will be critical for further development. Blending with other biopolymers, particularly the plant proteins should be considered to make the polysaccharides suitable for medical applications. Similarly, extensive *in vivo* and clinical studies should be conducted before any polysaccharide based biomaterial can be considered for practical use.

Acknowledgements

Narendra Reddy (author) expresses his gratitude to the Department of Biotechnology, Ministry of Science and Technology, Government of India for financial support through the Ramalingaswami Fellowship. Authors also thank the Center for Emerging Technologies at Jain University for their support to complete this work.

References

Andrade, F. K., S. M. G. Moreira, L. Domingues and F. M. P. Gama. 2010. Improving the affinity of fibroblasts for bacterial cellulose using carbohydrate binding modules fused to RGD. J. Biomed. Mater. Res. 92A: 9–17.

Arockianathan, P. M., S. Sekar, B. Kumaran and T. P. Sastry. 2012. Preparation, characterization and evaluation of biocomposite films containing chitosan and sago starch impregnated with silver nanoparticles. Intl. J. Biol. Macromol. 50: 939–646.

Azevedo, E. P., R. Retarekar, M. L. Raghavan and V. Kumar. 2013. Mechanical properties of cellulose: chitosan blends for potential use as a coronary artery bypass graft. J. Biomater. Sci. Polym. Ed. 24(3): 239–252.

Balmayor, E. R., K. Tuzlakoglu, H. S. Azevedo and R. L. Reis. 2009. Preparation and characterization of starch-poly-ε-caprolactone microparticles incorporating bioactive agents for drug delivery and tissue engineering applications. Acta Biomater. 5: 1035–1045.

Barbetta, A., A. Carrino, M. Costantini and M. Dentini. 2010. Polysaccharide based scaffolds obtained by freezing the external phase of gas-in-liquid foams. Soft Matter 6: 5213–5224.

Barralet, J. E., L. Wang, M. Lawson, J. T. Triffitt and P. R. Cooper. 2005. Comparison of bone marrow cell growth on 2D and 3D alginate hydrogels. J. Mater. Sci. Mater. Med. 16: 515–519.

Bidarra, S. J., C. C. Barrias, M. A. Barbosa, R. Soares and P. L. Granja. 2010. Immobilization of human mesenchymal stem cells withing RGD grafted alginate microspheres and assessment of their angiogenic potential. Biomacromol. 11: 1956–1964.

Carrick, C., M. Ruda, B. Pettersson, T. Larsson and L. Wagberg. 2013. Hollow cellulose capsules from CO_2 saturated cellulose solutions-their preparation and characterization. RSC Adv. 2: 2462–2472.

Chang, C. and M. Wang. 2013. Preparation of microfibrillated cellulose composites for sustained release of H_2O_2 or O_2 for biomedical applications. ACS Sust. Chem. Engg. 1: 1129–1134.

Chou, A. I. and S. B. Nicoll. 2009. Characterization of photocrosslinked alginate hydrogels for nucleus pulposus cell encapsulation. J. Biomed. Mater. Res. 91A: 187–194.

Chou, A. I., S. O. Akintoye and S. B. Nicoll. 2013. Photocrosslinked alginate hydrogels support enhanced matrix accumulation by nucleus pulposus cells *in vivo*. Osteoarthr. Cartilage 17: 1377–1384.

Dong, H., J. F. Snyder, K. S. Williams and J. W. Andzelm. 2013. Cation induced hydrogels of cellulose nanofibrils with tunable moduli. Biomacromol. 14: 3338–3345.

Erizal, D. P., B. Abbas and G. S. Sulistioso. 2014. Fast swelling superabsorbent hydrogels starch based prepared by gamma radiation techniques. Indo. J. Chem. 14(3): 248–252.

Filion, T. M., A. Kutikov and J. Song. 2011. Chemically modified cellulose fibrous meshes for use as tissue engineering scaffolds. Bioorg. Med. Chem. Lett. 21: 5067–5070.

Fundueanu, G., M. Constantin, P. Ascenzi and B. C. Simionescu. 2010. An intelligent multicompartmental system based on thermo-sensitive starch microspheres for temperature controlled release of drugs. Biomed. Microdev. 12: 693–704.

Gomez d'Ayala, G., A. Rosa, P. Laurienzo and M. Malinconico. 2007. Development of a new calcium sulphate based composite using alginate and chemically modified chitosan for bone regeneration. J. Biomed. Mater. Res. 81A: 811–820.

Grande, C. J., F. G. Torres, C. M. Gomez and M. C. Bano. 2009. Nanocomposites of bacterial cellulose/ hydroxyapatite for biomedical applications. Acta Biomater. 5: 1605–1615.

Guilherme, M. R., R. S. Oliveira, M. R. Mauricio, T. S. P. Cellet, M. Pereira, M. H. Kunita et al. 2012. Albumin release from a brain resembling superabsorbent magnetic hydrogel based on starch. Soft Matter 8: 6629–6639.

Jorfi, M., M. N. Roberts, E. J. Foster and C. Weder. 2013. Physiologically responsive, mechanically adaptive bionanocomposites for biomedical applications. ACS Appl. Mater. Interf. 5: 1517–1526.

Kim, G. and K. Park. 2009. Alginate nanofibers produced by an electrohydrodynamic process. Polym. Engg. 49: 2242–2248.

Kim, J., Z. Cai, H. S. Lee, G. S. Choi, D. H. Lee and C. Jo. 2011. Preparation and characterization of a bacterial cellulose chitosan composite for potential biomedical application. J. Polym. Res. 18: 739–744.

Kolakovic, R., T. Laaksonen, L. Peltonen, A. Laukkanen and J. Hirvonen. 2012. Spray dried nanofibrillar cellulose microparticles for sustained drug release. Intl. J. Pharm. 430: 47–55.

Kuo, C. K. and P. X. Ma. 2001. Ionically crosslinked alginate hydrogels as scaffolds for tissue engineering Part I. Structure, gelation rate and mechanical properties. Biomaterials 22: 511–521.

Lee, C., J. Shin, J. S. Lee, E. Byun, H. J. Ryu, S. H. Um et al. 2013. Bioinspired, calcium-free alginate hydrogels with tunable physical and mechanical properties and improved biocompatibility. Biomacromol. 14: 2004–2013.

Li, Y., Y. Tan, K. Xu, C. Lu, X. Liang and P. Wang. 2015. *In situ* crosslinkable hydrogels formed from modified starch and O-carboxymethyl chitosan. RSC Adv. 5: 30303–30310.

Ling, H., J. F. Snyder, K. S. Williams and J. W. Andzelm. 2013. Cation induced hydrogels of cellulose nanofibrils with tunable moduli. Biomacromol. 14: 3338–3345.

Liu, C., K. G. Desai, X. Meng and X. Chen. 2007. Sweet potato starch microparticles as controlled drug release carriers: preparation and *in vitro* drug release. Drying Technol. 25: 689–693.

Liu, K., Y. Wang, H. Li and Y. Duan. 2015. A facile on-pot synthesis of starch functionalized graphene as nanocarrier for pH sensitive and starch mediated drug delivery. Colloid. Surf. B: Biointer. 128: 86–93.

Liu, M., X. Zhang, B. Yang, Z. Li, F. Deng, Y. Yang et al. 2015. Fluorescent nanoparticles from starch: facile preparation, tunable luminescence and bioimaging. Carbohydrate Polym. 121: 49–55.

Machida-Sano, I., Y. Matsuda and H. Namiki. 2009. *In vitro* adhesion of human dermal fibroblasts on iron crosslinked alginate films. Biomed. Mater. 4: 025008.

Mallick, S. P., S. S. Sagiri, V. K. Singh, K. Pal, D. K. Pradhan and M. K. Bhattacharya. 2014. Effect of processed starches on the properties of gelatin based physical hydrogels: characterization, *in vitro* drug release and antimicrobial studies. Polym. Plast. Technol. Engg. 53: 700–715.

Mandal, A., S. Sekar, K. M. S. Meera, A. Mukherjee, T. P. Sastry and A. B. Mandal. 2014. Fabrication of collagen scaffolds impregnated with sago starch capped silver nanoparticles suitable for biomedical applications and their physiochemical studies. Phy. Chem. Chem. Phy. 16: 20175–20183.

Marques, A. P., R. L. Reis and J. A. Hunt. 2005. An *in vivo* study of the host response to starch based polymers and composites subcutaneously implanted in rats. Macromol. Biosci. 5: 775–785.

Martins, A., S. Chung, A. J. Pedro, R. A. Sousa, A. P. Marques, R. L. Reis et al. 2009. Hierarchial starch based fibrous scaffold for bone tissue engineering applications. J. Tissue Engg. Regen. Med. 3: 37–42.

Matricardi, P., M. Pontoriero, T. Coviello, M. A. Casadei and F. Alhaique. 2008. *In situ* crosslinkable novel alginate dextran methacrylate IPN hydrogels for biomedical applications: mechanical characterization and drug delivery properties. Biomacromol. 9: 2014–2020.

Moraes, M. A. and M. M. Beppu. 2013. Biocomposite membranes of sodium alginate and silk fibroin fibers for biomedical applications. J. Appl. Polym. Sci. 130: 3451–3457.

Morales, M. A., P. V. Finotelli, J. A. H. Coaquira, M. H. M. Rocha-Leao, C. Diaz-Aguila, E. M. Baggio-Saitovitch et al. 2008. *In situ* synthesis and magnetic studies of iron oxide nanoparticles in calcium alginate matrix for biomedical applications. Mater. Sci. Engg. C 28: 253–257.

Olderoy, M. O., M. Xie, J. Andreassen, B. L. Strand, Z. Zhang and P. Sikorski. 2012. Viscoelastic properties of mineralized alginate hydrogel beads. J. Mater. Sci. Mater. Med. 23: 1619–1627.

Onofrei, M. D., A. M. Dobos, S. Dunca, E. G. Ioanid and S. Ioan. 2015. Biocidal activity of cellulose materials for medical applications. J. Appl. Polym. Sci. 132: 41932.

Park, H. and K. Y. Lee. 2014. Cartilage regeneration using biodegradable oxidized alginate/hyaluronate hydrogels. J. Biomed. Mater. Res. Part A: 102A: 4519–4525.

Pertile, R., S. Moreira, F. Andrade, L. Domingues and M. Gama. 2012. Bacterial cellulose modified using recombinant proteins to improve neuronal and mesenchymal cell adhesion. Biotechnol. Prog. 28: 526–532.

Pescosolido, L., T. Vermonden, J. Malda, R. Censi, W. J. A. Dhert, F. Alhaique et al. 2011. *In situ* forming IPN hydrogels of calcium alginate and dextran-HEMA for biomedical applications. Acta Biomater. 7: 1627–1633.

Pooyan, P., R. Tannenbaum and H. Garmestani. 2012. Mechanical behavior of a cellulose reinforced scaffold in vascular tissue engineering. J. Mech. Beh. Biomed. Mater. 7: 50–59.

Pooyan, P., T. Kim, K. L. Jacob, R. Tannenbaum and H. Garmestani. 2013. Design of a cellulose based nanocomposite as a potential polymeric scaffold in tissue engineering. Polymer 54: 2105–2114.

Saboktakin, M. R., R. M. Tabatabaie, P. Ostovarazar, A. Maharramov and M. A. Ramazanov. 2012. Synthesis and characterization of modified starch hydrogels for photodynamic treatment of cancer. International J. Biol. Macromol. 51: 544–549.

Salgado, A. J., O. P. Coutinho and R. L. Reis. 2004. Novel starch based scaffolds for bone tissue engineering, cytotoxicity, cell culture and protein expression. Tissue Engg. 10(3/4): 465–474.

Salgado, A. J., O. P. Coutinho, R. L. Reis and J. E. Davies. 2007. *In vivo* response to starch based scaffolds designed for bone tissue engineering applications. J. Biomed. Mater. Res. Part A 80: 983–989.

Santander-Ortega, M. J., T. Stauner, B. Loretz, J. L. Ortega-Vinuesa, D. Bastos-Gonzalez, G. Wenz et al. 2010. Nanoparticles made from novel starch derivatives for transdermal drug delivery. J. Control. Rel. 141: 85–92.

Shen, W. and Y. Hsieh. 2014. Biocompatible sodium alginate fibers by aqueous processing and physical crosslinking. Carbohydrate Polym. 102: 893–900.

Shin, E. L., S. M. Choi, D. Singh, S. M. Zo, Y. H. Lee, J. H. Kim et al. 2014. Fabrication of cellulose based scaffold with microarchitecture using a leaching technique for biomedical applications. Cellulose 21: 3515–3525.

Sivoli, L., E. Perez, D. Caraballo, J. P. Rodriguez, D. Rodriguez, J. Moret et al. 2013. Cytocompatibility of a matrix of methylated cassava starch and chitosan. J. Cell. Plast. 49(6): 507–520.

Taheri, A. and M. Mohammadi. 2015. The use of cellulose nanocrystals for potential application in topical delivery of Hydroquinone. Chem. Biol. Drug Disc. 86: 102–106.

Thiele, C., D. Auerbach, G. Jung, L. Qiong, M. Schneider and G. Wenz. 2011. Nanoparticles of anionic starch and cationic cyclodextrin derivatives for the targeted delivery of drugs. Polym. Chem. 2: 209–215.

Torres, F. G., O. P. Troncoso, C. G. Grande and D. A. Diaz. 2011. Biocompatibility of starch based films from starch of Andean crops for biomedical applications. Mater. Sci. Engg. C. 31: 1737–1740.

Treenate, P., P. Monvisade and M. Yamaguchi. 2014. Development of hydroxyethylacryl chitosan/alginate hydrogel films for medical applications. J. Polym. Res. 21: 601–609.

Ul-Islam, M., W. A. Khattak, M. W. Ullah, S. Khan and J. K. Park. 2014. Synthesis of regenerated bacterial cellulose zinc oxide nanocomposite films for biomedical applications. Cellulose 21: 433–447.

Velasquz, D., G. P. Pavon-Djavid, L. Chaunier, A. Meddahi-Pelle and D. Lourdin. 2015. Effect of crystallinity and plasticizer on mechanical properties and tissue integration of starch based materials from two botanical origins. Carbohydrate Polym. 124: 180–187.

Wan, Y. Z., Y. Huang, C. D. Yuan, S. Raman, Y. Zhu, H. J. Jiang et al. 2007. Biomimetic synthesis of hydroxyapatite/bacterial cellulose nanocomposites for biomedical applications. Mater. Sci. Engg. C 27: 855–864.

Wang, J., J. Li, H. Yang, C. Zhu, J. Yang and F. Yao. 2015a. Preparation and characterization of protein resistant zwitterionic starches: the effect of substitution degrees. Starch 67: 920–929.

Wang, J., H. Sun, J. Li, D. Dong, Y. Zhang and F. Yao. 2015b. Ionic strength based hydrogels for the prevention of non-specific protein adsorption. Carbohydrate Polym. 117: 384–391.

Xiao, C. 2013. Current advances of chemical and physical starch based hydrogels. Starch 65: 82–86.

Xu, R., J. Zhang, P. Zhou, R. Yang, X. Feng and L. Xu. 2015. A novel artificial red blood cell substitute: grafted starch encapsulated hemoglobin. RSC Adv. 5: 43845–43853.

Yadav, V., B. J. Paniliatis, H. Shi, K. Lee, P. Cebe and D. L. Kaplan. 2010. Novel *In vivo* degradable cellulose chitin copolymer from metabolically engineered *Gluconacetobacter xylinus*. Appl. Environ. 76(18): 6257–6265.

Yadollahi, M., I. Gholamali, H. Namazi and M. Aghazadeh. 2015a. Synthesis and characterization of antibacterial carboxymethyl cellulose/ZuO nanocomposite hydrogels. Intl. J. Biol. Macromol. 74: 136–141.

Yadollahi, M., I. Gholamali, H. Namazi and M. Aghazadeh. 2015b. Synthesis and characterization of antibacterial carboxymethylcellulose/CuO bionanocomposite hydrogels. Intl. J. Biol. Macromol. 73: 109–114.

Yoo, S. M. and R. Ghosh. 2014. Fabrication of alginate fibers using a microporous membrane based molding technique. Biochem. Engg. J. 91: 58–65.

Zhang, H., X. Liu, M. Yang and L. Zhu. 2015. Silk fibroin/sodium alginate composite nanofibrous scaffold prepared through thermally induced phase separation (TIPS) method for biomedical applications. Mater. Sci. Engg. C 55: 8–13.

Zhang, L., C. Yang and L. Yan. 2005. Perspectives on strategies to fabricate starch based hydrogels with potential biomedical applications. J. Bioact. Compt. Polym. 20: 297–314.

Zhou, Z., J. Chen, C. Peng, T. Huang, H. Zhou, B. Ou et al. 2014. Fabrication and physical properties of gelatin/sodium alginate hyaluronic acid composite wound dressing hydrogel. J. Macromol. Sci. Part A Pure Appl. Chem. 51: 318–325.

4

Biopolymers in the Prevention of Dental Erosion

Javier Sotres[1,2]

Abstract

Dental erosion, that is, the loss of dental hard tissue induced by acids of non-bacterial origin, is currently recognized in many Western countries as the main factor responsible for tooth wear. Dental erosion results not only in aesthetic, orthodontic, and functional complications, but is also associated with sensitivity and pain. Its prevalence has become alarmingly high and continues to escalate. As a consequence, it is expected that dental erosion will have a major economic impact on dental services in the decades to come. Thus, it is not daring to place dental erosion as one of the biggest challenges in dentistry for the 21st century.

It is difficult to both diagnose dental erosion in early stages and to treat it in advanced stages. Thus, a considerable effort has been devoted to the development of prevention strategies. At present, most of such strategies focus on increasing the acid-resistance of the dentition and on weakening the erosive potential of erosive challenges, for example, acidic foods and beverages. Recently, it has been shown that different types of biopolymers can be used for these purposes. If topically applied, biopolymers can adsorb on

---
[1] Biomedical Science, Faculty of Health and Society, Malmö University, 20506 Malmö, Sweden.
[2] Biofilms-Research Center for Biointerfaces, Malmö University, 20506 Malmö, Sweden.
   E-mail: javier.sotres@mah.se

teeth increasing their acid-resistance. Additionally, the erosiveness of acidic beverages can be lowered if modified with biopolymers. Biopolymers present additional advantages over other anti-erosive compounds, for example, they do not possess health risks and, as expected from their wide use in the food industry, they may rise low consumer-acceptance concerns. This chapter aims at providing an overview of the potential of biopolymers in the prevention of dental erosion.

Dental Erosion—Introduction

Tooth wear, that is, the loss of dental hard tissue not caused by bacteria or trauma, is a growing concern in modern dentistry. While its prevalence over human history has notably decreased (Kaidonis 2008), it has recently rebounded as a result of changes in dietary habits and lifestyle (Gambon et al. 2012).

Tooth wear is an extremely complex process that can be originated by different mechanisms, mainly attrition, abrasion, and erosion. Attrition refers to the wear resulting from tooth-to-tooth contact, whereas abrasion involves contact between tooth surfaces and foreign material. Erosion refers instead to "loss of dental hard tissue by a chemical process that does not involve the influence of bacteria" (Pindborg 1970). It is accepted that, historically, tooth wear was mainly caused by abrasion, whereas erosion played a minor role (Kaidonis 2008). However, the prevalence of abrasion has been reduced due to the increasing consumption of processed softer foods. On the contrary, the prevalence of erosion has increased and it is currently acknowledged as the most common cause of tooth wear (Johansson et al. 2012).

Teeth are composed of different types of tissues. Enamel constitutes their outermost surface. Dentin, which accounts for most of the teeth portion, is found below the enamel. Both enamel and dentin consist of micro-meter sized mineral crystals embedded in a matrix formed by proteins, lipids, and water (Avery 2002). The mineral component of both tissues is also similar; a calcium-deficient carbonated hydroxyapatite (HAP) containing some fluoride. A simplified formula of tooth mineral composition is $Ca_{10-x}Na_n(PO_4)_{6-y}(CO_3)_z(OH)_{2-u}F_u$, which is different from that of stoichiometric HAP, i.e., $Ca_{10}(PO_4)_6(OH)_2$. Additionally, the mineral component in enamel and dentin is not identical. The carbonate content is significantly higher in dentin. Moreover, dentin is less mineralized than enamel. Despite these differences, for practical reasons HAP is often used as a model surface in dental erosion studies.

Exposure of teeth to acidic solutions leads to their dissolution (Fig. 1). In the field of dental erosion, the term "critical pH" is often found. This is the pH at which a solution is just saturated with respect to the mineral component in teeth. If the pH of the solution is above this value, the minerals in the solution will tend to precipitate on the surface, whereas if it is below the surface will tend to dissolve. Usually, a value of ~ 5.5 is found in the literature for the critical pH of teeth (the actual value depends on the concentration of tooth mineral components, for example, calcium and phosphate, in the surrounding medium (Dawes 2003)). Below the critical pH, dissolution results from the binding between the hydrogen ions (derived from the dissociation of acids in water) and the hydroxyl and phosphate groups on the HAP surface (Dorozhkin 1997).

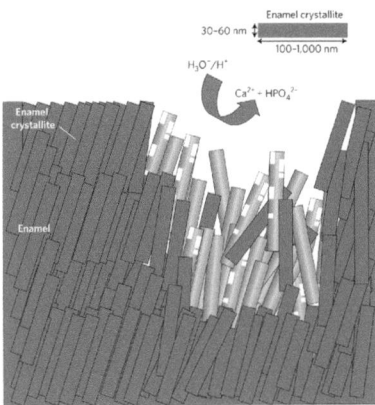

Fig. 1: Acidic solution, such as acidic beverages or gastric juices (pH 1–4), erode enamel and dentin crystals. As a result, Ca^{2+} and HPO_4^{2-} ions are released. Reprinted by permission from Macmillan Publishers Ltd. Nature Nanotechnology (Hannig and Hannig 2010), copyright 2010.

In the case of the mineral in enamel and dentin, the hydrogen ions can also combine with the carbonate ions on the surface. This makes enamel and dentin more acid soluble than HAP (Budz et al. 1987). The anions resulting from acid dissociation can also play a role in erosion by combining with calcium on the surface, this process being known as chelation (Featherstone and Lussi 2006). The initial mineral loss resulting from erosion causes an increase in roughness and in softness as the acid diffuses through the enamel matrix. In turn, enamel softening makes it more vulnerable to wear induced by mechanical impacts (Miller 1907).

The etiology of erosion is multifactorial. Factors leading to erosion are usually divided into extrinsic and intrinsic. Acids of extrinsic origin include those from acidic foods and beverages, as well as those from acidic medications (Zero 1996). Extrinsic factors also include environmental acid exposure in selected populations such as swimmers, workers in an environment with acidic industrial vapors, and professional wine tasters (Wiegand and Attin 2007). Dental erosion can also be caused by intrinsic factors, mainly disorders associated with the presence of gastric acid in the oral cavity (Bartlett 2006). The diagnosis of dental erosion is difficult and, subsequently, it is also difficult to determine its prevalence. It is difficult to detect early enamel erosion in routine dental practice as it causes no appreciable discoloration or softening. Additionally, patient symptoms are often absent in early stages. In the stages where wear is detectable, without information on the patient lifestyle, it is difficult to determine whether it is due mainly to erosion, to attrition, or to abrasion. Nevertheless, there is an agreement about the prevalence of dental erosion rapidly increasing in Western societies (Johansson et al. 2012). It is generally accepted that this is due to the recent increase of the level of prosperity in the Western world, which has led to a higher availability of acidic foods and beverages, i.e., acids of extrinsic origin (Gambon et al. 2012). Changes in lifestyle have also led to a growing number of people suffering from refluxes of gastric content, which constitute intrinsic acidic challenges for the denture (ten Cate and Imfeld 1996).

Dental erosion results not only in aesthetic, orthodontic, and functional complications (Fig. 2), but is also associated with sensitivity and pain for the patient. Moreover, it often requires restorative interventions. Because of its alarmingly high and continuously increasing prevalence, it is expected that dental erosion will have major economic impact on dental services in the decades to come. Thus, it is not daring to place dental erosion as one of the biggest challenges to dentistry for the 21st century.

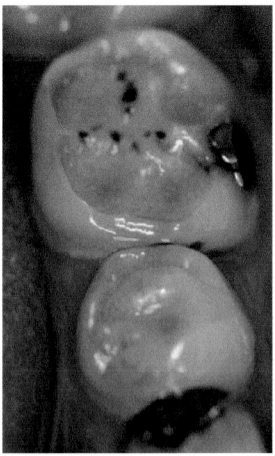

Fig. 2: Clinical appearance of erosive tooth wear in a frequent consumer of acidic drinks. Reprinted from (Johansson et al. 2012).

Saliva and Dental Erosion

Saliva plays a major role in dental erosion. Any erosive solution will interact with saliva, which is the biological fluid continuously secreted into the oral cavity by various salivary glands. Saliva is an aqueous fluid (water accounts for ca. 99% of its weight) containing mostly proteins (i.e., biopolymers) even though lipids and inorganic components are also present up to some extent (Humphrey and Williamson 2001). Indeed, one of the main functions of saliva is to counteract dental erosion. This is achieved by means of different mechanisms. For instance, saliva protects tooth surfaces from acids by diluting them (Hara and Zero 2014). The dilution effect is enhanced by several stimuli. Even before acids start to erode tooth surfaces, the salivary flow rate increases as a response to extra-oral stimuli such as odor or sight (Christensen and Navazesh 1984; Lee and Linden 1992). It has also been reported that vomiting is preceded by hypersalivation (Lee and Feldman 1998). Once the acid reaches the oral cavity, both intra-oral stimuli, due to chemical factors (for example, the presence of the acid itself) and mechanical factors (for example, mastication), also increase the salivary flow rate (Yeh et al. 2000; Engelen et al. 2003). Saliva stimulated by these mechanisms also has a higher buffering capacity as a result of a higher hydrogen carbonate content (Dawes 1969). Additionally, saliva is supersaturated with respect to calcium and phosphate, lowering the erosive critical pH and promoting remineralization (Hara and Zero 2014).

Saliva also protects tooth surfaces from acidic challenges by adsorbing on them, i.e., coating them with a film known as salivary pellicle (Lindh et al. 2014) which has acid resistance properties (Hannig and Hannig 2014). In a simplified scheme, salivary pellicles consist of an inner thin dense layer, formed mainly by proteins of relatively low molecular weight, and an outer thick diffuse layer, mainly composed by long and highly glycosylated mucins (Lindh et al. 2014) (Fig. 3). Even though more than 160 proteins and peptides form part of salivary pellicles (Siqueira et al. 2012), most of the pellicle mass can be attributed to only a few of them such as hystatin, cystatins, proline rich proteins, amylases, and mucins (Aroonsang et al. 2014; Yakubov et al. 2015).

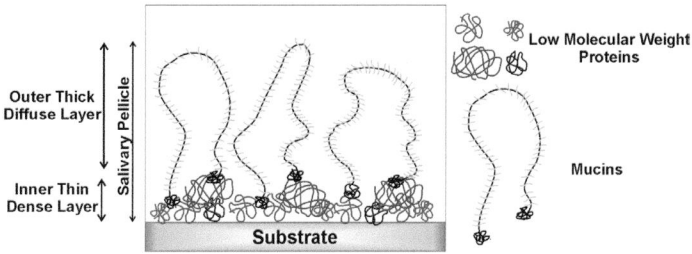

Fig. 3: Scheme of the two-layer model for salivary pellicles.

Exposure to a standard erosive acidic solution leads to an immediate removal of a fraction of the pellicle, mainly low molecular weight proteins from its innermost layer (Delvar et al. 2015). However, the pellicle is not completely removed and continues to homogeneously cover the underlying surface (Hannig and Balz 1999; Hannig et al. 2003; Delvar et al. 2015). The challenged pellicle reduces and retards the demineralization of the underlying HAP but does not prevent it completely. This indicates that the challenged pellicles can hamper but not fully prevent the interaction between the acid and the underlying HAP.

The mechanisms responsible for the anti-erosive properties of salivary pellicles are not yet clear. A mesh-like structure could confer the pellicle diffusion barrier properties (Hannig and Hannig 2014). Another possibility is that proteins bind different chemical groups on the tooth surfaces, stabilizing them against acid-induced dissociation (Van Kemenade and de Bruyn 1989). It has also been suggested that the components of the pellicle could act as a buffer by binding the acids that could attack tooth surfaces (Hannig and Joiner 2006).

The historical low prevalence of dental erosion suggests that the solution found by nature to protect teeth from erosion, i.e., saliva, was enough to counteract the acidic challenges humans were traditionally exposed to. However, the recent increase in this prevalence also indicates that saliva is not enough any longer to counteract the effects of the increasing number of acidic challenges associated with the modern lifestyle. Nevertheless, as in many other examples where biomimetic approaches have been used as starting points and sources of inspiration (Vincent et al. 2006), understanding and mimicking saliva is expected to originate novel and powerful strategies for counteracting dental erosion.

Preventive Strategies for Dental Erosion

It is difficult to both diagnose dental erosion in early stages and to treat it in advanced stages. This fact highlights the importance of prevention strategies.

Different strategies can be taken in order to address the different factors that can lead to dental erosion. Behavioral factors probably have a higher influence on dental erosion. A straight-forward strategy to prevent dental erosion would be to reduce the frequency and duration of acid exposures (Magalhães et al. 2009). That is, behaviors which promote erosion should be reduced or avoided. Examples include, for example, the in-take of acidic foods and beverages (Künzel et al. 2000; Dugmore and Rock 2004) and habits such as holding acidic drinks in the mouth prior to swallowing (Johansson et al. 2004). A lactovegetarian diet is also associated with a higher prevalence of dental erosion (Ganss et al. 1999). Different unhealthy lifestyle factors such as the consumption of drugs (Duxbury 1993) and alcohol (Robb and Smith 1990) may also promote erosion. Suggested preventive measures for environmental acid exposure include the use of protective equipment as well as adherence to threshold limit values recommended by occupational health legislations. Oral hygiene is also an aspect that should be considered. For instance, the resistance of teeth to abrasion caused by tooth brushing is diminished after exposure to erosive challenges (Attin et al. 2001). Dental erosion can also be caused by intrinsic factors, mainly disorders associated with the presence of gastric acid in the oral cavity. These disorders require a causal therapy (general medicine, psychological therapy) for a permanent reduction of the intrinsic acid exposure.

Dental erosion can also be originated by biological factors. A low salivary flow rate and buffering capacity is strongly associated with dental erosion (Hara et al. 2006). This is common, for example, in patients suffering from hyposalivation and xerostomia (dry mouth) whom are indeed more prone to suffer from dental erosion. These conditions require preventive measures such as salivary flow stimulation. This can be achieved by means of local stimulators, for example, chewing gums (Rios et al. 2006), or systematically, for example, by the administration of pilocarpine to xerostomia patients (Vivino et al. 1999). Patients suffering from salivary gland dysfunction often make use of salivary substitutes. They are basically water dilutions of biopolymers (for example, mucins or methylcelluloses) along with buffering agents similar to those found in natural saliva (Levine et al. 1987).

Excluding the situations where biological factors are present, the effective prevention of dental erosion would require addressing behavioral factors by means of lifestyle changes. However, attempts in this direction have been unsuccessful so far and further investigation and collaboration between different types of healthcare workers are needed. Therefore, considerable efforts in prevention have been devoted towards two directions: increasing the acid-resistance of the dentition and weakening the erosive potential of acidic challenges.

Assessment of preventive strategies for dental erosion

Before addressing specific preventive strategies for dental erosion, it is useful to consider some aspects of the current stage of the design of studies for assessing such strategies. At present, most published works on the evaluation of preventive measures for dental erosion are *in vitro* and *in situ* studies. *Ex vivo* studies and clinical trials are scarce (Hooper et al. 2007; Vashisht et al. 2010). In other words, research on preventive strategies for dental erosion can be considered to be in an early stage. The reasons for this might be that the prevalence of dental erosion and, therefore, the interest that it has attracted among the scientific community, has become significant only in recent times (Fig. 4a). Other possible reasons might be the difficulty of its diagnosis and the complexity of the experimental techniques needed for its assessment (Attin and Wegehaupt 2014).

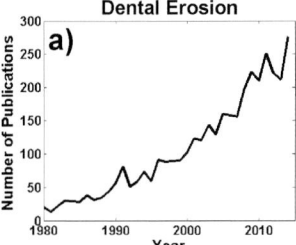 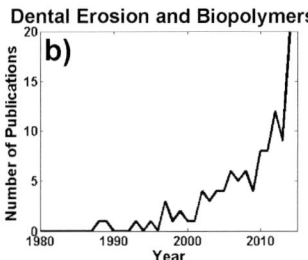

Fig. 4: Bibliometric summary showing an estimation of the number of scientific publications on (a) dental erosion and (b) the use of biopolymers in dental erosion for the last 35 years. Data corresponds to that provided by the ISI Web of Knowledge database for the search strings "(dental or tooth or teeth) and erosion" and "(dental or tooth or teeth) and erosion and (biopolymer or protein or polysaccharide or polyphosphate)" for (a) and (b) respectively.

In vitro and *in situ* studies on dental erosion are characterized by a high variation in study designs and experimental parameters (Wiegand and Attin 2011). For instance, different techniques are usually employed for assessing erosion (Attin 2006). Different techniques measure different properties and, therefore, it is difficult to compare their results. For instance, many studies focus on the use of different microscopies and profilometry to characterize topography modifications and eroded volume (Meurman and Frank 1991; Attin et al. 1997; Ablal et al. 2009) while many others focus on the characterization of HAP/tooth softening by means of indentation approaches (Attin et al. 1997; White et al. 2011). Other parameters that are subject of great variations between different studies, and which are expected to have a significant influence on the results, are the employed surface (for example, enamel, dentin, HAP) and experimental conditions such as the type of acid employed, pH temperature, agitation, exposure time, etc. Some attempts have been made to standardize these aspects of experimental studies (Shellis et al. 2011). However, the present situation is such that in most cases quantitative comparison between different anti-erosion preventive measures can only be made among results within the same study or, at best, between studies employing the same methodology. In the rest of cases, only qualitative comparisons are possible.

Topical application of anti-erosive compounds

Increasing the acid-resistance of the dentition can be achieved by topical application of anti-erosive compounds prior to its exposure to erosive challenges by using, for example, toothpastes, mouthwashes and varnishes. Those containing fluoride are the most well-known of such compounds. They interact with tooth surfaces by forming a fluorapatite layer on their surface which is more acid-resistant than biological apatites (Featherstone and Lussi 2006). Indeed, the efficiency of fluoride containing compounds against dental erosion has been extensively proved (for example (Mohammed and Dusara 2013)). Many studies have also focused on products delivering calcium and phosphate to tooth surfaces. While these compounds have been shown to harden tooth surfaces, their efficiency is below that of those containing fluoride (Buzalaf et al. 2014). Thus, topical fluoride is widely accepted as one of the most effective ways to prevent dental erosion. However, some concerns still exist on the health risks associated with the in-take of fluoride (Wong et al. 2010). Therefore, research on novel ways to protect teeth from erosion by means of topical application of non-hazardous compounds continues to be conducted (for example, Jager et al. 2013).

Modification of potentially erosive products

The modification of potentially erosive products, especially acidic soft drinks, in order to lower their erosiveness has also received significant attention. The acceptability of soft drinks is related to their acidity, so increasing their pH is not a viable option. The same applies to dilution with water, which would be otherwise an effective strategy as it reduces the titratable acidity of the drinks (Cairns et al. 2002). Adding fluoride to soft drinks is also a successful approach (Tahmassebi et al. 2006). However, it is forbidden in many Western countries due to the risk of fluorosis, i.e., the hypomineralization of teeth and bones. Most studies on reducing the erosive potential of drinks have focused instead on the addition of calcium and phosphate supplements. This approach has also proved to be successful (Tahmassebi et al. 2006) but, unfortunately, it leads to flavor deterioration as well (Grenby 1996). Because of health and consumer-acceptance concerns, plenty of research is devoted nowadays to find food-approved, non-hazardous substances with anti-erosive properties, being biopolymers obvious candidates.

It follows from the above discussion that the main disadvantage of addition of anti-erosive compounds to acidic beverages is flavor modification. This can lower consumer-acceptance and, therefore, the applicability of this strategy. Nevertheless, this strategy has a clear advantage over topical application. No topically applied anti-erosive compound has been shown to hamper indefinitely. In other words, the protective films that these compounds form on HAP are eventually removed upon exposure to acids. However, in the case where there is a bulk reservoir of anti-erosive compounds, for example, when they are included in acidic soft drinks, they will provide protection during the complete duration of the erosive challenge.

Use of biopolymers in preventive measures for dental erosion

Biopolymers (for example, proteins, peptides, polysaccharides, and polyphosphate chains) are promising agents for the prevention of dental erosion. An efficient anti-erosive performance of these compounds can be expected from the fact that they are the main components of the formulation used by nature to counteract dental erosion, that is, saliva. The fact that biopolymers do not possess health risks increases the interest of their use as anti-erosive agents. Moreover, their wide use in the food industry suggests that they may rise lower consumer-acceptance concerns than other compounds, for example those enriched with calcium and phosphate salts. Thus, it is no surprise that the use of biopolymers as anti-erosive performance is starting to attract significant attention within the dental erosion field (Fig. 4b).

One of the most noticeable outcomes of research in this field is that acid-induced dissolution of HAP can be counter-acted by biopolymers of very different properties. This has been shown both for cases where biopolymers were topically applied before exposure to the erosive challenge and for cases where erosive acidic solutions were modified with biopolymers. Effectively, anti-erosive properties have been reported for biopolymers of, for example, different structure, chemical composition and charge. For instance, both globular proteins such as albumins (Arends et al. 1986; Hemingway et al. 2008; Kosoric et al. 2010) and intrinsically-unstructured proteins such as caseins (White et al. 2011) have shown to prevent acid-induced dissolution of HAP. The role of the chemical composition of biopolymers in their anti-erosive properties is not clear either. For instance, it could be expected that phosphate-containing compounds would strongly interact with HAP surfaces via phosphate-calcium complexes hampering their dissolution. In fact, this could be concluded from an early study which reported that the anti-erosive properties of protein films was correlated with their number of phosphoserine residues (Reynolds et al. 1982). In addition, in a different study it was reported that the presence of phosphate groups in polymers was associated with a higher anti-erosive performance than the presence of other anionic moieties such as carboxyl, glucuronic, and pyruvic groups (Barbour et al. 2005). However, in a different study performed by the same group it was observed that a casein fraction containing several phosphorylated residues, the casein phosphopeptide (CPP) exhibited a similar anti-erosive performance than another casein fraction, the glycomacropeptide (GMP) which lacked these phosphorylated residues (White et al. 2011). Thus, even though different studies suggest that the presence of phosphate groups is correlated with the anti-erosive performance of a biopolymer, this has yet to be clarified. All the biopolymers mentioned so far have an overall negative charge at standard erosive pH values. However, cationic biopolymer such as chitosan have also shown to protect HAP from acid-induced dissolution (Delvar et al. 2015). Therefore, even though the charge influences the anti-erosive potential of a biopolymer (see below), it does not determine whether the biopolymer can counteract erosion.

Different mechanisms have been proposed to explain the anti-erosive properties of biopolymers. Most of these mechanisms involve the formation of adsorbed films. For instance, biopolymer films could counteract erosion by functioning as buffers (Reynolds and Storey 1979). Chemical groups in the adsorbed biopolymers susceptible to protonation would bind H^+ acid-derived groups increasing the pH at the surface.

Just the adsorption of the biopolymers could also be responsible for their anti-erosive properties, that is, adsorption on potential dissolution sites could block their accessibility by H$^+$ ions. The nature of dissolution sites of HAP is still under debate (Dorozhkin 2012). Nevertheless, it is worth discussing the more accepted ideas. Overall, the net positive surface charge of HAP under acidic conditions (Arends and Jongebloed 1977) indicates that the protonation of negatively charged surface groups (for example, hydroxyl and phosphate) exceeds the adsorption of the anions resulting from the acid onto positively charged surface groups (for example, calcium). Nevertheless, at some point during the dissolution process all the different chemical groups are removed from the surface. Most recent chemical descriptions on the acid-induced dissolution of HAP suggest that this process begins with the detachment of the protonated hydroxyl groups. This would be followed by the detachment of anion-calcium complexes. No variations in time have been observed for the surface charge of HAP in acid, which suggests that the detachment of calcium would immediately be compensated by additional proton adsorption. Calcium detachment would be followed by the detachment of phosphate groups. Independently of the accuracy of this scheme, the fact is that, for erosion to occur, all these processes, i.e., detachment of hydroxyl, phosphate and calcium groups, have to take place. Hampering these processes, for example, by means of adsorbing biopolymers on the surfaces, would result in the delay of the dissolution process.

Another possible explanation for the anti-erosive properties of biopolymer films is that they act as a permeable diffusion barrier against acids (Hannig and Hannig 2014). This mechanism would be of high relevance in the case of porous HAP structures, for example, enamel and dentin. In these cases it is likely that the biopolymers would penetrate into the pores. This is supported by a recent study where, by means of optical coherence tomography it was shown that chitosan applied on teeth could penetrate enamel up to the dentin-enamel junction (Arnaud et al. 2010). However, very little is known at present on the penetration of biopolymers on teeth and on the effect of this process on dental erosion.

The fact that biopolymers of very different properties can provide some degree of protection to HAP from acidic challenges suggests that all the processes mentioned above can take place. However, it is expected that the effective contribution of each of these mechanisms to the overall anti-erosive performance is highly influenced by the ionic character of the biopolymers. HAP surfaces exhibit a net positive charge under acidic conditions. However, this is just the average of a highly heterogeneous charge distribution of their surfaces which contain, for example, hydroxyl, phosphate, and calcium ions (Skartsila and Spanos 2007). This explains, as experimentally proved (Delvar et al. 2015), that both cationic and anionic biopolymers are able to adsorb on HAP and, therefore, block its potential dissolution sites. However, their effectiveness with respect to this mechanism will be different for anionic and cationic biopolymers. First, the charge of anionic biopolymers would be significantly lowered under acidic conditions and, therefore, they would be expected to develop weaker interactions with HAP surfaces than cationic biopolymers. In agreement with this, films of chitosan, that is, a cationic polymer, have shown to provide significant higher anti-erosive protection to HAP than films of carboxymethyl cellulose, that is, an anionic biopolymer

(Delvar et al. 2015). Moreover, films of anionic biopolymers could also act as buffers whereas films of cationic biopolymers would function as diffusion barriers.

The application of biopolymers in the field of dental erosion has not solely focused on their use for coating HAP. An example is the use of casein phosphopeptide stabilized amorphous calcium phosphate (CPP-ACP) both as an anti-erosive and a as remineralizing agent. CPP can stabilize over 100 times more calcium phosphate than is normally possible in an aqueous solution at neutral pH before spontaneous precipitation. The stabilized ACP, by being in dynamic equilibrium with free phosphate and calcium ions, maintains a high concentration of these ions close to the erosion lesion (Reynolds 1997). Moreover, dissociation of the CPP-bound ACP is facilitated by the acid generated during enamel remineralization, and this in turn increases the availability of phosphate and calcium ions for remineralization purposes (Reynolds 1997). CPP-ACP adsorbed on tooth surfaces can also counteract erosion, as a decrease in pH dissociates the CPP-ACP complex and subsequently ACP into free calcium and phosphate ions (Nongonierma and FitzGerald 2012). CPP-ACP has been used to modify the composition of acidic soft drinks. This resulted not only in a decrease of their erosiveness but also in higher levels of consumer-acceptance than the modification with bare calcium and phosphates (Ramalingam et al. 2005).

Studies on the anti-erosive performance of biopolymer films on clean HAP surfaces provide only incomplete information to understand their performance in *in vivo* situations. A parameter that is missing in many studies is the presence of saliva and, more specifically, of the salivary pellicle that is always present on tooth surfaces. Topical application of anti-erosive compounds will lead to the adsorption of the compounds onto the salivary pellicle. In the case where acidic solutions are modified with anti-erosive compounds, these compounds would also adsorb onto the salivary pellicles. In both scenarios, at the beginning of erosive challenges the acid will not interact with tooth surfaces but with the complex formed by the salivary pellicle and the anti-erosive compounds instead. Interaction between the acid and non-coated HAP will only take place at a later stage, when the eventual diffusion of the acid through this coating will erode the boundaries between HAP crystals resulting in their eventual release (along with the coating on their upper side).

As previously mentioned, because of both technical and ethical reasons, it is difficult to study dental erosion in *in vivo* conditions, that is, the conditions where a salivary pellicle will always be coating tooth surfaces. Nevertheless, dental erosion studies which take into account the presence of a salivary pellicle can be performed, for example, *in situ* by mounting test surfaces in removable intraoral splints (West et al. 2004). When inside the oral cavity, the surfaces will immediately acquire a pellicle, resembling those formed *in vivo*. Pellicles can also be formed *in vitro* by adsorbing previously collected saliva on the test surfaces (Delvar et al. 2015). While *in vitro* pellicles may differ from *in vivo* ones more than those formed *in situ*, *in vitro* experiments have the advantage of a higher control of the experimental conditions.

As in the case of non-coated HAP, many different biopolymers have been shown to provide some degree of protection to pellicle coated HAP from acid-induced dissolution. Examples include proteins such as albumins (Hemingway et al. 2010), caseins (Barbour et al. 2008) and mucins (Cheaib and Lussi 2011). Other examples are anionic polymers such as carboxymethyl cellulose and cationic polymers such as chitosan (Delvar et al. 2015). It is worth mentioning that not all biopolymers with the ability to counteract erosion of non-coated HAP have shown the same ability for pellicle coated HAP, that is, the protective performance of the pellicle was not improved by the presence of biopolymers. For instance, while the modification of acidic solutions with the anionic xanthan gum proved to lower their erosive potential in the absence of a pellicle (Barbour et al. 2005), the same was not observed in the presence of a pellicle (West et al. 2004; Scaramucci et al. 2011). However, it cannot be discarded that this was a consequence of methodological differences between the studies. The fact that the dissolution of pellicle coated HAP is reduced when the surrounding acid contains other anionic polymers, for example, carboxymethyl cellulose and polyphosphates, points in this direction (Hooper et al. 2007; Delvar et al. 2015). Overall, most studies published so far suggest that the anti-erosive performance of biopolymers is influenced by the presence of a pellicle coating the challenged HAP surfaces.

At present, very little is known on how biopolymers interact with pellicle coated HAP surfaces under acidic conditions. Following this research direction, recent advances have been made in understanding how the ionic character of biopolymers influences this interaction and, subsequently, the acid-induced dissolution of the underlying HAP (Delvar et al. 2015). If the acid solution contains anionic biopolymers, they penetrate the challenged pellicles (Fig. 5a). The ability of penetrating the pellicles could be facilitated by the anionic polyelectrolytes losing a significant fraction of their charge under acidic conditions, which would also imply a decrease of their effective size. Their incorporation into the challenged pellicles leads to a lower erosion rate than that observed in the absence of the biopolymers. The mechanisms responsible for this observation are not yet clear. Nevertheless, it is reasonable to expect that the incorporation of anionic biopolymers leads to more compact pellicles with a higher effectiveness as ionic diffusion barriers. In turn, cationic biopolymers interact with challenged pellicles by binding and crosslinking the anionic mucins present in their outermost layer (Fig. 5b). The positive charge of cationic biopolymers under acidic conditions enhances the diffusion barrier properties and, therefore, the anti-erosive properties of the modified pellicles, to a significantly higher extent than that achieved by means of the incorporation of anionic biopolymers.

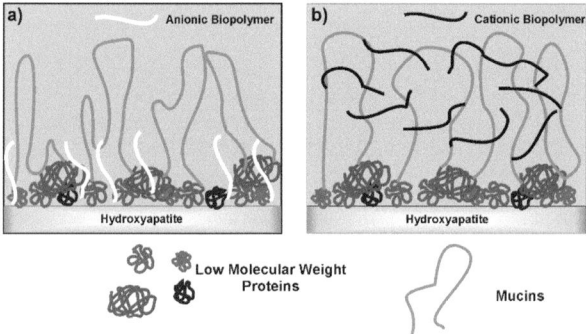

Fig. 5: Scheme of salivary pellicles modified with (a) anionic and (b) cationic biopolymers under acidic conditions.

Conclusions

The prevalence of dental erosion has become alarmingly high and continues to escalate. Significant efforts are devoted nowadays to develop preventive strategies for this condition. The effective prevention of dental erosion would require addressing behavioral factors by means of lifestyle changes. However, attempts in this direction have been unsuccessful so far. Therefore, considerable efforts in prevention have been devoted towards finding compounds with the ability of either increasing the acid-resistance of the dentition or weakening the erosive potential of acidic challenges. Recent research in this field points to biopolymers as interesting candidates. A wide variety of biopolymers have been shown to counteract, up to some extent, the acid-induced dissolution of the main mineral component of teeth, that is hydroxyapatite. Additionally, biopolymers present several practical advantages over other types of anti-erosive compounds, for example, the absence of health risks. Moreover, their wide use in the food industry suggests that biopolymer-containing erosive beverages and foods may raise lower consumer-acceptance concerns.

At present, a significant number of biopolymers with anti-erosive properties have been reported. However, very little is known about the mechanisms by which biopolymers slow down the erosion of teeth under acidic conditions. This knowledge is needed to design a priori strategies for finding novel and improved anti-erosive formulations. Nevertheless, recent findings suggest that the anti-erosive properties of biopolymers are highly influenced by their ionic character, cationic biopolymers exhibiting a higher anti-erosive performance than anionic ones. Finally, it is fair to mention both the current absence and the need of clinical trials in order to prove the efficacy of the use of biopolymers to protect teeth from erosive challenges in *in vivo* conditions.

Acknowledgments

Financial support from the Crafoord Foundation (grant 20140640) is acknowledged.

References

Ablal, M. A., J. S. Kaur, L. Cooper, F. D. Jarad, A. Milosevic, S. M. Higham et al. 2009. The erosive potential of some alcopops using bovine enamel: an *in vitro* study. J. Dent. 37: 835–839.

Arends, J. and W. L. Jongebloed. 1977. The enamel substrate-characteristics of the enamel surface. Swed. Dent. J. 1: 215–224.

Arends, J., J. Schuthof and J. Christoffersen. 1986. Inhibition of enamel demineralization by albumin *in vitro*. Caries Res. 20: 337–340.

Arnaud, T. M. S., B. de Barros Neto and F. B. Diniz. 2010. Chitosan effect on dental enamel de-remineralization: an *in vitro* evaluation. J. Dent. 38: 848–852.

Aroonsang, W., J. Sotres, Z. El-Schich, T. Arnebrant and L. Lindh. 2014. Influence of substratum hydrophobicity on salivary pellicles: organization or composition? Biofouling 30: 1123–1132.

Attin, T., U. Koidl, W. Buchalla, H. G. Schaller, A. M. Kielbassa and E. Hellwig. 1997. Correlation of microhardness and wear in differently eroded bovine dental enamel. Arch. Oral Biol. 42: 243–250.

Attin, T., S. Knöfel, W. Buchalla and R. Tütüncü. 2001. *In situ* evaluation of different remineralization periods to decrease brushing abrasion of demineralized enamel. Caries Res. 35: 216–222.

Attin, T. 2006. Methods for assessment of dental erosion. Monogr. Oral Sci. 20: 152–172.

Attin, T. and F. J. Wegehaupt. 2014. Methods for assessment of dental erosion. Monogr. Oral Sci. 25: 123–142.

Avery, J. K. 2002. Oral Development and Histology. Thieme, New York, NY.

Barbour, M. E., R. P. Shellis, D. M. Parker, G. C. Allen and M. Addy. 2005. An investigation of some food-approved polymers as agents to inhibit hydroxyapatite dissolution. Eur. J. Oral Sci. 113: 457–461.

Barbour, M. E., R. P. Shellis, D. M. Parker, G. C. Allen and M. Addy. 2008. Inhibition of hydroxyapatite dissolution by whole casein: the effects of ph, protein concentration, calcium, and ionic strength. Eur. J. Oral Sci. 116: 473–478.

Bartlett, D. 2006. Intrinsic causes of erosion. Monogr. Oral Sci. 20: 119–139.

Budz, J. A., M. Lore and G. H. Nancollas. 1987. Hydroxyapatite and carbonated apatite as models for the dissolution behavior of human dental enamel. Adv. Dent. Res. 1: 314–321.

Buzalaf, M. A. R., A. C. Magalhães and A. Wiegand. 2014. Alternatives to fluoride in the prevention and treatment of dental erosion. Monogr. Oral Sci. 25: 244–252.

Cairns, A. M., M. Watson, S. L. Creanor and R. H. Foye. 2002. The ph and titratable acidity of a range of diluting drinks and their potential effect on dental erosion. J. Dent. 30: 313–317.

Cheaib, Z. and A. Lussi. 2011. Impact of acquired enamel pellicle modification on initial dental erosion. Caries Res. 45: 107–112.

Christensen, C. M. and M. Navazesh. 1984. Anticipatory salivary flow to the sight of different foods. Apetite 5: 307–315.

Dawes, C. 1969. The effects of flow rate and duration of stimulation on the concentrations of protein and the main electrolytes in human parotid saliva. Arch. Oral Biol. 14: 277–294.

Dawes, C. 2003. What is the critical ph and why does a tooth dissolve in acid? J. Can. Dent. Assoc. 69: 722–724.

Delvar, A., L. Lindh, T. Arnebrant and J. Sotres. 2015. Interaction under acidic erosive conditions between polyelectrolytes and hydroxyapatite surfaces covered with salivary pellicles. ACS Appl. Mater. Interfaces 7: 21610–21618.

Dorozhkin, S. V. 1997. Surface reactions of apatite dissolution. J. Colloid Interface Sci. 191: 489–497.

Dorozhkin, S. V. 2012. Dissolution mechanism of calcium apatites in acids: a review of literature. World J. Methodol. 2: 1–17.

Dugmore, C. R. and W. P. Rock. 2004. A multifactorial analysis of factors associated with dental erosion. Br. Dent. J. 196: 283–286.

Duxbury, A. J. 1993. Ecstasy-dental implications. Br. Dent. J. 175: 38.

Engelen, L., R. A. de Wijk, J. F. Prinz, A. van der Bilt and F. Bosman. 2003. The relation between saliva flow after different stimulations and the perception of flavor and texture attributes in custard desserts. Physiol. Behav. 78: 165–169.

Featherstone, J. D. B. and A. Lussi. 2006. Understanding the chemistry of dental erosion. Monogr. Oral Sci. 20: 66–76.

Gambon, D. L., H. S. Brand and E. C. I. Veerman. 2012. Dental erosion in the 21st century: what is happening to nutritional habits and lifestyle in our society? Br. Dent. J. 213: 55–57.

Ganss, C., M. Schlechtriemen and J. Klimek. 1999. Dental erosions in subjects living on a raw food diet. Caries Res. 33: 74–80.

Grenby, T. H. 1996. Lessening dental erosive potential by product modification. Eur. J. Oral Sci. 104: 221–228.

Hannig, M. and M. Balz. 1999. Influence of *in vivo* formed salivary pellicle on enamel erosion. Caries Res. 33: 372–379.

Hannig, M., N. J. Hess, W. Hoth-Hannig and M. de Vrese. 2003. Influence of salivary pellicle formation time on enamel demineralization—an *in situ* pilot study. Clin. Oral Investig. 7: 158–161.

Hannig, M. and A. Joiner. 2006. The structure, function and properties of the acquired pellicle. Monogr. Oral Sci. 19: 29–64.

Hannig, M. and C. Hannig. 2010. Nanomaterials in preventive dentistry. Nat. Nano. 5: 565–569.

Hannig, M. and C. Hannig. 2014. The pellicle and erosion. Monogr. Oral Sci. 25: 206–214.

Hara, A. T., A. Lussi and D. T. Zero. 2006. Biological factors. Monogr. Oral Sci. 20: 88–99.

Hara, A. T. and D. T. Zero. 2014. The potential of saliva in protecting against dental erosion. Monogr. Oral Sci. 25: 197–205.

Hemingway, C. A., R. P. Shellis, D. M. Parker, M. Addy and M. E. Barbour. 2008. Inhibition of hydroxyapatite dissolution by ovalbumin as a function of ph, calcium concentration, protein concentration and acid type. Caries Res. 42: 348–353.

Hemingway, C. A., A. J. White, R. P. Shellis, M. Addy, D. M. Parker and M. E. Barbour. 2010. Enamel erosion in dietary acids: inhibition by food proteins *in vitro*. Caries Res. 44: 525–530.

Hooper, S., J. Hughes, D. Parker, M. Finke, R. G. Newcombe, M. Addy et al. 2007. A clinical study *in situ* to assess the effect of a food approved polymer on the erosion potential of drinks. J. Dent. 35: 541–546.

Humphrey, S. P. and R. T. Williamson. 2001. A review of saliva: normal composition, flow, and function. J. Prosthet. Dent. 85: 162–169.

Jager, D. H. J., A. Vissink, C. J. Timmer, E. Bronkhorst, A. M. Vieira and M. C. D. N. J. M. Huysmans. 2013. Reduction of erosion by protein-containing toothpastes. Caries Res. 47: 135–140.

Johansson, A.-K., P. Lingström, T. Imfeld and D. Birkhed. 2004. Influence of drinking method on tooth-surface ph in relation to dental erosion. Eur. J. Oral Sci. 112: 484–489.

Johansson, A.-K., R. Omar, G. E. Carlsson and A. Johansson. 2012. Dental erosion and its growing importance in clinical practice: from past to present. Int. J. Dent. 2012: 632907.

Kaidonis, J. A. 2008. Tooth wear: the view of the anthropologist. Clin. Oral Invest. 12: 21–26.

Kosoric, J., M. P. Hector and P. Anderson. 2010. The influence of proteins on demineralization kinetics of hydroxyapatite aggregates. J. Biomed. Mater. Res. A 94A: 972–977.

Künzel, W., M. S. Cruz and T. Fischer. 2000. Dental erosion in cuban children associated with excessive consumption of oranges. Eur. J. Oral Sci. 108: 104–109.

Lee, M. and M. Feldman. 1998. Nausea and vomiting. pp. 117–127. *In*: Feldman, M., M. H. Sleisenger and B. F. Scharschmidt (eds.). Sleisenger and Fordtran's Gastrointestinal and Liver Disease: Pathophysiology, Diagnosis, and Management, 6th ed. WB Saunders, Philadelphia.

Lee, V. M. and R. W. Linden. 1992. An olfactory-submandibular salivary reflex in humans. Exp. Physiol. 77: 221–224.

Levine, M. J., A. Aguirre, M. N. Hatton and L. A. Tabak. 1987. Artificial salivas: present and future. J. Dent. Res. 66: 693–698.

Lindh, L., W. Aroonsang, J. Sotres and T. Arnebrant. 2014. Salivary pellicles. Monogr. Oral Sci. 24: 30–39.

Magalhães, A. C., A. Wiegand, D. Rios, H. M. Honório and M. A. R. Buzalaf. 2009. Insights into preventive measures for dental erosion. J. Appl. Oral Sci. 17: 75–86.

Meurman, J. H. and R. M. Frank. 1991. Scanning electron microscopic study of the effect of salivary pellicle on enamel erosion. Caries Res. 25: 1–6.

Miller, W. D. 1907. Experiments and observations on the wasting of tooth tissue variously designed as erosion, abrasion, chemical abrasion, denudation, etc. Dent. Cosmos 49: 225–247.

Mohammed, A. and K. Dusara. 2013. What is the role of topical fluoride application in preventing dental erosion? Evid. Based Dent. 14: 59–62.

Nongonierma, A. B. and R. J. FitzGerald. 2012. Biofunctional properties of caseinophosphopeptides in the oral cavity. Caries Res. 46: 234–267.

Pindborg, J. J. 1970. Pathology of Dental Hard Tissues. Munksgaard, Köpenhamn, Denmark.

Ramalingam, L., L. B. Messer and E. C. Reynolds. 2005. Adding casein phosphopeptide-amorphous calcium phosphate to sports drinks to eliminate *in vitro* erosion. Pediatr. Dent. 27: 61–67.

Reynolds, E. C. and E. Storey. 1979. A review of the effect of milk on dental caries. Aust. J. Dairy Tech. 9: 175–179.

Reynolds, E. C., P. F. Riley and E. Storey. 1982. Phosphoprotein inhibition of hydroxyapatite dissolution. Calcif. Tissue Int. 34: S52–S56.

Reynolds, E. C. 1997. Remineralization of enamel subsurface lesions by casein phosphopeptide-stabilized calcium phosphate solutions. J. Dent. Res. 76: 1587–1595.

Rios, D., H. M. Honório, A. C. Magalhães, A. C. B. Delbem, M. A. A. M. Machado, S. M. B. Silva et al. 2006. Effect of salivary stimulation on erosion of human and bovine enamel subjected or not to subsequent abrasion: an *in situ/ex vivo* study. Caries Res. 40: 218–223.

Robb, N. D. and B. G. Smith. 1990. Prevalence of pathological tooth wear in patients with chronic alcoholism. Br. Dent. J. 169: 367–369.

Scaramucci, T., A. T. Hara, D. T. Zero, S. S. Ferreira, I. V. Aoki and M. A. P. Sobral. 2011. *In vitro* evaluation of the erosive potential of orange juice modified by food additives in enamel and dentine. J. Dent. 39: 841–848.

Shellis, R. P., C. Ganss, Y. Ren, D. T. Zero and A. Lussi. 2011. Methodology and models in erosion research: discussion and conclusions. Caries Res. 45: 69–77.

Siqueira, W. L., W. Custodio and E. E. McDonald. 2012. New insights into the composition and functions of the acquired enamel pellicle. J. Dent. Res. 91: 1110–1118.

Skartsila, K. and N. Spanos. 2007. Surface characterization of hydroxyapatite: potentiometric titrations coupled with solubility measurements. J. Colloid Interface Sci. 308: 405–412.

Tahmassebi, J. F., M. S. Duggal, G. Malik-Kotru and M. E. J. Curzon. 2006. Soft drinks and dental health: a review of the current literature. J. Dent. 34: 2–11.

ten Cate, J. M. and T. Imfeld. 1996. Dental erosion, summary. Eur. J. Oral Sci. 104: 241–244.

Van Kemenade, M. J. J. M. and P. L. de Bruyn. 1989. The influence of casein on the kinetics of hydroxyapatite precipitation. J. Colloid Interface Sci. 129: 1–14.

Vashisht, R., A. Kumar, R. Indira, M. R. Srinivasan and S. Ramachandran. 2010. Remineralization of early enamel lesions using casein phosphopeptide amorphous calcium phosphate: an *ex-vivo* study. Contemp. Clin. Dent. 1: 210–213.

West, N. X., J. A. Hughes, D. Parker, L. J. Weaver, M. Moohan, J. De'Ath et al. 2004. Modification of soft drinks with xanthan gum to minimise erosion: a study *in situ*. Br. Dent. J. 196: 478–481.

White, A. J., L. H. Gracia and M. E. Barbour. 2011. Inhibition of dental erosion by casein and casein-derived proteins. Caries Res. 45: 13–20.

Wiegand, A. and T. Attin. 2007. Occupational dental erosion from exposure to acids—a review. Occup. Med. 57: 169–176.

Wiegand, A. and T. Attin. 2011. Design of erosion/abrasion studies—insights and rational concepts. Caries Research 45: 53–59.

Vincent, J. F. V., O. A. Bogatyreva, N. R. Bogatyrev, A. Bowyer and A.-K. Pahl. 2006. Biomimetics: its practice and theory. J. R. Soc. Interface 3: 471–482.

Vivino, F. B., I. Al-Hashimi, Z. Khan, F. G. LeVeque, P. L. Salisbury, T. K. Tran-Johnson et al. 1999. Pilocarpine tablets for the treatment of dry mouth and dry eye symptoms in patients with sjögren syndrome: a randomized, placebo-controlled, fixed-dose, multicenter trial. Arch. Intern. Med. 159: 174–181.

Wong, M. C., A. M. Glenny, B. W. Tsang, E. C. Lo, H. V. Worthington and V. C. Marinho. 2010. Topical fluoride as a cause of dental fluorosis in children. Cochrane Database Syst. Rev. 20: CD007693.

Yakubov, G. E., L. Macakova, S. Wilson, J. H. C. Windust and J. R. Stokes. 2015. Aqueous lubrication by fractionated salivary proteins: synergistic interaction of mucin polymer brush with low molecular weight macromolecules. Tribol. Int. 89: 34–45.

Yeh, C. K., D. A. Johnson, M. W. Dodds, S. Sakai, J. D. Rugh and J. P. Hatch. 2000. Association of salivary flow rates with maximal bite force. J. Dent. Res. 79: 1560–1565.

Zero, D. T. 1996. Etiology of dental erosion—extrinsic factors. Eur. J. Oral Sci. 104: 162–177.

5

Drug Carriers by Liposomes Physically Coated with Peptides

Qiufen Zhang, Cuicui Su, Nan Wang and *Dehai Liang**

Introduction

Liposome has been demonstrated as one of the most clinically advanced drug-delivery systems (Lian and Ho 2001; Allen and Cullis 2013). Its applications include chemotherapy, vaccine, gene delivery, infectious diseases, and so on (Balazs and Godbey 2011; Soenen et al. 2011). Liposome is easy to prepare and is able to encapsulate both hydrophilic and hydrophobic drugs (Al-Jamal and Kostarelos 2011). However, liposome without surface modification, that is, naked liposome, is prone to be damaged or cleared by the components in blood stream, which accounts for its short circulation time, high drug leakage, and reduced pharmaceutical efficacy. Another disadvantage of naked liposome is the deficiency of targeting specific cells when administrated *in vivo*, causing strong side effects. Therefore, the surface of liposome is usually modified by agent of certain functions to solve one or more of the problems. For example, the circulation time of liposome in the blood stream is significantly prolonged with the attachment of polyethylene glycol (PEG) on the surface (Klibano et al. 1990; Blume and Cevc 1993; Blume et al. 1993). Besides PEG, polysaccharides, peptides, and other biocompatible molecules, have also been tested

Beijing National Laboratory for Molecular Sciences and the Key Laboratory of Polymer Chemistry and Physics of Ministry of Education, College of Chemistry and Molecular Engineering, Peking University, Beijing, China, 100871.
* Corresponding author: dliang@pku.edu.cn

with similar purposes (Sanko et al. 2011; Barea et al. 2010; Fukui and Fujimoto 2009; Fujimoto et al. 2007). Among these coating agents, peptides are of special interest because they can mimic the membrane proteins in cells, giving the systems many appealing properties. Targeting liposome towards specifics cell by attaching ligand peptides is probably the most-studied approach (Zhang et al. 2010; Zhao et al. 2009). In addition, cell-penetrating peptides (CPPs, such as octaarginine) (Schmidt et al. 2009) and pH-sensitive fusogenic peptides (such as GALA) (Li et al. 2004; Kakudo et al. 2004) have also been conjugated on the liposomal surface to enhance its pharmaceutical efficacy, by promoting endocytosis and membrane fusion, respectively.

The desired peptides are generally attached to the liposomal surface via covalent coupling, which can be divided into two categories: (1) directly conjugate peptides to the preformed liposomes via thioether bonds, disulfide bonds, hydrazone, amide, or carbamate bonds; (2) the peptides firstly conjugate to hydrophobic anchors, such as fatty acids and phospholipids, followed by insertion into liposomes during or after preparation (Khalil et al. 2007). For the liposomes with the surface modified by multiple agents, both approaches can be adopted at the same time. Torchilin and coworkers developed double-targeted pH-responsive drug carriers by attaching PEG, biotin, TAT peptide, and monoclonal antimyosin antibody 2G4 on the liposomal surface via covalent coupling (Sawant et al. 2006). The PEG was first attached to phosphatidylethanolamine via a pH-sensitive hydrazone bond, followed by the preparation of liposomes. The antibody was attached to the PEG chain via apNP group and incorporated into the preformed liposome later on.

The desired peptides can also attach to the liposomal surface via physical interactions. This strategy offers advantages over covalent coupling in terms of being low cost, more versatile, and less time-consuming. However, the vesicle structure is kinetically stable. The well-studied peptides, such as transmembrane peptides (Planque et al. 1998), CPPs (Khalil et al. 2007), fusion peptides (Langosch et al. 2001), and antimicrobial peptides (Ibrahim et al. 2000), have a strong capacity to rupture or disturb the bilayered membrane. Only the peptides with certain sequences are able to safely coat on the liposomal surface. In this chapter, we will focus the attention specifically on the coating peptides: their sequence design, the interactions with liposomes, and the enhancement on the coating of other peptides of certain functions. Finally, the performance of the liposomes physically coated by peptides of multiple functions as drug carriers will be briefly addressed.

Materials and Procedures

Design of coating peptides

The design of the coating peptides is dependent on the composition and physical properties of the liposomes. Since the cell membranes are negatively charged, the positively charged liposome may undergo non-specific interaction with the cell membrane, leading to a high cytotoxicity (Lappalainen et al. 1994). The neutral liposome is safer. However it cannot interact with peptides via electrostatic interaction, an important force binding them together. Therefore, we design positively charged peptides and study their coating ability on negatively charged liposome. The transition temperature (Tc), at which the lipid undergoes a gel-to-liquid crystalline phase transition, should also be considered. Since the liposome is more robust in a gel state, negative 1,2-dipalmitoyl-snglycero-3-phospho-(1'-rac-glycerol) (DPPG) and neutral1,2-dipalmitoyl-snglycero-3-phosphocholine (DPPC), whose Tc values are 41°C, are used to prepare liposomes at varying molar ratios. DPPG and DPPC are highly miscible. Their liposomes are in their gel state when used at 37°C.

Table 1 lists the peptides designed for coating on an anionic liposomal surface. They are divided into two groups. Group 1 includes three peptides, W2K3, W2R3, and W2G3, which are used to study the coating mechanisms (Su et al. 2014). Each of them contains two tryptophan (W) residues in the C-terminal for anchoring in the interfacial region of lipid bilayers (Wimley and White 1996), and three hydrophilic asparagine (N) residues in the N-terminal for hindering the aggregation of liposomes. In between are three positively charged lysine (K, W2K3) residues or arginine (R, W2R3) residues to facilitate the binding of peptides on liposomes via electrostatic interactions. W2G3, which contains no positively charged residues, is used as a control. A spacer, served as two glycine (G) residues, is inserted in between the charged segment and the N-segment. Glycine is an achiral amino acid with a side chain of only one hydrogen atom. It can fit in both hydrophilic and hydrophobic environments, preventing the formation of secondary structures. The W residue not only serves as an "anchor", its side chain is a fluorophore whose fluorescence emission spectrum is very sensitive to the polarity change of environment. It acts as a good indicator, denoting whether peptides are inserted into the membrane surface (Christiaens et al. 2002; Clark et al. 2003).

Table 1: Sequence of the peptides.

	Name	Sequence
[1]Group 1	W2K3	Ac-WWKKKGGNNN-NH2
	W2R3	Ac-WWRRRGGNNN-NH2
	W2G3	Ac-WWGGGGGNNN-NH2
Group 2	W2R4	Ac-WWRRRRGGNNN-NH2
	W2NGR	Ac-WWRRRRGNGRG-NH2
	W2TAT	Ac-WWRKKRRQRRR-NH2

[1]from Ref. Su et al. 2014

Group 2 in Table 1 also includes three peptides. They are used to test the coating of the liposome by peptides of different functions. As a coating peptide, W2R4 follows the design of W2R3, except that the length of the charged segment increased by one arginine residue. W2NGR starts with a WWRRRR—segment to achieve effective coating on the surface of anionic liposomes. Its terminal sequence is replaced by GNGRG, which can specifically recognize aminopeptidase N (APN)/ CD13 on tumor vessels (Vives et al. 2008). This peptide can function as a ligand. A common cell penetrating peptide (CPP) sequence—RKKRRQRRR—, named TAT, is introduced to the third peptide (Cao et al. 2002). Since it already contains enough positively charged amino acid residues, the original—RRRR—is removed. This peptide is correspondingly named as W2TAT, and it is used to enhance the cellular uptake efficiency.

Materials

All peptides with > 98% purity were purchased from GL Biochem (Shanghai) Ltd. (Shanghai, China). Drypowder of DPPC and chloroform solution of DPPG (sodium salt) were purchased from Avanti Polar Lipids, Inc. (USA). Hepes was purchased from Sino-American Biotechnology Co. Triton-X100 (98%) was purchased from Xilong Chemical Inc. (China). Doxorubicin hydrochloride (DOX-HCl, > 98% purity) was purchased from Adamas Reagent, Ltd. (Switzerland). The reagents used for cell experiments were purchased from life technologies Co. (Shanghai). Milli-Q water (18.2 MΩ.cm) was used in all the experiments. The vials used in the experiment were carefully washed and sterilized.

Liposome preparations

The large unilamellar vesicles (LUV) formed by DPPC and DPPG were prepared by the lipid film method, followed by several cycles of extrusion. Briefly, a chloroform solution of the lipid mixture with desired composition was added to a 50 mL pyriform flask together with some Teflon beads. The solvent was removed by a rotary evaporator at 50°C. The formed thin film was further dried under vacuum overnight. The dry film was then hydrated with HB buffer (pH 7.4, 20 mMHepes, 0.1 mM EDTA) or HBS buffer (pH 7.4, 20 mMHepes, 0.1 mM EDTA, 150 mMNaCl) at 50°C for 1 h by a rotary evaporator (no vacuum). Occasional vortex for 10 s was conducted during the hydration process. The resulting suspension was then pushed through a polycarbonate membrane with a pore diameter of 100 nm at 50°C for 21 times using a mini-extruder (Avanti Polar Lipids, Inc.).

Liposomes encapsulating calcein were prepared by following above procedures but using 80 mM calcein in water as the hydration solution. The free calcein molecules were removed by gel filtration on a Sepharose CL-4B column equilibrated in HBS buffer. The final concentration of liposome was determined by modified Bartlett method (Bartlett 1959).

The DOX-loaded liposomes were prepared by pH-gradient method. The lipid film was hydrated with citrate buffer (300 mM, pH 4.0) instead of HBS buffer. The extruded liposomes were passed through a Sephadex G50 gel-filtration column pre-equilibrated in the HBS buffer to exchange the external phase. The liposome was then pre-heated to 65°C and a proper amount of 2 mg/ml DOX solution was added. The solution was further incubated at 65°C for 30 min with gentle stirring. The final DOX/liposome molar ratio (D/L) was 1:5. Sephadex G50 gel-filtration column was used to remove unloaded DOX. The final concentration of liposomes was determined by the modified Bartlett method. The loading efficiency was calculated by using the UV adsorption data at 480 nm.

Laser Light Scattering (LLS)

A commercialized spectrometer from Brookhaven Instruments Corporation (BI-200SM Goniometer, Holtsville, NY) was used to perform both static light scattering (SLS) and dynamic light scattering (DLS) over a scattering angular range of 20°−120°. A vertically polarized, 17 mW He-Ne laser (Newport, USA) operating at 633 nm was used as the light source, and a BI-TurboCo digital correlator (Brookhaven Instruments Corp.) was used to collect and process data. In SLS, for a very dilute solution, the weight-averaged molar mass (M_w) and the root mean-square radius of gyration (R_g) are obtained on the basis of

$$HC / R_{vv}(\theta) = (1/M_w)\left[1 + (1/3)R_g^2 q^2\right] + 2A_2 C \tag{1}$$

where $H = 4\pi^2 n^2 (dn/dC)^2/(N_A \lambda^4)$ and $q = 4\pi n/\lambda \sin(\theta/2)$ with N_A, n, dn/dC, and λ being Avogadro's number, the solvent refractive index, the specific refractive index increment, and the wavelength of light in a vacuum, respectively. The dn/dC values of peptide and liposome are very close, both are ~ 0.154 ml/g (Vacklin et al. 2005). Since the scattered intensity from the peptide was negligible compared with that from the liposome, and the weight ratio of peptide coated on the liposome was less than 10 wt % in all the studied conditions, the concentration of pure liposome was used to calculate the size and molecular weight.

In DLS, the intensity−intensity time correlation function $G^{(2)}(\tau)$ in the self-beating mode was measured. A Laplace inversion program, CONTIN, was used to process the data to obtain the line width distribution and diffusion coefficient. The diffusion coefficient D can be further converted into the hydrodynamic radius R_h by using the Stokes−Einstein equation

$$D = k_B T/6\pi\eta R_h \tag{2}$$

where k_B, T, and η are the Boltzmann constant, the absolute temperature, and the viscosity of the solvent, respectively. For each sample, we measured the correlation functions at five angles covering 30°−90°. Only the CONTIN analysis at 30° or 90° was shown if the results were similar. But the calculation on hydrodynamic radius ($R_{h,app}$) was based on the extrapolation to zero angle.

The aqueous solutions of peptides and liposomes were filtered through 0.45 µm filters (Sartorius stedim Biotech, Goettingen, Germany) to remove dust. The +/− charge ratio of peptides to liposomes was denoted as $\rho_{p/l}$. To calculate the coating amounts of peptides, liposomes were added to peptides at 25°C instantly. This time point was set as t_0. The mixture was vortexed at 1200 rpm for 20 s and then monitored by laser light scattering. To measure the pH sensitivity of liposomes coated with peptides, 60 µL of calcein-loaded liposomes at 500 µM was added to 100 µL peptide solutions at 40 µM ($\rho_{p/l} = 1$). The mixture was then vortexed at 1200 rpm for 3 min, followed by incubating at 37°C for 15 min. The mixed solutions was then heated to 50°C and stayed for 30 min. After being cooled to 37°C, the mixed solution (50 µL) was evenly distributed into the buffers (2.0 mL) at varying pHs and monitored by laser light scattering at 37°C for a week.

Fluorescence measurements

Peptide–phospholipid interactions were studied by monitoring the changes in the Trp fluorescence emission spectra of the peptides. Intrinsic fluorescence of the Trp residues of the coated peptides was measured before and after the addition of phospholipid liposomes to peptide solutions. Trp fluorescence was measured in a spectrofluorometer equipped with a temperature controller. Emission spectra were recorded between 300 and 450 nm with an excitation wavelength of 280 nm. Correction for light scattering was carried out by subtracting the corresponding spectra of the liposomes.

Zeta Potential Analysis

Electrophoretic mobility was measured using a zeta potential analyzer (ZetaPALS, Brookhaven Instruments, Holtsville, NY). Each sample was measured three times. The zeta potential ξ was calculated using the Smoulokowski model

$$\xi = \frac{\mu \eta}{\varepsilon} \tag{3}$$

where μ is the electrophoretic mobility ($m^2 \mu s^{-1} V^{-1}$), ε is the dielectric constant, and η is the viscosity of the solvent.

Transmission Electron Microscopy (TEM)

For approximately 30 s, 10 μL of the sample was applied to a copper grid covered with a carbon film support (T10023, Beijing Xinxing Braim Technology C., Ltd.). The excess sample solution was removed by filter paper. A drop of 1.0% phosphotungstic acid was then placed on the grid, and the excess stain was wicked away 30 s later. The samples were viewed on a H-9000NAR transmission electron microscope after they had dried.

Controlled Release of Calcein

30 μL of calcein-loaded liposomes at 500 μM was added to 50 μL of peptide solutions at 40 μM ($\rho_{p/l} = 1$). The mixture was then vortexed at 1200 rpm for 3 min. The mixed solution containing coated liposomes (50 μL) was evenly distributed into the buffers (2.0 mL) at varying pHs. After being incubated at 37°C for 5 min, each sample was heated to 50°C at a heating rate of 0.1°C/min and then cooled to 37°C at 0.2°C/min. After the heating and cooling cycle, Triton X-100 was added to release all the calcein from the liposome. The released calcein was determined by measuring the fluorescence at $\lambda_{ex} = 490$ and $\lambda_{em} = 520$ nm. The percentage of calcein leakage was calculated according to the equation

$$F = (I_{pH} - I_0)/(I_X - I_0) \tag{4}$$

with I_0, I_{pH} and I_X being the initial fluorescence before the heating, the corrected intensity at different pHs before and after the addition of Triton X-100, respectively.

Drug effect assays

Human fibrosarcoma cells HT1080 (purchased from Cancer Hospital, Chinese Academy of Medical Sciences, Beijing, China) were cultured in RPMI 1640 medium containing antibiotics (100 U/mL penicillin, 100 mg/mL streptomycin) and 10% fatal bovine serum at 37°C in humidified air with 5% CO_2 before use. Sulforhodamine B (SRB) assay was used to determine the cytotoxicity of peptides modified liposomal carriers. HT1080 cells were seeded into 96-well plates (5×10^3 cells/well, 100 µl/well). 100 µl of the liposome coated with peptides at varying mixing ratios were added to 96-well plates and incubated with cells for 48 h at 37°C. After removal of the medium, the cell viability was tested by SRB assay, and the UV absorbance at 540 nm was collected. Survival % = (A_{540} for the treated cells/A_{540} for the control cells) × 100%.

Cellular uptake of liposomes

HT1080 cells (2 ml) were seeded on glass plates (~ 9 cm^2) 1 day prior to evaluation. The prepared anionic liposomes were added to peptide solutions and incubated for 0.5 h. The resulted coated liposomes were then added to glass plates and incubated for 4 h at 37°C. The final DOX concentration in medium was 15 µM. After washing the cells with PBS buffer twice, they were lysed by 4% paraformaldehyde. Hoechst 33258 was used for nuclear staining. The cellular uptake efficiency was determined by confocal laser light scanning microscope.

Results and Discussion

Coating mechanisms by W2K3, W2R3 and W2G3

The coating of the positively charged peptides on anionic liposome is determined by several parameters, including temperature, mixing ratio, charge density, and salt concentration. Figure 1A shows the stability of DPPC/DPPG (60:40) liposome itself in HB buffer at 25°C. At 50 and 250 h, the sample is heated to 50°C (above the T_c) for 30 min and then cooled back to 25°C. The hydrodynamic radius $R_{h,app}$ (the subscript "app" denotes apparent value) and the radius of gyration $R_{g,app}$ is almost constant at 25°C in the studied time period, suggesting that the liposome is stable even with the occasional thermal treatment. The $R_{g,app}$ and $R_{h,app}$ values of the uncoated liposome are also close to each other. The ratio of $R_{g,app}/R_{h,app}$ can be used to determine the conformation of a particle. It is well established that the ratio is 1.0 for a vesicle (Burchard 1983). The determined $R_{g,app}$ and $R_{h,app}$ values confirm the integrity of the liposome even with heating treatment. Clearly, the heating treatment does not affect the morphology or the stability of the uncoated liposomes. Figure 1A also shows that the $R_{h,app}$ and $R_{g,app}$ of the liposome at 50°C are 10−15 nm larger than those at 25°C. The swelling at high temperature is caused by the gel-to-liquid crystalline phase transition (Taylor and Morris 1995).

The behavior of the liposome coated with peptides is quite different. As shown in Fig. 1B, a heavy aggregation of the liposomes occurs in the presence of W2K3. The $R_{g,app}$ reaches about 180 nm in 6 h. However, the aggregation is alleviated as the sample

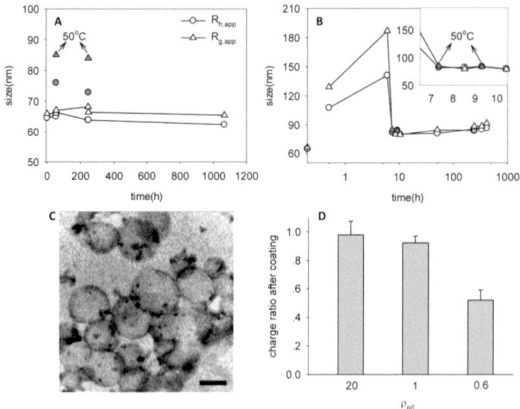

Fig. 1: Time dependence of the sizes of DPPC/DPPG liposomes (60:40 m/m ratio) (A) before and (B) after added into W2K3 ($\rho_{p/l}$ = 20) in HB buffer. Temperature: 25°C. The filled symbols show the results at 50°C. The inset in Panel (B) magnifies the data in the 7–10 h range. Panel (C) shows the electronic micrographs of W2K3-coated liposomes. The samples were stained with 1% phosphotungstic acid. $\rho_{p/l}$ = 20. Scale bar: 100 nm. Panel (D) shows the charge ratio of coated W2K3 to DPPC/DPPG liposomes (60:40 m/m ratio) at different mixing $\rho_{p/l}$ values. From Ref. Su et al. 2014.

is heated to 50°C for half an hour and cooled back to 25°C at ~ 8 h. The $R_{h,app}$ and $R_{g,app}$ are about 80 nm, only slightly larger than the liposome without coating. The two values are close to each other, implying that the liposome maintains its integrity. The TEM image also confirms the vesicle structure (Fig. 1C). No prominent change is observed in the studied time period after the first heating treatment. Further heating, as indicated in the inset in Fig. 1B, causes no effect on the size of the coated liposome. This suggests that the coated peptides hinder the swelling of the liposome at temperatures above T_c. One possible explanation is that the lipids are laterally immobile at temperatures below T_c, which prevents the W residues from being inserted into the interfacial region of the bilayer. The immobility also deteriorates the electrostatic interaction between DPPG and W2K3 because their charge densities are different. Inter particles interaction, which leads to the aggregation of liposomes, is thus dominant at temperatures below T_c. This situation is improved when the lipids start to diffuse above T_c. The close contact of the peptide with the bilayer via both anchoring and electrostatic interaction facilitates the coating of the peptide on the liposome. Therefore, a thermal treatment at 50°C for 30 min is conducted in the following experiments unless stated otherwise.

Mixing ratio is another parameter affecting the coating efficiency. The amount of the coated peptide can be determined from the molecular weight difference of the liposome before and after coating. Figure 1D compares the charge ratio of the coated peptide W2K3 to DPPG at different mixing molar ratios (denoted by $\rho_{p/l}$). At $\rho_{p/l}$ = 20, the coated W2K3/DPPG charge ratio is only 0.98, suggesting that more than 95% of the peptides are not coated.

With decreasing $\rho_{p/l}$ to 1.0 and 0.60, the coated ratios are 0.92 and 0.52, respectively, indicating that most of the peptides are coated on the liposomal surface. This implies that the electrostatic attraction not only serves as the major driving force for the coating, but also determines the saturated amount of W2K3 on DPPC/DPPG liposomes.

The role of electrostatic interaction is further investigated by comparing the coating behavior of W2K3, W2R3, and W2G3 on DPPC/DPPG liposomes of different charge ratios (Figs. 2A and 2B) even in the presence of 150 mM NaCl (Fig. 2C). The $\rho_{p/l}= 20$ is chosen to ensure the amount of peptide is high enough. Firstly, W2G3, which contains no charges, exhibits a negligible amount of the coating compared with W2K3 and W2R3 under the same conditions (Fig. 2A). This further demonstrates the importance of charged amino acid residues during the coating process. Secondly, the comparison of Figs. 2B and 2C shows that the amount of coated W2R3 or W2K3 decreases in the presence of 150 mMNaCl. According to Stradner et al. (Stradner et al. 2004), the electrostatic interaction between cationic peptides and anionic liposomes can be divided into two categories: the long-ranged electrostatic repulsion force between peptides and the short-ranged electrostatic attraction force between DPPG and peptides. The addition of NaCl screens both of the electrostatic interactions. But the screening of the short-ranged electrostatic attraction dominates at the studied salt concentration, which deteriorates the coating of the peptides on liposomal surface. Figure 2 also

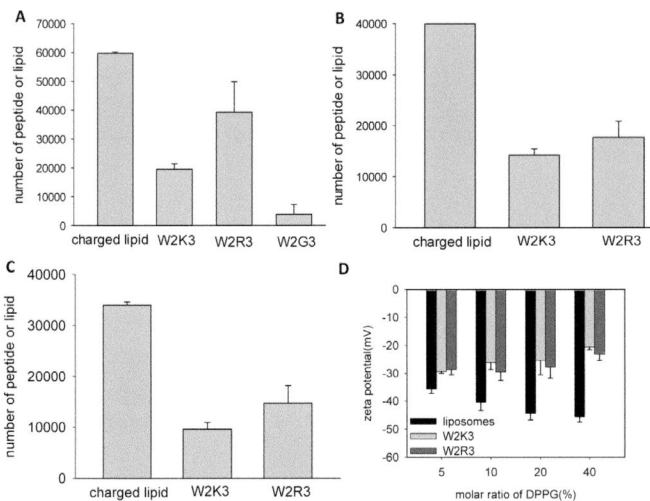

Fig. 2: Number of coated peptides on (A) DPPC/DPPG liposomes (60:40 m/m ratio) in HB buffer, (B) DPPC/DPPG liposomes (80:20 m/m ratio) in HB buffer, and (C) DPPC/DPPG liposomes (80:20 m/m ratio) in HBS buffer. The first bar in panels A to C represents the number of charged lipids in each liposome. Panel (D) shows the zeta potential of DPPC/DPPG liposomes with and without coated peptides in HB buffer. $\rho_{p/l} = 20$. Temperature = 25°C. From Ref. Su et al. 2014.

shows that the coated amount of W2R3 is always larger than that of W2K3 under all the studied conditions, even though they carry the same amount of charges. It has been reported that the delocalized charge of the guanidinium group of arginine is able to mediate the translocation of arginine-rich oligo/polymers across bulk and lipid bilayer membranes (Sakai and Matile 2003; Stromstedt et al. 2010). The multivalent nature of the guanidinium group allows arginine to simultaneously interact with both phosphate and glycerol groups and thus enhance the attraction between the peptide and the lipid (Wu et al. 2013). On the other hand, the strong interaction may change the phase behavior of peptide–lipid mixtures. This suggests that the intermolecular interactions other than electrostatic attraction can also play a role during the coating of peptide on liposome.

The effective coating of cationic peptides on the liposomal surface would neutralize the charges, resulting in a higher zeta potential. For the naked liposome, its zeta potential decreases from −34 to −48 mV as the DPPG content increases from 5% to 40% (Fig. 2D). As expected, the coating of peptides leads to an increase in the negative zeta potential. The liposome with higher content of DPPG has the capacity to absorb a larger amount of peptides, as demonstrated by the lower absolute zeta potential values. The zeta potential values also confirm that the coated amount of W2R3 is larger than that of W2K3 under the same conditions. Interestingly, no charge reversal is observed in all the studied conditions even though each peptide carries three charges. We attributed it to the screening caused by the hydrophilic N-terminal segment. The coating of the peptide is caused by the presence of tryptophan residues and charged groups at the C-terminal. The binding of the peptide on the liposomal surface will leave the neutral–GGNNN segment facing outward, which effectively screens the surface charges of the liposome. This is similar to the screening effect of attached poly(ethylene glycol) (Phillips et al. 1996; Levchenko et al. 2002).

The role of tryptophan residues during coating is evaluated by fluorescence emission spectra. Without liposome, the maximum emission wavelength (λ_{max}) of W2K3 or W2R3 is 355 ± 1 nm in HB buffer, and it is independent of the peptide sequence. The λ_{max} shifts to a lower wavelength with the addition of DPPC/DPPG liposomes. The degree of the shift is dependent on the content of DPPG in the liposome. Results (Su et al. 2014) show that the λ_{max} values of W2R3 and W2K3 shift by 6–8 nm and 5 nm, respectively, in the presence of a liposome containing 40% DPPG. The level of wavelength shift is similar to the values reported in the literature (Chen and Barkley 1998). The blue-shift is attributed to the interaction of the indole group in the tryptophan residue with the polar solvent. It has been reported that higher solvent polarity results in emission at lower energies or longer wavelengths, while lower solvent polarity results in blue-shift (Strickland et al. 1972). The λ_{max} shift of W2R3 or W2K3 in the presence of DPPC/DPPG liposome indicates that the environment of Trp residues becomes more hydrophobic, that is, the Trp residues reach the interface region of the bilayer, functioning as anchors. Both the blue shift of λ_{max} and the coated amount suggest that the coating ability of W2R3 is better than that of W2K3.

Physical properties of liposome coated with W2K3 or W2R3

The coated peptides endow the liposome with some new features. Since W2K3 or W2R3 carry basic amino acids, which are deprotonated as the pH values are lowered to a certain value, the coated liposome exhibits new pH-response behavior. As shown in Fig. 3A, the naked DPPC/DPPG liposome (60:40 m/m ratio) is stable in the HBS buffer at pH values ranging from 5.5 to 7.4. When it is coated with W2K3 or W2R3,

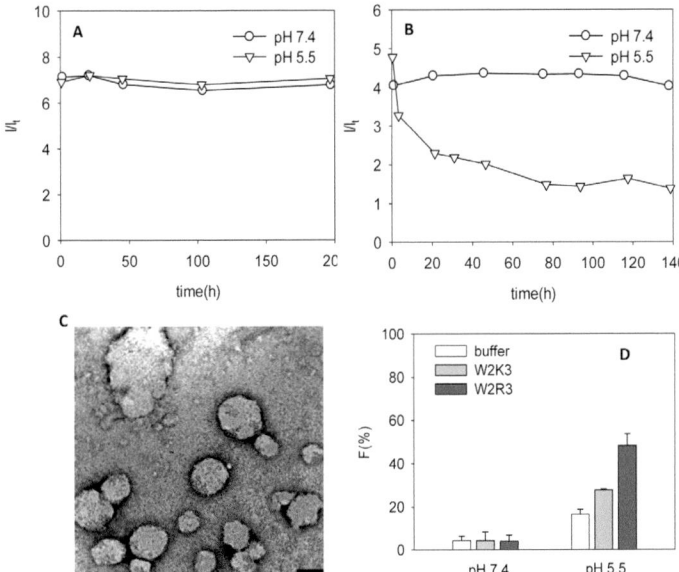

Fig. 3: Time dependence of the intensity of DPPC/DPPG liposomes (60:40 m/m ratio) itself (A) and coated with (B) W2K3 at different pHs in HBS buffer. Panel (C) shows the electronic micrographs of liposomes at ~ 24 h after mixing with W2K3 at pH = 5.5. The samples were stained with 1% phosphotungstic acid. Scale bar: 100 nm. Panel (D) compares the percentage of the calcein released from naked liposomes (white bar) and the liposomes coated with W2K3 (gray bar) or W2R3 (black bar) at pH 7.4 and pH 5.5. $\rho_{p/l}$ = 1.0. Temperature = 37°C. From Ref. Su et al. 2014.

the stability is deteriorated at low pH. Figure 3B compares the behavior of DPPC/DPPG liposome (60:40 m/m ratio) coated with W2K3 at $\rho_{p/l}$ = 1.0. The amount of the uncoated peptides is small, and their effect is negligible at such conditions. At neutral pH, such as 7.4, the peptide coated liposome dose not exhibit prominent change at the studied time period, as demonstrated by the size and the excess scattered intensity. However, the scattered intensity sharply decreases by a factor of four in ~ 80 h at pH 5.5. The size distribution is also broadened with time. The decrease in scattered intensity and the broadening in size distribution suggest that some of the liposomes are ruptured. TEM images (Fig. 3C) confirm this conclusion. The rupture of the liposome and even phase separation are more obvious at higher mixing ratios, such as $\rho_{p/l}$ = 20. The behavior of the liposome coated with W2R3 is similar to that of the liposome coated with W2K3 at varying pH, except that the former exhibits a broader distribution right after coating even at pH 7.4. We attribute it to a lateral phase separation caused by strong binding of arginine to the liposomal surface (Mbamala et al. 2005).

The rupture and deformation of the bilayer caused by coated peptide can be used to release the cargo as trigged by pH. This idea is tested by using calcein as the model drug and fluorescence label. The calcein is encapsulated in liposomes before they are coated with peptides. The concentration of loaded calcein is controlled at 80 mM, at which its fluorescence is self-quenched (Allen and Cleland 1980). The release of calcein from the liposome results in an increase in fluorescence, which can be used to determine the concentration. A heating and cooling cycle is conducted on the sample to enhance the release of calcein. Figure 3D compares the amount of released calcein from the naked liposome, and the liposomes coated with W2K3 or W2R3 under the same conditions. At pH 7.4, the released amount of calcein from the three liposomes is similar, all are about 4%. This suggests that the permeability of uncoated liposomes is low at neutral pH, and the coated peptides exhibit negligible effect. At pH 5.5, however, the percentage of the released calcein increases to 16.5%, 27.7%, and 48.3% for the naked liposome, the liposome coated with W2K3, and the liposome coated with W2R3, respectively. Clearly, the permeability of the liposome itself is higher at lower pH. The coating of W2K3 or W2R3 further enhances the permeability, and W2R3 is stronger than W2K3 in disturbing the lipid membrane at pH 5.5. The leakage of calcein from the liposome during the heating and cooling cycle is closely monitored. For the naked liposome and the liposome coated with W2K3, a dramatic change influorescence intensity occurs at $41-42°C$, around the T_c of the liposome. As for the liposome coated with W2R3, besides a heavy leakage at $41-42°C$, a continued leakage is also observed at temperatures above the transition point. These results imply that the coated peptide does not change the transition temperature of the liposomes. The enhanced release of the calcein from the coated liposome can be explained by the defects caused by lipids and peptides within the membranes (Papahadjopoulos et al. 1973; Cruzeirohansson et al. 1989). Since W2K3 or W2R3 carries more charges than DPPG, the strong electrostatic interaction between the peptide and DPPG will cause a lateral redistribution of the charged lipids to fulfill charge neutralization. The redistribution occurs only around or above T_c. The redistribution of charged lipids leads to domains rich with charged lipids and peptides, which can be treated as lateral microphase separation. This has been confirmed by using giant unilamellar vesicles (Su et al. 2014). The periphery of such domains contains defects, which serves as the passage of the cargo. W2R3 penetrates even deeper in the bilayer, causing a heavy leakage even at temperatures above T_c.

Liposome coated with multiple peptides

A successful drug carrier is able to overcome multiple barriers along the delivery pathway. The surface of the liposome, therefore, should be coated by multiple peptides, each having different functions. On the basis of the above studies, the coating peptide W2R4, the targeting peptide W2NGR, and the cell penetrating peptides W2TAT, are designed and used for coating on DPPC/DPPG liposome. W2R4 follows a similar design as W2R3, except that W2R4 has four arginine residues.

The coating ability of W2R4 is first evaluated. The peptide over liposome molar charge ratio, $\rho_{p/l}$, is a crucial parameter determining not only the coating efficiency, but also the saturated amount of coated peptides. Zeta potential analysis is applied to evaluate the coating of W2R4 on liposomes of DPPC and DPPG at 60:40 and 80:20 (m/m ratio), separately. Since the salt concentration affected the measurement of the zeta potential, the HB buffer is used in the experiment. As shown in Fig. 4A, the zeta potential of the DPPC/DPPG (60:40) liposome before peptide coating is more negative than that of DPPC/DPPG (80:20) liposome at the same conditions. This is

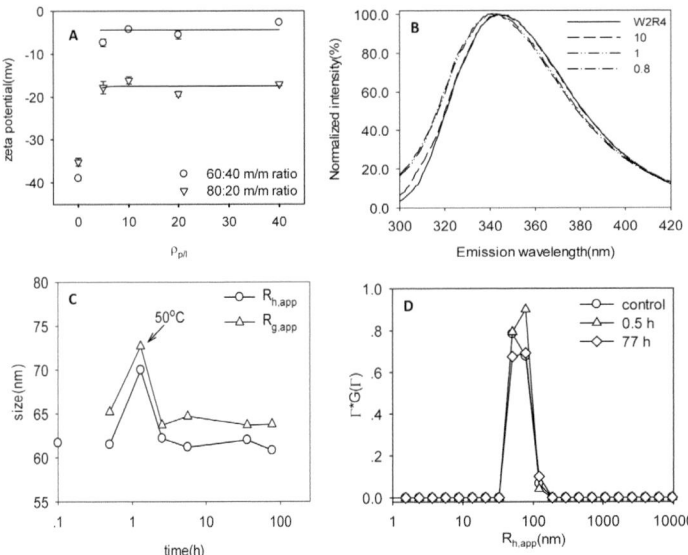

Fig. 4: The coating behavior of W2R4 on DPPC/DPPG liposome. (A) Zeta potential of DPPC/DPPG liposomes coated with W2R4 at different $\rho_{p/l}$ ratios in HB buffer; (B) fluorescence emission spectra of W2R4 after mixed with DPPC/DPPG (60:40) liposome at different $\rho_{p/l}$ ratios in HBS buffer. λex = 280 nm; (C) size and (D) size distribution of DPPC/DPPG liposomes (60:40 m/m ratio) with time after added to W2R4 solutions in HBS buffer. Scattering angle: 30°, $\rho_{p/l}$ = 1. Temperature: 25°C.

reasonable since the former liposome contained more of the negatively charged lipid DPPG. The absolute zeta potential values decreases with the absorption of positively charged W2R4. The values reached a plateau at $\rho_{p/l}$ = 5 in both cases, suggesting that the absorption of W2R4 on the liposome surface is saturated. However, the zeta potential at plateau for DPPC/DPPG (60:40) liposome is close to zero, while the value for DPPC/DPPG (80:20) liposome is still highly negatively charged (−18 mV). This demonstrates that the liposome with higher charge density has the capacity to absorb a larger amount of peptides. Even though W2R4 only has one more positive charge than W2R3 or W2K3, the zeta potential values of the liposome coated with W2R4 are much smaller than those coated with W2R3 or W2K3 under the same conditions (Fig. 2D), indicating that the number of charged residue is the key for coating. Figure 4A also shows that no charge reversal is observed in the studied conditions. This can also be attributed to the screening caused by the hydrophilic N-terminal segment.

Figure 4B shows the Trp fluorescence emission curve at different $\rho_{p/l}$ = 1 ratios. At $\rho_{p/l} \geq 2$, the average blue shift of Trp is only about 1 nm. This is caused by the free peptides in solution, which covers the effect of coated peptides. At $\rho_{p/l}$ = 1, the blue shift of λ_{max} increases to ~ 5 nm and remains unchanged as the $\rho_{p/l}$ continued to decrease to 0.8, indicating that W2R4 molecules on liposomal surfaces are almost saturated with Trp residues "anchored" in the interface region of the bilayer (Chen and Barkley 1998).

The DPPC/DPPG (60:40) liposome coated with W2R4 at $\rho_{p/l}$ = 1 is further characterized by LLS. As shown in Fig. 4C, the apparent hydrodynamic radius $R_{h,app}$

of the naked DPPC/DPPG (60:40) liposome is 62 nm at 25°C. It is barely changed after coated with W2R4. A swelling occurs when the sample is heated to 50°C, as demonstrated by an increase in size by 10 nm. This is a normal behavior of the liposome (Taylor and Morris 1995). Figure 4C also shows that the size of the liposome is recovered and maintained for ~ 100 h as the sample is cooled back to 25°C. The $R_{g,app}$ and $R_{h,app}$ values exhibit a similar trend. They are close to each other at the studied conditions. The $R_{g,app}/R_{h,app}$ ratio is close to 1, suggesting that the liposome maintains its vesicle structure (Burchard 1983) after coated with W2R4. Moreover, the size distribution is kept almost unchanged during the whole process (Fig. 4D). The calculation on the excess scattered intensity indicates that the molecular mass of the liposome before and after coating is 8.2×10^7 and 9.2×10^7 g/mol, respectively. The coating efficiency of W2R4 in HBS buffer is thus determined to be ~ 60%.

The targeting peptide W2NGR alone does not exhibit good coating ability under the same conditions. As shown in Fig. 5A, W2NGR induces aggregation of DPPC/ DPPG (60:40) liposomes at 25°C at $\rho_{p/l} = 1$. Upon mixing W2NGR peptides with liposomes, the $R_{h,app}$ increased from 60 nm to 100 nm in 0.1 hr. The heating treatment at 50ºC for half an hour only temporarily alleviates the aggregation. When the temperature is recovered to 25°C after 2 h, the aggregation continues and the size of the aggregate reaches about 1 μm in 38 h (Fig. 5B), indicating the occurrence of phase separation and precipitation. The situation is improved when W2NGR and W2R4 are mixed together. Figure 5C shows the coating results of W2R4 and W2NGR at an equal molar ratio. No prominent aggregation is observed during the whole coating process at $\rho_{p/l} = 1$. The size of the liposome is increased by 8 nm right after mixing. Heating at 50ºC caused

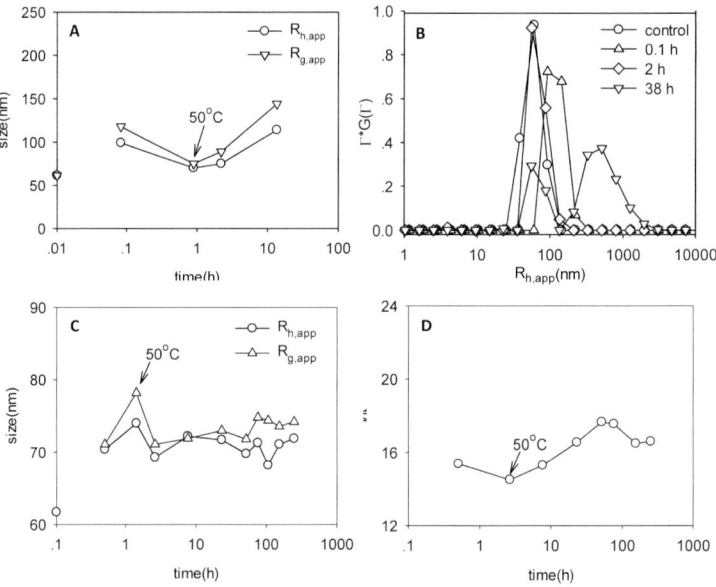

Fig. 5: Size (A) and size distribution (B) of DPPC/DPPG liposomes (60:40 m/m ratio) in the presence of W2NGR; Size (C) and intensity (D) of DPPC/DPPG liposomes (60:40 m/m ratio) in the presence of W2R4/ W2NGR (1:1, m/m). HBS buffer, $\rho_{p/l} = 1$. Scattering angle: 30°.

only swelling. The size is recovered to 70 nm after cooling, and kept constant in the next 250 h. The scattered intensity shows a similar result (Fig. 5D). The molecular weights of the liposome before and after coating are determined to be 8.2×10^7 and 1.0×10^8 g/mol, respectively. The increase in molecular weight suggests that nearly all the W2R4 and W2NGR are adsorbed onto the liposomal surface. The amount is about twice that of W2R4 alone. Therefore, the mixing of W2R4 and W2NGR at 1:1 ratio not only alleviates the aggregation of liposome induced by W2NGR, but also enhances the coating efficiency of W2R4. A synergistic effect between W2R4 and W2NGR could exist upon coating onto the liposomal surface.

As a cell penetrating peptide, TAT has the intrinsic property to disturb lipid membranes (Piantavigna et al. 2011). As expected, W2TAT does not exhibit any coating capacity, but destroys the liposome instead. As shown in Fig. 6A, a heavy aggregation of DPPC/DPPG (60:40) liposomes is observed 0.1 hr after they are mixed with W2TAT at $\rho_{p/l} = 1$. The size of the aggregate reaches the micrometer level and a precipitation on the bottom of the vial is visible to the eye within 0.5 h. The addition of W2R4 also improves the coating of W2TAT. However, the disruption of liposome is not completely prevented even when the molar ratio of W2R4 to W2TAT reaches 9:1. As shown in Fig. 6B, the $R_{h, app}$ and $R_{g, app}$ of the liposome are 140 and 300 nm, respectively, at W2R4 to W2TAT ratio of 9:1 after mixing. Both values are much larger than the size of individual liposome (62 nm). The $R_{g, app}/R_{h, app}$ ratio much larger than 1 also suggests that the particles are not vesicles. Heating at 50°C for half an hour only temporarily alleviated the situation. Aggregation of the liposome continues after the temperature is turned to 25°C. At the ending stage, both the size and the excess scattered

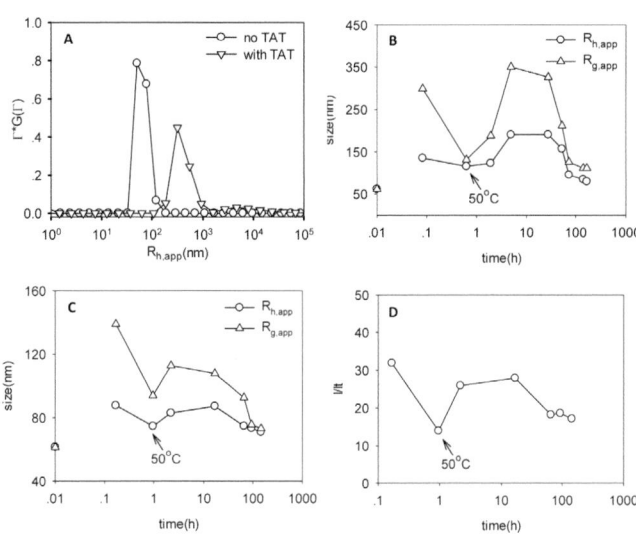

Fig. 6: Size distribution (A) of liposomes before and after mixed with W2TAT; Size (B) of liposomes in the presence of W2TAT/W2R4 (9:1, m/m); size (C) and excess scattered intensity (D) of liposomes after coated with mixtures of W2R4/W2NGR/W2TAT (50:45:5, m/m). DPPC/DPPG liposomes (60:40 m/m ratio) in HBS buffer, $\rho_{p/l} = 1$. Scattering angle: 30°.

intensity decrease with time. The $R_{g, app}$ and $R_{h,app}$ of the liposome are 110 nm and 80 nm, respectively, both of which are still larger than the size (62 nm) of liposome itself. The excess scattered intensity is also higher than that of the liposome before coating. A broad size distribution is observed. All these suggested that the liposomes coated with W2R4 and W2TAT at 9:1 are not in ideal vesicle structures.

The situation is further improved when all the three peptides are mixed together. Figures 6C and 6D show the DPPC/DPPG (60:40) liposomes coated with W2R4/W2NGR/W2TAT at molar ratios of 50:45:5. The final $\rho_{p/l} = 1$. Only a weak aggregation occurs after the heating treatment at 50°C, as demonstrated by the changes in size and excess scattered intensity. The $R_{g,app}$ and $R_{h,app}$ of the coated liposome at final stage are 73 nm and 71 nm, respectively. Their ratio is close to 1, suggesting that the coated liposome maintains its vesicle structure. In addition, the coated liposome exhibits a narrow distribution during the whole process. The molecular weight of the coated liposome at final stage is determined to be 1.0×10^8 g/mol, indicating that almost all the peptides are coated on the liposomal surface.

Liposome coated with peptides as a drug carrier

The performance of the coated liposome as a drug carrier is tested with DOX as the model drug. DOX is loaded into anionic liposomes DPPC/DPPG (60:40 m/m ratio) by pH gradient method. Human fibrosarcoma cells HT1080, which can specifically recognize the NGR sequence, is selected for cell experiment. Free drug is used as the control. Four groups of peptides or mixtures, that is, W2R4, W2R4/W2NGR (1:1), W2R4/W2TAT (95:5), and W2R4/W2NGR/W2TAT (50:45:5), are chosen to study the effect of coating peptides on liposomal drug delivery efficiency. Figure 7 compares the drug uptake amount by HT1080 cells after 4 hr of medication. The fluorescence intensity of free DOX (Fig. 7A) is relatively strong, while uncoated liposomes display a much lower uptake efficiency (Fig. 7B). The liposomes coated with one or two different types of peptides (Figs. 7C–7E) exhibit similar or slightly better uptake compared with that of an uncoated liposome. However, their performances are worse than free DOX. The exception is the liposome coated with three different peptides of W2R4/W2NGR/W2TAT (50:45:5). Its uptake efficiency (Fig. 7F) is comparable to free DOX. Since the diameter of liposome (~ 130 nm) is several orders higher than that of DOX (< 1 nm), the coated W2NGR together with W2TAT enhance the uptake of the liposome. Moreover, the overlapping of the red channel representing the drug and the blue channel representing the cell nucleus suggests that the majority of the drugs enter the cell nucleus.

Figure 8 quantitatively compares the effect of different DOX carriers. Free DOX exhibits a low drug effect in spite of its relatively high drug uptake efficiency. Entrapment in liposome clearly enhances the pharmacokinetics of DOX, as demonstrated by the higher drug effect of free or coated liposomes. The effect of W2R4/W2TAT coated liposome is nearly the same as that of W2R4 coated one, suggesting that the enhancement produced by W2TAT is limited. However, the introduction of W2NGR promotes the drug effect to a large extent. This is probably due to the less amount of W2TAT, which is only 1/9 of W2NGR. Figure 8 also shows that the performance of the liposomes coated with W2R4/W2NGR (1:1) is similar to

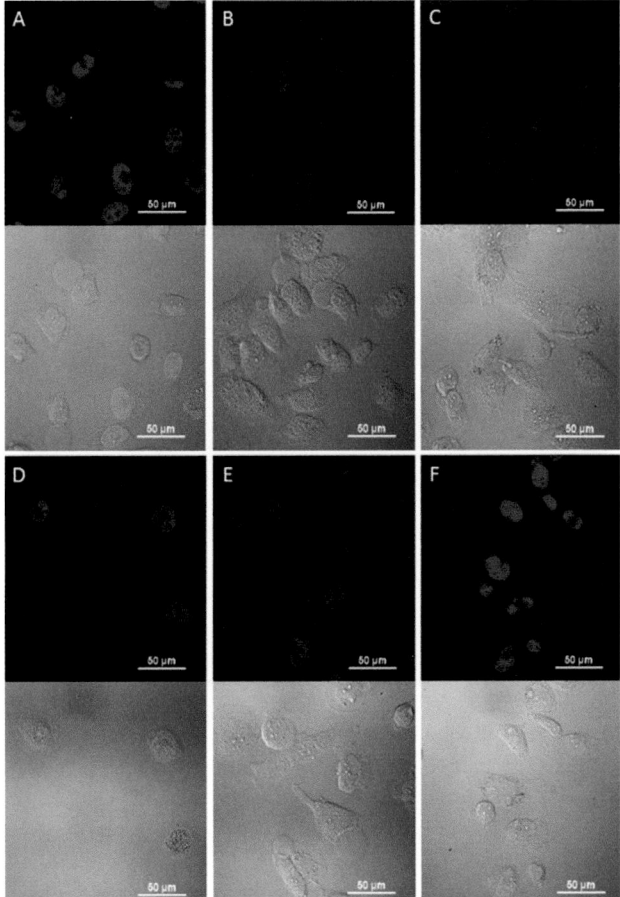

Fig. 7: Confocal images of the HT1080 cells incubated with 15 μM (A) free DOX, (B) uncoated liposomes, and liposomes coated with (C) W2R4, (D) W2R4/W2NGR (1:1), (E) W2R4/W2TAT (95:5), and (F) W2R4/W2NGR/W2TAT (50:45:5) for 4 h. In each set, the images on the top and on the bottom show the DOX fluorescence and overlays of the images of DOX fluorescence and the blue fluorescence of the cell nucleus, respectively. Scale: 50 μm.

that of the liposome coated with W2R4/W2NGR/W2TAT (50:45:5). Considering that the cell uptake of the liposome coated with W2R4/W2NGR/W2TAT is much higher than that of W2R4/W2NGR, the drug effect is not necessarily caused by the peptide coated liposomes inside the cell, but also by those outside the cell. The behaviors of free DOX and the DOX loaded free liposome are another proof. The former has a much higher cell uptake efficacy (Fig. 7), but its drug effect is lower (Fig. 8). Therefore, the drug effect is a collaboration of DOX, peptides, and liposomes starting from the surface of the cell, and the operation is probably maintained during the delivery pathway. As a cell penetrating peptide, TAT sequence improves the cellular uptake (Amand et al. 2011), but fails to enhance the drug effect of peptide coated liposomes, implying that a certain barrier or mechanism plays a role in the interactions between the peptides and cell.

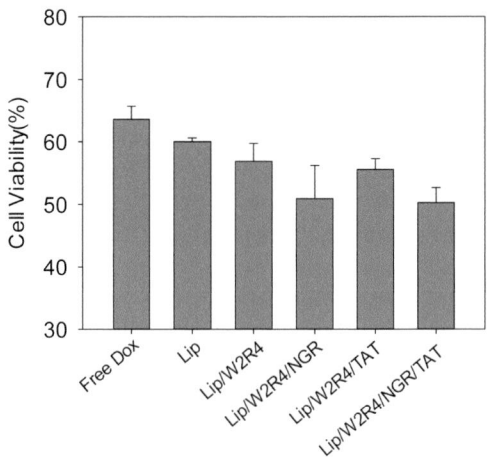

Fig. 8: Cell viability of HT1080 cells incubated with DOX carriers for 48 h.

Conclusions

We have demonstrated that cationic peptides of W2K3, W2R3, and W2R4 can successfully attach to the anionic liposomal surface via electrostatic interaction and the "anchoring" of Trp residuals in the interfacial region of lipid bilayers. The attachment of peptides is able to tune the permeability of the bilayer and to render the liposome some new features, such as pH responsibility. Using W2R4 as an example, we also demonstrate that it can synergistically improve the coating of targeting peptides W2NGR and cell penetrating peptide W2TAT, both of which cause strong aggregation and precipitation of liposomes when used alone. This is an attractive feature of the coating peptides because the development of smart drug carriers requires liposome with multiple functions. And most of the functional peptides, such as targeting peptides and cell penetrating peptides, are intrinsic to deform or destroy the lipid bilayers.

We also briefly tested the performance of the liposome coated with peptide as a drug carrier. The DOX-loaded liposome coated with mixed peptides of different functions exhibits intriguing results on *in vitro* cell uptake and drug effect. For example, the liposome coated with W2R4, W2NGR, and W2TAT enhances the cell uptake, but fails to cause a strong effect in drug effect compared with the liposome coated with W2R4 and W2NGR at similar concentrations. This suggests that cell uptake and drug effect are not strongly correlated. The liposome physically coated with peptides of multi-functions not only offers a practical approach to fabricate high performance drug delivery vehicles, it is also helpful to probe the mechanism of cell bioactivities.

Acknowledgement

Financial support of this work from the National Natural Science Foundation of China (21174007) is gratefully acknowledged.

References

Al-Jamal, W. T. and K. Kostarelos. 2011. Liposomes: from a clinically established drug delivery system to a nanoparticle platform for theranostic nanomedicine. Acc. Chem. Res. 44: 1094–1104.

Allen, T. M. and L. G. Cleland. 1980. Serum-induced leakage of liposome contents. Biochim. Biophys. Acta. 597: 418–426.

Allen, T. M. and P. R. Cullis. 2013. Liposomal drug delivery systems: from concept to clinical applications. Adv. Drug Del. Rev. 65: 36–48.

Amand, H. L., C. L. Bostrom, P. Lincoln, B. Norden and E. K. Esbjoerner. 2011. Binding of cell-penetrating penetratin peptides to plasma membrane vesicles correlates directly with cellular uptake. Biochim. Biophys. Acta.-Biomembranes 1808: 1860–1867.

Balazs, D. A. and W. Godbey. 2011. Liposomes for use in gene delivery. J. Drug Deliv. 2011: 326497.

Barea, M. J., M. J. Jenkins, M. H. Gaber and R. H. Bridson. 2010. Evaluation of liposomes coated with a pH responsive polymer. Int. J. Pharm. 402: 89–94.

Bartlett, G. R. 1959. Phosphorus assay in column chromatography. J. Biol. Chem. 234: 466–468.

Blume, G. and G. Cevc. 1993. Molecular mechanism of the lipid vesicle longevity *in vivo*. Biochim. Biophys. Acta. 1146: 157–168.

Blume, G., G. Cevc, M. Crommelin, I. Bakkerwoudenberg, C. Kluft and G. Storm. 1993. Specific targeting with poly(ethylene glycol)-modified liposomes—coupling of homing devices to the ends of the polymeric chains combines effective target binding with long circulation times. Biochim. Biophys. Acta. 1149: 180–184.

Burchard, W. 1983. Static and dynamic light-scattering from branched polymers and bio-polymers. Adv. Polym. Sci. 48: 1–124.

Cao, G. D., W. Pei, H. L. Ge, Q. H. Liang, Y. M. Luo, F. R. Sharp et al. 2002. *In vivo* delivery of a Bcl-xL fusion protein containing the TAT protein transduction domain protects against ischemic brain injury and neuronal apoptosis. J. Neurosci. 22: 5423–5431.

Chen, Y. and M. D. Barkley. 1998. Toward understanding tryptophan fluorescence in proteins. Biochemistry 37: 9976–9982.

Christiaens, B., S. Symoens, S. Verheyden, Y. Engelborghs, A. Joliot, A. Prochiantz et al. 2002. Tryptophan fluorescence study of the interaction of penetratin peptides with model membranes. Eur. J. Biochem. 269: 2918–2926.

Clark, E. H., J. M. East and A. G. Lee. 2003. The role of tryptophan residues in an integral membrane protein: diacylglycerol kinase. Biochemistry 42: 11065–11073.

Cruzeirohansson, L., J. H. Ipsen and O. G. Mouritsen. 1989. Intrinsic molecules in lipid-membranes change the lipid-domain interfacial area—cholesterol at domain interfaces. Biochim. Biophys. Acta. 979: 166–176.

Fujimoto, K., T. Toyoda and Y. Fukui. 2007. Preparation of bionanocapsules by the layer-by-layer deposition of polypeptides onto a liposome. Macromolecules 40: 5122–5128.

Fukui, Y. and K. Fujimoto. 2009. The preparation of sugar polymer-coated nanocapsules by the layer-by-layer deposition on the liposome. Langmuir. 25: 10020–10025.

Ibrahim, H. R., Y. Sugimoto and T. Aoki. 2000. Ovotransferrin antimicrobial peptide (OTAP-92) kills bacteria through a membrane damage mechanism. Biochim. Biophys. Acta. 1523: 196–205.

Kakudo, T., S. Chaki, S. Futaki, I. Nakase, K. Akaji, T. Kawakami et al. 2004. Transferrin-modified liposomes equipped with a pH-sensitive fusogenic peptide: an artificial viral-like delivery system. Biochemistry 43: 5618–5628.

Khalil, I. A., K. Kogure, S. Futaki, S. Hama, H. Akita, M. Ueno et al. 2007. Octaarginine-modified multifunctional envelope-type nanoparticles for gene delivery. Gene Ther. 14: 682–689.

Klibanov, A. L., K. Maruyama, V. P. Torchilin and L. Huang. 1990. Amphipathic polyethylene glycols effectively prolong the circulation time of liposomes. FEBS Lett. 268: 235–237.

Langosch, D., J. M. Crane, B. Brosig, A. Hellwig, L. K. Tamm and J. Reed. 2001. Peptide mimics of SNARE transmembrane segments drive membrane fusion depending on their conformational plasticity. J. Mol. Biol. 311: 709–721.

Lappalainen, K., I. Jääskeläinen, K. Syrjänen, A. Urtti and S. Syrjänen. 1994. Comparison of cell proliferation and toxicity assays using two cationic liposomes. Pharm. Res. 11: 1127–1131.

Levchenko, T. S., R. Rammohan, A. N. Lukyanov, K. R. Whiteman and V. P. Torchilin. 2002. Liposome clearance in mice: the effect of a separate and combined presence of surface charge and polymer coating. Int. J. Pharm. 240: 95–102.

Li, W. J., F. Nicol and F. C. Szoka. 2004. GALA: a designed synthetic pH-responsive amphipathic peptide with applications in drug and gene delivery. Adv. Drug Del. Rev. 56: 967–985.

Lian, T. and R. J. Y. Ho. 2001. Trends and developments in liposome drug delivery systems. J. Pharm. Sci. 90: 667–680.

Mbamala, E. C., A. Ben-Shaul and S. May. 2005. Domain formation induced by the adsorption of charged proteins on mixed lipid membranes. Biophys. J. 88: 1702–1714.

Papahadjopoulos, D., K. Jacobson, S. Nir and T. Isac. 1973. Phase-transitions in phospholipid vesicles—fluorescence polarization and permeability measurements concerning effect of temperature and cholesterol. Biochim. Biophys. Acta. 311: 330–348.

Phillips, N. C., C. Heydari and M. Saoud. 1996. Reduction of cationic liposome zeta (zeta) potential by amphiphilic poly(ethylene glycol) derivatives. Eur. J. Pharm. Sci. 4: S43–S43.

Piantavigna, S., G. A. McCubbin, S. Boehnke, B. Graham, L. Spiccia and L. L. Martin. 2011. A mechanistic investigation of cell-penetrating Tat peptides with supported lipid membranes. Biochim. Biophys. Acta.-Biomembranes 1808: 1811–1817.

Planque, M. R. R. D., D. V. Greathouse, R. E. Koeppe, H. Schäfer, D. Marsh and J. A. Killian. 1998. Influence of lipid/peptide hydrophobic mismatch on the thickness of diacylphosphatidylcholine bilayers: A ^{2}H NMR and ESR study using designed transmembrane α-helical peptides and gramicidin A. Biochemistry 37: 9333–9345.

Sakai, N. and S. Matile. 2003. Anion-mediated transfer of polyarginine across liquid and bilayer membranes. J. Am. Chem. Soc. 125: 14348–14356.

Sanko, N., S. J. Alund, M. Hiorth, A.-L. Kjoniksen and G. Smistad. 2011. Studies on pectin coating of liposomes for drug delivery. Colloids Surf. B. 88: 664–673.

Sawant, R. M., J. P. Hurley, S. Salmaso, A. Kale, E. Tolcheva, T. S. Levchenko et al. 2006. "Smart" drug delivery systems: double-targeted ph-responsive pharmaceutical nanocarriers. Bioconjugate Chem. 17: 943–949.

Schmidt, N., A. Mishra, G. H. Lai and G. C. L. Wong. 2009. Arginine-rich cell-penetrating peptides. FEBS Lett. 584: 1806–1813.

Soenen, S. J., G. Vande Velde, A. Ketkar-Atre, U. Himmelreich and M. De Cuyper. 2011. Magnetoliposomes as magnetic resonance imaging contrast agents. Wiley Interdiscip. Rev. Nanomed. Nanobiotechnol. 3: 197–211.

Stradner, A., H. Sedgwick, F. Cardinaux, W. C. K. Poon, S. U. Egelhaaf and P. Schurtenberger. 2004. Equilibrium cluster formation in concentrated protein solutions and colloids. Nature 432: 492–495.

Strickland, E. H., C. Billups and E. Kay. 1972. Effects of hydrogen-bonding and solvents upon tryptophanyl 1-l-a absorption-band—studies using 2,3-dimethylindole. Biochemistry 11: 3657–3662.

Stromstedt, A. A., L. Ringstad, A. Schmidtchen and M. Malmsten. 2010. Interaction between amphiphilic peptides and phospholipid membranes. Curr. Opin. Colloid Interface Sci. 15: 467–478.

Su, C., Y. Xia, J. Sun, N. Wang, L. Zhu, T. Chen et al. 2014. Liposomes physically coated with peptides: preparation and characterization. Langmuir. 30: 6219–6227.

Taylor, K. M. G. and R. M. Morris. 1995. Thermal-analysis of phase-transition behavior in liposomes. Thermochim. Acta. 248: 289–301.

Vacklin, H. P., F. Tiberg, G. Fragneto and R. K. Thomas. 2005. Phospholipase A(2) hydrolysis of supported phospholipid bilayers: a neutron reflectivity and ellipsornetry study. Biochemistry 44: 2811–2821.

Vives, E., J. Schmidt and A. Pelegrin. 2008. Cell-penetrating and cell-targeting peptides in drug delivery. Biochim. Biophys. Acta.-Rev. Cancer 1786: 126–138.

Wimley, W. C. and S. H. White. 1996. Experimentally determined hydrophobicity scale for proteins at membrane interfaces. Nat. Struct. Biol. 3: 842–848.

Wu, Z., Q. Cui and A. Yethiraj. 2013. Why do arginine and lysine organize lipids differently? Insights from coarse-grained and atomistic simulations. J. Phys. Chem. B. 117: 12145–12156.

Zhang, Y., J. Wang, D. Bian, X. Zhang and Q. Zhang. 2010. Targeted delivery of RGD-modified liposomes encapsulating both combretastatin A-4 and doxorubicin for tumor therapy: *In vitro* and *in vivo* studies. Eur. J. Pharm. Biopharm. 74: 467–473.

Zhao, H., J. Wang, Q. Sun, C. Luo and Q. Zhang. 2009. RGD-based strategies for improving antitumor activity of paclitaxel-loaded liposomes in nude mice xenografted with human ovarian cancer. J. Drug Targeting 17: 10–18.

6

Biopolymers for *In Vitro* Tissue Model Biofabrication

Aleksander Skardal

Introduction

Three decades ago, tissue engineering and regenerative medicine (TERM) emerged as promising interdisciplinary fields with vast potential to revolutionize medical practices (Oerlemans et al. 2014). New approaches, such as construction of biological tissue substitutes for diagnostic and research applications, as well as replacement tissues or regenerative therapies for injured tissues, were touted as the next major breakthroughs. However in practice, translation to commercially robust clinical products has been a slow and difficult process (Berthiaume et al. 2011). In many cases long-term success rates have not been optimal, and costs associated with the regulatory process to bring these technologies to accepted clinical practice that can be reimbursed through health insurance plans have been staggering. This is not to say that progress has not been made. There are examples of successful clinical translation in skin (Han et al. 2014; Maver et al. 2015), cartilage (Fulco et al. 2014; Adachi et al. 2014), and bladder (Atala et al. 2006) repair or replacement, and while limited in patient number, recent studies have successfully implanted vaginal and urethral tissues in humans (Raya-

Wake Forest Institute for Regenerative Medicine, Wake Forest School of Medicine, Medical Center Boulevard, Winston-Salem, NC 27157; Department of Cancer Biology, Wake Forest School of Medicine, Medical Center Boulevard, Winston-Salem, NC 27157; Virginia Tech-Wake Forest School of Biomedical Engineering and Sciences, Wake Forest School of Medicine, Medical Center Boulevard, Winston-Salem, NC 27157; Comprehensive Cancer Center of Wake Forest Baptist Medical Center, Medical Center Boulevard, Winston-Salem, NC 27157.

Rivera et al. 2011; Raya-Rivera et al. 2014). Additionally, countless prototype tissues and organs have been engineered but have yet to be implanted regularly in humans.

Despite the fact that the full promise of tissue engineering and regenerative medicine has not been completely realized yet, there have been incredible advances in the many tools in the TERM toolkit that researchers leverage in their work, including cells, stem cells, biomaterials, signaling molecules, bioreactors, and the many platform technologies that have come to exist, such as biofabrication, growth factor delivery, microfabrication and microfluidics, nanotechnology, and genetics (Berthiaume et al. 2011; Kaul and Ventikos 2015). These advancements have resulted in an acceleration of the development and implementation of microphysiological tissue engineered constructs, or "organoids", in *in vitro* applications, such as diagnostics, drug and toxicology screening, and disease modeling (Benam et al. 2015a; Polini et al. 2014). These *in vitro* biological systems do not aim to be implanted into patients, and as such, they do not suffer from the same regulatory and clinical hurdles that traditional "full-scale" replacement organs or regenerative therapies suffer from. Therefore, a multitude of *in vitro* tissue model systems and "organ-on-a-chip" platforms have been explored in recent years, many of which leverage the same toolkit components as described above. In particular, cutting edge cell, biomaterial, and bio- and micro-fabrication technologies have allowed researchers to generate miniaturized biological tissue organoids with remarkable levels of function that in some cases can mimic actual human organs in a scaled-down fashion.

In the majority of these advanced model systems, biofabrication technologies are employed to deposit or encapsulate cells within 3D biopolymer materials in order to create 3D architectures. Biopolymers represent a wide range of different materials, yet are only one category within the larger collection of materials considered to be biomaterials. Other categories include metals, ceramics, synthetic polymers, as well as some types of nanoparticles. In general, biopolymers consist of naturally derived polysaccharides or proteins, although hybrid natural-synthetic materials as well as blends of synthetic and natural polymers exist as well (Williams 2011, 2009). Biopolymers lend themselves naturally to biofabrication technologies as, in general, they initially exist as soluble components of aqueous solutions that can be used to easily encapsulate cells and other biological components, after which a variety of chemical or physical manipulations can induce crosslinking, paired with the particular biofabrication strategy, generated solidified—often in gel form—cell-containing tissue-like constructs. This cell-compatible multi-step encapsulation and fabrication process is not supported by metal and ceramic materials. Some, but not all, synthetic polymer systems are compatible with this process. For example, a variety of water-soluble crosslinkable synthetic polymer chains can be used to form 3D hydrogel constructs quite readily, while many other synthetic polymers require high temperatures to perform melt-curing processes for 3D fabrication. The latter is not cell-friendly (Skardal et al. 2015a).

In the context of biopolymers for 3D biofabrication, biopolymers generally take an end state of a hydrogel. If designed appropriately, these water-swollen networks of polysaccharides, peptides, and occasionally synthetic components can provide environments that mimic the natural extracellular matrix of the body, although often in a reductionist manner. This capability to recapitulate aspects of natural tissues, paired with the readiness of many biopolymers to be integrated with biofabrication hardware, is what sets these materials apart for engineering of model tissues for *in vitro* applications. In this chapter, we will discuss the benefits of 3D architectures that biopolymer biofabrication can provide, and how these environments are often superior to the traditional 2D cell culture methods of the past. Additionally, we will describe several common biofabrication technologies and how biopolymers are integrated with the corresponding hardware. Lastly, we will highlight a variety of biofabricated *in vitro* models and organ-on-a-chip technologies, and their demonstrated and potential areas of application.

3D versus 2D Culture Environments

Development of new and effective drugs for a wide range of pathologies has been limited due to the inability to accurately model tissue phenotype, function, and signaling mechanisms in a controlled environment. Animal models allow only limited manipulation and study of these mechanisms, and are not necessarily predictive of results in humans. Traditional *in vitro* 2D cultures fail to recapitulate the 3D microenvironment of *in vivo* tissues (Fig. 1) (Kunz-Schughart et al. 2004). Drug diffusion kinetics vary dramatically, drug doses effective in 2D are often ineffective when scaled to patients, and cell–cell/cell-matrix interactions are inaccurate (Ho et al. 2010; Drewitz et al. 2011). Tissue culture dishes have three major differences from the tissue where cells were originally isolated: surface topography, surface stiffness, and most importantly, a 2D rather than 3D architecture. As a consequence, plastic 2D culture places a selective pressure on cells that has the potential to significantly alter their molecular and phenotypic properties. The resulting functional differences between 2D cultures and 3D constructs has been shown repeatedly in many tissue types and pathologies, and in general 3D systems outperform 2D cultures in recapitulating *in vivo* function and response to drugs and toxins (Nam et al. 2015). In the drug development pipeline (Fig. 2A), this lack of *in vivo* accuracy in traditional 2D cultures has resulted in countless discrepancies between *in vitro* toxicology outcomes and performance in patients (McKim 2010). In fact, we recently demonstrated that on 2D tissue culture dishes, metastatic colon carcinoma cells appeared epithelial, but when transitioned into a tumor foci form factor inside a 3D liver organoid host environment, they "switched" to a phenotype that appeared more mesenchymal and metastatic (Skardal et al. 2015b). These kinds of bioengineered construct technologies have evolved to the point that they can better mimic the structure, cellular heterogeneity, and function of *in vivo* tissue, and are more suitable for mimicking human physiology than traditional 2D cell cultures. These model organs can be viable for longer periods of time and are cultured to develop functional properties similar to native tissues. This approach has the potential to recapitulate the dynamic role of cell–cell, cell–ECM, and mechanical interactions inside tissues. Subsequently, these relatively new technologies are vastly superior than their predecessors for drug and toxicology testing and personalized medicine applications.

Fortunately, the general concept of performing research using 3D versus 2D cultures has gained significant traction over the last decade. However, there remain hurdles and challenges to overcome. Two-dimensional cell culture is an established practice that will certainly remain a widely used tool for many years to come, because

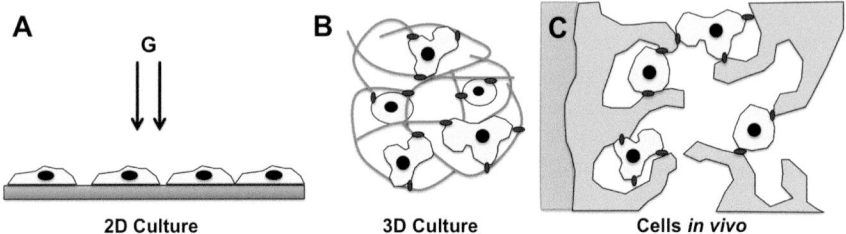

Fig. 1: Cells in (A) 2D and (B) 3D *in vitro* culture environments. (B) 3D culture in biopolymer networks provides cells with a surrounding microenvironment more similar to that of many (C) *in vivo* tissues.

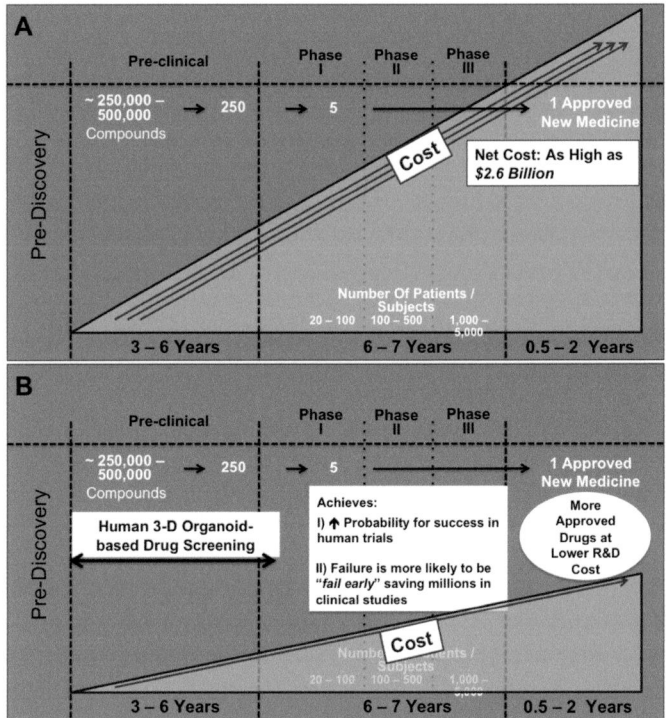

Fig. 2: (A) The current drug development pipeline requires many years and multiple billions of dollars to bring a drug to market. (B) Plugging in human-based biofabricated organoids into pre-clinical stages, can potentially improve the efficiency of the drug development pipeline.

it is far too easy and inexpensive for a complete paradigm shift from 2D to 3D to occur. The same reasons that make 2D culture attractive and widespread, are what have delayed adaptation to 3D systems. In general, employing 3D systems is more complicated. It requires understanding how to employ the innate characteristics of new technologies such as biomaterial development and biofabrication techniques. Following successful establishment of cultures with 3D environments, simple processes such as cell harvesting and cell passaging, trivial steps in 2D cell cultures, can be quite complex, and sometimes not possible without causing harm to the cells. For example, if cells are cultured within a 3D hydrogel construct, one must effectively dissolve the matrix away to remove the cells. Some hydrogel systems support this by building such a feature into the material chemistry (Zhang 2008), but most do not, instead requiring enzymatic dissolution. Furthermore, traditional imaging techniques have mostly been developed for 2D cell cultures in which the cells are confined to a narrow focal plane. High quality imaging in 3D may require confocal or macro-confocal imaging, expensive tools that not all researchers have access to. Additionally, employing 3D tissue culture can result in more research costs for materials, presenting another challenge depending on funding. More advanced biomaterial systems that have been engineered to be user friendly are more expensive than tissue culture plastic. Although, it should be noted that there are some inexpensive materials that can be deployed if users are educated in the field. When it comes to microfluidic organ-on-a-chip technologies, unless the devices and components needed are available commercially, researchers must fabricate this hardware themselves prior to implementation. Fabrication techniques, such as micro-molding, soft lithography, and machining, require additional skill sets and equipment, and bring their own respective costs.

However, in the end, when data is critically assessed, a common conclusion is often reached; results attained from studies employing 3D systems or dynamic on-a-chip platforms often vastly surpass those in static 2D environments (Nam et al. 2015), more closely mimicking physiology of the human body. As a result, these newer, more capable 3D platforms have immense potential to influence the drug development pipeline—decreasing development costs, increasing success of drug candidates in human clinical trials, and perhaps just as important, forcing non-optimal drug candidates to fail early, before human trials (Fig. 2B). To create these viable and functional 3D tissue systems and on-a-chip 3D environments, a variety of biopolymer biomaterial types, fabrication techniques, and engineering approaches are combined, resulting in the more broad category termed biofabrication.

Biofabrication Technologies

A number of biofabrication approaches have been explored in recent years, encompassing the use of inkjet-like printers, extrusion deposition devices, laser-assisted patterning devices, and 3D stereolithography. In general, these approaches are able to physically manipulate biopolymers, forming 3D constructs. To better understand the essential components required for successful biofabrication of viable tissue and organ structures, here we will describe some of the most common fabrication modalities currently being employed in biopolymer biofabrication (Fig. 3).

3D Encapsulation

The most basic approach to biopolymer-supported tissue construct biofabrication is by 3D cell encapsulation. Cell encapsulation is performed by suspending cells within a polymer network that is crosslinked, thereby providing cells with a 3D environment in which to reside instead of a 2D surface (Hunt and Grover 2010). This approach is the most simplistic and most general technique within the overall group of biofabrication types, and it should be noted that the other techniques we describe almost always

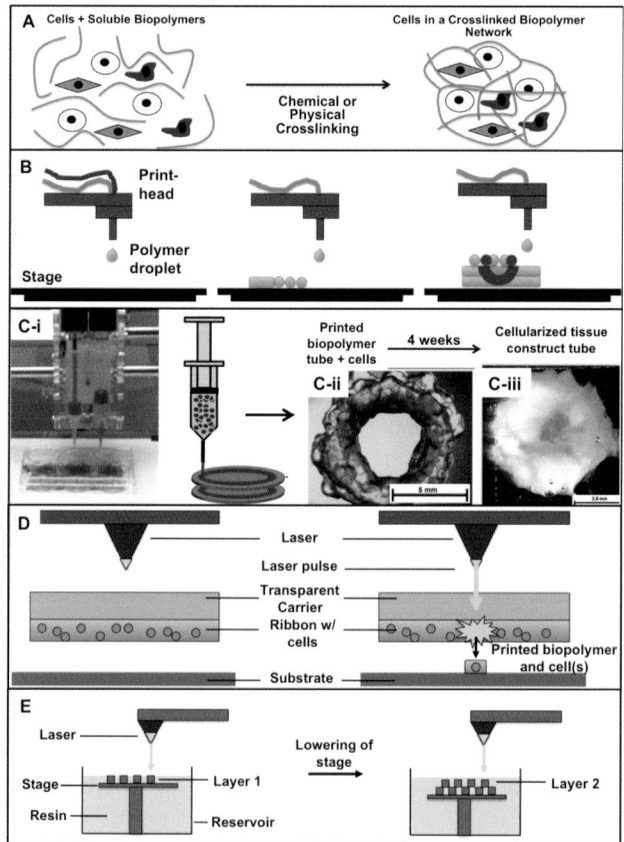

Fig. 3: Biofabrication strategies employing biopolymers. (A) 3D cell encapsulation; (B) Inkjet droplet or drop-by-drop printing; (C) Extrusion bioprinting; and (D) Laser-induced forward transfer (LIFT)-based deposition. (E) 3D stereolithography fabrication. (C-i) A syringe-based extrusion printer; (C-ii) Extruded cell-hydrogel tubes that (C-iii) mature over time into cellularized ECM-containing tubes.

employ 3D encapsulation in their procedures, resulting in cellularized 3D constructs. However, we wish to highlight 3D encapsulation on its own, as it can be a simple and straightforward way for researchers with fewer fabrication and engineering resources to still generate 3D tissue constructs that can be significantly superior to 2D cultures.

In general, 3D encapsulation is performed with two primary sets of components. The first is the population or multiple populations of cells that will be encapsulated. The second is the set of polymers and reagents required to initiate crosslinking into a 3D insoluble network. The particular protocol for performing encapsulation varies based on the polymer in questions, but normally takes one of several forms. In one form, the polymer reagents are used to suspend the cells, after which spontaneous chemical or physical crosslinking occurs. Often, the cell suspension-polymer solution is pipetted as droplets into tissue culture wells or into well inserts and allowed to crosslink. Alternatively, some of the chemical reactions employed are stimuli sensitive, requiring a change in temperature or introduction of light (ultraviolet being most prevalent) to initiate the reaction (Nguyen and West 2002; Tan et al. 2009; Yeon et al. 2013).

In these instances, the user can induce formation of the 3D constructs at will, often saving valuable time. In another form, crosslinking occurs quickly after two of the reagents are mixed. While effective, this reduces manipulation time available for controlling construct shape and size, and reduces time available for distributing multiple constructs throughout well plates. Instead, drop encapsulation is often used. In this technique, often performed with fast-gelling materials such as sodium alginate, cells are suspended in one solution, and introduced dropwise into a second solution. As each cell-containing drop reaches the second solution, the reactions occur, resulting in near-spherical micro-capsules containing cells. As stated, which of these very general approaches is employed is highly dependent on the chemical nature of the polymer systems employed and the kinetics of crosslinking (Nicodemus and Bryant 2008). Examples of these materials, their chemistries, and how they are used in biofabrication of *in vitro* constructs will be discussed further at a later point in this chapter.

Inkjet printing

Inkjet printing, which can also referred to as "drop-by-drop" bioprinting, is one biofabrication approach that has been explored for creating 3D biological structures for some time, and is closely related to technologies used for protein or cell patterning. Where basic patterning creates a 2D pattern comprised of proteins, cells, or both, on a 2D surface, by incorporating a hydrogel that can be deposited by the device, 3D cellularized structures can be fabricated in a drop by drop manner (Catros et al. 2011; Guillotin and Guillemot 2011). These types of bioprinters often use a cartridge-based delivery system mounted on a XYZ plotting system. The cartridge system is similar to that used in traditional inkjet printing such that cells and biomaterial components can be loaded into individual cartridges for computer controlled deposition. In fact, early versions of these devices were actual inkjet printers that were repurposed to deposit cells and other biological materials. The drop-by-drop approach relies on being able to quickly polymerize or stabilize the printed material in place, so that subsequent droplets can be added to the growing structure, increasing the size of the construct drop by drop. The polymerization rates of the dropped material is a direct result of the various crosslinking chemistries inherent to materials used, and is essential for successful deposition and 3D construct biofabrication. The requirement for a fast-gelling material places a limitation on the types of biopolymers that are appropriate for this type of fabrication. One challenge with this approach is scalability. As the printed droplets are typically very small volumes, scaling up fabrication to a large human-sized organ structure is a challenge. On the other hand, the small droplet volumes can support high resolution printing of intricate structures and precise architectures.

Extrusion-based biofabrication

Extrusion-based biofabrication, which usually deposits material using a device with syringe-like printheads, is another relatively common approach to 3D bioprinting that also relies on the physical and chemical properties of the biopolymer materials being printed. In this approach, the properties of the biopolymer or hydrogel are used to facilitate extrusion through a syringe tip, often driven by pneumatic pressure or mechanical pistons controlled by the device software. Generally, the material needs to be soft or sheer thinnable enough to allow passage through a small diameter printhead nozzle, but must also support its 3D shape after deposition. One common approach is employing melt-curable polymers such as polycaprolactone, which when heated can be deformed and printed at relatively high resolutions, and cool down to a solid material. However, melt-cure extrusion cannot be performed with cells due to the heat or solvents required to dissolve the polymer. Instead, cell-based extrusion biofabrication is usually performed using crosslinkable hydrogels. Printing with hydrogels via extrusion can be difficult when working with materials that rely on extended periods of time for crosslinking to occur. Mistiming the extrusion process and crosslinking dynamics can result in structures that collapse because crosslinking has not occurred quickly enough, or clogging of the printhead as a result of polymerization or crosslinking too quickly. Fortunately, a wide variety of studies have developed novel crosslinking chemistries and techniques to improve spatial and temporal control over biopolymers that can contain encapsulated cells for fabricating cell-containing 3D structures (Skardal et al. 2010b; Skardal et al. 2010c; Pescosolido et al. 2011).

Scaffold-free printing

"Scaffold-free" bioprinting technology is an approach to biofabrication that some might consider a type of extrusion printing. However, this specific method has a bulk of established work behind it, and has even yielded a commercial bioprinting entity. Scaffold-free bioprinting is based on the principles of tissue liquidity and tissue fusion. Preformed aggregates or rods comprised entirely of cells are printed in geometric patterns or architectures and allowed to fuse after printing to form larger constructs (Jakab et al. 2008). Generally, multiple layers of aggregates or rods are printed, and after the fusion period, singular 3D structures are formed. In pioneering 3D printing work, this technique was used to build branched vascular structures (Norotte et al. 2009), followed by nerve graft structures (Marga et al. 2012). It should be noted that this type of bioprinting still relies on biomaterial scaffolds for support. Often, the cell aggregates and rods are printed into a biopolymer or additively stacked using space-holding biomaterials such as agarose or other non-cell adherent hydrogels to preserve the appropriate structures during the tissue fusion and maturation process (Jakab et al. 2008; Norotte et al. 2009; Jakab et al. 2006; Mironov et al. 2009). These space-holders are usually removed when the construct has fused and has the mechanical and physical properties to support itself. The advantage of this approach to biofabrication lies is its high cellularity and cell density, which accelerates fusion between each of the printed pieces. However, relatively tedious preparation times, printing speeds, and building material volumes limit its scalability to large scale bioprinting. However, it is quite appropriate for small-sized *in vitro* constructs. This method has been explored extensively and is the basis for commercially available technologies.

Laser-induced forward transfer deposition

Laser-induced forward transfer (LIFT)-based biofabrication is a relatively new technology that has been translated to bioengineering from other fields (Bohandy et al. 1986; Barron et al. 2004). LIFT technology was first developed for high resolution patterning of metals in applications like computer chip fabrication. In recent years it has been adapted to micropatterning peptides, DNA, and cells. LIFT devices are comprised of a laser that is pulsed on demand and donor material comprised of a printable material that is usually referred to as the "ribbon". The ribbon supported on a transport layer such as gold or titanium that can absorb the laser energy and transfer it to the ribbon. When the laser pulses on the ribbon, the focused energy generates a small, high-pressure micro-bubble that propels a droplet of the ribbon material down onto a collecting substrate. By moving the stage or the laser in relation to the ribbon, material can be pattered into desired conformations on the stage (Chrisey 2000; Colina et al. 2005; Dinca et al. 2008). In LIFT-based biofabrication, the ribbon may be comprised of a biopolymer or protein, and can contain cells within. In this scenario the laser pulse induces droplets that contain cells to be deposited in a pattern on the substrate to create cellular structures and patterns. The lack of a nozzle in LIFT biofabrication is a major difference from other biofabrication methods, doing away with clogging issues. This results in increased flexibility in the printing materials, as long as they can be transferred to the substrate by the energy supplied by the laser. Studies have shown few negative effects on cell viabily (Hopp et al. 2005; Gruene et al. 2010; Koch et al. 2010) and the ability to print nearly a single cell per droplet suggests that LIFT has much potential as an effective biofabrication strategy in the future (Guillotin et al. 2010). The incredibly high resolution of LIFT is directed by a number of parameters, including the laser power, the biopolymer material properties, the relative hydrophilic and hydrophobic natures of the substrate material and the printable material, cell density, and the distance between the ribbon and the collecting stage (Guillemot et al. 2010). There are also several challenges that need to be overcome. The high resolution translates into small printing volumes per laser pulse, and printing requires fast gelation kinetics of the printable material, and a fast moving stage for fabricating larger structures quickly. Furthermore, to create structures of size, multiple ribbons are often employed, requiring reloading during the printing process.

Stereolithography and projection patterning

Stereolithography is a solid free form fabrication technique that uses a reservoir containing a photopolymerizable polymer solution, a laser with control in the X-Y plane, and a stage with vertical Z-axis control. Fabrication occurs at the polymer solution surface. The stage lowers incrementally, allowing polymerization of layers on top of each other, thereby creating 3D structures in a step-by-step manner. Resolution can be manipulated by focusing the laser and altering the laser energy. Traditionally, stereolithography has been used to create cell-free scaffolds, but with the development of biopolymers and proteins that can be photo-crosslinked on demand, stereolithography has been adapted for tissue engineering applications. Some examples of biomaterials that are compatible with this technique are methacrylated or acrylated materials such as gelatin-methacrylate, hyaluronic acid-methacrylate, polyethylene glycol diacrylate (PEGDA), and polyethylene glycol dimethacrylate (PEGDMA) (Billiet et al. 2012; Soman et al. 2013; Hribar et al. 2014). More recent developments have led to stereolithography that uses visible light as a curing source for cell-laden materials, thereby minimizing any cell damage from exposure to the UV light or laser (Lin et al. 2013). Stereolithography has also been multiplexed by using digital mirror devices that allow UV light to be applied to the polymer solutions as projections of millions of individual points or pixels at once, facilitating curing of entire layers of the 3D constructs at once, significantly increasing fabrication speed (Zhang et al. 2012; Gou et al. 2014).

Biopolymer Integration in Biofabrication

One of the integral components of biofabrication, and tissue engineering in general, is biomaterials—in particular functional biopolymer hydrogels that allow crosslinking manipulation for biofabrication protocols, cell encapsulation, cell-biopolymer interaction, and soluble cytokine loading and release (Buwalda et al. 2014). While much attention has been paid to biofabrication hardware, such as bioprinting devices that have been developed over the past 10 years, and the many new commercial entities selling these hardware platforms currently, significantly less attention has been given to the biomaterials these devices actually manipulate. These biomaterials are arguably the lynchpin in realizing successful biofabrication applications, as the physical and chemical properties of these materials directly influence whether or not a particular biofabrication approach will work (Malda et al. 2013). Specifically, tight control over the mechanical properties of a biopolymer preparation is required in order to support a fluid state for initial mixing with cells and other components such as growth factors or drugs followed by a more robust state after biofabrication that retains a 3D architecture. Furthermore, the transient state between liquid and solid (or gelled) states needs to be fluid enough to allow for the physical demands of depositions (such as extrusion in the case of bioprinting) and crosslink or set up quick enough to hold its shape, as indicated prior. Importantly, during these mechanical property manipulations, which are generally controlled by physical or chemical crosslinking processes, environmental conditions must be such that the viability and function of any cells that are incorporated remains sufficiently high to result in viable and function tissue constructs (Skardal and Atala 2015). Realization of successful tissue construct biofabrication can be a delicate orchestration of biological, chemical, and physical aspects of biopolymer hydrogels.

As described above, there are a variety of commonly employed biopolymer types—the most common being collagen, gelatin, alginate, hyaluronic acid, fibrin, and silk. However, it should be noted that other biopolymers exist and are employed quite successfully. Additionally, it is important to understand that while some of the biopolymers listed above can be employed in their near natural or "raw" forms to form polymer networks and 3D systems (e.g., collagen and alginate), often, synthetic chemical modifications are introduced to provide necessary functional groups for more effective crosslinking control (Burdick and Prestwich 2011). Furthermore, in the case of some biopolymers, they do not innately contain motifs for cell attachment. Often, additional covalent modifications are made to adhere peptides or other components to allow for increased interaction with cells within the biopolymer environments (Skardal and Atala 2015). In the following section, we highlight the biopolymer types listed above, and provide basic background information for each— understanding that this short list is but a limited snapshot of the many biopolymer systems that exist.

Collagen

Collagen is one of the most frequently used biopolymers in biomedical research and cell cultures, since it is the most abundant component of the ECM in most types of tissues (Hesse et al. 2010). Isolation and purification of collagen is well established, particularly for collagen type I. Using collagen as a surface coating for tissue culture plates and to make simple gels for cell culture has become common practice. Collagen biomaterial matrices are indeed useful and have yielded many important biological advances. However, in normal tissue and ECM, collagen is but one of many components. The lack of other common ECM components such as elastin, fibrinogen, laminin, and glycosaminoglycans, may result in biological signaling that can induce unanticipated cellular changes. Furthermore, collagen fibers and gels primarily contain hydrophobic peptide motifs. As a result, when used as implants or cell delivery agents, collagen gels can exclude water and contract, potentially resulting in decreased diffusion of nutrients and gases. Despite this limitation, collagen is still used extensively in tissue culture.

Gelatin

Gelatin is a mixture of peptide sequences derived from collagen that has undergone hydrolytic degradation. This product can be dissolved in aqueous solutions more easily than collagen, while still maintaining the ability to form simple gels through hydrophobic crosslinking when brought to low temperatures. Unfortunately, the gelation/melt temperature of gelatin solutions/gels lies between 30 and 35°C, which limits is use in this gel form to applications that are at or above physiological temperatures, in which case the gelled solutions dissolve. Due to this limitation, gelatin often requires additional chemical modification, alternative crosslinking techniques, or integration with other proteins or polymers for implementation in 3D culture applications.

Alginate

Alginate is a natural polysaccharide derived not from the extracellular matrix, but rather from algae or seaweed. It has been a common material in regenerative medicine and tissue engineering applications due to the ease at which it can form a hydrogel. Crosslinking is achieved via an almost instantaneous sodium-calcium ion exchange reaction. This has resulted in alginate being the material of choice for microencapsulation of cells, in which easily available and inexpensive alginic sodium salt, or sodium alginate, which is unmodified, quickly gels into calcium alginate hydrogel microspheres (Santos et al. 2010). These gel capsules have been employed extensively for creating micro-capsules containing trapped liver cells or pancreatic islets (Opara et al. 2010). However, without chemical modification, alginate is mostly inert, and use for cell and tissue culture is limited without incorporating additional cell-adherent motifs through covalent modification. Additionally, the reagents generally used for crosslinking, such as $CaCl_2$, as well as sodium citrate and ethylenediaminetetraacetic acid (EDTA), commonly used chelators, have been shown to have detrimental effects on cell viability during the encapsulation process in some cases (Cohen et al. 2011). However, because of the ease and simplicity with which alginate capsules can be formed, it remains popular in applications requiring cell encapsulation.

Hyaluronic acid

Hyaluronic acid (HA), or hyaluronan, is a versatile glycosaminoglycan (GAG) polysaccharide that is present in tissues as a major component of the ECM. HA has shown great potential in regenerative medicine (Allison and Grande-Allen 2006; Knudson and Knudson 2001). Unmodified HA has been used clinically for over three decades (Kuo 2006), in applications such as treatment and lubrication of damaged joints (Galus et al. 2006; Schiavinato et al. 2002). More recently, HA has been chemically modified with a variety of functional groups to become a more useful and robust biomaterial that can be crosslinked or loaded with cells or other biomolecules (Prestwich and Kuo 2008). HA hydrogels can be formed by photocrosslinking methacrylate groups that have been added to the HA chains. These groups can undergo free radical polymerization when exposed to ultraviolet (UV) irradiation to form soft hydrogels. These photocrosslinkable MA-HA hydrogels have been used in many applications, from cutaneous and corneal wound healing (Miki et al. 2002) to 3D extrusion bioprinting (Skardal et al. 2010b). Thiol-modification of HA also yields another variety of HA that can form hydrogels through Michael-type addition crosslinking. Like the MA-HA variety of HA, thiol-modified HA, particularly a thiolated carboxymethyl HA (CMHA-S), has been implemented in many applications in regenerative medicine such as wound healing (Kirker et al. 2004), generation of tumor models (Liu et al. 2007), and bioprinting of cellularized structures (Skardal et al. 2010c; Skardal et al. 2015a).

Fibrin

Another naturally-occurring material for generating biopolymer hydrogels is fibrin, which has been employed in tissue culture for various cell and tissues types. Fibrin is comprised of fibrinogen monomers that are joined by thrombin-mediated cleavage, exposing crosslinking sites. In the human body, it plays a key role in blood clotting, wound healing, and tumor growth. It is often prepared in a concentrated glue-like form, which has been used extensively in the clinic as a hemostatic agent, sealant, and surgical glue. Less concentrated fibrin gels have been used as a tissue engineering scaffold for regenerative medicine applications due to its fast crosslinking rates (Ahmed et al. 2008). In the context of biopolymer bioprinting, our laboratory has used a fibrin-collagen blend to generate printable hydrogels that can encapsulate stem cells and rapidly cover and treat full thickness wounds, accelerating skin regeneration after injury (Skardal et al. 2012a).

Silk

Silk fibroin is a unique silk-based insoluble protein that due to its biomechanical properties is substantially different from the majority of other naturally derived biopolymer materials. It has proven to be remarkably versatile, having been implemented in a wide variety of applications including solid implants, hydrogels, threads and sutures, and drug delivery vehicles. In nature, silk fibroin is bound to hydrophilic sericin proteins, forming what we know of as silk. Sericins can induce unwanted immune or inflammatory responses, and are therefore generally separated from silk fibroin before use in biomedical applications. Silk fibroin chains themselves are comprised of block polymer-like alternating hydrophilic and hydrophobic regions, giving the material amphiphilic characteristics and the capability to form semi-crystalline structures through hydrophobic interactions and crosslinking. A variety of processing techniques have generated a variety of forms of silk fibroin that have been implemented in regenerative medicine, including treatment of wounds and bioengineering of tissues (Meinel and Kaplan 2012).

In vitro Models

There is a critical need for improved bioengineered tissue models to predict efficacy, pharmacokinetics, and potential toxicity for candidate drugs. *In vivo* animal models have long served as the gold standard for preclinical testing, but the drawbacks that are associated with animal models are contributors to the high cost and uncertainty in translating a candidate drug from bench to clinical and commercial implementation. *In vitro* cellular platforms comprised of actual human-derived cells are preferable from a predictive point of view (Greenhough et al. 2010). However, in order to accurately reflect human physiology and be effective for drug screening, cells must retain their *in vivo* functions and be stable in culture for extended periods of time. These requirements are critical for widespread adoption in pharmacokinetic and toxicity testing.

Liver

Often, the liver is the first tissue to be critically assessed for toxicity during drug and toxicology screening due to its role in metabolism. *In vitro* cultured primary hepatocytes are the optimal choice for screening studies in the pharmaceutical industry (Gomez-Lechon et al. 2010). However, there is still a need for new culture systems that improve the long-term maintenance of hepatocytes with retention of high levels of liver function for *in vitro* drug screening. *In vitro* liver models have been employed extensively in the realm of drug testing by researchers in academia and within the pharmaceutical industry. Traditionally, liver-derived cell lines such as HepG2 cells were often employed, since primary hepatocytes were difficult to maintain in culture until relatively recently. Unfortunately, HepG2 cells were derived from a hepatoma, and therefore, despite being robust and easy to maintain in culture, they do not retain full hepatocyte functionality. HepG2 cells express an incomplete subset of cytochrome p450 isoforms, limiting their use in drug metabolism studies. Furthermore, with the robust and easy to culture nature comes a decreased sensitivity to environmental stimuli and toxins. Despite these shortcomings, they remain a useful model cell type, and remain a common choice for proof-of-concept work, particularly in the development of new 3D liver systems and biofabrication technologies. However, with new approaches that increase ease of hepatocyte culture, primary human hepatocytes are becoming the industry standard for most liver-based screening studies. Only several years ago, it was very difficult to maintain hepatocytes in culture for more than a week, while retaining viability and function, thereby limiting their use in long-term studies.

Fortunately, a variety of 3D cell culture and organoid fabrication strategies have been established that have enabled formation of and extended maintenance of relatively high functioning hepatocyte-based tissue constructs with high viability. For example, hanging drop and RWV bioreactor cultures have successfully supported generation of primary hepatocyte spheroids (Chang and Hughes-Fulford 2014). Hanging drop techniques and the resulting liver spheroids are now used widely, and are even commercially available as fully formed spheroids. These spheroids have been shown to have significantly improved lifetimes and metabolic functionality than traditional cultures (Kim et al. 2015; Messner et al. 2013). Likewise, RWV-generated hepatocyte spheroids are superior to 2D systems in terms of gene expression, liver function, and cell phenotype (Chang and Hughes-Fulford 2014).

A variety of other approaches have been implemented that employ biomaterials, such as biopolymer hydrogels used to encapsulate and support hepatocytes in culture. In particular, materials derived from or containing decellularized liver tissue have been explored using several methods to form liver-like environments that increase lifetime and function hepatocyte cultures. In one such approach, porcine liver was decellularized through the vasculature using a detergent, after which a discs were cut from the cell-free ECM. When cultured on the liver ECM discs, which retained key molecular components native to the liver, hepatocytes expressed increased albumin levels compared to cells on tissue culture plastic and in collagen gels. Notably, these cultures could be maintained for three weeks, a length of time dramatically longer than traditional 2D cultures could support (Lang et al. 2011). Building on this use of native liver ECM, our group further solubilized decellularized liver and incorporated it into a hyaluronic acid hydrogel system. The resulting liver-specific hydrogel material could be prepared in a fashion more compatible with high throughput screening studies. Notably, we extended viability and function out to 28 days, and achieved increased albumin and urea production, increased viability, superior morphology, and importantly, increased drug metabolism (Skardal et al. 2012b).

Heart

In drug screening scenarios, together with liver, cardiac tissue is often assessed for toxic effects. However, since few cardiac models that accurately recapitulate *in vivo* function have existed until recently, drug screening procedures have been inadequate in terms of identifying cardiac toxicity (Natarajan et al. 2011; Grosberg et al. 2011). As a result, several drugs made it to market, were available commercially for a time, but were later withdrawn by the FDA (Nordt et al. 2010; Bhise et al. 2014). For example, astemizole, an anti-psychotic produced by Janssen Pharmaceutica was commercially available for 11 years before being recalled for slowing potassium channel function, causing torsade de pointes, and causing long QT syndrome. Rofecoxib, known more commonly as Vioxx, an NSAID produced by Merck, was commercially available for five years before being recalled for increased risk of heart attack or stroke, and being linked to over 27,500 heart attacks or sudden cardiac arrests. Several other drugs that were recalled for cardiac side effects include pergoglide (Permax), cisapride (Propulsid), Valdecoxib (Bextra), and terodiline (Micturin). These, and other drugs recalled due to cardiac side effects, were not recalled for causing cell toxicity specifically, but rather for inducing functional problems that resulted in detrimental changes in beating behavior (e.g., long QT syndrome, beat rate slowing, ventricular tachycardia, torsade de pointes, etc.). As such, there is an important need for cardiac models to accurately support baseline cardiac function—primarily beating-associated actions—and respond appropriately to function altering drugs and stimuli.

Initially, the majority of cardiac models have been engineered using rat cardiomyocytes, but more recently human cardiomyocytes, derived from induced pluripotent stem (iPS) cells, have emerged as a more appropriate cell source for human-specific applications (Zanella et al. 2014). In addition to providing human-specific models for drug screening, the use of iPS technology allows fabrication of patient-specific models that are incredibly useful for establishing models of cardiac tissue with specific genetic disorders that effect the heart, such as Duchenne muscular dystrophy.

A variety of strategies have been explored to engineer cardiac models, including patches, micropatterned surfaces, hydrogels, and mechanical property customization (Cimetta et al. 2013). Cell sheet technology, which employs a temperature-sensitive polymer to release cell monolayers, has been employed to create cardiac patches. These cardiac monolayers could then be stacked layer-by-layer, forming 3D cardiac patch constructs that beat spontaneously and in a concerted fashion (Shimizu et al. 2002). Several biopolymers have been explored for creating cardiac constructs. For example, methacrylated varieties of gelatin and tropoelastin were tailored to cardiomyocyte cultures. The researchers found that cell attachment and alignment depended heavily on the type of hydrogel employed. However, beating activity was more dependent on the physical stiffness of the hydrogel (Annabi et al. 2013). This study highlighted the type of manipulations of biopolymer systems that can be performed to influence function of engineered tissue constructs. In addition to the approaches described above, some researchers have explored the use of natural extracellular matrix materials, which are comprised of the natural biopolymers in cardiac tissue. For this approach, hearts were decellularized by perfusion of detergents, preserving the ECM structure and the vascular architecture. Using this intact network, cardiac or endothelial cells could re-introduced into the constructs, and then maintained in bioreactors. The resulting cardiac constructs could beat successfully, albeit at a much reduced rate compared to physiological levels (Ott et al. 2008). This type of approach could yield cardiac tissue constructs that functioned for 120 days in culture, while presenting appropriate cell morphology, contractile forces, and electrical conduction (Guyette et al. 2015). Cardiac constructs have also been developed for increased throughput studies. On such system consisted of arrays of PDMS films, patterned with fibronectin, in which 40 independent cardiac films could be monitored in real-time (Agarwal et al. 2013). Other similar approaches have allowed monitoring of the effects of calcium dynamics within cardiomyocyte microfluidic devices (Martewicz et al. 2012).

Cancer

In addition to normal tissue models for screening applications, the same advances in tissue engineering that support fabrication of tissue constructs such as liver can be employed to fabricate models of cancer. Cancer is one of the leading causes of deaths around the world. Tumor growth in a given tissue can cause decreased function, and can eventually result in metastasis and patient death, thus necessitating development of more effective treatments. However, to develop such drugs and therapies, better test platforms for conducting research are needed. Additionally, with advances in tissue engineered organoid systems, one can expand into disease modeling, allowing study of pathologies in settings that are easier to manipulate and observe.

Cancer models have ranged in complexity, and application. In one study, the effect of peroxisome proliferator-activated receptor activation on hepatocellular carcinoma (HCC) cell migration and invasion was tested first in a simple 2D wound assay, and subsequently in a 3D Matrigel hydrogel-based invasion assay. These assays demonstrated that certain drugs could reduce or prevent invasive behavior (Shen et al. 2012). A separate HCC Matrigel invasion model was employed to demonstrate cell invasion tracking using quantum dot nanoparticles and several imaging modalities. This platform was able to assess invasive phenotypes, reversal of cell senescence prior to invasion, and quantum dot-highlighted expression of MT1-MMP in filopodia, or invadopodia, of the cells (Fang et al. 2013). In addition to assessing migration in invasion models, cancer models are being employed to investigate progression phenomena such as epithelial-to-mesenchymal transition (EMT), which is an integral event in the progression from a more benign phenotype towards metastatic states. Co-culture models have been developed that provide the cellular components of the tumor microenvironment that would normally interact with tumor cells. For example, when Bel-7402 HCC cells were co-cultured together with normal epithelial cells or normal vascular endothelial cells, the cells actually underwent an "MET" (mesenchymal-to-epithelial transition), becoming less invasive and motile. On the other hand, when co-cultured with conditioned media from mesenchymal fibroblast cells, they underwent an EMT-like transition, becoming elongated, motile, and more invasive (Ding et al. 2013). These results demonstrate the importance of the tumor microenvironment, including surrounding cells of the host tissue, in cancer model systems. In addition to stromal cells, the ECM is an integral component of the tumor microenvironment. For example, when HepG2 cells were formed into 3D heterospheroids together with stromal fibroblasts and embedded in collagen, the cells became significantly more resistant to chemotherapy compared to cells not embedded in collagen (Yip and Cho 2013). Our group recently created a liver organoid system with colon carcinoma tumor foci using biopolymer hydrogel microcarriers and a rotating wall vessel bioreactor system. We could recapitulate tumor growth in the micro-livers over time and demonstrated dose dependent responses to the drug 5-fluorouracil. We were also able to manipulate the Wnt signaling pathway using small molecule drugs to increase or decrease drug resistance to the drug (Skardal et al. 2015b). As they continue to advance, versatile cancer model systems such as these will likely provide useful diagnostic and drug screening platforms.

Body on a Chip Models

In recent years, advances in biotechnology areas such as tissue engineering, biomaterials, and micro- and biofabrication, have allowed derivation of new biological systems with massive potential as test platforms. Researchers have developed a wide variety of human-derived *in vitro* models that can be used as specific normal tissues for testing drugs, toxins, and drug candidates (Skardal et al. 2010a; Prestwich 2008; Prestwich 2007). Furthermore, through the use of genetics as well as external environmental manipulations, these systems can be employed as specific disease models (Benam et al. 2015a; Barrila et al. 2010; Nickerson and Ott 2004; Nickerson et al. 2007). Further integration with engineering, microfabrication, and microfluidic technology has resulted in dynamic micro-devices that support cell and organoid culture, fluid flow, multi-tissue interactions, high-throughput testing, and environmental sampling and biosensing. These versatile organ-on-a-chip platforms are being widely explored for applications such as drug discovery (Polini et al. 2014), and purport to significantly impact the future of medicine.

Liver

"On-a-chip" are often microfluidic systems with fluid channels and housing for cells, organoids, or diagnostics. Initially on-a-chip devices were simpler; sometimes the chip was just a device or piece of hardware with patterns or wells used to create multicellular organoids. An example of this concept is the use of microwells of various shapes and sizes containing cell-adherent collagen or non-adherent polyethylene glycol. Based on the well parameters, HepG2 cells or rat hepatocytes could be formed into either spheroids or cylindrical constructs in a highly controlled manner. These 3D constructs maintained better liver function than 2D controls (Mori et al. 2008; Fukuda et al. 2006). In another example, HepG2 spheroids were created using an array of channels and pyramid-shaped micro-wells to generate functional HepG2 spheroids, which could then be employed in the same device for multi-drug screening (Torisawa et al. 2007). Newer liver-on-a-chip devices often direct fluid flow for improving diffusion, circulating nutrients, drugs, or toxins, aliquot sampling, or even connecting liver constructs to other tissue types forming multi-organoid devices.

In one liver-on-a-chip, hydrogel matrices were used to embed HepG2 and NIH-3T3 cells within fluid arrays. These 3D organoids had better functioning than 2D control cultures, and responded appropriately to acetaminophen in toxin screening (Au et al. 2014). Similarly, our group recently took advantage of a versatile photopolymerizable HA biopolymer system to perform *in situ* device photopatterning to generate HepG2 liver organoids inside parallel channel PDMS fluidic devices that had been fabricated by soft lithography and molding techniques. We demonstrated toxicity screening in a parallel manner using multiple alcohol concentrations, which resulted in dose dependent decreases in viability and function with increasing doses, as expected (Skardal et al. 2015c). We are currently modifying this approach by combining *in situ* organoid biofabrication with screening systems to be significantly miniaturized further to increase throughput in experiments on single devices the size of traditional microscope slides. Microfabrication approaches can be employed to generate more intricate structures, such as liver sinusoids. For example, precise layering of rat hepatocytes and endothelial cell co-cultures with fluid flow can generate sinusoid-like models (Kang et al. 2015). In another example, a device with two distinct chambers separated by a porous membrane with human hepatocytes and endothelial cells was demonstrated to maintain increased albumin and urea secretion under flow conditions compared to traditional static cultures (Prodanov et al. 2015).

Lung

The lungs serve as one of most common ports of entry for drugs, toxins, and pathogens in the human body. Therefore, lung-on-a-chip devices have been under development for nearly a decade (Huh et al. 2007). The majority of these biomimetic lung devices consist of lung epithelial-endothelial interfaces that are generally comprised of cell monolayers on either side of a semi-permeable membrane. These interfaces often separate an airway channel and a fluid channel, forming a barrier that can facilitate transport across the interface under the appropriate conditions. By engineering additional pneumatic channels into the devices, programmed cyclic wall stretch paired with fluid dynamics in the fluid channel can support the mechanical cues resembling breathing (Douville et al. 2011; Huh et al. 2010). These "functional" models have been able to serve as mimics of lung pathologies, including inflammation, pulmonary edema, mucus plug rupture, and epithelial damage, and have begun to be explored for drug screening (Benam et al. 2015b; Huh et al. 2012; Tavana et al. 2011; Hu et al. 2015). These on-a-chip lung models typically rely on this bilayer construction, rather than a 3D bulk construct morphology in which cells would be encapsulated inside biopolymer networks. However, most of these systems do still rely on certain biopolymers for providing cell attachment and communication cues from the membrane component of the devices. Often, ECM components, such as fibronectin or laminin, are employed to coat the membranes prior to introduction of the lung cells.

Vascular

The very term "microfluidics" indicates that this technology is naturally capable of fluid handling. As such, microfluidic chips are a natural fit for creating vascular models and systems. Additionally, since some drugs are introduced directly to the blood stream, and most other drugs arrive in the drug stream shortly after introduction through other means, fluidic systems that mimic vasculature are an important component of drug screening technologies. Many vascular-like fluidic devices have been fabricated, taking a variety of form factors, including both straight channels (Kim et al. 2014; Korin et al. 2012) and more complex branched features (Lamberti et al. 2013; Doshi et al. 2010). A key feature of the vascular system beyond transport from one tissue to another, is transport of drugs and other materials through the endothelium into adjacent tissues. Many vascular microfluidic devices have been created to recapitulate this endothelial transport feature. In one such example, a device was fabricated that was comprised of two individual channels placed perpendicular to one another, with one channel passing under the other. At this location, a semi-permeable membrane on which endothelial cells were seeded formed the only barrier between channels. Using fluorescently labeled albumin, transport through the endothelium could be measured in the outflow channel using a laser for quantification. This general schematic could be adapted to many other soluble agents to asses their endothelium permeability. Another endothelial device, capable of regulated shear stress conditions, was used to assess the influence of shear stress mechanical properties on changes in nanoparticle uptake by the cells, demonstrating the ability to modulate flow and shear stress to mimic different zones of vasculature in the body that may respond differently to administered agents (Young et al. 2010). Likewise, other microfluidic endothelial devices have been employed to assess how changing the shape of drugs and nanoparticles can influence the rate at which these agents can adhere to and pass through endothelium (Kolhar et al. 2013). As stated above, one function of vasculature is to allow transport between tissues and organs throughout the body. As organ-on-a-chip platforms grow in complexity, and multiple organ types are incorporated onboard a single platform, vascular components will be necessary-both for serving as connecting vascular and acting as responsive vascular tissue analogs.

Cancer

Many biofabricated *in vitro* cancer models, such as those described in the previous section, have the potential to be even more powerful and user friendly if integrated with microfabrication, microfluidic, and sensor technologies, thereby providing tumor-on-a-chip platforms for more substantial *in vitro* applications with more capabilities. The microenvironments of tumors are complex, with varying levels of vascularization, pressures, and mass transport. These physical characteristics are parameters that can be monitored and controlled using microfluidic and microfabrication strategies. Cancer-on-a-chip systems can be employed for general drug development screening, dose testing, and to test treatment regimens on a patient-by-patient basis (Wlodkowic and Cooper 2010; Young 2013).

Early systems often employed the chip and fluidic components to facilitate measurement taking and diagnostics. Examples include paper-based microreactors for integrating cancer cells with immunoassays (Lei and Huang 2014), quantification of apoptosis of tumor cells (Ye et al. 2007), and electrical impedance measurements of cells to determine cell death as an effect of drugs and toxins (Yeon and Park 2005). Additionally, a variety of devices have been developed to collect and assess circulating tumor cells, as early-diagnosis tools (Kang et al. 2012; Kirby et al. 2012; Dong et al. 2013; Li et al. 2013).

More recent advancements include development of devices designed for integration with additional high complexity, advanced technologies such as imaging or microarray analyses, allowing more novel investigation, and detailed observation and quantification to be performed. The small size scale of on-a-chip systems has been shown to play a significant role in cell metabolism, based on the bioavailability of oxygen. This metabolomics-on-a-chip demonstrated that the microfluidic environment provided more access to oxygen compared to Petri dish cultures, resulting in increases in Krebs cycle activity and decreased expression of hypoxia-regulated factor-1 (Ouattara et al. 2012). A device comprised of multiple drug gradient mixers and parallel cell culture chambers was developed to support multi-concentration drug screens paired with cell-labeling and high content imaging data collection on-chip (Ye et al. 2007). In another device, HCT-116 colon carcinoma cells and HepG2 cells (used as a liver model), were encapsulated in Matrigel cultures in separate chambers, while myeloblasts (bone marrow model) were encapsulated in alginate an additional chamber, so that the cytotoxic effects of the 5-FU prodrug Tegafur could be tested on each cell type. Interestingly, in 3D, the liver constructs were able to metabolize Tegafur to 5-FU, resulting in cell death in the other 3D constructs, while cells in 2D could not metabolize the prodrug to its active form (Sung and Shuler 2009).In another example of increased complexity, microscale bioreactors were prepared that housed hepatocytes, non-parenchymal cells (NPCs), and breast cancer cells with the goal to model the hepatic niche. The device contained oxygen sensors, micropumps for controlling nutrient distribution, and real-time sampling (Wheeler et al. 2013). This work resulted in observation of spontaneous dormancy of the breast cancer cells within the hepatic niche, determined to be due to microenvironment cytokine profiles that were altered by the NPCs. Additionally, breast cancer has been studied using a recently developed mammary duct-on-a-chip and breast cancer-on-a-chip systems (Vidi et al. 2014; Yang et al. 2015). Lung tumors have also been evaluated using microfluidic platforms. In one example, human non-small cell lung cancer was assessed for sensitivity to several common chemotherapy agents versus 2D controls in a parallel channel device for increasing throughput and simplifying drug administration (Xu et al. 2013). In another example, lung cancer spheroids were formed from either cell lines or patient-derived lung cancer cells, with and without pericyte co-cultures, and screened for susceptibility to cisplatin. Interestingly, co-culture systems demonstrated higher chemoresistance, demonstrating the explorations that can be performed that investigate multi-cellular systems and their effects on drug efficacy (Ruppen et al. 2015). These more complex examples of cancer-on-a-chip systems demonstrate the beginnings of the kinds of studies and findings that are projected to be possible in the near future as these systems gain popularity and become widespread within cancer research.

Conclusions

The future impact that *in vitro* tissue models and organ-on-a-chip systems may have on drug development, disease modeling, and personalized medicine is highly promising (Fig. 4). However, there currently remain limitations that if overcome will improve

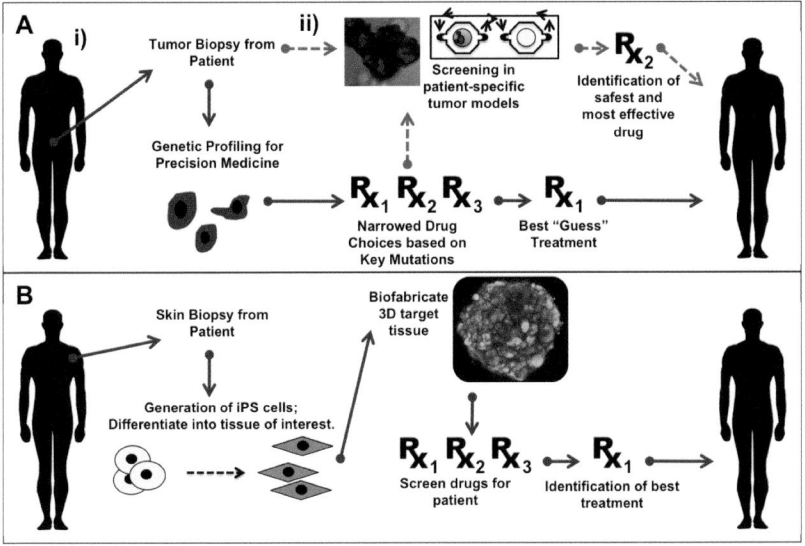

Fig. 4: Employing biofabricated tissues in personalized medicine. (A) In precision medicine for cancer patients, cells from tumor biopsies can be used to create *in vitro* tumor models specific to a given patient. Potentially effective drug therapies can then be screened in the models, thereby identifying the safest and most effective drug therapy for that patient. (B) In genetic diseases such as cystic fibrosis of muscular dystrophy, cells can be harvested from alternative tissues, such as skin, turned into induced pluripotent stem cells, differentiated into cells of the tissue of interest (e.g., lung or heart), and biofabricated into 3D organoids, after which drugs can be screened for the original patient.

the overall effectiveness of these systems, including physiological accuracy, response to drugs, and more logistical aspects such as scalability. Implementation of primary cells instead of cell lines, combined with 3D architectures containing extracellular matrix components and supporting cells, appears to be a general framework for improving both construct function, as well as capturing the *in vivo* accuracy of tumor components in such models. Incorporating tumor cells derived from patients will drive development and testing on platforms that are geared towards specific patients, which will almost certainly result in more accurate and effective diagnoses, prognoses, and chemotherapy regimens in the clinic, as well as development of more nuanced and targeted drugs. Combining these high functioning models with platform technologies such as miniaturized devices, automated sensing, and data collection systems, will serve to dramatically increase the throughput of the studies that can be performed. These advances will most likely save researchers significant amounts of time and reduce the currently massive costs associated with bringing new drugs to patients and the market.

On-a-chip technologies have gained significant momentum in recent years, finding use in many research areas and biomedical applliations. While relatively new technologies, many are already showing promise in the hands of researchers. Systems of increased biological complexity have begun to emerge that feature other organoids in addition to the liver (Atac et al. 2013; Maschmeyer et al. 2015; Materne et al. 2015; Wagner et al. 2013). These multi-organoid devices, termed "body-on-a-chip" systems, have vast potential in a variety of applications, but to date have been primarily comprised of cell lines, not fully functional hepatocytes, and as such require additional work to demonstrate their ability to accurately mimic human physiology and responses to environmental factors. As these systems improve and become established and more commonplace, we expect that clinicians and the industry will begin implementing them in day to day operations, resulting in dramatically improved diagnostics, prognostics, and pharmaceutical screening platforms. Ultimately, implementation of these systems will result in improved patient quality of life. Two of the key tools we as researchers have, on which many of these examples of engineered tissue models are built, are biopolymer/biomaterial science and biofabrication technologies. These materials and devices have allowed us to create high functioning 3D tissue constructs that more and more resemble *in vivo* human tissue. To date, no single biomaterial or biofabrication technique is perfect. These will continue to improve; and with them, so will physiological accuracy of engineered tissues and their deployment into biomedical applications.

References

Adachi, N., M. Ochi, M. Deie, A. Nakamae, G. Kamei, Y. Uchio et al. 2014. Implantation of tissue-engineered cartilage-like tissue for the treatment for full-thickness cartilage defects of the knee. Knee surgery, sports traumatology, arthroscopy: Official Journal of the ESSKA 22: 1241–1248, doi:10.1007/s00167-013-2521-0.

Agarwal, A., J. A. Goss, A. Cho, M. L. McCain and K. K. Parker. 2013. Microfluidic heart on a chip for higher throughput pharmacological studies. Lab Chip 13: 3599–3608, doi:10.1039/c3lc50350j.

Ahmed, T. A., E. V. Dare and M. Hincke. 2008. Fibrin: a versatile scaffold for tissue engineering applications. Tissue Eng. Part B Rev. 14: 199–215, doi:10.1089/ten.teb.2007.0435.

Allison, D. D. and K. J. Grande-Allen. 2006. Review. Hyaluronan: a powerful tissue engineering tool. Tissue Eng. 12: 2131–2140, doi:10.1089/ten.2006.12.2131.

Annabi, N., S. Selimovic, J. P. Acevedo Cox, J. Ribas, M. Afshar Bakooshli, D. Heintze et al. 2013. Hydrogel-coated microfluidic channels for cardiomyocyte culture. Lab Chip 13: 3569–3577, doi:10.1039/c3lc50252j.

Atac, B., I. Wagner, R. Horland, R. Lauster, U. Marx, A. G. Tonevitsky et al. 2013. Skin and hair on-a-chip: in vitro skin models versus *ex vivo* tissue maintenance with dynamic perfusion. Lab Chip 13: 3555–3561, doi:10.1039/c3lc50227a.

Atala, A., S. B. Bauer, S. Soker, J. J. Yoo and A. B. Retik. 2006. Tissue-engineered autologous bladders for patients needing cystoplasty. Lancet 367: 1241–1246, doi:10.1016/S0140-6736(06)68438-9.

Au, S. H., M. D. Chamberlain, S. Mahesh, M. V. Sefton and A. R. Wheeler. 2014. Hepatic organoids for microfluidic drug screening. Lab Chip 14: 3290–3299, doi:10.1039/c4lc00531g.

Barrila, J., A. Radtke, S. Sarker, A. Crabbé, M. M. Herbst-Kralovetz, C. M. Ott et al. 2010. 3-D cell culture models: Innovative and predictive platforms for studying human disease pathways and drug design. Nat. Rev. Microbiol. (In press).

Barron, J. A., B. R. Ringeisen, H. Kim, B. J. Spargo and D. B. Chrisey. 2004. Application of laser printing to mammalian cells. Thin Solid Films 453: 383–387.

Benam, K. H., S. Dauth, B. Hassell, A. Herland, A. Jain, K. J. Jang et al. 2015a. Engineered *in vitro* disease models. Ann. Rev. Path. 10: 195–262, doi:10.1146/annurev-pathol-012414-040418.

Benam, K. H., R. Villenave, C. Lucchesi, A. Varone, C. Hubeau, H. H. Lee et al. 2015b. Small airway-on-a-chip enables analysis of human lung inflammation and drug responses *in vitro*. Nat. Methods, doi:10.1038/nmeth.3697.

Berthiaume, F., T. J. Maguire and M. L. Yarmush. 2011. Tissue engineering and regenerative medicine: history, progress, and challenges. Annu. Rev. Chem. Biomol. Eng. 2: 403–430, doi:10.1146/annurev-chembioeng-061010-114257.

Bhise, N. S., J. Ribas, V. Manoharan, Y. S. Zhang, A. Polini, S. Massa et al. 2014. Organ-on-a-chip platforms for studying drug delivery systems. J. Control Release 190: 82–93, doi:10.1016/j.jconrel.2014.05.004.

Billiet, T., M. Vandenhaute, J. Schelfhout, S. Van Vlierberghe and P. Dubruel. 2012. A review of trends and limitations in hydrogel-rapid prototyping for tissue engineering. Biomaterials 33: 6020–6041, doi:10.1016/j.biomaterials.2012.04.050.

Bohandy, J., B. Kim and F. Adrian. 1986. Metal deposition from a supported metal film using an excimer laser. J. Appl. Phys. 60: 1538.

Burdick, J. A. and G. D. Prestwich. 2011. Hyaluronic acid hydrogels for biomedical applications. Adv. Mater. 23: H41–56, doi:10.1002/adma.201003963.

Buwalda, S. J., K. W. Boere, P. J. Dijkstra, J. Feijen, T. Vermonden and W. E. Hennink. 2014. Hydrogels in a historical perspective: from simple networks to smart materials. J. Control Release 190: 254–273, doi:10.1016/j.jconrel.2014.03.052.

Catros, S., J. C. Fricain, B. Guillotin, B. Pippenger, R. Bareille, M. Remy et al. 2011. Laser-assisted bioprinting for creating on-demand patterns of human osteoprogenitor cells and nano-hydroxyapatite. Biofabrication 3: 025001, doi:S1758-5082(11)79099-610.1088/1758-5082/3/2/025001.

Chang, T. T. and M. Hughes-Fulford. 2014. Molecular mechanisms underlying the enhanced functions of three-dimensional hepatocyte aggregates. Biomaterials 35: 2162–2171, doi:10.1016/j.biomaterials.2013.11.063.

Chrisey, D. B. 2000. Materials processing: the power of direct writing. Science 289: 879–881, doi:10.1126/science.289.5481.879.

Cimetta, E., A. Godier-Furnemont and G. Vunjak-Novakovic. 2013. Bioengineering heart tissue for *in vitro* testing. Curr. Opin. Biotechnol. 24: 926–932, doi:10.1016/j.copbio.2013.07.002.

Cohen, J., K. L. Zaleski, G. Nourissat, T. P. Julien, M. A. Randolph and M. J. Yaremchuk. 2011. Survival of porcine mesenchymal stem cells over the alginate recovered cellular method. J. Biomed. Mater. Res. A 96: 93–99, doi:10.1002/jbm.a.32961.

Colina, M., P. Serra, J. M. Fernandez-Pradas, L. Sevilla and J. L. Morenza. 2005. DNA deposition through laser induced forward transfer. Biosens. Bioelectron. 20: 1638–1642, doi:10.1016/j.bios.2004.08.047.

Dinca, V., E. Kasotakis, J. Catherine, A. Mourka, A. Ranella, A. Ovsianikov et al. 2008. Directed three-dimensional patterning of self-assembled peptide fibrils. Nano Letters 8: 538–543, doi:10.1021/nl072798r.

Ding, S., W. Zhang, Z. Xu, C. Xing, H. Xie, H. Guo et al. 2013. Induction of an EMT-like transformation and MET *in vitro*. Journal of Translational Medicine 11: 164, doi:10.1186/1479-5876-11-164.

Dong, Y., A. M. Skelley, K. D. Merdek, K. M. Sprott, C. Jiang, W. E. Pierceall et al. 2013. Microfluidics and circulating tumor cells. The Journal of Molecular Diagnostics : JMD 15: 149–157, doi:10.1016/j.jmoldx.2012.09.004.

Doshi, N., B. Prabhakarpandian, A. Rea-Ramsey, K. Pant, S. Sundaram and S. Mitragotri. 2010. Flow and adhesion of drug carriers in blood vessels depend on their shape: a study using model synthetic microvascular networks. J. Control Release 146: 196–200, doi:10.1016/j.jconrel.2010.04.007.

Douville, N. J., P. Zamankhan, Y. C. Tung, R. Li, B. L. Vaughan, C. F. Tai et al. 2011. Combination of fluid and solid mechanical stresses contribute to cell death and detachment in a microfluidic alveolar model. Lab Chip 11: 609–619, doi:10.1039/c0lc00251h.

Drewitz, M., M. Helbling, N. Fried, M. Bieri, W. Moritz, J. Lichtenberg et al. 2011. Towards automated production and drug sensitivity testing using scaffold-free spherical tumor microtissues. Biotechnol. J. 6: 1488–1496, doi:10.1002/biot.201100290.

Fang, M., C. W. Peng, S. P. Liu, J. P. Yuan and Y. Li. 2013. *In vitro* invasive pattern of hepatocellular carcinoma cell line HCCLM9 based on three-dimensional cell culture and quantum dots molecular imaging. Journal of Huazhong University of Science and Technology. Medical sciences = Hua zhong ke ji da xue xue bao. Yi xue Ying De wen ban = Huazhong keji daxue xuebao. Yixue Yingdewen ban 33: 520–524, doi:10.1007/s11596-013-1152-5.

Fukuda, J., Y. Sakai and K. Nakazawa. 2006. Novel hepatocyte culture system developed using microfabrication and collagen/polyethylene glycol microcontact printing. Biomaterials 27: 1061–1070, doi:10.1016/j.biomaterials.2005.07.031.

Fulco, I., S. Miot, M. D. Haug, A. Barbero, A. Wixmerten, S. Feliciano et al. 2014. Engineered autologous cartilage tissue for nasal reconstruction after tumour resection: an observational first-in-human trial. Lancet 384: 337–346, doi:10.1016/S0140-6736(14)60544-4.

Galus, R., M. Antiszko and P. Wlodarski. 2006. Clinical applications of hyaluronic acid. Pol. Merkur. Lekarski 20: 606–608.

Gomez-Lechon, M. J., J. V. Castell and M. T. Donato. 2010. The use of hepatocytes to investigate drug toxicity. Methods Mol. Biol. 640: 389–415, doi:10.1007/978-1-60761-688-7_21.

Gou, M., X. Qu, W. Zhu, M. Xiang, J. Yang, K. Zhang et al. 2014. Bio-inspired detoxification using 3D-printed hydrogel nanocomposites. Nature communications 5: 3774, doi:10.1038/ncomms4774.

Greenhough, S., C. N. Medine and D. C. Hay. 2010. Pluripotent stem cell derived hepatocyte like cells and their potential in toxicity screening. Toxicology 278: 250–255, doi:S0300-483X(10)00291-10.1016/j.tox.2010.07.012.

Grosberg, A., P. W. Alford, M. L. McCain and K. K. Parker. 2011. Ensembles of engineered cardiac tissues for physiological and pharmacological study: heart on a chip. Lab Chip 11: 4165–4173, doi:10.1039/c1lc20557a.

Gruene, M., A. Deiwick, L. Koch, S. Schlie, C. Unger, N. Hofmann et al. 2010. Laser printing of stem cells for biofabrication of scaffold-free autologous grafts. Tissue Eng. Part C Methods, doi:10.1089/ten.TEC.2010.0359.

Guillemot, F., A. Souquet, S. Catros and B. Guillotin. 2010. Laser-assisted cell printing: principle, physical parameters versus cell fate and perspectives in tissue engineering. Nanomedicine (Lond) 5: 507–515, doi:10.2217/nnm.10.14.

Guillotin, B., A. Souquet, S. Catros, M. Duocastella, B. Pippenger, S. Bellance et al. 2010. Laser assisted bioprinting of engineered tissue with high cell density and microscale organization. Biomaterials 31: 7250–7256, doi:10.1016/j.biomaterials.2010.05.055.

Guillotin, B. and F. Guillemot. 2011. Cell patterning technologies for organotypic tissue fabrication. Trends Biotechnol. 29: 183–190, doi:S0167-7799(10)00220-910.1016/j.tibtech.2010.12.008.

Guyette, J. P., J. Charest, R. W. Mills, B. Jank, P. T. Moser, S. E. Gilpin et al. 2015. Bioengineering human myocardium on native extracellular matrix. Circ. Res., doi:10.1161/CIRCRESAHA.115.306874.

Han, S. K., S. Y. Kim, R. J. Choi, S. H. Jeong and W. K. Kim. 2014. Comparison of tissue-engineered and artificial dermis grafts after removal of basal cell carcinoma on face—a pilot study. Dermatologic surgery : official publication for American Society for Dermatologic Surgery [et al.] 40: 460–467, doi:10.1111/dsu.12446.

Hesse, E., T. E. Hefferan, J. E. Tarara, C. Haasper, R. Meller, C. Krettek et al. 2010. Collagen type I hydrogel allows migration, proliferation, and osteogenic differentiation of rat bone marrow stromal cells. J. Biomed. Mater. Res. A 94: 442–449, doi:10.1002/jbm.a.32696.

Ho, W. J., E. A. Pham, J. W. Kim, C. W. Ng, J. H. Kim, D. T. Kamei et al. 2010. Incorporation of multicellular spheroids into 3-D polymeric scaffolds provides an improved tumor model for screening anticancer drugs. Cancer Science 101: 2637–2643, doi:10.1111/j.1349-7006.2010.01723.x.

Hopp, B., T. Smausz, N. Kresz, N. Barna, Z. Bor, L. Kolozsvari et al. 2005. Survival and proliferative ability of various living cell types after laser-induced forward transfer. Tissue Eng. 11: 1817–1823, doi:10.1089/ten.2005.11.1817.

Hribar, K. C., P. Soman, J. Warner, P. Chung and S. Chen. 2014. Light-assisted direct-write of 3D functional biomaterials. Lab. Chip. 14: 268–275, doi:10.1039/c3lc50634g.

Hu, Y., S. Bian, J. Grotberg, M. Filoche, J. White, S. Takayama et al. 2015. A microfluidic model to study fluid dynamics of mucus plug rupture in small lung airways. Biomicrofluidics 9: 044119, doi:10.1063/1.4928766.

Huh, D., H. Fujioka, Y. C. Tung, N. Futai, R. Paine, 3rd, J. B. Grotberg et al. 2007. Acoustically detectable cellular-level lung injury induced by fluid mechanical stresses in microfluidic airway systems. Proc. Natl. Acad. Sci. U S A 104: 18886–18891, doi:10.1073/pnas.0610868104.

Huh, D., B. D. Matthews, A. Mammoto, M. Montoya-Zavala, H. Y. Hsin and D. E. Ingber. 2010. Reconstituting organ-level lung functions on a chip. Science 328: 1662–1668, doi:10.1126/science.1188302.

Huh, D., D. C. Leslie, B. D. Matthews, J. P. Fraser, S. Jurek, G. A. Hamilton et al. 2012. A human disease model of drug toxicity-induced pulmonary edema in a lung-on-a-chip microdevice. Science Translational Medicine 4: 159ra147, doi:10.1126/scitranslmed.3004249.

Hunt, N. C. and L. M. Grover. 2010. Cell encapsulation using biopolymer gels for regenerative medicine. Biotechnology Letters 32: 733–742, doi:10.1007/s10529-010-0221-0.

Jakab, K., B. Damon, A. Neagu, A. Kachurin and G. Forgacs. 2006. Three-dimensional tissue constructs built by bioprinting. Biorheology 43: 509–513.

Jakab, K., C. Norotte, B. Damon, F. Marga, A. Neagu, C. L. Besch-Williford et al. 2008. Tissue engineering by self-assembly of cells printed into topologically defined structures. Tissue Eng. Part A 14: 413–421.

Kang, J. H., S. Krause, H. Tobin, A. Mammoto, M. Kanapathipillai and D. E. Ingber. 2012. A combined micromagnetic-microfluidic device for rapid capture and culture of rare circulating tumor cells. Lab. Chip. 12: 2175–2181, doi:10.1039/c2lc40072c.

Kang, Y. B., T. R. Sodunke, J. Lamontagne, J. Cirillo, C. Rajiv, M. J. Bouchard et al. 2015. Liver sinusoid on a chip: long-term layered co-culture of primary rat hepatocytes and endothelial cells in microfluidic platforms. Biotechnol. Bioeng., doi:10.1002/bit.25659.

Kaul, H. and Y. Ventikos. 2015. On the genealogy of tissue engineering and regenerative medicine. Tissue Eng. Part B Rev. 21: 203–217, doi:10.1089/ten.TEB.2014.0285.

Kim, D., S. Finkenstaedt-Quinn, K. R. Hurley, J. T. Buchman and C. L. Haynes. 2014. On-chip evaluation of platelet adhesion and aggregation upon exposure to mesoporous silica nanoparticles. The Analyst 139: 906–913, doi:10.1039/c3an01679j.

Kim, J. Y., D. A. Fluri, R. Marchan, K. Boonen, S. Mohanty, P. Singh et al. 2015. 3D spherical microtissues and microfluidic technology for multi-tissue experiments and analysis. J. Biotechnol. 205: 24–35, doi:10.1016/j.jbiotec.2015.01.003.

Kirby, B. J., M. Jodari, M. S. Loftus, G. Gakhar, E. D. Pratt, C. Chanel-Vos et al. 2012. Functional characterization of circulating tumor cells with a prostate-cancer-specific microfluidic device. PLoS One 7: e35976, doi:10.1371/journal.pone.0035976.

Kirker, K. R., Y. Luo, S. E. Morris, J. Shelby and G. D. Prestwich. 2004. Glycosaminoglycan hydrogels as supplemental wound dressings for donor sites. J. Burn Care Rehabil. 25: 276–286.

Knudson, C. B. and W. Knudson. 2001. Cartilage proteoglycans. Semin. Cell Dev. Biol. 12: 69–78.

Koch, L., S. Kuhn, H. Sorg, M. Gruene, S. Schlie, R. Gaebel et al. 2010. Laser printing of skin cells and human stem cells. Tissue Eng. Part C Methods 16: 847–854, doi:10.1089/ten.TEC.2009.0397.

Kolhar, P., A. C. Anselmo, V. Gupta, K. Pant, B. Prabhakarpandian, E. Ruoslahti et al. 2013. Using shape effects to target antibody-coated nanoparticles to lung and brain endothelium. Proc. Natl. Acad. Sci. U S A 110: 10753–10758, doi:10.1073/pnas.1308345110.

Korin, N., M. Kanapathipillai, B. D. Matthews, M. Crescente, A. Brill, T. Mammoto et al. 2012. Shear-activated nanotherapeutics for drug targeting to obstructed blood vessels. Science 337: 738–742, doi:10.1126/science.1217815.

Kunz-Schughart, L. A., J. P. Freyer, F. Hofstaedter and R. Ebner. 2004. The use of 3-D cultures for high-throughput screening: the multicellular spheroid model. J. Biomol. Screen 9: 273–285, doi:10.1177/1087057104265040.

Kuo, J. W. 2006. Practical Aspects of Hyaluronan Based Medical Products. CRC/Taylor & Francis, Boca Raton.

Lamberti, G., Y. Tang, B. Prabhakarpandian, Y. Wang, K. Pant, M. F. Kiani et al. 2013. Adhesive interaction of functionalized particles and endothelium in idealized microvascular networks. Microvasc. Res. 89: 107–114, doi:10.1016/j.mvr.2013.03.007.

Lang, R., M. M. Stern, L. Smith, Y. Liu, S. Bharadwaj, G. Liu et al. 2011. Three-dimensional culture of hepatocytes on porcine liver tissue-derived extracellular matrix. Biomaterials 32: 7042–7052, doi:S0142-9612(11)00670-310.1016/j.biomaterials.2011.06.005.

Lei, K. F. and C. H. Huang. 2014. Paper-based microreactor integrating cell culture and subsequent immunoassay for the investigation of cellular phosphorylation. ACS Appl. Mater. Interfaces 6: 22423–22429, doi:10.1021/am506388q.

Li, P., Z. S. Stratton, M. Dao, J. Ritz and T. J. Huang. 2013. Probing circulating tumor cells in microfluidics. Lab. Chip. 13: 602–609, doi:10.1039/c2lc90148j.

Lin, H., D. Zhang, P. G. Alexander, G. Yang, J. Tan, A. W. Cheng et al. 2013. Application of visible light-based projection stereolithography for live cell-scaffold fabrication with designed architecture. Biomaterials 34: 331–339, doi:10.1016/j.biomaterials.2012.09.048.

Liu, Y., X. Z. Shu and G. D. Prestwich. 2007. Tumor engineering: orthotopic cancer models in mice using cell-loaded, injectable, cross-linked hyaluronan-derived hydrogels. Tissue Eng. 13: 1091–1101.

Malda, J., J. Visser, F. P. Melchels, T. Jungst, W. E. Hennink, W. J. Dhert et al. 2013. 25th anniversary article: engineering hydrogels for biofabrication. Adv. Mater. 25: 5011–5028, doi:10.1002/adma.201302042.

Marga, F., K. Jakab, C. Khatiwala, B. Shepherd, S. Dorfman, B. Hubbard et al. 2012. Toward engineering functional organ modules by additive manufacturing. Biofabrication 4: 022001, doi:10.1088/1758-5082/4/2/022001.

Martewicz, S., F. Michielin, E. Serena, A. Zambon, M. Mongillo and N. Elvassore. 2012. Reversible alteration of calcium dynamics in cardiomyocytes during acute hypoxia transient in a microfluidic platform. Integr Biol. (Camb) 4: 153–164, doi:10.1039/c1ib00087j.

Maschmeyer, I., A. K. Lorenz, K. Schimek, T. Hasenberg, A. P. Ramme, J. Hubner et al. 2015. A four-organ-chip for interconnected long-term co-culture of human intestine, liver, skin and kidney equivalents. Lab. Chip. 15: 2688–2699, doi:10.1039/c5lc00392j.

Materne, E. M., I. Maschmeyer, A. K. Lorenz, R. Horland, K. M. Schimek, M. Busek et al. 2015. The multi-organ chip—a microfluidic platform for long-term multi-tissue coculture. J. Vis. Exp., e52526, doi:10.3791/52526.

Maver, T., U. Maver, K. S. Kleinschek, I. M. Rascan and D. M. Smrke. 2015. Advanced therapies of skin injuries. Wiener klinische Wochenschrift, doi:10.1007/s00508-015-0859-7.

McKim, J. M., Jr. 2010. Building a tiered approach to *in vitro* predictive toxicity screening: a focus on assays with *in vivo* relevance. Comb. Chem. High Throughput Screen 13: 188–206.

Meinel, L. and D. L. Kaplan. 2012. Silk constructs for delivery of musculoskeletal therapeutics. Adv. Drug Deliv. Rev. 64: 1111–1122, doi:S0169-409X(12)00121-410.1016/j.addr.2012.03.016.

Messner, S., I. Agarkova, W. Moritz and J. M. Kelm. 2013. Multi-cell type human liver microtissues for hepatotoxicity testing. Arch. Toxicol. 87: 209–213, doi:10.1007/s00204-012-0968-2.

Miki, D., K. Dastgheib, T. Kim, A. Pfister-Serres, K. A. Smeds, M. Inoue et al. 2002. A photopolymerized sealant for corneal lacerations. Cornea 21: 393–399.

Mironov, V., R. P. Visconti, V. Kasyanov, G. Forgacs, C. J. Drake and R. R. Markwald. 2009. Organ printing: tissue spheroids as building blocks. Biomaterials 30: 2164–2174, doi:S0142-9612(09)00005-210.1016/j.biomaterials.2008.12.084.

Mori, R., Y. Sakai and K. Nakazawa. 2008. Micropatterned organoid culture of rat hepatocytes and HepG2 cells. J. Biosci. Bioeng. 106: 237–242, doi:10.1263/jbb.106.237.

Nam, K. H., A. S. Smith, S. Lone, S. Kwon and D. H. Kim. 2015. Biomimetic 3D tissue models for advanced high-throughput drug screening. J. Lab. Autom. 20: 201–215, doi:10.1177/2211068214557813.

Natarajan, A., M. Stancescu, V. Dhir, C. Armstrong, F. Sommerhage, J. J. Hickman et al. 2011. Patterned cardiomyocytes on microelectrode arrays as a functional, high information content drug screening platform. Biomaterials 32: 4267–4274, doi:10.1016/j.biomaterials.2010.12.022.

Nguyen, K. T. and J. L. West. 2002. Photopolymerizable hydrogels for tissue engineering applications. Biomaterials 23: 4307–4314.

Nickerson, C. A. and C. M. Ott. 2004. A new dimension in modeling infectious disease (Invited Review). ASM News 70: 169–175.

Nickerson, C. A., E. G. Richter and C. M. Ott. 2007. Studying host-pathogen interactions in 3-D: organotypic models for infectious disease and drug development. J. Neuroimmune Pharmacol. 2: 26–31, doi:10.1007/s11481-006-9047-x.

Nicodemus, G. D. and S. J. Bryant. 2008. Cell encapsulation in biodegradable hydrogels for tissue engineering applications. Tissue Eng. Part B Rev. 14: 149–165, doi:10.1089/ten.teb.2007.0332.

Nordt, S. P., A. Minns, C. Tomaszewski, F. L. Cantrell and R. F. Clark. 2010. Retrospective review of digoxin exposures to a poison control system following recall of Digitek(R) tablets. Am. J. Cardiovasc. Drugs 10: 261–263, doi:10.2165/11537640-000000000-00000.

Norotte, C., F. S. Marga, L. E. Niklason and G. Forgacs. 2009. Scaffold-free vascular tissue engineering using bioprinting. Biomaterials 30: 5910–5917, doi:S0142-9612(09)00640-110.1016/j.biomaterials.2009.06.034 [doi].

Oerlemans, A. J., M. E. van Hoek, E. van Leeuwen and W. J. Dekkers. 2014. Hype and expectations in tissue engineering. Regen. Med. 9: 113–122, doi:10.2217/rme.13.89.

Opara, E. C., S. H. Mirmalek-Sani, O. Khanna, M. L. Moya and E. M. Brey. 2010. Design of a bioartificial pancreas(+). J. Investig. Med. 58: 831–837, doi:10.231/JIM.0b013e3181ed3807.

Ott, H. C., T. S. Matthiesen, S. K. Goh, L. D. Black, S. M. Kren, T. I. Netoff et al. 2008. Perfusion-decellularized matrix: using nature's platform to engineer a bioartificial heart. Nat. Med. 14: 213–221, doi:10.1038/nm1684.

Ouattara, D. A., J. M. Prot, A. Bunescu, M. E. Dumas, B. Elena-Herrmann, E. Leclerc et al. 2012. Metabolomics-on-a-chip and metabolic flux analysis for label-free modeling of the internal metabolism of HepG2/C3A cells. Molecular bioSystems 8: 1908–1920, doi:10.1039/c2mb25049g.

Pescosolido, L., W. Schuurman, J. Malda, P. Matricardi, F. Alhaique, T. Coviello et al. 2011. Hyaluronic acid and dextran-based semi-IPN hydrogels as biomaterials for bioprinting. Biomacromolecules 12: 1831–1838, doi:10.1021/bm200178w.

Polini, A., L. Prodanov, N. S. Bhise, V. Manoharan, M. R. Dokmeci and A. Khademhosseini. 2014. Organs-on-a-chip: a new tool for drug discovery. Expert Opin. Drug Discov. 9: 335–352, doi:10.1517/17460441.2014.886562.

Prestwich, G. D., Y. Liu, B. Yu, X. Z. Shu and A. Scott. 2007. 3-D culture in synthetic extracellular matrices: new tissue models for drug toxicology and cancer drug discovery. Adv. Enzyme Regul. 47: 196–207, doi:S0065-2571(06)00070-710.1016/j.advenzreg.2006.12.012.

Prestwich, G. D. 2008. Evaluating drug efficacy and toxicology in three dimensions: using synthetic extracellular matrices in drug discovery. Acc. Chem. Res. 41: 139–148.

Prestwich, G. D. and J. W. Kuo. 2008. Chemically-modified HA for therapy and regenerative medicine. Curr. Pharm. Biotechnol. 9: 242–245.

Prodanov, L., R. Jindal, S. S. Bale, M. Hegde, W. J. McCarty, I. Golberg et al. 2015. Long term maintenance of a microfluidic 3-D human liver sinusoid. Biotechnol. Bioeng., doi:10.1002/bit.25700.

Raya-Rivera, A., D. R. Esquiliano, J. J. Yoo, E. Lopez-Bayghen, S. Soker and A. Atala. 2011. Tissue-engineered autologous urethras for patients who need reconstruction: an observational study. Lancet 377: 1175–1182, doi:10.1016/S0140-6736(10)62354-9.

Raya-Rivera, A. M., D. Esquiliano, R. Fierro-Pastrana, E. Lopez-Bayghen, P. Valencia, R. Ordorica-Flores et al. 2014. Tissue-engineered autologous vaginal organs in patients: a pilot cohort study. Lancet 384: 329–336, doi:10.1016/S0140-6736(14)60542-00.

Ruppen, J., F. D. Wildhaber, C. Strub, S. R. Hall, R. A. Schmid, T. Geiser et al. 2015. Towards personalized medicine: chemosensitivity assays of patient lung cancer cell spheroids in a perfused microfluidic platform. Lab. Chip. 15: 3076–3085, doi:10.1039/c5lc00454c.

Samuel, S. P., N. Jain, F. O'Dowd, T. Paul, D. Kashanin, V. A. Gerard et al. 2012. Multifactorial determinants that govern nanoparticle uptake by human endothelial cells under flow. Int. J. Nanomedicine 7: 2943–2956, doi:10.2147/IJN.S30624.

Santos, E., J. Zarate, G. Orive, R. M. Hernandez and J. L. Pedraz. 2010. Biomaterials in cell microencapsulation. Adv. Exp. Med. Biol. 670: 5–21.

Schiavinato, A., M. Finesso, R. Cortivo and G. Abatangelo. 2002. Comparison of the effects of intra-articular injections of Hyaluronan and its chemically cross-linked derivative (Hylan G-F20) in normal rabbit knee joints. Clin. Exp. Rheumatol. 20: 445–454.

Shen, B., E. S. Chu, G. Zhao, K. Man, C. W. Wu, J. T. Cheng et al. 2012. PPARgamma inhibits hepatocellular carcinoma metastases *in vitro* and in mice. Br. J. Cancer 106: 1486–1494, doi:10.1038/bjc.2012.130.

Shimizu, T., M. Yamato, Y. Isoi, T. Akutsu, T. Setomaru, K. Abe et al. 2002. Fabrication of pulsatile cardiac tissue grafts using a novel 3-dimensional cell sheet manipulation technique and temperature-responsive cell culture surfaces. Circ. Res. 90: e40.

Skardal, A., S. F. Sarker, A. Crabbe, C. A. Nickerson and G. D. Prestwich. 2010a. The generation of 3-D tissue models based on hyaluronan hydrogel-coated microcarriers within a rotating wall vessel bioreactor. Biomaterials 31: 8426–8435, doi:S0142-9612(10)00890-210.1016/j.biomaterials.2010.07.047.

Skardal, A., J. Zhang, L. McCoard, X. Xu, S. Oottamasathien and G. D. Prestwich. 2010b. Photocrosslinkable hyaluronan-gelatin hydrogels for two-step bioprinting. Tissue Eng. Part A 16: 2675–2685, doi:10.1089/ten.TEA.2009.0798.

Skardal, A., J. Zhang, L. McCoard, S. Oottamasathien and G. D. Prestwich. 2010c. Dynamically crosslinked gold nanoparticle—hyaluronan hydrogels. Adv. Mater. 22: 4736–4740, doi:10.1002/adma.201001436.

Skardal, A., D. Mack, E. Kapetanovic, A. Atala, J. D. Jackson, J. Yoo et al. 2012a. Bioprinted amniotic fluid-derived stem cells accelerate healing of large skin wounds. Stem Cells Transl. Med. 1: 792–802, doi:sctm.2012-008810.5966/sctm.2012-0088.

Skardal, A., L. Smith, S. Bharadwaj, A. Atala, S. Soker and Y. Zhang. 2012b. Tissue specific synthetic ECM hydrogels for 3-D *in vitro* maintenance of hepatocyte function. Biomaterials 33: 4565–4575, doi:S0142-9612(12)00321-310.1016/j.biomaterials.2012.03.034.

Skardal, A. 2015. Bioprinting essentials of cell and protein viability. pp. 1–17. Essentials of 3D Biofabrication and Translation. *In*: A. Atala and J. J. Yoo (eds.). Elsevier. London Wall, UK.

Skardal, A. and A. Atala. 2015. Biomaterials for integration with 3-D bioprinting. Annals of Biomedical Engineering 43(3): 730–746, doi:10.1007/s10439-014-1207-1.

Skardal, A., M. Devarasetty, H. W. Kang, I. Mead, C. Bishop, T. Shupe et al. 2015a. A hydrogel bioink toolkit for mimicking native tissue biochemical and mechanical properties in bioprinted tissue constructs. Acta Biomater. 25: 24–34, doi:10.1016/j.actbio.2015.07.030.

Skardal, A., M. Devarasetty, C. Rodman, A. Atala and S. Soker. 2015b. Liver-tumor hybrid organoids for modeling tumor growth and drug response *in vitro*. Ann. Biomed. Eng. 43(10): 2361–2373.

Skardal, A., M. Devarasetty, S. Soker and A. R. Hall. 2015c. *In situ* patterned micro 3-D liver constructs for parallel toxicology testing in a fluidic device. Biofabrication 7(3): 031001.

Soman, P., P. H. Chung, A. P. Zhang and S. Chen. 2013. Digital microfabrication of user-defined 3D microstructures in cell-laden hydrogels. Biotechnol. Bioeng. 110: 3038–3047, doi:10.1002/bit.24957.

Sung, J. H. and M. L. Shuler. 2009. A micro cell culture analog (microCCA) with 3-D hydrogel culture of multiple cell lines to assess metabolism-dependent cytotoxicity of anti-cancer drugs. Lab. Chip. 9: 1385–1394, doi:10.1039/b901377f.

Tan, H., C. M. Ramirez, N. Miljkovic, H. Li, J. P. Rubin and K. G. Marra. 2009. Thermosensitive injectable hyaluronic acid hydrogel for adipose tissue engineering. Biomaterials 30: 6844–6853, doi:10.1016/j.biomaterials.2009.08.058.

Tavana, H., P. Zamankhan, P. J. Christensen, J. B. Grotberg and S. Takayama. 2011. Epithelium damage and protection during reopening of occluded airways in a physiologic microfluidic pulmonary airway model. Biomed. Microdevices 13: 731–742, doi:10.1007/s10544-011-9543-5.

Torisawa, Y. S., A. Takagi, Y. Nashimoto, T. Yasukawa, H. Shiku and T. A. Matsue. 2007. Multicellular spheroid array to realize spheroid formation, culture, and viability assay on a chip. Biomaterials 28: 559–566, doi:10.1016/j.biomaterials.2006.08.054.

Vidi, P. A., T. Maleki, M. Ochoa, L. Wang, S. M. Clark, J. F. Leary et al. 2014. Disease-on-a-chip: mimicry of tumor growth in mammary ducts. Lab. Chip. 14: 172–177, doi:10.1039/c3lc50819f.

Wagner, I., E. M. Materne, S. Brincker, U. Sussbier, C. Fradrich, M. Busek et al. 2013. A dynamic multi-organ-chip for long-term cultivation and substance testing proven by 3D human liver and skin tissue co-culture. Lab. Chip. 13: 3538–3547, doi:10.1039/c3lc50234a.

Wheeler, S. E., J. T. Borenstein, A. M. Clark, M. R. Ebrahimkhani, I. J. Fox., L. Griffith et al. 2013. All-human microphysical model of metastasis therapy. Stem Cell Res. Ther. 4 Suppl. 1: S11, doi:10.1186/scrt372.

Williams, D. 2011. The continuing evolution of biomaterials. Biomaterials 32: 1–2, doi:S0142-9612(10)01245-710.1016/j.biomaterials.2010.09.048.

Williams, D. F. 2009. On the nature of biomaterials. Biomaterials 30: 5897–5909, doi:S0142-9612(09)00726-110.1016/j.biomaterials.2009.07.027.

Wlodkowic, D. and J. M. Cooper. 2010. Tumors on chips: oncology meets microfluidics. Curr. Opin. Chem. Biol. 14: 556–567, doi:10.1016/j.cbpa.2010.08.016.

Xu, Z., Y. Gao, Y. Hao, E. Li, Y. Wang, J. Zhang et al. 2013. Application of a microfluidic chip-based 3D co-culture to test drug sensitivity for individualized treatment of lung cancer. Biomaterials 34: 4109–4117, doi:10.1016/j.biomaterials.2013.02.045.

Yang, Y., X. Yang, J. Zou, C. Jia, Y. Hu, H. Du et al. 2015. Evaluation of photodynamic therapy efficiency using an *in vitro* three-dimensional microfluidic breast cancer tissue model. Lab. Chip. 15: 735–744, doi:10.1039/c4lc01065e.

Ye, N., J. Qin, W. Shi, X. Liu and B. Lin. 2007a. Cell-based high content screening using an integrated microfluidic device. Lab. Chip. 7: 1696–1704, doi:10.1039/b711513j.

Ye, N., J. Qin, X. Liu, W. Shi and B. Lin. 2007b. Characterizing doxorubicin-induced apoptosis in HepG2 cells using an integrated microfluidic device. Electrophoresis 28: 1146–1153, doi:10.1002/elps.200600450.

Yeon, B., M. H. Park, H. J. Moon, S. J. Kim, Y. W. Cheon and B. Jeong. 2013. 3D culture of adipose-tissue-derived stem cells mainly leads to chondrogenesis in poly(ethylene glycol)-poly(L-alanine) diblock copolymer thermogel. Biomacromolecules 14: 3256–3266, doi:10.1021/bm400868j.

Yeon, J. H. and J. K. Park. 2005. Cytotoxicity test based on electrochemical impedance measurement of HepG2 cultured in microfabricated cell chip. Analytical Biochemistry 341: 308–315, doi:10.1016/j.ab.2005.03.047.

Yip, D. and C. H. Cho. 2013. A multicellular 3D heterospheroid model of liver tumor and stromal cells in collagen gel for anti-cancer drug testing. Biochem. Biophys. Res. Commun. 433: 327–332, doi:10.1016/j.bbrc.2013.03.008.

Young, E. W., M. W. Watson, S. Srigunapalan, A. R. Wheeler and C. A. Simmons. 2010. Technique for real-time measurements of endothelial permeability in a microfluidic membrane chip using laser-induced fluorescence detection. Analytical Chem. 82: 808–816, doi:10.1021/ac901560w.

Young, E. W. 2013. Cells, tissues, and organs on chips: challenges and opportunities for the cancer tumor microenvironment. Integr. Biol. (Camb) 5: 1096–1109, doi:10.1039/c3ib40076j.

Zanella, F., R. C. Lyon and F. Sheikh. 2014. Modeling heart disease in a dish: from somatic cells to disease-relevant cardiomyocytes. Trends Cardiovasc. Med. 24: 32–44, doi:10.1016/j.tcm.2013.06.002.

Zhang, A. P., X. Qu, P. Soman, K. C. Hribar, J. W. Lee, S. Chen et al. 2012. Rapid fabrication of complex 3D extracellular microenvironments by dynamic optical projection stereolithography. Adv. Mater. 24: 4266–4270, doi:10.1002/adma.201202024.

Zhang, J., A. Skardal and G. D. Prestwich. 2008. Engineered extracellular matrices with cleavable crosslinkers for cell expansion and easy cell recovery. Biomaterials 29: 4521–4531, doi:S0142-9612(08)00565-610.1016/j.biomaterials.2008.08.008.

7

Medical Application of Polyampholytes

Kazuaki Matsumura,* Robin Rajan, Sana Ahmed and
Minkle Jain

Introduction

Polyampholytes from Bio-based Polymers

Polyampholytes are polymers that carry both positive and negative charges. There are two types of polyampholytes: one in which the existence of positive and negative charges is owing to the presence of anionic and cationic monomers, and one in which the presence of a zwitterion is responsible for both charges. The term polyampholytes refers to a broad array of polymers including both types mentioned above; however, in recent times, zwitterionic polymers in themselves have emerged as a new class of polymers. The main difference between the two types of polyampholytes is that in the former case, the charge of the polymer backbone can be easily changed or tuned by changing the ratio of the two monomers. Thus, in these polymers, one charge can dominate and the net charge of the polymer may be either positive, negative or zero. However, in zwitterionic polyampholytes, the net charge is usually zero under normal conditions because of the presence of an equal number of positive and negative charges. This type of polyampholyte displays a hybrid-like property profile owing to

School of Materials Science, Japan Advanced Institute of Science and Technology 1-1 Asahidai, Nomi, Ishikawa, 923-1292, JAPAN.
* Corresponding author: mkazuaki@jaist.ac.jp

the presence of a high population of polymer-bound ion pairs attached to the polymer chain (Laschewsky 2014).

Because of their properties, polyampholytes have been receiving increased research attention, as evidenced by the increasing number of research articles (Fig. 1). Protein is one class of polyampholytes, and multiple bio-based polyampholytes such as polypeptide- and polysaccharide-derived polymers have been synthesized and characterized for various types of biomaterial applications (Kudaibergenov 2002). The biomedical applications of polyampholytes in various fields like tissue engineering, non-fouling agents, drug delivery, and membrane applications, have been reviewed by Zurick and Bernards (2014).

Polyampholytes as cryoprotectants

Cryopreservation of living cells is crucial in biological, medical, and agricultural research fields and in the clinical practice of reproductive medicine. Recently, Matsumura and Hyon (2009) showed that polyampholytes can be effective cryoprotective agents (CPAs). CPAs are additives provided to cells before freezing to enhance post-thaw survival. They introduced a negative charge in a cationic bio-based polymer, ε-poly-L-lysine (ε-PLL), by using succinic anhydride (SA). ε-PLL is an L-lysine homopolymer biosynthesized by *Streptomyces* species. It is used as a food additive owing to its antimicrobial activities ascribed to the cationic charge density of its side-chain α-amino groups. At an appropriate cation to anion charge ratio (65% of the α-amino groups were converted into carboxyl groups), the polyampholytes showed remarkable CPA efficacy and cells exhibited a viability after freezing that was significantly higher than that with dimethyl sulfoxide (DMSO). Moreover, due to the inherently lower osmotic pressure of carboxylated PLL (COOH-PLL) (even after neutralization with HCl or NaOH) than that of DMSO, higher concentrations of COOH-PLL can be employed without significant loss of cell viability (Fig. 2).

COOH-PLL also showed excellent biocompatibility, as evident from the retention of proliferation ability of the cells after cryopreservation in the presence of COOH-PLL. Cytotoxicity studies revealed that DMSO has far greater cytotoxicity than COOH-PLL. The use of COOH-PLL eliminates the need to immediately remove the CPA after thawing, a problem persistent with DMSO due to its high cytotoxicity. Preliminary analysis of the antifreeze properties of the polymer revealed that it suppresses ice recrystallization.

Matsumura et al. (2010) established that this polyampholyte can be used for cryopreservation of various types of cells, including primary cells, derived cells, adhesive and floating cells, etc. In another study, the authors showed that COOH-PLL enables long-term cryopreservation. They were able to successfully cryopreserve human bone marrow cells (hBMSCs) for up to 24 months, suggesting that COOH-PLL does not affect the phenotypic characteristics and proliferative ability of the cells (Matsumura et al. 2013).

To ascertain the requirement for both charges in the polymer and to determine whether cryopreservation is a property of PLL alone or is a general property of polyampholytes, they synthesized another polyampholyte: aminated polyacrylic

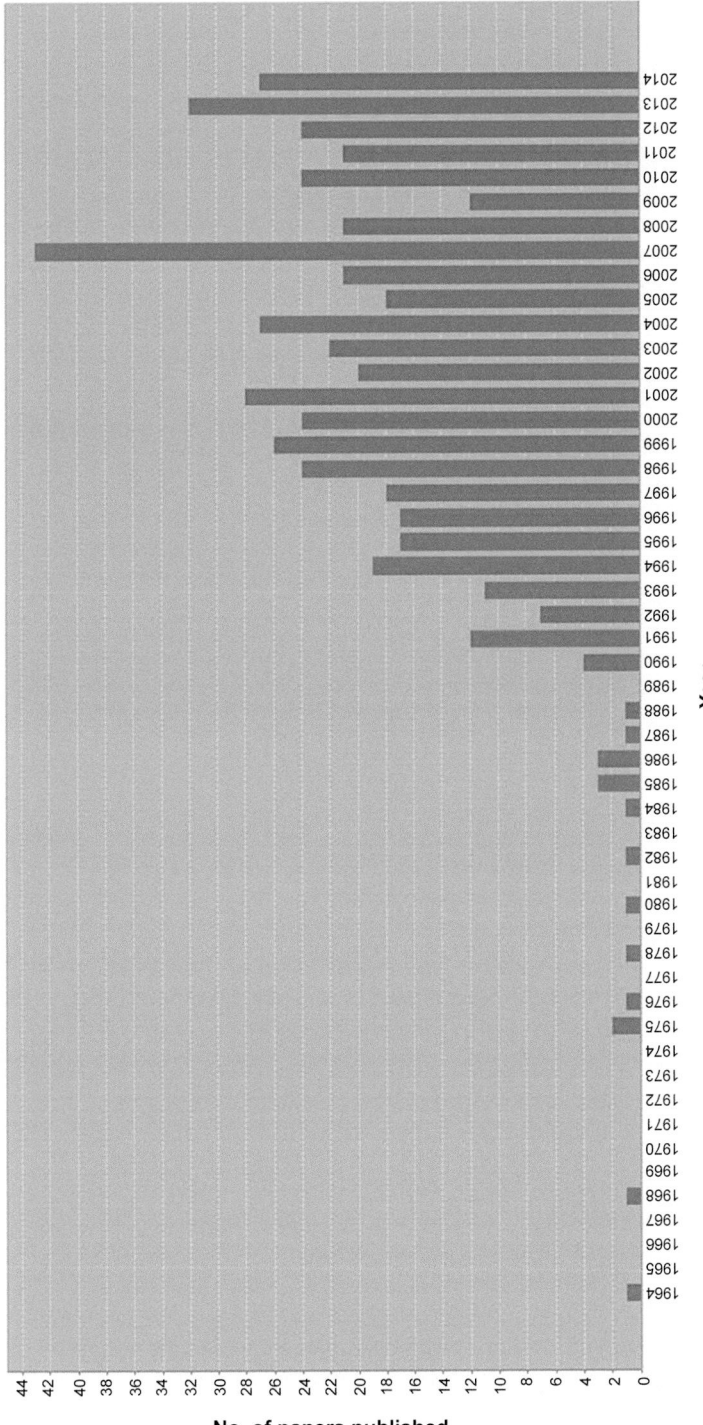

Fig. 1: Comparison of the number of publications related to polyampholytes in the period 1964–2014 (Data collected on the basis of title search from Web of Science, Thomson Reuters).

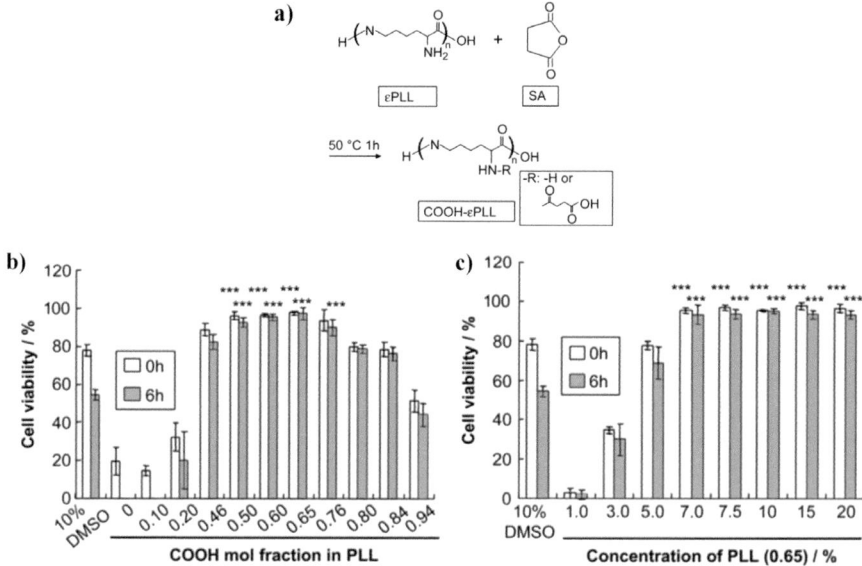

Fig. 2: (a) Schematic representation of the PLL succinylation reaction. Cryoprotective properties of COOH-PLLs. (a) L929 cells were cryopreserved with 10% DMSO and 7.5% (w/w) PLL with different ratios of introduced COOH. Cell viability immediately (white bars), and 6 h (gray bars) after thawing at 37°C. (b) L929 cells were cryopreserved with various concentrations of PLL (0.65). Cell viability immediately (white bars), and 6 h (gray bars) after thawing at 37°C. Data are expressed as the mean ± SD for three independent experiments (five samples each). ***P < 0.001 vs. 10% DMSO for the corresponding time period (0 or 6 h) (From Matsumura and Hyon 2009 with permission).

acid (NH$_2$-PAAc). The use of unaminated PAAc resulted in very low cell viability; however, when the NH$_2$ group was introduced, cell viability enhanced significantly.

The above-mentioned findings have led to the development of multiple polyampholytes for cryopreservation. Rajan et al. (2013) developed a completely synthetic polyampholyte via reversible addition fragmentation chain transfer (RAFT) polymerization. To this end, the authors prepared a 1:1 equimolar mixture of random copolymer of methacrylic acid and 2-(dimethylamino) ethyl methacrylate. This copolymer showed remarkable cryoprotective efficiency, and this study established the universal acceptability of polyampholytes as cryoprotectants. Because of the synthetic nature of this polyampholyte and the resultant ease of modification, various hydrophobic and hydrophilic groups were introduced to the copolymer. The results highlighted the significance of hydrophobicity of a polyampholyte in the cryopreservation process. With the increase in hydrophobicity, cell viability increased significantly and more than 96% viability was obtained with a meagre amount of hydrophobic moiety (5% introduction) at 10% polymer concentration. Analogous to COOH-PLL, this polyampholyte showed excellent biocompatibility. A preliminary mechanistic study with the synthetic polyampholyte revealed that it protects the cell membrane during freezing and prevents membrane rupture, and introduction of hydrophobicity further assisted in the membrane protection. The mechanism of cell protection may be related to cell membrane absorption of polyampholytes, which may reduce freezing damage to cell membranes. It was revealed that the concentrations of COOH-PLL that exhibit the cryoprotective activities described above also possess anti-freeze protein (AFP)-like properties. It has been reported that some AFP-like proteins have membrane protective properties. AFPs prevent freezing and induce freeze tolerance by binding to the surface of ice crystals to lower the freezing point of water noncolligatively and inhibit ice recrystallization (Griffith and Yaish 2004).

Matsumura et al. (2011) implemented this strategy to vitrify human induced pluripotent (iPS) cells using COOH-PLL, and they showed that the cells retained their pluripotency. Additionally, using this polyampholyte eliminated the need to add DMSO or serum proteins. The versatility of this polyampholyte was further demonstrated by Maehara et al. (2013), who vitrified a cell sheet in liquid nitrogen vapor using a vitrification solution containing DMSO, ethylene glycol (EG), sucrose, and 10% COOH-PLL. Vitrification refers to the process of transformation of any substance into a glassy state, involves cooling at very fast rate, and causes an enormous increase in viscosity. By averting mechanical damage caused by ice crystals and resisting the change in salt concentration, vitrification prevents major damage to cells. Fracturing of the fragile cell sheet after vitrification and rewarming was prevented by coating the cell sheet with a viscous vitrification solution, which contained both permeable and non-permeable CPAs (Maehara et al. 2013). The vitrification process did not damage the macro- and microstructures of the cell sheets, and hence, possesses excellent potential for applications related to clinical cell sheet therapy (Fig. 3).

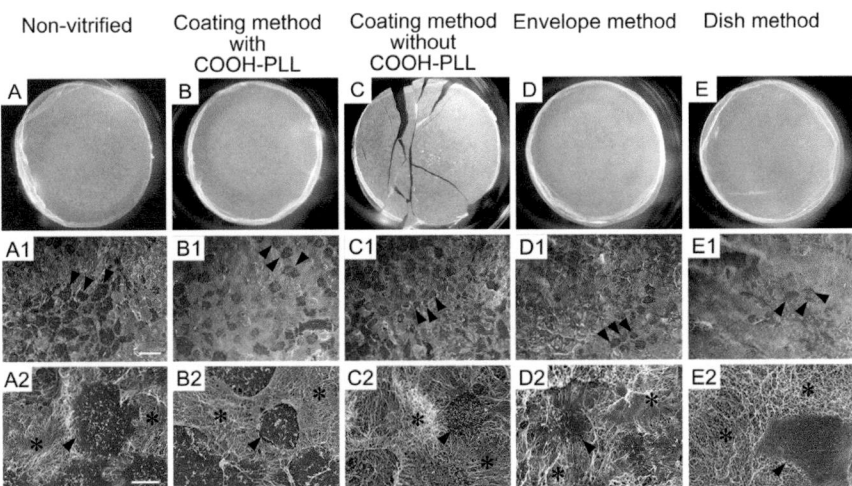

Fig. 3: Macro- and microstructures of triple-layered rabbit chondrocyte sheets after vitrification. A-E: Morphological appearance of chondrocyte sheets after vitrification and rewarming. A1–E2: Scanning electron microscopic images of the surfaces of cell sheets recovered after vitrification and rewarming. A1–E1: ×300, Scale bar = 50 μm; A2–E2: ×2,000, Scale bar = 10 μm. The surfaces (A1–E2) are irregular, featuring pavement-like cell populations (arrowheads in A1–E1 indicate representative three cells) and well-developed extracellular matrices with a dense fibrous structure (*). The microstructures of cell sheets vitrified by any of the methods described in this report were similar to those of the non-vitrified control sample (From Maehara et al. 2013 with permission).

Present-day cryopreservation methods work well for cells but are less effective for large cell-biomaterial constructs. Thus, new strategies need to be developed for construction of "off-the-shelf" tissue-engineered products for clinical development. To this end, Jain et al. (2014) developed a cryoprotective hydrogel based on polyampholytes in which cells can be encapsulated for cryopreservation. The authors utilized crosslinking chemistry that not only eliminated the concerns regarding cytotoxicity but also provided a convenient route to develop *in-situ* hydrogels. In the first step, they functionalized dextran with azide groups (azide-Dex) to incorporate crosslinking sites, followed by reaction with PLL to introduce positive charges in the system. Negative charges were added by reacting with SA, which resulted in the formation of dextran polyampholyte (azide-Dex-PA). In the next step, they synthesized alkyne-functionalized dextran with dibenzylcyclooctyne (DBCO-Dex). Then, azide-Dex-PA and DBCO-Dex were mixed with cells to form *in-situ* hydrogels with azide-alkyne Cu-free click chemistry. This hydrogel could successfully cryopreserve cells, enabling long-term storage and making it a suitable off-the-shelf tissue-engineered product.

This potential of the cryoprotective polyampholyte was extended to other biological systems including oocytes. Watanabe et al. (2013) vitrified mouse oocytes using COOH-PLL and were successful in producing live offspring. They showed that a solution of EG and COOH-PLL maintained the developmental ability of the oocytes *in vitro*. Vitrification with this mixture at certain concentrations resulted in significantly improved *in vivo* development, which may result in increased developmental ability beyond the blastocyst stage *in vivo*.

Vorontsov et al. (2014) investigated the characteristics and mechanism of the antifreeze effect of COOH-PLL on the growth of ice crystals by studying the crystallization of ice in the presence of COOH-PLL in free-growth experiments. To this end, they designed a growth cell with various degrees of supercooling. They observed hysteresis of the growth rate and depression of the freezing point, in addition to the transformation of ice crystals to a dendritic morphology. They used the Gibbs–Thomson law and the Langmuir's adsorption isotherm to explain the inhibitory effect of COOH-PLL on crystal growth and proposed that the adsorption of large biological molecules has a non-steady-state character and occurs at a slower rate than the embedding of crystal growth units.

Ice growth or recrystallization during thawing is one of the major reasons of cell death (Fowler and Toner 2005); hence, the ability to inhibit ice recrystallization is a desirable property of cryoprotectants. AFPs exhibit ice recrystallization inhibition (IRI) activity by binding to ice crystals to cause a non-colligative freezing point depression (McKown and Warren 1991). Mitchell et al. 2014, characterized the IRI efficacy of polyampholytes by using a splat assay in which a polymer sample was dropped onto a chilled glass slide, transferred to a microscope maintained at –6°C, and analyzed after 30 min. They analyzed polyampholytes (50% COOH substitution) along with a synthetic polyampholyte composed of poly(aminoethyl methacrylate) and SA (PAEMA-co-SA). The mean largest grain size (MLGS) of the ice crystals relative to a phosphate-buffered saline (PBS) control was determined. The results showed that the polyampholytes had significant IRI activity. To confirm that the IRI activity was due to the presence of both the charges and the neutral nature of the polyampholyte, polyampholytes with different ratios of COOH substitution were

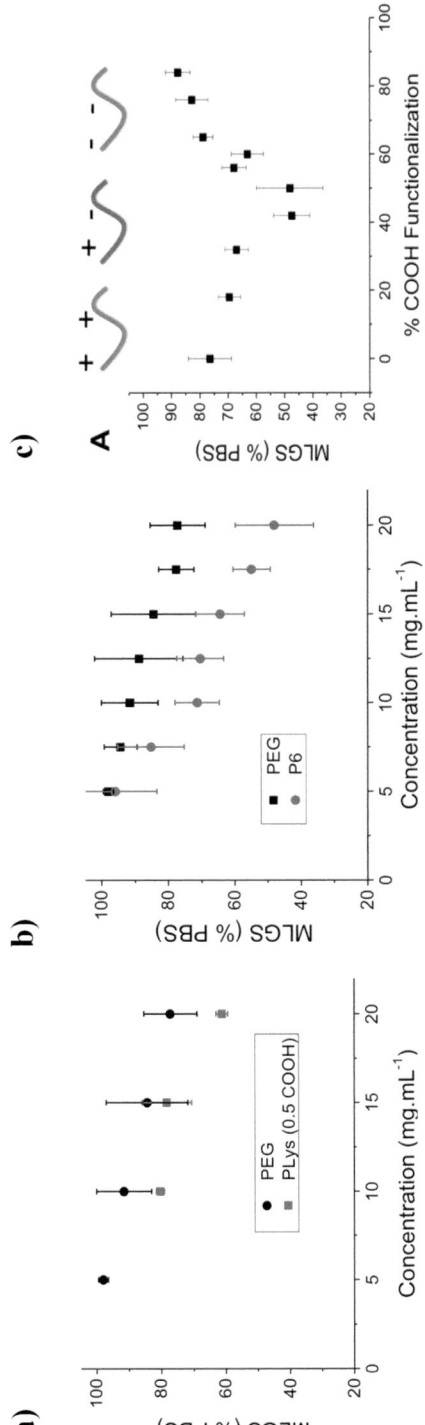

Fig. 4: Ice recrystallization inhibition by poly(ampholytes). (A) Comparison of PEG and carboxylated poly(lysine). (A) Comparison of polyethylene glycol (PEG) to PAEMA-co-succinic anhydride (50% functionality), and (C) IRI activity of PAEMA-derived polymers measured at 20 mg mL^{-1} and effect of degree of carboxylation on activity. Error bars represent ± SD from a minimum of three repeats. MLGS = mean largest grain size relative to phosphate buffered saline control (From Mitchell et al. 2014 with permission).

prepared. Maximum IRI activity was observed at around 50% substitution (Fig. 4). On the basis of this observation, the authors suggested that the charge balance is crucial for high IRI activity. The mechanism of inhibition is apparently different from that of other IRI-active polymers, which need hydroxyl groups (ice-bonding motifs) to inhibit recrystallization, as COOH-PLL does not contain hydroxyl groups. Detailed study is needed to uncover the exact underlying mechanism, which would enable the development of more robust systems.

Betaine as a protein aggregation inhibitor

Proteins are of the most complex biomolecules and are essential for almost all functions in the body. They are aptly called the building blocks. For proteins to be functional, they must properly fold into their native states. Any defect in the protein folding or unfolding from its native state leads to protein instability, which usually manifests as protein aggregation. In research environments, aggregation can pose great technical challenges, while in industries like pharmaceutical and biotechnological industries, they can also lead to economic problems. In humans, it manifests in several dreadful diseases, primarily neurodegenerative conditions like Parkinson's and Alzheimer's diseases, prions, etc. (Ross and Poirier 2004). Misfolding of newly synthesized proteins can be extremely lethal to cells; in such instances, molecular chaperones come into play to inhibit aggregation and simultaneously stimulate proper folding (Hartl et al. 2011).

Betaine polymers exhibit remarkable anti-biofouling properties and highly resist nonspecific protein adsorption and cell adhesion (Zhang Z. et al. 2006; Tada et al. 2009). It was known that zwitterionic betaine polymers have great potential in making materials biocompatible, owing to their excellent anti-biofouling property. A study by Kitano et al. (2005) revealed that betaine polymers do not significantly alter the hydrogen bonding between water molecules, and therefore, the water structure is maintained at the interface between the polymer and the material, due to the charge balance.

Rajan et al. (2015) reported that the zwitterionic polymer poly-sulfobetaine (poly-SPB) showed very high activity in inhibiting the thermal aggregation of lysozyme. This was the first report of a zwitterionic polymer being used to suppress *in vitro* protein aggregation. The polymer was synthesized using a facile synthetic route involving RAFT polymerization. When lysozyme in PBS buffer was heated at 90°C for 30 min, comprehensive aggregation was observed. On the contrary, when lysozyme was mixed with poly-SPB, aggregation was completely suppressed. The nature of the aggregates was established via transmission electron microscopy (TEM), which revealed the formation of amyloid-like fibrils in aggregation. This fibrillation process was arrested by the presence of poly-SPB. Quantification of the fibrillation using thioflavin T showed that the aggregation inhibition activity of poly-SPB was remarkably higher than that of previously known reagents including arginine. The authors analyzed whether the polymer inhibits only the physical aggregation or whether it has the ability to prevent the loss of enzymatic activity. The results again demonstrated that poly-SPB shows extremely high efficiency and lysozyme retained almost full activity. Preliminary mechanistic studies using infrared and circular dichroism spectroscopy showed that poly-SPB prevented any change in the secondary structure. Conformation studies using ¹H-NMR revealed that the polymer partially stabilizes higher-order structure of lysozyme during heating with all amino acid residues present in the secondary structure being retained (Fig. 5), which in turn leads to the solubility of lysozyme at such elevated temperature. Therefore, the authors suggested that poly-SPB shows weak and reversible interaction with proteins, enabling it to act as a molecular shield, reducing collisions between aggregating species, and maintaining the water structure.

The research group of Rabilloud has done extensive work on the role of non-detergent sulfobetaines (NDSB) as stabilizing and solubilizing agents for proteins

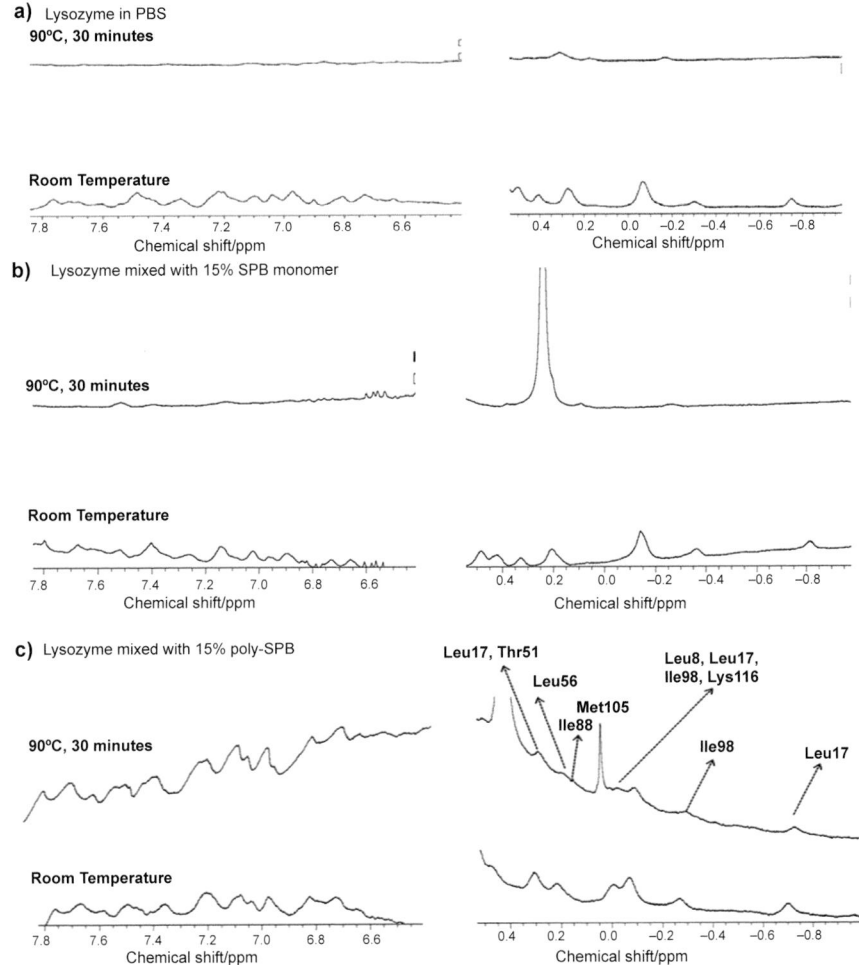

Fig. 5: ¹H NMR spectra of a mixture of (a) lysozyme in PBS, (b) lysozyme mixed with monomer SPB, and (c) lysozyme mixed with poly-SPB at room temperature and after heating to 90°C for 30 min. When no additive was used, all the peaks disappeared suggesting that lysozyme is transformed into a random coil state and has lost its secondary structure. When SPB monomer was used, only few peaks were retained. On the other hand, when poly-SPB was used, resulted in many signals over a wide range of chemical shifts and almost all the peaks were retained (From Rajan and Matsumura 2015 with permission).

(Vuillard et al. 1995a,b, 1996; Goldberg et al. 1996). They found that NDSBs can aid in the formation of protein crystals and suggested this to be due to the ability of NDSBs to prevent amorphous aggregation. Moreover, with the addition of NDSBs to protein solution, the amount of active protein recovered in *in-vitro* folding experiments was substantially increased.

Glycine betaine is one of the most well-known and studied osmoprotectants. It elevates the osmotic pressure in the cytoplasm and stabilizes proteins and membranes under conditions of adverse salt levels or temperatures (McNeil et al. 1999). Glycine betaine was shown to restore the activity of malate dehydrogenase (Pollard and Jones 1979). Caldas et al. (1999) showed that glycine betaine at low concentrations protects β-galactosidase and citrate synthase against thermodenaturation *in vitro*. Additionally, it triggers citrate synthase renaturation after urea denaturation. Over the years, multiple organic compounds like arginine (Taneja and Ahmed 1994; Asano et al. 2002; Das et al. 2004), proline (Samuel et al. 2000), cyclodextrins (Karuppiah and Sharma 1995), polyamines (Kudou et al. 2003), and a whole array of other small compounds have been employed to prevent protein folding.

Drug Delivery by Polyampholytes

Nanocarriers

In the past centuries, a vast number of life-threatening diseases have been identified, some of which are still incurable and pose a challenge in finding effective remedies. At the beginning of the 21st century, a wide variety of peptides, proteins, and DNA analogs are available to be used as drugs, which can prove to be milestones in the treatment of deadly diseases such as cancer, cardiovascular diseases, and immunedisorders. However, no significant improvements have been made in the prevention of fatal diseases. Current advancements in nanotechnology for biomedical applications and more specifically, drug delivery have instigated an accelerated growth in very promising nanomaterials (Gu et al. 2013). The development of drug delivery technology in the field of nanomedicine has revolutionized treatments (Shi et al. 2010). Various types of nanocarriers such as liposomes, metallic nanoparticles (NPs), etc. are widely used for efficient targeting of drugs (De Jong and Borm 2008). Despite the enormous advances in the development of drug nanocarriers (Sawant and Torchilin 2012), there is a pressing need for the development of multifunctional therapeutic delivery carriers.

Polymeric NPs hold great potential for use as biomaterials in therapeutic delivery. Since the last few decades, multifarious work has been conducted to develop highly effective nanomedicines from biocompatible polymers. Nanomedicines play a significant role in enhancing the efficacy and specificity of drugs and protecting them from degradation. Various polymers have been approved by the U.S. food and drug administration for clinical healthcare depending upon their physicochemical characteristics. Poly(D,L-lactide-co-glycolide), polylactic acid, chitosan, and gelatin are the polymers the most commonly used for drug vehicles (Solaro et al. 2010). These NPs can be employed in various routes for delivery such as oral, nasal, transdermal, pulmonary, and ocular delivery. However, in some cases, nanocarriers are not able to cross the biological barriers and are easily degraded, resulting in rapid clearance from the body. During the last decades, the development of novel polymeric NPs for use in therapeutic delivery systems has received increasing research attention, and various approaches to designing new polymeric NP systems have been taken. Novel NPs should possess high stability, enhanced drug adsorption efficacy, and improved therapeutic efficacy. There remains a pressing need for the development of facile, stable, non-toxic nanocarriers that show high efficiency for therapeutic delivery.

Evolution of self-assembled polyampholyte NPs

Polyampholytes have shown tendency to self-assemble and form into NPs. They are of growing interest and relevance for applications in biomedical and pharmaceutical fields. A polymeric system based on using poly(ethylene oxide)-block-poly(aspartic acid) (PEO-PAA)–adriamycin drug conjugate was shown to self-assemble into micelles in aqueous media, which can be used in biomedical applications (Yokoyama et al. 1992). These amphiphilic block copolymers form a core-shell structure in which the core is hydrophobic while the outer layer is in hydrophilic in nature (Zhang et al. 2006). The polymers self-organize due to specific interactions such as intermolecular, hydrogen-bonding, or hydrophobic interactions in solution.

Poly(amino acid)-based self-assembled NPs such as poly(γ-glutamic acid)-graft-(L-arginine) (γ-PGA-arg) and poly(γ-glutamic acid)-graft-(L-lysine) (γ-PGA-Lys) have been developed (Shen et al. 2012). Recently, a unique self-assembled polyampholyte-based nanocarrier was established by the reaction of a small amount of hydrophobic alkyl chains, dodecylsuccinic anhydride (DDSA; 3% or 5%), and 35% or 65% degree of substitution of SA on PLLin a single polymeric backbone as shown in Scheme 1 (Ahmed et al. 2014). SA was introduced into PLL to achieve two types of NPs with anionic and cationic surface charges that were termed PLL-DDSA (3 or 5)-SA(35 or 65). This NP contains charged hydrophobic systems in the PLL owing to the presence of wide-ranging cross-linking sites. In general, the hydrophobic and electrostatic interactions act as a driving force for self-complexation in this kind of systems. The properties of polyampholyte NPs are similar to those of nanogels, which are aggregated through intermolecular forces to some extent (Akiyoshi et al. 1993). Various self-assembled nanocarriers are still being developed based on the interactions of amino acid residues.

Drug loading onto and encapsulation into polyampholyte NPs

Aggregation, degradation, and denaturation are the main hurdles for protein-based drugs. To achieve safe, sustained, and targeted delivery, it is important for therapeutic molecules to reach their target without any hindrance (Mitragotri et al. 2014). Thus, the use of nanocarriers to deliver drugs across biological barriers while protecting them from metabolism and excretion are in high demand. Efficient drug loading onto carriers is essential in establishing sustained-drug delivery systems. The most indispensable characteristics of nanocarriers are (i) high stability or long circulation time, (ii) targeted delivery, and (iii) effective protection/encapsulation.

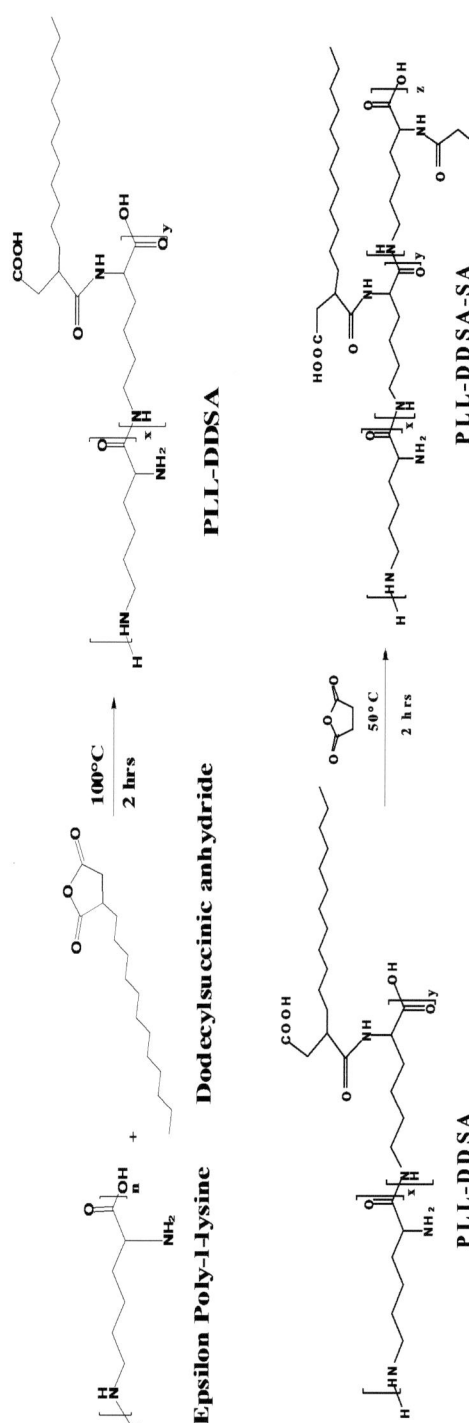

Scheme 1: Scheme of the preparation of self-assembled polyampholyte NPs (From Ahmed et al. 2014 with permission).

Nanocarriers such as liposomes, polymeric micelles, and dendrimers have been extensively utilized as targeted drug carrier systems because of the ability to encapsulate medicinal drugs, proteins, genes, or other therapeutic molecules. However, liposomes and other carriers display an intrinsic instability, resulting in low shielding of the drugs and fast release under physiological conditions (Immordino et al. 2006). This highlights the importance of intermolecular interactions such as electrostatic or hydrophobic interactions, which play a crucial role in the uptake and adsorption of drugs inside the amphoteric carrier. The use of polyampholyte NPs has greatly enhanced the protein adsorption efficacy (Ahmed et al. 2014). Polyampholyte NPs containing both positively and negatively charged units have the ability to strongly bind to oppositely charged particles due to electrostatic interactions. There currently are two main types of protein-based drug carriers, based on lysozyme (cationic protein) or bovine serum albumin (BSA; anionic protein). Lysozyme shows high adsorption efficacy towards anionic polyampholyte NPs. However, the like charges between polyampholyte and protein in the conjugate weaken the adsorption efficacy. Therefore, oppositely charged polyampholyte–drug conjugate enhances the ionic character because polyampholytes are responsive to pH and ionic strength under physiological conditions.

With regard to the size of NPs for therapeutic applications, numerous studies have shown that smaller NPs show longer blood circulation than larger ones. The nano-size (10–100 nm) diameter is required for efficient cytoplasmic delivery (Kievit and Zhang 2011). Polymeric NPs have a size range of 10–1000 nm, depending on their physicochemical characteristics. For example, micelles self-assembled in aqueous media under physiological conditions generally have a small size. Similarly, self-assembled polyampholyte NPs exhibit a narrow size distribution (15–20 nm), are uniform in size, and can disperse well (Ahmed et al. 2014). This might be attributed to the compact packing owing to hydrophobic moieties and electrostatic charges present in the polymeric chains.

Morphology and surface characters are important factors in nanocarriers for effective and efficient cellular uptake of therapeutics in targeted delivery systems. TEM is one of the versatile techniques that is widely used to determine the morphology of NPs. Most nanocarriers including polyampholytes are spherical (Fig. 6). Spherical NPs are internalized inside the cells at a higher rate than rod- or disk-shaped NPs (Chithrani et al. 2006).

Cytotoxicity becomes the major issue for nanocarriers in sustained delivery. Toxicological studies of nanocarriers are very rare although they are crucial for application of nanocarrier systems in drug delivery and other biomedical applications. The cytotoxicity of nanocarriers is greatly influenced by their surface charges. Multiple studies have revealed that cationic groups on NPs may profoundly influence the cytotoxicity. Cationic melamine-based dendrimers tended to interact with cells unfavorably and showed increased toxicity. These adverse effects were attributed to lower targeting specificity towards cells (Chen et al. 2004). Negatively charged polyampholyte NPs are generally less toxic than positively charged (Ahmed et al. 2014). Therefore, anionic nanocarriers might be better candidates for therapeutic use.

PLL-DDSA(5)-SA(35)

PLL-DDSA(5)-SA(65)

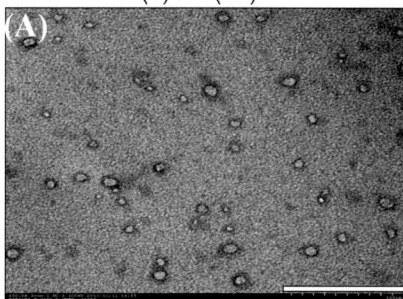
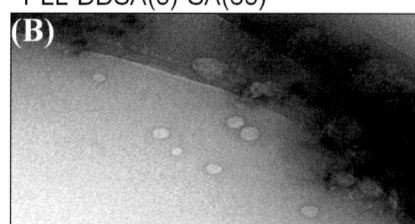

Fig. 6: TEM images showing the morphology of polyampholyte NPs. Bars = 100 nm. (A) Cationic polyampholytes, (B) anionic polyampholytes (From Ahmed et al. 2014 with permission).

Polyampholyte NPs with long circulation time

Nanocarrier stability is one of the most desirable features for therapeutic delivery. It can lead to increased circulation time and thus, increased exposure of and continuous delivery to the affected area. DLS (dynamic light scattering) has been used to determine the colloidal stability of NP suspensions based on monitoring of changes in the NP size. Self-assembled, cholesterol-based, brush-like block copolymers were stable under physiological condition (Tran et al. 2014). The small-sized polyethylene glycol (PEG) NPs have long blood circulation times (Perrault et al. 2009). Similarly, PLL-based polyampholyte NPs showed little changes in size even after one week and had long circulation times (Ahmed et al. 2014).

Design of polyampholyte NPs for cytoplasmic delivery

Various techniques including electroporation and ultrasonication have been formulated for immunotherapy or gene therapy based on the internalization of a drug, antibody, gene, or any other moiety inside cells, and they have been used for effective treatment of diseases such as cancer. However, these techniques pose numerous challenges hampering effective treatment. These include ineffective drug concentration reaching the target site, life-threatening side effects caused by non-specific tissue distribution of anticancer agents in cancer immunotherapy, and acquired resistance of the cancer cells against the chemicals used in chemotherapy triggering cross-resistance.

Numerous studies have been carried out to explore the use of amphiphilic polymers in therapies. In an attempt to improve cytoplasmic delivery, polyampholyte NPs with improved cell membrane penetration have been developed. Ahmed et al. (2014) reported for the first time the use of a combination of polyampholyte carrier NPs and a novel strategy termed "freeze concentration" for protein delivery. Freeze concentration is a physical phenomenon involving phase separation during freezing, in which unfrozen solutes (e.g., protein-based drugs) are concentrated (Bhatnagar et al. 2008). The basic mechanism relies on the use of low temperature-mediated protein delivery with the aid of polyampholyte NPs, which help to increase the diffusion of

(A)

(B)

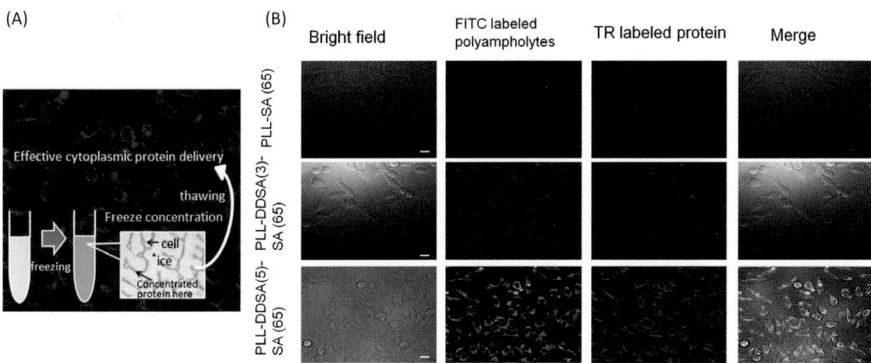

Fig. 7: Schematic image of the concept of protein cytoplasmic delivery via freeze concentration (A) and confocal microscopic images (B) shows the internalization of lysozyme protein loaded PLL-SA(65) or PLL-DDSA(3 or 5)-SA(65) polyampholyte NPs with 10% PLL-SA(65) as a cryoprotectant. Bars = 10 μm (From Ahmed et al. 2014 with permission).

proteins inside the cell. Because of the phase separation of solute molecules, they are easily delivered inside the plasma membrane (Fig. 7(a)). In the study of Ahmed et al. (2014), the solution containing protein and the cells were frozen to –80°C. Cell stability was maintained by the use of the polyampholyte as a CPA. DMSO is a well-known cryoprotective agent but due to its high cytotoxicity and differentiation effects on cells such as neurons and cardiac myocytes, which are the major targets of many drugs, its use is limited. COOH-PLL is merely cytotoxic and has little or no effect on the differentiation, structure, or normal functioning of cells. The PLL-DDSA(5)-SA(65)-based NPs were condensed on the peripheral cell membrane because of the high affinity between the NPs and the membrane at low temperature. It has been shown that internalization efficiency increased when lysozyme protein was loaded onto hydrophobic polyampholyte NPs (Fig. 7(b)). This study resulted in the development of a facile and effective protein-based drug delivery method using self-assembled amphiphilic polyampholyte.

Various studies have shown that the use of amphiphilic polymer has stead fastly increased in the nanomedicine and biomedical engineering fields. For cancer immunotherapy applications, therapeutic molecules must escape from endosomes after entry inside the cells via endocytosis to protect them from lysosomal degradation.

Self-assembled NPs have been explored for the development of vaccine delivery systems. Akagi et al. (2007) reported on an amphiphilic poly-(γ-glutamic acid) phenylalanine NP-based vaccine system that generated an immune response against various diseases. The hydrophobic moieties of the NP led to disruption of the endosomal membrane resulting in more effective escape (Akagi et al. 2011). Thus, these amphiphilic polymeric NPs exhibit great potential for immunotherapy (Akagi et al. 2007).

The use of self-assembled polyampholyte nanocarriers in gene therapy has been considered in many reports. Various viral carriers such as retroviruses and adenoviruses are being used for plasmid delivery. However, viral carriers have the disadvantage that they can integrate randomly into the host genome (Gould and Favorov 2013), often rendering them unsuitable for the treatment of genetic disorders. These issues stimulated the development of self-assembled NPs as non-viral carriers. In the case of non-viral carriers, there is very little chance of mutagenic events in transformed cells and, moreover, they can deliver genes to a higher extent.

In one report, plasmid delivery to bone marrow dendritic cells (BMSCs) was achieved with high transfection efficacy by using self-assembled amphiphilic PLL modified with palmitic acid (PA) (Clements et al. 2007). Moreover, a PLL-graft-HA comb-type copolymer that forms complexes with DNA has been developed. This PLL-graft-HA-based polyampholyte can dissociate into ions under high ionic strength and exhibit intermolecular poly-ion complex. This carrier tends to encapsulate DNA more efficiently and thus, can be utilized for DNA targeting in gene therapy (Asayama et al. 1998).

So, there is growing interest of usage of self-assembled nanocarrier in cancer immunotherapy. Therefore, polyampholyte NPs are expected to be a good candidate as biomaterials and also can be used into clinical studies in future.

Conclusion and Future Perspectives

Rationally designed polyampholytes have been shown to be promising cryoprotective agents and drug carriers for effective and safe therapeutic delivery. With regard to cryoprotective properties, although mechanisms have to be further investigated, polyampholytes showed similar effects to anti-freezing proteins. Additionally, owing to their low toxicity, polyampholytes can replace the toxic DMSO developed half a century ago as a freezing injury inhibitor. And their applications must be for broader field in the biomaterials including tissue engineering. In the application of self-assembled NPs for materials delivery, various factors such as size, surface properties, specificity towards cells, and most importantly, endosomal escape property could play a pivotal role in successful outcome of drug therapy. In addition, self-assembled polyampholyte nanocarriers show good biocompatibility, excellent stability, and high drug adsorbance. These carriers are easy to modify, have high responsiveness, and ability to deliver drugs to their target site across biological barriers, and can prolong the circulation time of the encapsulated drugs. The development of polyampholyte-based biomaterials will continue to attract much interest and the NPs possess good potential in various biomedical treatments and basic technologies in future.

References

Ahmed, S., F. Hayashi, T. Nagashima and K. Matsumura. 2014. Protein cytoplasmic delivery using polyampholyte nanoparticles and freeze concentration. Biomaterials 35: 6508–6518.

Akagi, T., X. Wang, T. Utob, M. Baba and M. Akashi. 2007. Protein direct delivery to dendritic cells using nanoparticles based on amphiphilic poly(amino acid) derivatives. Biomaterials 28: 3427–3436.

Akagi, T., F. Shima and M. Akashi. 2011. Intracellular degradation and distribution of protein-encapsulated amphiphilic poly(amino acid) nanoparticles. Biomaterials 32: 4959–4967.

Akiyoshi, K., S. Deguchi, N. Moriguchi, S. Yamaguchi and J. Sunamoto. 1993. Self aggregates of hydrophobized polysaccharides in water. Formation and characteristics of nanoparticles. Macromolecules 26(1993): 3062–3068.

Asano, R., T. Kudo, K. Makabe, K. Tsumoto and I. Kumagai. 2002. Antitumor activity of interleukin-21 prepared by novel refolding procedure from inclusion bodies expressed in *Escherichia coli*. FEBS Lett. 528: 70–76.

Asayama, S., M. Nogawa, Y. Takei, T. Akaike and A. Maruyama. 1998. Synthesis of novel polyampholyte comb-type copolymers consisting of a poly(L-lysine) backbone and hyaluronic acid side chains for a DNA carrier. Bioconjugate Chem. 9: 476–481.

Bhatnagar, B. S., M. J. Pikal and R. H. Bogner. 2008. Study of the individual contribution of ice formation and freeze-concentration on isothermal stability of lactate dehydrogenase during freezing. J. Pharm. Sci. 97: 798–814.

Caldas, T., N. D.-Caulet, A. Ghazi and G. Richarme. 1999. Thermoprotection by glycine betaine and choline. Microbiology 145: 2543–2548.

Chen, H. T., M. F. Neerman, A. R. Parrish and E. E. Simanek. 2004. Cytotoxicity, hemolysis and acute *in vivo* toxicity of dendrimers based on melamine, candidate vehicles for drug delivery. J. Amer. Chem. Soc. 126: 10044–10048.

Chithrani, B. D., A. A. Ghazani and W. C. Chan. 2006. Determining the size and shape dependence of gold nanoparticles uptake into mammalian cells. Nano Lett. 6: 662–668.

Clements, B. A., V. Incanib, C. Kucharskia, A. Lavasanifarb, B. Ritchiec and H. Uludag. 2007. A comparative evaluation of poly-L-lysine-palmitic acid and lipofectamine™ 2000 for plasmid delivery to bone marrow stromal cells. Biomaterials 28: 4693–4704.

Das, D., J. Kriangkum, L. P. Nagata, R. E. Fulton and M. R. Suresh. 2004. Development of a biotin mimic tagged ScFv antibody against western equine encephalitis virus: bacterial expression and refolding. Virol. Methods 2004: 117: 169–177.

De Jong, W. H. and P. J. A. Borm. 2008. Drug delivery and nanoparticles: applications and hazards. Int. J. Nanomedicine 3: 133–149.

Fowler, A. and M. Toner. 2005. Cryo-Injury and Biopreservation. Ann. N.Y. Acad. Sci. 1066: 119–135.

Goldberg, M. E., N. Expert-Bezançon, L. Vuillard and T. Rabilloud. 1996. Non-detergent sulphobetaines: a new class of molecules that facilitate *in vitro* protein renaturation. Folding Des. 1: 21–27.

Gould, D. J. and P. Favorov. 2013. Vectors for the treatment of autoimmune disease. Gene therapy 10: 912–927.

Griffith, M. and M. W. Yaish. 2004. Antifreeze proteins in overwintering plants: a tale of two activities. Trends. Plant Sci. 9: 399–405.

Gu, W., C. Wu, J. Chen and Y. Xiao. 2013. Nanotechnology in the targeted drug delivery for bone diseases and bone regeneration. Int. J. Nanomedicine 8: 2305–2317.

Hartl, F. U., A. Bracher and M. Hayer-Hartl. 2011. Molecular chaperones in protein folding and proteostasis. Nature 475: 324–332.

Immordino, M. L., F. Dosio and L. Catter. 2006. Stealth liposomes: review of the basic science, rationale and applications, existing and potential. Int. J. Nanomedicine 1: 297–315.

Jain, M., R. Rajan, S. H. Hyon and K. Matsumura. 2014. Hydrogelation of dextran-based polyampholytes with cryoprotective properties via click chemistry. Biomater. Sci. 2: 308–317.

Karuppiah, N. and A. Sharma. 1995. Cyclodextrins as protein folding aids. Biophys. Res. Commun. 211: 60–66.

Kievit, F. M. and M. Zhang. 2011. Cancer nanotheranostics: improving imaging and therapy by targeted delivery across biological barriers. Adv. Mater. 23: 217–247.

Kitano, H., T. Mori, Y. Takeuchi, S. Tada, M. Gemmei-Ide, Y. Yokoyama et al. 2005. Structure of water incorporated in sulfobetaine polymer films as studied by ATR-FTIR. Macromol. Biosci. 5: 314–321.

Kudaibergenov, S. E. 2002. Polyampholytes: Synthesis, Characterization, and Application. Kluwer Academic/Plenum Publishers, New York.

Kudou, M., K. Shiraki, S. Fujiwara, T. Imanaka and M. Takagi. 2003. Prevention of thermal inactivation and aggregation of lysozyme by polyamines. Eur. J. Biochem. 270: 4547–4554.

Laschewsky, A. 2014. Structures and synthesis of zwitterionic polymers. Polymers 6: 1544–1601.

Maehara, M., M. Sato, M. Watanabe, H. Matsunari, M. Kokubo, T. Kanai et al. 2013. Development of a novel vitrification method for chondrocyte sheets. BMC Biotechnol. 13: 58.

Matsumura, K. and S. H. Hyon. 2009. Polyampholytes as low toxic efficient cryoprotective agents with antifreeze protein properties. Biomaterials 30: 4842–4849.

Matsumura, K., J. Y. Bae and S. H. Hyon. 2010. Polyampholytes as cryoprotective agents for mammalian cell cryopreservation. Cell Transplantat. 19: 691–699.

Matsumura, K., J. Bae, H. Kim and S.H. Hyon. 2011. Effective vitrification of human induced pluripotent stem cells using carboxylated ε-poly-L-lysine. Cryobiology 63: 76–83.

Matsumura, K., F. Hayashi, T. Nagashima and S.H. Hyon. 2013. Long term cryopreservation of human mesenchymal stem cells using carboxylated poly-l-lysine without the addition of proteins or dimethyl sulfoxide. J. Biomater. Sci. Polym. Edn. 24: 1484–1497.

McKown, R. L. and G. J. Warren. 1991. Enhanced survival of yeast expressing an antifreeze gene analogue after freezing. Cryobiology 28: 474–482.

McNeil, S. D., M. L. Nuccio and A. D. Hanson. 1999. Betaines and related osmoprotectants. Targets for metabolic engineering of stress resistance. Plant Physiol. 120: 945–50.

Mitchell, D. E., M. Lilliman, S. G. Spain and M. I. Gibson. 2014. Quantitative study on the antifreeze protein mimetic ice growth inhibition properties of poly(ampholytes) derived from vinyl-based polymers. Biomater. Sci. 2: 1787–1795.

Mitragotri, S., P. A. Burke and R. Langer. 2014. Overcoming the challenges in administering biopharmaceuticals: formulation and delivery strategies. Nat. Rev. Drug. Discov. 13: 655–672.

Perrault, S. D., C. Walkey, T. Jennings, H. C. Fischer and W. C. W. Chan. 2009. Mediating tumor targeting efficiency of nanoparticles through design. Nano Lett. 9: 1909–1915.

Pollard, A. and R. G. W. Jones. 1979. Metabolic engineering of glycine betaine synthesis. Planta 144: 291–298.

Rajan, R., M. Jain and K. Matsumura. 2013. Cryoprotective properties of completely synthetic polyampholytes via reversible addition-fragmentation chain transfer (RAFT) polymerization and the effects of hydrophobicity. J. Biomater. Sci. Polym. Edn. 24: 1767–1780.

Rajan, R. and K. Matsumura. 2015. A zwitterionic polymer as a novel inhibitor of protein aggregation. J. Mater. Chem. B 3: 5683–5689.

Ross, C. A. and M. A. Poirier. 2004. Protein aggregation and neurodegenerative disease. Nat. Med. 10: S10–S17.

Samuel, D., G. Ganesh, P.-W. Yang, M.-M. Chang, S.-L. Wang, K.-C. Hwang et al. 2000. Proline inhibits aggregation during protein refolding. Protein Sci. 9: 344–352.

Sawant, R. R. and V. P. Torchilin. 2012. Multifunctional nanocarriers and intracellular drug delivery. Curr. Opin. Solid State Mater. Sci. 16: 269–275.

Shen, H., T. Akagi and M. Akashi. 2012. Polyampholyte nanoparticles prepared by self complexation of cationized poly(γ-glutamic acid) for protein carriers. Macromol. Biosci. 12: 1100–1105.

Shi, J., A. R. Vatruba, O. C. Farokhzad and R. Langer. 2010. Nanotechnology in drug delivery and tissue engineering: from discovery to application. Nano Lett. 10: 3223–3230.

Solaro, R., F. Chiellini and A. Battisti. 2010. Targeted delivery of protein drugs by nanocarriers. Materials 3: 1928–1980.

Tada, S., C. Inaba, K. Mizukami, S. Fujishita, M. Gemmei-Ide, H. Kitano et al. 2009. Anti-Biofouling properties of polymers with a carboxybetaine moiety. Macromol. Biosci. 9: 63–70.

Taneja, S. and F. Ahmad. 1994. Increased thermal stability of proteins in the presence of amino acids. Biochem. J. 303: 147–153.

Tran, T. H., C. T. Nguyen, L. Gonzalez-Fajardo, D. Hargrove, D. Song, P. Deshmukh et al. 2014. Long circulating self assembled nanoparticles from cholesterol-containing brush-like block copolymers for improved drug delivery to tumors. 2014. Biomacromolecules 15: 4363–4375.

Vorontsov, D., G. Sazaki, S. H. Hyon, K. Matsumura and Y. Furukawa. 2014. Antifreeze effect of carboxylated ε-poly-L-lysine on the growth kinetics of ice crystals. J. Phys. Chem. B 118: 10240–10249.

Vuillard, L., D. Madern, B. Franzetti and T. Rabilloud. 1995a. Halophilic protein stabilization by the mild solubilizing agents nondetergent sulfobetaines. Anal. Biochem. 230: 290–294.

Vuillard, L., C. Braun-Breton and T. Rabilloud. 1995b. Non-detergent sulphobetaines: a new class of mild solubilization agents for protein purification. Biochem. J. 305: 337–343.

Vuillard, L., B. Baalbaki, M. Lehmann, M. Roth, P. Legrand and S. Norager. 1996. Protein crystallography with non-detergent sulfobetaines. J. Cryst. Growth 168: 150–154.

Watanabe, H., N. Kohaya, M. Kamoshita, K. Fujiwara, K. Matsumura, S. H. Hyon et al. 2013. Efficient production of live offspring from mouse oocytes vitrified with a novel cryoprotective agent, carboxylated e-poly-L-lysine. PLoS ONE 8: 1–5.

Yokoyama, M., G. S. Kwon, T. Okano, Y. Sakurai, T. Seto and K. Kataoka. 1992. Preparation of micelle-forming polymer-drug conjugates. Bioconjugate Chem. 3: 295–301.

Zhang, P., Q. Liu, A. Qing, J. Shi and M. Lu. 2006. Synthesis and characterization of core-shell-type polymeric micelles from diblock copolymers via reversible addition-fragmentation chain transfer. J. Polym. Sci. A Polym. Chem. 44: 3312–3320.

Zhang, Z., T. Chao, S. Chen and S. Jiang. 2006. Superlow fouling sulfobetaine and carboxybetaine polymers on glass slides. Langmuir 22: 10072–10077.

Zurick, K. M. and M. T. Bernards. 2014. Recent biomedical advances with polyampholyte polymers. J. Appl. Polym. Sci. 131: 40069.

8

Biomedical Applications of Recombinant Proteins and Derived Polypeptides

Francisco Javier Arias,* Sergio Acosta-Rodríguez, Tatjana Flora and *Sofía Serrano-Dúcar*

Abstract

Significant research efforts are currently being focused on the development of innovative biomedical devices. In this regard, one of the most important challenges is the development of better biomaterials that combine the advantages of conventional natural and chemically synthesized materials while improving their properties. Recombinant proteins derived from natural proteins and genetically engineered polymers represent valuable alternatives due to their biocompatibility, biodegradability, non-toxic nature, and non-immunogenic properties. Furthermore, such biomaterials are able to mimic different physiological tissue components and environments, a property that is much sought after in tissue regeneration, and are excellent candidates in controlled drug- or gene-release due to their multi-responsive behavior and their ability to carry therapeutic agents to specific targets.

BIOFORGE Research Group (Group for Advanced Materials and Nanobiotechnology), CIBER-BBN, University of Valladolid, 47011 Valladolid, Spain.
* Corresponding author: arias@bioforge.uva.es

This review summarizes the most recent developments in biomedical fields in which various biomaterials, for example recombinant proteins based on natural proteins such as elastin, tropoelastin, silk and collagen, or their genetically engineered derivatives (elastin-like, silk-like and silk-elastin-like recombinamers), are used. As will be discussed in this review, these materials are excellent candidates for biomedical applications such as tissue engineering and drug or gene delivery.

Introduction

Numerous efforts have been made over the past couple of decades to develop efficient strategies for producing biomaterials that actively participate in the formation of functional tissues. However, as restoration of the functions of dysfunctional or damaged tissues requires the whole architecture and complexity of native organs and tissues to be mimicked, the success of such strategies depends crucially on the biomaterial used (Yang et al. 2001; Nichol and Khademhosseini 2009). In this regard, both naturally derived and synthetic materials have been extensively studied with the aim of providing provisional scaffolds that are able to interact biomolecularly with cells that control their function, thus guiding the spatially and temporally complex multicellular processes of tissue formation and regeneration. Synthetic polymers have been widely investigated as they can be manufactured reproducibly on a large scale with controlled strengths, degradation rates, and microstructures (Hubbell 1995). However, such polymers exhibit different disadvantages, such as undesirable degradation products or the need to use toxic organic solvents during their synthesis (Meilander and Bellamkonda 2004). In contrast, naturally derived materials have the potential advantage of biological recognition, although they can be difficult and expensive to obtain as they present several limitations, including the possibility of an immunogenic response post-implantation and the invariability in molecular structure associated with animal sources (Hodde 2002). These limitations can be overcome by using recombinant protein expression technologies, which allow for greater control over their properties and tissue responses. Indeed, recombinant technology allows the production of biomaterials while combining the advantages of natural and synthetic approaches. Indeed, it is possible to produce biocompatible and tunable materials that guarantee a high reproducibility (Sengupta and Heilshorn 2010). Indeed, the development of recombinant proteins allows us to obtain biomaterials based on extremely complex structures and specific interactions performed by nature over millennia. Thus, the numerous examples reported to date clearly demonstrate that these materials, such as recombinant biomaterials based on the sequence of fibrous (elastin, collagen, silks, or resilin) or globular proteins (albumin) (McGann et al. 2013; Weimer et al. 2013; Fagerholm et al. 2014; de Torre et al. 2015; Huang et al. 2015), are optimal candidates for controlled drug and gene delivery, tissue engineering, and other biomedical applications.

This review discusses the most recent recombinant materials based on the sequence of natural fibrous proteins such as collagen, tropoelastin, elastin and silk, or based on engineered sequences derived from the combination or modification of conserved motifs present in these proteins, such as elastin-like recombinamers (ELRs), silk-elastin-like proteins or recombinamers (SELRs), and silk-like proteins or recombinamers (SLRs). All these materials present minimal or no toxicity and low immunogenicity, and it is also possible to control their biodegradability. Furthermore, they self-assemble into complex structures with outstanding mechanical properties (Gomes et al. 2012; Annabi et al. 2013a).

Collagen is the most abundant protein in mammals (1/3 of the protein of humans) and the main protein in connective tissue (3/4 of the dry weight of skin; (Chattopadhyay and Raines 2014)). As such, it is an important material in terms of the development of tissue engineering devices because it plays a crucial structural role in those tissues where it is present, and because of its cell interactivity as collagen modulates chemotaxis, cell adhesion, and migration,and is involved in cell differentiation and morphogenesis (Myllyharju and Kivirikko 2004). Elastin is the second most abundant extracellular matrix protein in mammals and is responsible for the elasticity of multiple tissues, such as skin, ligaments, lungs, or blood vessels. It has the unique mechanical property of allowing repeated extensibility followed by elastic recoil (Gosline et al. 2002). The natural precursor of elastin, namely tropoelastin (TE), is a 60 kD anonglycosylated protein encoded by a single gene in humans. It is soluble and secreted into the extracellular matrix, where it is deposited onto microfibrils stabilized by cross-linking (Mithieux et al. 2013). From a tissue engineering point of view, TE has a lower turnover and the important characteristic of self-assembling into elastic fibers by coacervation, a process characterized by an inverse temperature transition (ITT) and an aqueous phase-separation (Urry 2007; Wise and Weiss 2009). Another well-studied fibrous protein-based material is silk. Silk fibroin polymers are produced by two main groups of insects—larvae of the order *Lepidoptera* (the species *Bombyxmori* is particularly important), and members of the class *Arachnida*—and has long been of industrial and medical interest because of its unique mechanical properties. Fibroin is the most interesting silk protein for biomedical applications because of its hydrophobicity and its hierarchical self-organization into nano-crystals (β-sheet structures) that can self-assemble supramolecularly into fibers that combine strength, elasticity, and hypoallergenic properties (Vepari and Kaplan 2007). Although numerous examples of recombinant materials based on these natural proteins have been described, it is also important to note the family of recombinant engineered polymers based on the repetition of conserved motifs of these natural proteins, such as ELRs, SELRs, and SLRs. The design of recombinant polymers allows the production of a large number of different smart materials, thus meaning that more applications can be obtained. The most common domains are VPGXG (in the case of ELRs), which provides the characteristic of TE, thus allowing variation of the monomers and giving rise to a greater versatility for biomaterials applications, GAGAGs (for SLRs), and the combination of both for SELRs, which combine the high tensile strength of silks with the resilience of elastin (Qiu et al. 2010; Rodríguez-Cabello et al. 2012; Włodarczyk-Biegun et al. 2014).

This review provides an overview of various recombinant proteins used in tissue engineering and drug-delivery devices, as well as for applications in gene delivery. We highlight the use of recombinant proteins, and finally discuss more sophisticated recombinant biomaterials that can interact with their biological environment, thus allowing them to actively participate in tissue-regeneration and drug-delivery pathways.

Recombinant Proteins for Tissue Engineering

Tissue engineering is an interdisciplinary field that requires an in-depth understanding of the development and sustainability of tissues or organs, and of the materials that sustain and support them. The key to tissue engineering is the interaction between the cellular environment and biomaterials, which must exhibit several biological features as well as mechanical rigidity or flexibility, a porous environment for adequate diffusion of nutrients, and the retention and presentation of biochemical factors (Chapekar 2000; Vacanti 2010).

Recent progress in tissue engineering has resulted in the necessary increase in appropriate and compatible biomaterials. In this regard, protein-based materials are a valuable alternative due to their ability to mimic different tissue environments, their versatile structure and design, the lack of toxic degradation products, and their ability to incorporate specific recognition motifs and interact with cells (Werkmeister and Ramshaw 2012).

Skin tissue regeneration

Human skin is the largest multifunctional organ of the body and plays an important role in protecting the body against microbial, chemical, physical, or mechanical damage. It also helps to maintain many physiological parameters, such as body temperature or water content (Wysocki 1999). Severe acute and chronic skin wounds due to burns, abrasions, lesions, or leg ulcers result in a substantial loss of dermal tissues. According to the WHO, 300,000 deaths per year are attributed to burn injuries, while 6 million patients worldwide suffer from burns every year. Additionally, more than 6 million individuals suffer from chronic skin ulcers (Yildirimer et al. 2012). Skin has the ability to heal itself, with injury triggering a complex signaling cascade that leads to hemostasis, inflammation, cell migration, proliferation, and maturation in order to repair the damaged tissue and to restore the protective skin barrier (Mutsaers et al. 1997). The wound-repair process involves the combined activity of inflammatory, vascular, connective tissue, and epithelial cells. Furthermore, the extracellular matrix plays an important role by facilitating cell signaling and cell migration, thus helping to support the healing process (Vedrenne et al. 2012; Zgheib et al. 2014). Various approaches to skin substitution have been introduced over the last few years (Wang et al. 2013a). Thus, although autologous skin grafting remains the "gold standard" in these scenarios, it has its own complications, especially the fact that donor sites are limited and it results in general scar formation and prolonged hospital stays (Ruszczak 2003; van der Veen et al. 2010; Pereira et al. 2013). Recombinant biomaterials have been shown to be a promising alternative for skin regeneration, thus resulting in the replacement of some current therapies (Rnjak-Kovacina et al. 2012; Annabi et al. 2013a; Annabi et al. 2013b; Shilo et al. 2013; Wang et al. 2013b; Woodley et al. 2013; Wang et al. 2015b).

Although natural collagen is one of the most widely used biomaterials in dermal substitutes because of its physical, mechanical, and biological properties, its use remains restricted by its lack of elasticity and the fact that elastic scaffolds are required to develop functional dermal substitutes (Chevallay and Herbage 2000; Rnjak et al. 2011). Thus, Rnjak-Kovacina et al. have combined natural collagen with rhTE in order to better mimic the native composition of skin and to control its physical and mechanical properties. These authors fabricated easily manipulated scaffolds with different proportions of rhTE and collagen and showed a relationship between collagen proportion and electrospinning efficiency, with more concentrated collagen solutions leading to a lower electrospinning efficiency. They also demonstrated cell infiltration *in vitro* and noted that a 100 per cent rhTE electrospun scaffold enabled the infiltration of fibroblasts at a lower level than 80 per cent rhTE-20 per cent collagen electrospun scaffolds. Consequently, 80 per cent rhTE-20 per cent collagen electrospun scaffolds were tested *in vivo* to determine the implantation response in a mouse model. The results showed that combining both materials into the same scaffold provides synergic properties. Thus, in addition to the tolerance and persistence of the composite, this device allowed fibroblast infiltration and angiogenesis while maintaining a mild inflammatory response and exhibiting improved scaffold handling and manipulation (Rnjak-Kovacina et al. 2012). In a similar study, microfiber scaffolds based only on electrospun rhTE were used as vehicles for adipose-derived stem cells (ADSC) in the treatment of dermal wounds. The effectiveness of these membranes in improving skin wound closure and restoring a normal epithelium in mice was demonstrated (Machula et al. 2014).

rhTE has also been used to enhance the properties of synthetic devices for tissue regeneration. Thus, Weiss' group has recently demonstrated the transfer of benefits, such as cell interaction and low thrombogenic properties, from TE to synthetic materials when combined (Bax et al. 2014). The most widely accepted synthetic skin substitute for skin tissue regeneration in burn patients is Integra Dermal Regeneration Template (IDRT) (Integra Life Sciences Corporation, NJ), a skin substitute based on a bilayer membrane. One of these layers is made of a porous matrix of cross-linked bovine tendon collagen and glycosaminoglycan fibers and is intended for dermal substitution, whereas the other one is made of thin polysiloxane and is intended for epidermal replacement. However, this device has some limitations, such as the lack of vascularization of the regenerated tissue. As such, a novel skin regeneration template, known as tropoelastin dermal regeneration template (TDRT), which incorporates rhTE to enhance the properties of the device for the treatment of severe skin wounds, has been developed. This new device was obtained by covalently crosslinking rhTE with glutaraldehyde in a type I collagen (chondroitin-6-sulfate matrix platform) and was extensively evaluated *in vivo* using mouse and pig models. A comparison of the two devices (IDRT and TDRT) showed that the TDRT enabled tissue vascularization while maintaining and even surpassing the mechanical properties and fibroblast colonization (Wang et al. 2015b).

Other hybrid scaffolds have also been developed using rhTE. Thus, Annabi et al. have prepared 3D hydrogels and 2D films based on methacrylated tropoelastin photocrosslinked by UV light that are suitable for cell encapsulation or cell seeding. The rhTE provides interesting mechanical properties to the hydrogels, which exhibit high extensibility, reversible deformation with low energy loss, and high resilience upon stretching (Annabi et al. 2013b).

The potential for using rhTE-based devices for skin tissue regeneration is evident, therefore new recombinant approaches based on other proteins have been described in the last few years. In this regard, important progress has been made in the treatment of skin diseases with recombinant human collagen type VII (rhC7). Type VII collagen is an ECM protein that plays a crucial role as an adhesion molecule in the dermal-epidermal junction zone (DEJZ) (Ko and Marinkovich 2010). C7 has been shown to be vital for the maintenance of skin integrity and also for skin wound closure. Indeed, due to its role in laminin-332 deposition and integrin $\alpha_6\beta_4$ expression, C7 is a pivotal protein for epidermal re-epithelization and dermal granulation tissue during closure (Nyström et al. 2013). For this reason, therapies for skin wound healing that include rhC7 have been tested. For example, Wang et al. have produced rhC7 from dermal fibroblasts and used it in full-thickness wounds in athymic nude mouse models. These studies demonstrated that the simple topical application of rhC7 promoted wound healing as rhC7 was stably incorporated into the DEJZ of the healing wounds, thereby improving the re-epithelialization process. Moreover, topical rhC7 inhibited fibrosis of the wounded skin and the restoration of hC7 expression in RDEB mouse models was observed (Wang et al. 2013b). Recessive dystrophic epidermolysisbullosa (RDEB) is a disorder associated with a defect in both alleles of the *COL7A1* gene, one of the exons that encodes the alpha chains of hC7 (Christiano et al. 1994). RDEB patients exhibit skin fragility, skin blistering, erosions, nail loss, joint contractures, trauma-induced blisters, and aggressive squamous cell carcinomas that lead to premature death (Fine et al. 2008). Unfortunately, there is currently no reliable treatment for RDEB. Recombinant hC7 has been studied as a protein-based therapy for the treatment of RDEB both topically and intravenously. Woodley et al. (2013) have studied re-localization of the injected rhC7 and reversion of the RDEB skin phenotype in a mouse model. They found restored hC7 expression and effectively demonstrated correct migration of the injected rhC7 to wounded tissues and correction of the major structural abnormality of RDEB mouse skin. Indeed, rhC7 was incorporated into the DEJZ and formed anchoring fibril structures without any adverse effects being observed (Woodley et al. 2013).

Other recombinant collagen types have also been used to treat cutaneous lesions. Thus, a flowable hydrogel made of recombinant human type I collagen (rhC1), produced in tobacco plants, has been developed and its ability to treat acute, chronic, and tunneled cutaneous lesions tested. In this regard, Shilo et al. (2013) formed saline rhC1 hydrogel matrices and compared their effects in wound healing with bovine and cadaveric human C1. Application of rhC1 hydrogels resulted in faster lesion closure and accelerated the healing process, with an earlier angiogenic response in comparison with controls (Shilo et al. 2013).

In summary, although skin tissue is able to self-regenerate, in some cases (severe wounds or burns) a scaffold that enables regeneration of the different cell types in the skin, supporting cell growth and cell interaction, is required. Recombinant scaffolds have been shown to promote skin regeneration since it is possible to produce 3D matrices that perfectly mimic the dermal ECM, its structure and its biochemical properties.

Vascular regeneration

Cardiovascular disease is currently one of the leading causes of mortality in the world due to the lack of healthy substitutes. To overcome these limitations, several different approaches, including autologous autografts, biodegradable synthetic polymer-based constructs, endothelial cells seeded on synthetic grafts, etc., have been investigated (Cleary et al. 2012).

A combination of natural and synthetic polymers may give rise to homogeneous and reproducible structures that promote excellent cell adhesion, growth and migration. Furthermore, the fact that such polymers are often biodegradable means that host cells can produce their own extracellular matrix to replace the degraded scaffold (Furth et al. 2007). In this regard, Cosgriff-Hernandez et al. (2012) combined the

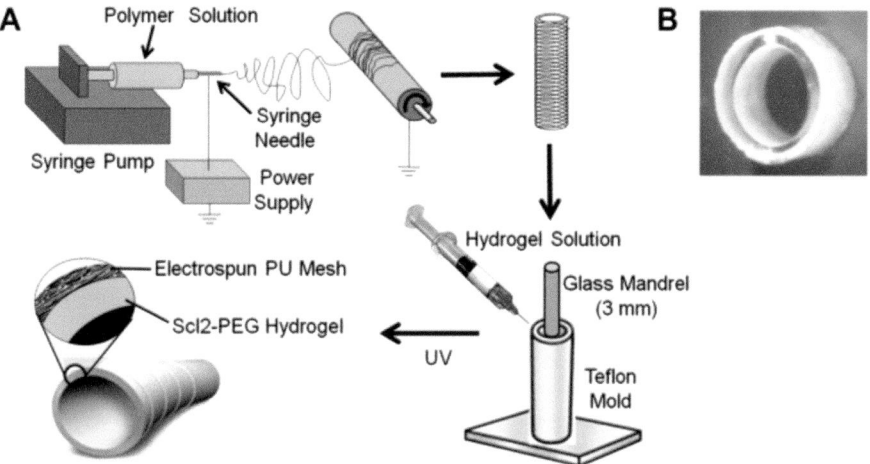

Fig. 1: Representation of multilayer graft fabrication (A) and multilayer graft (B). Reproduced from (Browning et al. 2012).

biomechanical properties of a poly(ethylene glycol) (PEG) hydrogel and *Scl2-2* (collagen-mimetic protein derived from group A Streptococcus) to develop a bioactive hydrogel that binds to endothelial cells (ECs) and resists platelet adhesion. This hydrogel was subsequently reinforced with an electrospun polyurethane mesh to improve its biomechanical properties. *In vitro* tests demonstrated that tuning the migration speed by altering the protein concentration in the PEG-Scl2 hydrogels promoted higher migration speeds than those found in PEG-collagen analogs (Browning et al. 2012).

Mechanical properties are critical to the success of the implant. Thus, the biostability of many scaffolds depends on several factors such as strength, elasticity, absorption at the material interface, and its chemical degradation. It is therefore essential to retain the mechanical strength of the scaffold structure post-implantation in order to be able to reconstruct hard, load-bearing tissues (Griffith and Naughton 2002).

In light of the above, Caves et al. (2010) generated an acellular arterial substitute comprising synthetic collagen microfibers and a recombinant elastin-like protein to improve the mechanical properties of the scaffolds and subsequently assessed their structural and mechanical properties. Reinforcing the vascular graft with collagen microfibers should modulate suture retention strength, burst strength, and compliance. By exploiting the non-thrombogenic features of elastin, the resulting acellular constructs exhibited favorable performance as implanted vascular grafts (Caves et al. 2010). The development of vascular grafts has focused on finding a biomaterial that is non-thrombogenic, minimizes intimal hyperplasia, matches the mechanical properties of native vessels, and allows for regeneration of arterial tissue. Indeed, the importance of establishing an elastic fiber structure in a vascular scaffold that is similar to the arterial wall has long been recognized as the depletion or loss of elastin has been correlated to both aneurysmal progression and severe smooth muscle cell hyperplasia in both animals and humans (Hoerstrup et al. 2001).

The generation of protein polymers that mimic native structural proteins and adopt the characteristics of the arterial wall offers a unique approach to the development of a vascular graft. Ultimately, the success of this approach is the manipulation of proteins that constitute the architecture of the native ECM (Ratcliffe 2000). Given their bioactive properties, natural materials exhibit better interactions with cells that allow them to enhance the performance of cells in biological systems. This was nicely demonstrated by McKenna et al. (2012), who developed an electrospun small-diameter vascular graft containing recombinant human tropoelastin produced in *E. coli* to impart critical cell signaling to the biomaterial and which, when cross-linked, mimics native elastin fibers. This electrospun tubular vascular scaffold demonstrated physical and mechanical properties similar to extracted arterial elastin with a controlled length and diameter. Moreover, it supported smooth muscle cell attachment, spreading, and growth (McKenna et al. 2012). An alternative method for producing vascular stents is the use of coated stents comprising a bare metal stent covered with a layer of natural materials to prevent immunogenic responses and which should support endothelialization to achieve physiological hemocompatibility (Nakayama et al. 2003). The material used to coat the stent should have stable mechanical characteristics under physiological pressure and flow conditions. Gonzalez et al. (2015) were able to develop a method for coating vascular stents with elastin-like recombinamer-based catalyst-free click gels. These recombinamers presented a universal cell-adhesion epitope known as RGD (arginine, glycine, aspartic acid), an REDV (arginine, glutamic acid, aspartic acid, valine) cell-adhesion domain that is more specific for endothelial cells, and a structural recombinamer lacking any bioactive sequence. The catalyst-free click gels were produced by modifying the ELRs using the Huisgen 1,3-dipolar cycloaddition of azides and alkynes according to the concepts of click chemistry (Huisgen 1963; Kolb et al. 2001). The bare metal stents were embedded in the ELR gels by injection molding and subsequently were endothelialized under dynamic pressure and flow conditions in a bioreactor. Finally, the stents were exposed to blood in a Chandler loop for one hour. The results showed that the presence of the RGD cell-adhesion sequence elicits a higher adhesion and proliferation rate of endothelial cells with respect to the stents coated with REDV-ELR. *In vitro* endothelialization of the devices prior to implantation *in vivo* resulted in improved mechanical stability, physiological hemocompatibility, and a reduced risk of thrombosis as a result of minimal platelet adhesion (de Torre et al. 2015).

Bone regeneration

Significant research effort has been dedicated to improving the mechanisms of bone regeneration and the remodeling process for native bone extracellular matrix in recent years (Agarwal and García 2015). Numerous diseases and injuries, including osteoarthritis, osteogenesis imperfecta, and traumatic processes, can adversely affect the musculoskeletal system and consequently restrict quality of life. Although autografting and allografting have been the standard strategies for repairing bone defects, they nevertheless present some drawbacks, such as limited quantities of donor tissue, donor-site morbidity, immune response in the host tissue, etc. (Polo-Corrales et al. 2014). To date, the generation of living tissue constructs that are structurally, functionally, and mechanically comparable to natural bone remains a challenge. Other approaches have focused on improving the efficacy of bone grafts or other scaffolds by using recombinant proteins, which offer a much higher level of tunability, spatiotemporal control, bioactivity, and stimulation of bone formation (Hollister 2005). An ideal bone graft or scaffold should comprise biomaterials that imitate the structure and properties of natural bone ECM and provide all the necessary environmental milestones found in natural bone (Hutmacher 2000) have developed and characterized a novel class of ECM-based composite scaffolds that combine the compatibility of the polymers collagen and ELR in order to create a homogeneous network structure that could support osteoblast adhesion, growth, and differentiation. Differentiation of the pre-osteoblast was assessed in ELR-collagen and collagen gels for a period of 21 days. The results demonstrated that ELR-collagen scaffolds were suitable substrates for cell culture by allowing pre-osteoblast cell attachment, differentiation, and subsequent mineralization over a period of three weeks. The ELR-collagen scaffolds showed equivalent biocompatibility and cell-interaction properties to those of collagen scaffolds (Amruthwar and Janorkar 2013). Along similar lines, and exploiting the features presented by ELRs, Tejeda-Montes et al. (2014) created a periosteal graft for enhanced bone regeneration using bioactive ELR membranes containing four bioactive peptides in order to promote mesenchymal stem cell adhesion (RGDS from fibronectin and other ECM proteins), endothelial cell adhesion (REDV from fibronectin), mineralization (SN$_A$15), and both cell adhesion and mineralization (RGDS-SN$_A$15). These authors found that the amino acid sequence of the SN$_A$15 fragment induced osteoblastic differentiation and mineralization. Mineralization of the membrane in the presence of cells was similar under both static and dynamic culture conditions. Indeed, the SN$_A$15 fragment had a strong effect on the mineralization of membranes (Tejeda-Montes et al. 2014). Bone regeneration was subsequently assessed in a critical size rat calvarial defect model, which showed that animals implanted with HAP membranes had the highest mean volume of ossified tissue and exhibited an osteoid matrix with active osteoblasts within the defect. The analog of the SN15 fragment of statherin, in which aspartate (D) residues substitute the original phosphoserines and whose bioactivity is equivalent to the SN15 fragment of statherin, led to cellular signaling that stimulated progenitor cells and enhanced the growth of osteoblasts *in vivo* (Raj et al. 1992).

Amongst the many natural biomaterials available, silk-based polymer scaffolds are a promising candidate for the development of tissue grafts that can be used for bone regeneration as silk fibroin presents optimal mechanical properties, biodegradability, cytocompatibility, low immunogenicity, and controllable porosity (Sofia et al. 2001; Mottaghitalab et al. 2015). Moisenovich et al. (2012) compared two porous scaffolds made from different silk proteins. The first scaffold comprised fibroin from *Bombyxmori* and the other was a recombinant analog of *Nephilaclavipes spidroin 1*, known as rS1/9, which was expressed in yeast. Their biocompatibility and degradability were assessed *in vitro* and *in vivo*. The *in vitro* results indicated that the cell growth of mouse fibroblasts was similar for both scaffolds. They were subsequently implanted into the subcutaneous spaces of Balb/c mice and found to be well tolerated by the host animals, with no signs of inflammation, rejection, or other abnormal conditions. After eight weeks, both types of scaffolds had been adhered to by subcutaneous tissues but maintained their original shape and were easily distinguishable (Moisenovich et al. 2012).

Nervous system regeneration

One billion people worldwide are affected by neurological diseases (WHO 2006), and an estimated 6.8 million people die every year as a result of neurological disorders. These numbers will increase substantially in the near future in the developed world as a result of population aging. Despite the availability of numerous and varied treatments for neurological diseases, complete recovery is rare and many disorders have limited therapeutic options and no cure. The main reason for the lack of effective treatment is the limited development of technologies aimed at regenerating the central nervous system (Case and Tessier-Lavigne 2005). After a neuronal injury, the potential to regenerate the neurons responsible for signal transmission is limited, and large-scale tissue defects can rarely be restored (Liu et al. 2011). As a result, there have been many efforts to develop biomaterials that promote neurite growth.

Various parameters must be taken into consideration in neural cell culture. For example, a bioactive scaffold with the appropriate mechanical properties is required in order to sustain the cells and specific protein domains that enable neurite growth and neural differentiation from neural stem cells. In this regard, the ability of matrices based on cross-linked ELRs to support neurite growth has been demonstrated recently. Thus, an integrin-binding ligand involved in neurite elongation during neuronal cell differentiation and associated with adhesion-mediated cell migration was incorporated into ELR scaffolds containing the bioactive peptide RGD (Rogers et al. 1987; Sedaghati and Seifalian 2015). Subsequently, Jeon et al. manufactured recombinant ELR matrices and demonstrated that the adhesion, spreading morphology, and migration speed of Neuro-2a cells reached similar levels in 2D ELR matrices to those seen on fibronectin-coated surfaces *in vitro* (Jeon et al. 2012). Furthermore, elastin-like hydrogels allow the development of 3D matrices, which in turn allow the effect of biomechanics and biochemistry on neural behavior to be assessed *in vitro*. For example, Heilshorn's group have described 3D scaffolds made of chemically cross-linked RGD-ELRs suitable for studying neurite outgrowth and the various cell morphologies present in the behavior of dorsal root ganglia (DRG), a common model for peripheral nerve regeneration, *in vitro*. These matrices have allowed the relationship between RGD-ligand density and neurite growth to be determined, thereby helping to optimize the stiffness of 3D hydrogels (Lampe et al. 2013). Moreover, such systems can be studied incombination with the effect of neurotrophins. It is wellknown that regeneration of the peripheral nervous system is a complex process in which the matrix, cell culture, and different growth factors all play a very specific role, as is the case in nature (Son and Thompson 1995; Fu and Gordon 1997; Macaya and Spector 2012). In order to try to elucidate the interaction between 3D RGD-ELRs hydrogels and different neurotrophic factors in neurite behavior, chick DRG explants were cultured on these bioactive matrices supplemented with a neural growth factor (NGF) gradient such that two important parameters could be determined. Firstly, an increase in RGD-ligand concentration enhanced neurite outgrowth in both the presence and absence of NGF (Romano et al. 2015a). However, even more importantly, a synergistic effect between the 3D RGD-EL matrices and NGF treatment on neurite outgrowth was demonstrated, with outgrowth in the 3D matrix containing a high concentration of RGD-ligand being enhanced upon treatment with NGF (Romano et al. 2015b).

Other 3D matrices for neural tissue regeneration based on different recombinant biomaterials, such as recombinant spider silk matrices, have also been developed. The use of natural spider silk fibers as guides for nerve regeneration has already been demonstrated in animal testing in sheep with promising results (Radtke et al. 2011). In order to elucidate the mechanisms behind the interaction between neuron cells and the silk matrices, various recombinant spider silk matrices have been developed. Thus, Lewicka et al. designed matrices based on the recombinant spider silk protein 4RepCT, which provides an efficient substrate for neural stem cell (NSC) differentiation without affecting cell viability (Lewicka et al. 2012). Similarly, Kaplan's group studied matrices based on other different recombinant spider silk proteins, especially major ampullatespidroind 1 (MaSp1) and 2 (MaSp2), and demonstrated the ability of MaSp1 silk protein-based matrices to regulate neuron growth by interacting with neuron receptors and upregulating NCAM expression (An et al. 2015). Kaplan's group has also manufactured composites comprising rhTE and natural silk. These composites were formed by taking advantage of charge and hydrophobic-hydrophilic interactions between rhTE and natural silk, followed by autoclaving to crosslink the silk fibroin chains (Hu et al. 2013). The resulting composites were used to create 3D matrices with differently charged regions, thus allowing neuron cell culture and regulation of the growth and formation of charge-sensitive cell networks. Also in the field of peripheral nerve regeneration, silk-rhTE films have been developed for the study of peripheral neuron and Schwann cell growth (White et al. 2015), and it has been reported that the use of patterned films allows the growth direction of neurites and Schwann cells to be controlled without negatively affecting the cell culture.

In conclusion, recombinant biomaterials are excellent candidates as scaffolds for neural tissue regeneration as they can incorporate specific motifs that promote neurite growth, without being chemically modified. In addition, their tunable mechanical properties means that they allow the diffusion of neurotrophic factors, which is extremely important for controlling the growth direction.

Corneal tissue regeneration

The cornea is an avascular and transparent connective tissue which is roughly 500 μm thick (Liu et al. 1999). The cornea has two main functions: protection of the eye by serving as a barrier against external objects and refraction of light. Indeed, it is the main optical element of the eye, refracting 70 per cent of the light entering the eye for vision (McLaughlin et al. 2009; White et al. 2015). In 2010, the WHO estimated the number of visually impaired people in the world to be around 285 million, with 39 million of these being blind. Corneal blindness represents 5.1 per cent of all cases, and it is estimated that approximately 1.5 million new cases are diagnosed each year (Pascolini and Mariotti 2011). The treatment of irreversible corneal tissue damage is basically reduced to two main approaches, namely allogenic transplants or synthetic materials. Allogenic transplantation is the most effective treatment for corneal blindness, and many forms of irreversible corneal blindness are treatable by corneal transplantation using donated tissue. However, the main problem of this approach is the availability of cadaveric corneas, with demand far exceeding the number of donors, especially in the developing world (Whitcher et al. 2002). Moreover, allogenic transplantation can lead to transplant rejection and therefore long-term steroid-based immunosuppression, and it also represents a risk of transmissible diseases (e.g., HIV) or infections (e.g., fungal and herpes simplex virus keratitis). Furthermore, in many cases cadaveric corneas are not suitable for transplantation due to aging of the population and the increasing number of refractive surgery patients (Panda et al. 2007; Tan et al. 2012). Consequently, alternative pathways, such as the use of synthetic materials, are needed. In this regard, recombinant biomaterials that mimic the corneal extracellular matrix (ECM) and promote endogenous regeneration of corneal tissue are a promising option.

One of the most widely studied recombinant materials for this purpose is collagen, which is the main protein in the human cornea (approx. 70 per cent dry weight). Recombinant collagen allows the formation of robust and biodegradable 3D hydrogels as a result of its triple-helix structure and, although these hydrogels can be degraded by collagenases, chemical cross-linking delays their biodegradation (Liu et al. 2006). Fagerholm's group has developed various 3D hydrogels based on recombinant human collagen (rhC) suitable for corneal tissue regeneration. In addition, they have demonstrated that chemically cross-linked hydrogels based on recombinant human collagen type I (rhC1) and type III (rhC3) support *in vitro* epithelium and nerve culture and that these hydrogels have appropriate optical properties and tensile strength for use as corneal substitutes (Liu et al. 2008). The hydrogels were made by cross-linking rhC solutions with 1-ethyl-3-(3-dimethylaminopropyl) carbodiimide (EDC) and *N*-hydroxysuccinimide (NHS), and although neither of them reached the strength values of natural cornea, the bioactive, mechanical, and optical properties of rhC3 hydrogels showed such satisfactory results in animal testing that they were subsequently tested in humans. Phase I clinical studies of rhC3 cross-linked hydrogels in humans over four years revealed that these materials allow tissue regeneration by endogenous cell recruitment. Furthermore, the neo-corneas are stable, and no patient showed implant rejection or the need for long-term immunosuppression treatment (Fagerholm et al. 2014). However, the characteristics of these hydrogels still needed to be improved further in order to facilitate surgical manipulation and to reduce costs for the manufacture of implants on a larger scale. Thus, different cross-linking strategies were studied, and two main approaches were found to significantly improve the properties of the 3D rhC3 chemical cross-linked hydrogels. Thus, rhC3 hydrogels cross-linked with other carbodiimide reagents, such as *N*-cyclohexyl-*N'*-(2-morpholinoethyl) carbodiimidemetho-*p*-toluenesulfonate (CMC). In comparison with the initial rhC3-EDC hydrogels, the resulting rhC3-CMC hydrogels gelled at ambient temperature, were stiffer and showed a superior collagenase resistance (Ahn et al. 2013). Similarly, 3D hydrogels based on the combination of rhC3 and phosphorylcholine have also been developed. In this case, the collagen network was reinforced with a second network made from 2-methacryloyloxyethylphosphorylcholine (MPC) to give rise to lamellae-like layers of rhC3-MPC interconnected with fiber-like structures (Fig. 2). The resulting hydrogels had higher mechanical strength, thus making them feasible for post-fabrication modification using laser cutting and microcontact printing (Hayes et al. 2015; Islam et al. 2015).

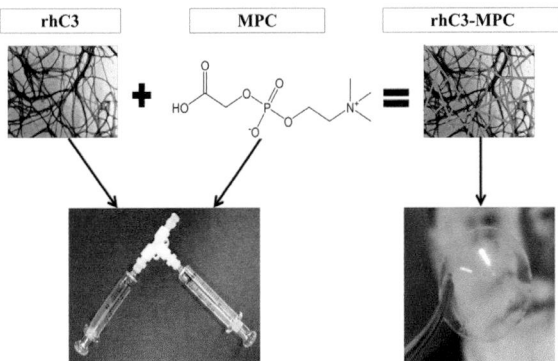

Fig. 2: Schematic representation of the formation process of interpenetrating networks of recombinant human collagen. Adapted from (Buznyk et al. 2015).

rhC3-MPC implants were initially studied in a small sample population (three patients), and the remarkable results obtained suggested the potential use of these devices to repair corneal damage in patients with severe pathologies (Buznyk et al. 2015). However, rhC-based scaffolds are not the only recombinant approach as other strategies have been employed to obtain scaffolds suitable for corneal tissue regeneration. Thus, Kilic et al. assembled micropatterned natural collagen-ELR films into multi-layered 3D scaffolds by dehydrothermal cross-linking. The resulting translucent multi-film devices mimicked the ordered and densely packed structure of corneal collagen fibrils, supporting keratocyte attachment and proliferation (Kilic et al. 2014). The ability of ELR scaffolds to provide an appropriate environment for the adhesion and growth of other ocular tissues, such as conjunctival epithelial cells (Martinez-Osorio et al. 2009) and retinal pigment epithelial (RPE) cells, has also been demonstrated for the treatment of age-related macular degeneration, a disease associated with degeneration of the RPE cells in the macula that affects up to 8 per cent of the population older than 65 years in the developed world. The only effective treatment to cure this disease is the transplantation of autologous RPE cells, and to this end a biointeractive scaffold is crucial. Accordingly, ELR surfaces have been shown to be excellent candidates as transplantation vehicles in humans as these devices both stimulate cell adhesion and cell growth and maintain the characteristics of the RPE phenotype (Srivastava et al. 2011; Singh et al. 2014).

In summary, recombinant biomaterials appear to be one of the most promising alternatives to the lack of viable human corneas and for regenerating other ocular tissues. Indeed, various examples of recombinant scaffolds developed recently have enabled the successful regeneration of different ocular tissues.

Cartilage regeneration

Cartilage is a connective tissue consisting of a dense matrix of collagen and elastic fibers embedded in a rubbery ground substance (Buckwalter and Mankin 1997). It has a limited regenerative capacity due to the absence of nerves and blood vessels. Although traditional methods such as autografts and allografts have been employed clinically to treat joint cartilage lesions, these therapies have their own inherent problems (Grande et al. 1997). Consequently, tissue engineering may provide alternative solutions for joint cartilage repair and regeneration by developing biomimetic tissue substitutes with the mechanical properties required to resist the loads to which joints are subjected (Chung and Burdick 2008). In this regard, considerable progress has been made in the development of methods to modify the mechanical properties of substitutes, for example by modifying the quantity of ECM components produced by chondrocytes by mechanical or chemical stimulation, adjusting the internal scaffold structure, and choosing appropriate scaffold materials or their combinations (Grande et al. 1997). For example, Jia et al. (2013) developed a 3D biodegradable porous scaffold combining the biological characteristics of human-like collagen (HLC) produced by recombinant *E. coli* and the mechanical properties of nano-hydroxyapatite (nHA). nHA presents excellent bioactivity, high biocompatibility, strong plasticity and outstanding mechanical properties (Huang et al. 1997). As such, a combination of these materials could improve the wettability and permeability of the resulting materials and enhance the mechanical properties of the resulting scaffolds. A comparison of HLC/nHA scaffolds with the control group showed that the compression stress in the former was about 2.67 ± 0.37 MPa higher than in the latter. Rabbit chondrocytes were subsequently seeded on the composite porous scaffolds and cultured for 21 days, thereby demonstrating that chondrocytes attached to and proliferated on the surface of the scaffold and formed a dense layer of cells, presenting a homogeneous distribution and abundant glycosaminoglycan synthesis and maintaining natural chondrocyte morphology compared to control scaffolds (Jia et al. 2013).

Different collagens in a variety of scaffolds have been used as a biomaterial-based scaffold for chondrocytes in joint cartilage repair and tissue engineering. Collagen, especially type II collagen, forms a natural environment for the chondrocytes since it is the predominant matrix molecule in cartilage (Wakitani et al. 1989; Newman 1998). In this regard, Pulkkinen et al. (2012) analyzed a new recombinant human type II collagen (rhC2) biomaterial in a nude mouse model *in vivo* and demonstrated that the rhC2-gel seeded with chondrocytes formed a tissue with abundant presence of collagen and proteoglycans when grown subcutaneously for six weeks in the backs of nude mice. The use of an animal component-free rhC2 gel as a scaffold for chondrocytes resulted in better maintenance of the construct shape compared with the cells without a scaffold. A soft gel material lacking synthetic or animal-derived additives results in a safe and reproducible way by which more structural competence can be added to the implantation of chondrocytes (Pulkkinen et al. 2013).

Particular interest has been raised as regards biodegradable hydrogels that can act as a temporary support for the deposition of a neo-cartilaginous matrix. The incorporation of hydrolytically or enzymatically cleavable substrates is the most common approach used to impart biodegradability to hydrogel systems (Bryant et al. 2004). However, the major drawback of such hydrogels is the lack of control over degradation kinetics since the degradation mechanism is not specific (Bahney et al. 2011). Specific enzyme-sensitive peptides, for example, can be included in the hydrogel network to enable localized cell-induced degradation. Matrix metalloproteinases (MMPs) are often targeted as the most suitable route for enzymatic degradation since they are known to be involved in the cleavage of ECM components during native tissue remodeling. MMP7 is thought to play a role in chondrogenesis by controlling the bioavailability of chondrogenic factors and facilitating the maturation of collagen type II (Bryant et al. 2004). In this regard, Parmar et al. (2015) developed MMP7-degradable hydrogels based on recombinant Streptococcal collagen-like 2 (Scl2) proteins and functionalized with GAG-binding peptides, which can be easily tailored to recreate the biochemical microenvironment of joint cartilage. In this study, a blank slate Scl2 protein was cross-linked with the MMP7-sensitive peptide to form hydrogels and functionalized with peptides that bind hyaluronic acid (HA) and chondroitin sulfate (CS). The authors subsequently investigated how GAG-binding peptides affect the chondrogenic differentiation of human mesenchymal stem cells encapsulated within the hydrogels that could then be implanted to treat focal defects, MMP7 gene expression and activity. HA bind MMP7-Scl2 hydrogels were found to direct the largest increase in gene expression and lead to the highest overall collagen and sGAG accumulation (Parmar et al. 2015).

Drug Delivery

Recombinant protein-based devices with the same nature as cellular components also represent interesting carriers for drug delivery due to their biocompatibility, biodegradability, and the fact that their sequence can be controlled genetically (Shi et al. 2014; Doblhofer and Scheibel 2015). Their monodispersity is another relevant characteristic for drug-delivery applications (Kopeček 2003) as it enables pharmacokinetic profiles to be generated and structure-function relationships to be determined, which is often not possible for statistically defined polymer systems. Chemically synthesized polymers, especially more complicated and longer chain length polymers, which often generate statistical distributions of polymer lengths, cannot achieve this precision (Hench and Polak 2002; Price et al. 2014).

The bio-engineering process allows these recombinant proteins to be modified by adding cell-specific ligands that confer active targeting abilities (Price et al. 2014). The use of recombinant proteins in drug delivery allows drugs to be stabilized and their release controlled, thus meaning that they can be applied in targeted drug administration to enhance treatment possibilities and avoid diffusion of the drug throughout the human body, thereby minimizing undesirable effects in healthy tissues.

This section of the review provides an overview of the most recent research published over the last few years on the delivery of genes and drugs. In this regard, the main types of recombinant polymers that will be described are: ELRs, SLRs, and SELRs.

Elastin-like recombinamers for drug delivery

Recombinant polypeptides derived from the elastin sequence have been widely used in drug delivery applications to treat several diseases. The versatility of ELRs makes them an excellent option for the construction of various structures, such as nanoparticles, hydrogel, depots, etc. (MacEwan and Chilkoti 2014a; Price et al. 2014; Rodriguez-Cabello et al. 2015). Furthermore, these materials may be suitable for applications in targeted drug delivery or as a result of their smart behavior, by way of which they can respond to environmental stimuli such as temperature, pH, and light, amongst others (Price et al. 2014).

Although there are a huge number of innovative methods involving ELRs in fields as diverse as maternal-fetal medicine, ophthalmology, and cardiovascular or infectious diseases, the highest number of novel advances are in anti-cancer therapies (Despanie et al. 2015). According to the WHO, over 14 million new cases and 8.2 million cancer-related deaths are diagnosed every year (Cancer 2014). This has motivated researchers to develop innovative anti-cancer treatments, and ELRs are an emerging tool in this field (McDaniel et al. 2010; Raucher and Ryu 2015). Most systemically delivered anticancer treatments must pass through barriers to prevent clearance of drug from the circulation, enhance the penetration, and accumulation of drug at the tumor site, and achieve internalization of drug in cancer cells, a major barrier that intracellular therapeutic targets have to overcome (MacEwan and Chilkoti 2014b). The challenge of increasing the uptake of a drug by a tumor cell can be overcome using ELRs (McDaniel et al. 2010; Price et al. 2014; Raucher and Ryu 2015; Ryu and Raucher 2015), as can be seen from the following recent examples.

Based on a previous study in which an ELR was fused with a poly-aspartic acid tail (named ELR-D) with an ability to form nanoparticles (Fujita et al. 2009), Matsumoto et al. (2014) have designed a new targeted nanoparticle (ELR-D-E) combining this ELR-D with the EGF (epidermal growth factor) sequence with the aim of allowing its exposure on the surface. The resulting nanoparticles (around 30 nm) present a specific cellular interaction, as revealed by *in vitro* results in A549 cells, a human lung adenocarcinoma epithelial cell line that overexpresses the EGF receptor. This system was also shown to be a good candidate for drug-delivery applications by the loading of paclitaxel, a well-known anti-cancer drug, which was found to be internalized into A549 cells and to induce cell death (Matsumoto et al. 2014).

The same group designed an advanced approach for loading a single-chain vascular endothelial growth factor (scVEGF$_{121}$)-derived polypeptide into nanoparticles. With the aim of providing noncovalent tethering upon formation of a heterodimer coiled-coil structure, two peptides known to establish this structural motif, one containing basic (helixB) and the other acid (helixA) residues, were fused to the former ELR-D and the scVEGF$_{121}$, respectively. When combined with paclitaxel (PTX), this VEGF-tethered ELR-D-helixB construct exhibits enhanced cytotoxicity levels compared with ELR-D-helixB against HeLa cells, showing considerable cell death only 6 h post-treatment. Moreover, although its cytotoxic capability is similar to that of free PTX applied directly to culture cells, this nanostructure reduces renal clearance effects and allows a more specific delivery. These results suggest that both components combine their properties to allow ELR-D-nanoparticle formation and helixA-scVEGF$_{121}$ recognition via binding to the VEGF receptor. Furthermore, the combination of coiled-coil heterodimers that are able to form nanoparticles with targeted drug delivery enhances tumor suppression and increases apoptotic cell death (Assal et al. 2015).

Taken together, these two studies demonstrate that customized drug-delivery systems that target different cell types and receptors can be constructed using ELRs.

Based on previous studies (Massodi et al. 2010; Walker et al. 2014), Ryu et al. described the effects of an ELR fused with a p21-derived cell cycle inhibitory peptide (p21) and a Bac cell-penetrating peptide (Fig. 3), combined with hyperthermia or hyperthermia and gemcitabine, a chemotherapy agent widely used to treat pancreatic cancer. Hyperthermia, or local mild heating (40–43°C) of the tumor site, has been widely used clinically (Dewhirst et al. 1997). Although local mild hyperthermia

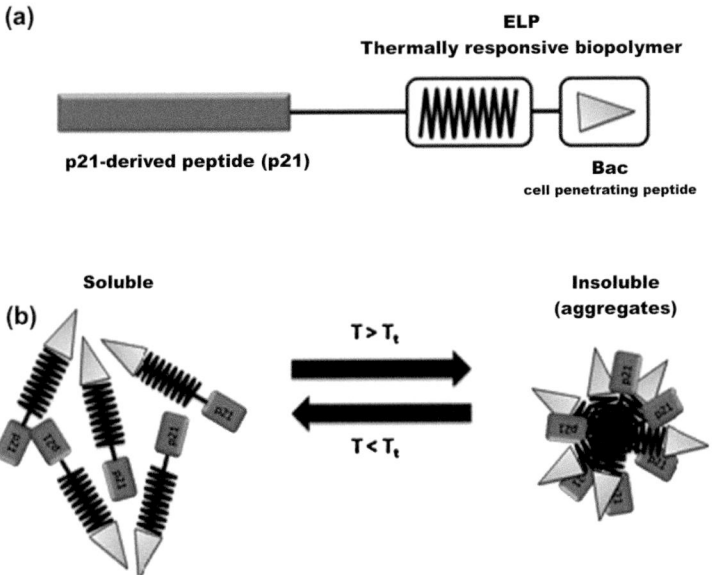

Fig. 3: Schematic diagrams of an ELR-CPP drug-delivery system. (a) The delivery system consists of the p21, an anticancer cargo molecule at the N-terminus, followed by the thermally responsive elastin-like polypeptide and Bac cell penetrating peptide. (b) Thermally responsive property of ELR. Aggregation of ELR at high temperature (T > Tt) can increase of the tumor accumulation of anticancer cargo molecule, p21. Reprinted with permission from (Ryu and Raucher 2014).

does not directly kill tissue, it has been shown to sensitize the tumor to anti-cancer therapies as well as to increase vascular permeability and tumor blood flow compared with normal vasculature, thereby enhancing intracellular trafficking into the tumor cells (Andrew Mackay and Chilkoti 2008; McDaniel et al. 2010). The thermo-responsive property of ELRs allows the use of a local mild hyperthermia to target tumors for the transport of chemotherapeutics while reducing the toxicity of the drug and allowing the lowest possible dose with the best effectiveness. *In vitro* and *in vivo* results show that p21-ELR-Bac combined with hyperthermia inhibits growth of three pancreatic cancer cell lines and in a pancreatic tumor xenograft mouse model by mimicking the effects of wildtype p21, thus leading to arrest at the G1 and G2 or S phase of the cell cycle. However, the best effect was obtained when p21-ELR$_1$-Bac was combined with hyperthermia and gemcitabine. This resulted in an enhancement of both the *in vitro* cytotoxicity and tumor growth inhibition in the animal model from values of around 34 per cent and 58 per cent, respectively, achieved using p21-ELR$_1$-Bac and gemcitabine, to 81 per cent for the combined treatment (Ryu and Raucher 2014).

Over the past few years, topical ocular administration has been considered as a possible application of ELR-based nanoparticles in some treatments, especially as regards the development of new release mechanisms given the high incidence of ocular-associated diseases (Olthoff et al. 2005; Shukla et al. 2008).

A new strategy in this regard involves the combination of an ELR-based nanoparticle comprising a block copolymer with hydrophilic (serine-containing) and hydrophobic (isoleucine-containing) domains with a mitogen protein known as lacritin (Lacrt). This structure is able to self-assemble at 37°C to expose Lacrt at the surface, thus allowing it to come into contact with the ocular surface. *In vitro* studies revealed that Lacrt-ELR had the ability to trigger calcium-dependent cell signaling, could be internalized into the cells and facilitated scratch closure in monolayers of a human corneal epithelial cell line. Furthermore, *in vivo* experiments in a murine corneal abrasion model (non-obese diabetic (NOD) mice mimicking photorefractive keratectomy) showed that the topical application of Lacrt-ELR to the ocular surface promoted complete wound healing at only 24 h post-treatment, whereas the ELR alone and the untreated group still showed a significant wound area. Another important aspect of this construct is that Lacrt-ELR nanoparticles produced complete corneal epithelium regeneration whereas another ELR fused to Lacrt, which did not undergo thermally mediated assembly, did not (Wang et al. 2014a).

With the aim of enhancing the treatment of dry eye, the same biopharmaceutical protein component of human tears mentioned above (Lacrt) was fused to another ELR comprising 96 repetitions of the VPGVG pentapetide. This resulted in a new device with the ability to form an intra-lacrimal depot at physiological temperature, thus allowing greater control of the drug localization and maintaining Lacrt-mediated cell signaling pathways. *In vitro* studies showed that Lacrt-ELR had the ability to enhance β-hexosaminidase secretion and actin remodeling in isolated primary cultured lacrimal gland acinar cells from female New Zealand white rabbits. Furthermore, *in vivo* results showed an enhancement in tear secretion in both male and female NOD mice (around 40.9 per cent and 50.9 per cent respectively) compared with the ELR or free Lacrt alone, which had an effectiveness of 29.6 per cent in males and 42.9 per cent in females (Wang et al. 2015a).

With regard to similar applications, a considerable number of disorders, such as dry eye due to lymphocytic infiltration and loss of function of the lacrimal gland (LG), can be involved in Sjögren's syndrome (SjS) (da Costa et al. 2006; Li et al. 2010). Consequently, the same diblock ELR copolymer proposed by Wang et al. (2014a) has been functionalized with FK506 binding protein 12 (FKBP), which is the binding partner of the small molecule drug rapamycin (Rapa) (Shah et al. 2013). Rapa, which is a potent immunosuppressant with high toxicity for the treatment of SjS, was both encapsulated in the hydrophobic core of the ELR nanoparticle and in the corona bound to the FKBP. Systemic administration of both free Rapa and Rapa encapsulated into FKBP-ELR to NOD mice by intravenous injection showed that the latter system released the drug at a very slow rate, thereby allowing the drug to be retained during circulation *in vivo* and reducing lymphocyte infiltration into the LG of NOD mice and renal exposure of the drug, minimizing the toxicity associated with the free drug. The nanoparticle-based system was also found to have an effect on inflammation and mTOR pathway genes and to be more effective at reducing a tear biomarker related with tear secretion in SjS, namely cathepsin S (CATS), compared with the free drug (Shah et al. 2013). Long-term objectives for this system include the encapsulation of Rapa into an ELR nanoparticle containing targeting motifs for other tissues in order to enhance cell-specific treatments, as has previously been demonstrated for a knob domain of the fibre capsid protein of an adenovirus serotype 5-targeting nanoparticle with the same ELR backbone. This latter system has been shown to improve internalization into hepatocytes, to bind to the coxsackie virus and adenovirus receptor-expressing hepatocyte cell lines, and to allow cellular uptake, thus indicating that the knob domain of adenovirus serotype 5 fiber protein is a critical factor for facilitating targeted cellular internalization of the fusion protein nanoparticles (Sun et al. 2011).

Age-related macular degeneration (AMD) is another ocular disease whose treatment is currently being studied. In this regard, Wang et al. have combined the aforementioned diblock copolymer and another soluble ELR with an sHSPs mini-peptide, which is a 20 amino acid peptide derived from αB-crystallin (Wang et al. 2014b). This protein is a chaperone with anti-apoptotic and anti-inflammatory activity that is apically secreted in exosomes by polarized human retinal pigment epithelial cells (RPE), thus protecting them from oxidative stress (Arrigo et al. 2007; Sreekumar et al. 2010), a process which is involved in the progression of AMD. Like the sHSPs mini-peptide, *in vitro* results revealed that both soluble and nanoparticulate ELRs fused with sHSPs exhibit anti-apoptotic activity in RPE cells, whereas the ELR controls do not.

A novel application of ELRs developed for the treatment of post-traumatic arthritis (PTA) involves the development of a cross-linked ELR (xELR) drug depot combined with IL1Ra (IL1 receptor antagonist) and TNFRII (TNFα inhibitor) for intra-articular delivery thereof. Although these cytokines provide potential therapeutic targets for PTA, intra-articular injections of anti-cytokine therapies have proven difficult owing to rapid clearance from the joint space. *In vivo* results have shown that inhibition of IL-1 significantly reduces the severity of cartilage degeneration and synovitis. Moreover, inhibition of TNF-α alone, or with IL1Ra, led to deleterious effects on bone morphology, articular cartilage degeneration, and synovitis. These findings suggest that IL-1 plays a critical role in the pathogenesis of PTA following articular fracture, and sustained intra-articular cytokine inhibition may provide a therapeutic approach for reducing or preventing joint degeneration following trauma. The use of xELR combined with IL-1a for sustained intra-articular delivery allows clearance from the joint space to be reduced, thereby enhancing the effects of IL-1a and reducing the dose and frequency of the injection (Kimmerling et al. 2015).

Although new proposals and perspectives are needed to increase the number of recombinant polymers reaching clinic trials, their numerous preclinical applications show that these polymers can be a powerful approach for developing biomedical applications in the fields of tissue engineering and drug delivery.

Silk-like recombinamers for drug delivery

Unlike the consensus sequence used in most ELR constructs, silk and silk-like proteins (SLRs) contain a number of commonly used sequences from several species of silk worms and spiders. Thus, the silk fibroin derived from the silkworm *Bombyxmori*, which is extracted from natural sources rather than being synthesized using recombinant techniques, has been widely used for controlled release of drugs from films, gels, implants, and nanoparticles (Price et al. 2014). Alternatively, recombinant silks from two species of spider, namely *Nephilaclavipes* and *Araneusdiadematus*, are widely mimicked due to their favorable properties and the difficulty of isolating them from natural sources. Spider silk is well known to have a high tensile strength and high elasticity (Huang et al. 2015). Given the possibility of recombinant production of spider silk proteins, technical applications of spider silk materials are nowadays feasible (Price et al. 2014; Shi et al. 2014).

The engineered recombinant spider silk protein eADF4(C16) is based on the dragline silk sequence of ADF4 (*Araneusdiadematus* fibroin). With the aim of creating a delivery model based on silk capsules that avoids the use of toxic toluene (commonly used to produce spider silk capsules), Blüm et al. developed a new capsule-formation technique involving the use of medical grade silicon oil, with an additional processing step involving a water/ethanol bath to structurally stabilize the silk capsules. These microcapsules are mechanically stable and can be used as a transport system for higher molecular weight compounds such as enzymes or other drugs. The resulting eADF4(C16) capsules were subsequently tested as a protective device for delivering an inactive β-galactosidase precursor, with α-complementation being used to activate this precursor on demand. The encapsulated enzymes remain active even in the presence of site-specific proteases in the surrounding medium, and enzyme precursors/intermediates can be activated inside the capsules using external triggers. These results suggest that eADF4(C16) capsules could be an excellent device for the protection of enzymes, drugs, load, etc. (Blüm et al. 2014).

A new positively charged variant of eADF4(C16) was developed by the same group with the aim of creating a polycationic spider silk protein eADF4(κ16) that allows the incorporation of negatively charged substances, such as nucleic acids. Nucleic acids bound to eADF4(κ16) are released more slowly in the presence of salts than low molecular weight substances, which undergo a burst release under the same conditions. eADF4(C16) shows a slow and linear but salt-dependent release. Indeed, the presence of kosmotropic salts along with the much slower release can result in collapse of the particle. An interesting insight was obtained upon combining eADF4(κ16) particles with eADF4(C16), which allows the release of small molecular substances to be slowed and controlled (Doblhofer and Scheibel 2015).

Nanoscale complexes of recombinant silk polymers containing tumor homing peptides (THP) combined with DNA have been designed with the objective of reducing their non-selective cytotoxicity and targeting specific gene carriers. In initial studies, Kaplan's group proposed new bioengineered silk-based ionic complexes derived from the native sequence of the dragline protein MaSp1 from the spider *Nephilaclavipes* in combination with a poly(L-lysine) domain to interact with pDNA and a THP that specifically binds to nucleolin, which is expressed in tumor cells. The resulting silk-based nanocomplex had a diameter of around 90 nm and exhibited a relatively high target specificity and transfection efficiency in a melanoma cancer cell line (Numata et al. 2011). Further studies based on these results were performed with the aim of comparing the effectiveness of two different THPs, namely F3 peptide and Lyp1, combined with the same silk-based poly(L-lysine). Three different cell lines (melanoma, human breast tumor, and non-tumorigenic mammary epithelial cells as negative control) were transfected. The results demonstrated that silk-based pDNA nanocomplexes containing higher amounts of THPs showed greater specificity for tumor cells. Indeed, Lyp1 presented some degree of cytotoxicity in the non-tumorigenic cell line, reducing cell viability to 80 per cent compared with the F3 nanocomplex, thus making this the best candidate for targeted delivery to tumorigenic cells (Numata et al. 2012).

Silk elastin-like recombinamers for drug delivery

SELRs are chimeric recombinant polymers whose sequence contains selected domains from the structural proteins silk and elastin. As such, they combine specific properties of both native proteins, thereby displaying unique mechanical properties that combine the high strength of silk with the resilience of elastin while incorporating its multi-responsive sensitivity. This versatile behavior provided by the silk and elastin blocks makes SELRs a promising biomaterial for nanocarriers and injectable drug-release systems (Gustafson et al. 2009; Greish et al. 2010; Huang et al. 2015).

A recent example of the versatility of these materials has been described by Price et al. in a study based on previous work from the same group (Gustafson et al. 2013). The initial SELR was modified to introduce a lysine in position 815 and longer silk and elastin units, thus giving SELR185K. This combination enhanced the ability for localized release of adenoviruses (Gustafson and Ghandehari 2010) and meant that the elastin domains could facilitate enhanced bioactive agent release from the hydrogels while the longer silk blocks were able to maintain robust cross-linking.

Further studies were performed with the aim of modifying the SELR185K sequence by introducing an MMP-responsive sequence at three different positions of the construct to give SELR815K-RS1, SELR815K-RS2, and SELR815K-RS5, respectively (Price et al. 2015). *In vitro* results revealed that these three new MMP-responsive SELRs are more easily degraded than the original SELR815K in the presence of MMP-2. Moreover, the degradation kinetics depends on the location of the MMP-responsive motif in the silk domain, as revealed by the 20 per cent decrease in degradation of SELR815K-RS5. These results were verified by way of *in vivo* experiments in a mouse model of solid head and neck tumors. The composition in which the MMP sequence did not affect the silk or elastin domains, namely SELR815K-RS1, provided the most effective cancer treatment as a matrix for mediating viral gene therapy, increasing mice survival from 29 per cent to 100 per cent over 50 days compared with the control group. Furthermore, histological examination of the hydrogels postmortem revealed evidence for the degradation of MMP-responsive SELRs but not for SELP815K.

In another interesting study on the synergism derived from block combination, a series of SELRs (SE8Y, S2E8Y, and S4E8Y) with various silk-to-elastin recombinant block ratios was constructed by Kaplan's group with the aim of determining their ability to form micellar-like nanoparticles upon thermal stimulus, as well as the influence of each recombinamer (Xia et al. 2011). Two different steps in micellar-like formation were studied (Fig. 4). Firstly, the ability of SELRs to spontaneously assemble was found to depend on the silk-to-elastin ratio, with larger nanoparticles being formed in those cases in which the silk block was longer (S2E8Y and S4E8Y) than in SE8Y. However, thermo-responsive micellar formation of the SELRs triggered by the elastin blocks was masked by a high content of silk domains in the polymer, which may affect the reversibility of the conformational changes. It is therefore crucial to achieve an optimal ratio between silk and elastin units in order to allow the ordered association of SELR-based molecules.

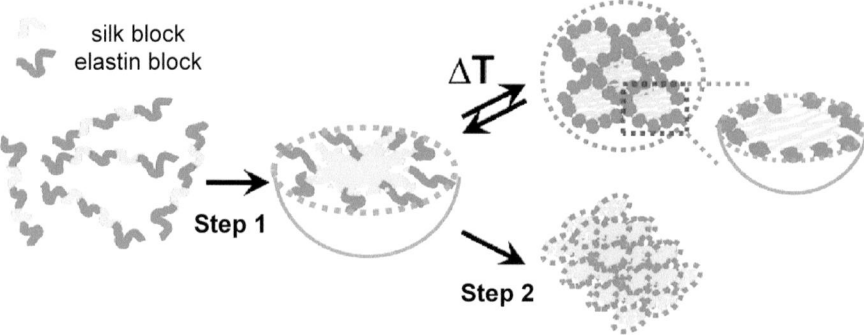

Fig. 4: Proposed Two-Step Self-Assembly of SELR. Step 1: spontaneous formation of micellar-like particles. Step 2: thermal responsive self-assembly of the particles into reversible coacervates or irreversible gel states. Reprinted with permission from (Xia et al. 2011).

On the basis of this study, these authors subsequently combined the SELRs with doxorubicin (Dox, a hydrophobic antitumor drug) to achieve an efficient loading of the drug, with the highest loading being achieved for SE8Y (this construct presented a silk-to-elastin ratio of 1:8, with a larger proportion of elastin blocks than in S2E8Y and S4E8Y). These results demonstrated the dominant role of hydrophobic interactions in drug encapsulation and in the stability of drug-loaded nanoparticles. Interestingly, Dox-SE8Y and Dox-S2E8Y nanoparticles exhibited a similar cytotoxicity, which was 1.8-fold higher than for the free drug. The lower cytotoxicity of Dox-S4E8Y was related to its inability to release Dox completely. Given the higher drug loading capacity of SE8Y and the cytotoxic nature of its Dox-loaded nanoparticles, the intracellular trafficking of nanoparticles was studied. The results suggested significant cellular uptake by endocytosis and a nuclear localization four hours post-treatment (Xia et al. 2014).

Innovative developments in the field of drug delivery have been reported in recent years. Given their excellent properties and versatile behavior, these three genetically engineered polymers are promising materials for increasing the variety of devices, including nanoparticles, depots, or hydrogels. Additionally, these materials can be targeted to specific ligands and can respond to environmental stimuli, thus meaning that they can be used to treat a wide range of diseases.

Conclusions

Recombinant technology allows us to develop new biomaterials with an enormous complexity and valuable functionalities that mimic natural structures. Thus, it is possible to produce biocompatible materials with improved mechanical properties and with much more specific biological functions, via the incorporation of bioactive domains, without needing to use chemical methods. As a result, the use of devices based on recombinant materials has increased considerably in the biomedical field over the past few years. In tissue engineering, for example, recombinant approaches such as collagen, tropoelastin, silk, or ELRs have provided new scaffolds and surfaces that interact specifically with the tissues to provide a suitable microenvironment for cell colonization and the subsequent regeneration of damaged tissue. In addition, recombinant technology has enabled the development of a broad range of recombinant polymers based on the combination or modification of conserved motifs derived from natural proteins. Such polymers are widely applied in controlled drug delivery due to their versatile ability to form nanoparticles, depots, or hydrogels depending on their composition. Furthermore, when combined with bioactive domains, they can be targeted to specific ligands or respond to environmental stimuli for the treatment of cancer, ocular or other important diseases.

Although new proposals and perspectives are necessary to increase the number of recombinant materials entering clinic trials, their numerous preclinical applications show that these biomaterials can be a powerful approach for the development of biomedical applications in the fields of tissue engineering and drug delivery.

Acknowledgements

The authors are grateful for ERDF funding from the EU and MINECO (PRI-PIBAR-2011-1403, MAT2012-38043, MAT2013-42473-R, and MAT2013-41723-R), the JCyL (projects VA152A12, VA155A12, and VA313U14), the CIBER-BBN, the JCyL and the Instituto de Salud Carlos III under the "Network Center of Regenerative Medicine and Cellular Therapy of Castilla and Leon." This project has received funding from the "European Union's Seventh Framework Programme for research, technological development, and demonstration under grant agreement number 317304."

References

Agarwal, R. and A. J. García. 2015. Biomaterial strategies for engineering implants for enhanced osseointegration and bone repair. Adv. Drug Deliv. Rev. 94: 53–62.

Ahn, J.-I., L. Kuffova, K. Merrett, D. Mitra, J. V. Forrester, F. Li et al. 2013. Crosslinked collagen hydrogels as corneal implants: effects of sterically bulky vs. non-bulky carbodiimides as crosslinkers. Acta Biomater. 9: 7796–7805.

Amruthwar, S. S. and A. V. Janorkar. 2013. *In vitro* evaluation of elastin-like polypeptide–collagen composite scaffold for bone tissue engineering. Dent. Mater. 29: 211–220.

An, B., M. D. Tang-Schomer, W. Huang, J. He, J. A. Jones, R. V. Lewis et al. 2015. Physical and biological regulation of neuron regenerative growth and network formation on recombinant dragline silks. Biomaterials 48: 137–146.

Annabi, N., S. M. Mithieux, G. Camci-Unal, M. R. Dokmeci, A. S. Weiss and A. Khademhosseini. 2013a. Elastomeric recombinant protein-based biomaterials. Biochem. Eng. J. 77: 110–118.

Annabi, N., S. M. Mithieux, P. Zorlutuna, G. Camci-Unal, A. S. Weiss and A. Khademhosseini. 2013b. Engineered cell-laden human protein-based elastomer. Biomaterials 34: 5496–5505.

Arrigo, A. P., S. Simon, B. Gibert, C. Kretz-Remy, M. Nivon, A. Czekalla et al. 2007. Hsp27 (HspB1) and αB-crystallin (HspB5) as therapeutic targets. FEBS Lett. 581: 3665–3674.

Assal, Y., Y. Mizuguchi, M. Mie and E. Kobatake. 2015. Growth factor tethering to protein nanoparticles via coiled-coil formation for targeted drug delivery. Bioconjug. Chem. 26: 1672–1677.

Bahney, C. S., C. W. Hsu, J. U. Yoo, J. L. West and B. Johnstone. 2011. A bioresponsive hydrogel tuned to chondrogenesis of human mesenchymal stem cells. FASEB J. 25: 1486–1496.

Bax, D. V., A. Kondyurin, A. Waterhouse, D. R. McKenzie, A. S. Weiss and M. M. Bilek. 2014. Surface plasma modification and tropoelastin coating of a polyurethane co-polymer for enhanced cell attachment and reduced thrombogenicity. Biomaterials 35: 6797–6809.

Blüm, C., A. Nichtl and T. Scheibel. 2014. Spider silk capsules as protective reaction containers for enzymes. Adv. Funct. Mater. 24: 763–768.

Browning, M. B., D. Dempsey, V. Guiza, S. Becerra, J. Rivera, B. Russell et al. 2012. Multilayer vascular grafts based on collagen-mimetic proteins. Acta Biomater. 8: 1010–1021.

Bryant, S. J., R. J. Bender, K. L. Durand and K. S. Anseth. 2004. Encapsulating chondrocytes in degrading PEG hydrogels with high modulus: engineering gel structural changes to facilitate cartilaginous tissue production. Biotechnol. Bioeng. 86: 747–755.

Buckwalter, J. and H. Mankin. 1997. Articular cartilage: tissue design and chondrocyte-matrix interactions. Instr. Course. Lect. 47: 477–486.

Buznyk, O., N. Pasyechnikova, M. M. Islam, S. Iakymenko, P. Fagerholm and M. Griffith. 2015. Bioengineered corneas grafted as alternatives to human donor corneas in three high-risk patients. Clin. Transl. Sci. 8: 558–562.

Cancer, I. A. f. R. o. 2014. World Cancer Report 2014. WHO, Geneva.

Case, L. C. and M. Tessier-Lavigne. 2005. Regeneration of the adult central nervous system. Curr. Biol. 15: R749–R753.

Caves, J. M., V. A. Kumar, A. W. Martinez, J. Kim, C. M. Ripberger, C. A. Haller et al. 2010. The use of microfiber composites of elastin-like protein matrix reinforced with synthetic collagen in the design of vascular grafts. Biomaterials 31: 7175–7182.

Cleary, M. A., E. Geiger, C. Grady, C. Best, Y. Naito and C. Breuer. 2012. Vascular tissue engineering: the next generation. Trends. Mol. Med. 18: 394–404.

Chapekar, M. S. 2000. Tissue engineering: challenges and opportunities. J. Biomed. Mater. Res. A 53: 617–620.

Chattopadhyay, S. and R. T. Raines. 2014. Review collagen-based biomaterials for wound healing. Biopolymers 101: 821–833.

Chevallay, B. and D. Herbage. 2000. Collagen-based biomaterials as 3D scaffold for cell cultures: applications for tissue engineering and gene therapy. Med. Biol. Eng. Comput. 38: 211–218.

Christiano, A. M., G. G. Hoffman, L. C. Chung-Honet, S. Lee, W. Cheng, J. Uitto et al. 1994. Structural organization of the human type VII collagen gene (COL7A1), composed of more exons than any previously characterized gene. Genomics 21: 169–179.

Chung, C. and J. A. Burdick. 2008. Engineering cartilage tissue. Adv. Drug Deliv. Rev. 60: 243–262.

da Costa, S. R., K. Wu, M. MacVeigh, M. Pidgeon, C. Ding, J. E. Schechter et al. 2006. Male NOD mouse external lacrimal glands exhibit profound changes in the exocytotic pathway early in postnatal development. Exp. Eye Res. 82: 33–45.

de Torre, I. G., F. Wolf, M. Santos, L. Rongen, M. Alonso, S. Jockenhoevel et al. 2015. Elastin-like recombinamer-covered stents: towards a fully biocompatible and non-thrombogenic device for cardiovascular diseases. Acta Biomater. 12: 146–155.

Despanie, J., J. P. Dhandhukia, S. F. Hamm-Alvarez and J. A. MacKay. 2015. Elastin-like polypeptides: therapeutic applications for an emerging class of nanomedicines. J. Control. Release. 2015, In press.

Dewhirst, M. W., L. Prosnitz, D. Thrall, D. Prescott, S. Clegg, C. Charles et al. 1997. Hyperthermic treatment of malignant diseases: current status and a view toward the future. Semin. Oncol. 24: 616–625.

Doblhofer, E. and T. Scheibel. 2015. Engineering of recombinant spider silk proteins allows defined uptake and release of substances. J. Pharma. Sci. 104: 988–994.

Fagerholm, P., N. S. Lagali, J. A. Ong, K. Merrett, W. B. Jackson, J. W. Polarek et al. 2014. Stable corneal regeneration four years after implantation of a cell-free recombinant human collagen scaffold. Biomaterials 35: 2420–2427.

Fine, J.-D., R. A. Eady, E. A. Bauer, J. W. Bauer, L. Bruckner-Tuderman, A. Heagerty et al. 2008. The classification of inherited epidermolysis bullosa (EB): Report of the Third International Consensus Meeting on Diagnosis and Classification of EB. J. Am. Acad. Dermatol. 58: 931–950.

Fu, S. Y. and T. Gordon. 1997. The cellular and molecular basis of peripheral nerve regeneration. Mol. Neurobiol. 14: 67–116.

Fujita, Y., M. Mie and E. Kobatake. 2009. Construction of nanoscale protein particle using temperature-sensitive elastin-like peptide and polyaspartic acid chain. Biomaterials 30: 3450–3457.

Furth, M. E., A. Atala and M. E. Van Dyke. 2007. Smart biomaterials design for tissue engineering and regenerative medicine. Biomaterials 28: 5068–5073.

Gomes, S., I. B. Leonor, J. F. Mano, R. L. Reis and D. L. Kaplan. 2012. Natural and genetically engineered proteins for tissue engineering. Prog. Polym. Sci. 37: 1–17.

Gosline, J., M. Lillie, E. Carrington, P. Guerette, C. Ortlepp and K. Savage. 2002. Elastic proteins: biological roles and mechanical properties. Philos. Trans. R. Soc. Lond., B, Biol. Sci. 357: 121–132.

Grande, D. A., C. Halberstadt, G. Naughton, R. Schwartz and R. Manji. 1997. Evaluation of matrix scaffolds for tissue engineering of articular cartilage grafts. J. Biomed. Mater. Res. A 34: 211–220.

Greish, K., J. Frandsen, S. Scharff, J. Gustafson, J. Cappello, D. Li et al. 2010. Silk-elastinlike protein polymers improve the efficacy of adenovirus thymidine kinase enzyme prodrug therapy of head and neck tumors. J. Gene. Med. 12: 572–579.

Griffith, L. G. and G. Naughton. 2002. Tissue engineering—current challenges and expanding opportunities. Science 295: 1009–1014.

Gustafson, J., K. Greish, J. Frandsen, J. Cappello and H. Ghandehari. 2009. Silk-elastinlike recombinant polymers for gene therapy of head and neck cancer: from molecular definition to controlled gene expression. J. Control. Release 140: 256–261.

Gustafson, J. A. and H. Ghandehari. 2010. Silk-elastinlike protein polymers for matrix-mediated cancer gene therapy. Adv. Drug Deliv. Rev. 62: 1509–1523.

Gustafson, J. A., R. A. Price, J. Frandsen, C. R. Henak, J. Cappello and H. Ghandehari. 2013. Synthesis and characterization of a matrix-metalloproteinase responsive silk-elastinlike protein polymer. Biomacromolecules 14: 618–625.

Hayes, S., P. Lewis, M. M. Islam, J. Doutch, T. Sorensen, T. White et al. 2015. The structural and optical properties of type III human collagen biosynthetic corneal substitutes. Acta Biomater. 25: 121–130.

Hench, L. L. and J. M. Polak. 2002. Third-generation biomedical materials. Science 295: 1014–1017.

Hodde, J. 2002. Naturally occurring scaffolds for soft tissue repair and regeneration. Tissue Eng. 8: 295–308.

Hoerstrup, S. P., G. Zünd, R. Sodian, A. M. Schnell, J. Grünenfelder and M. I. Turina. 2001. Tissue engineering of small caliber vascular grafts. Eur. J. Cardiothorac. Surg. 20: 164–169.

Hollister, S. J. 2005. Porous scaffold design for tissue engineering. Nat. Mater. 4: 518–524.

Hu, X., M. D. Tang-Schomer, W. Huang, X. X. Xia, A. S. Weiss and D. L. Kaplan. 2013. Charge-tunable autoclaved silk-tropoelastin protein alloys that control neuron cell responses. Adv. Funct. Mater. 23: 3875–3884.

Huang, H. Y., Z. H. Liu and T. Feng. 1997. *In vivo* evaluation of porous Hydroxylapatite ceramic as cervical vertebra substitute. Clin. Neurol. and Neurosurg. 99: S20–S21.

Huang, W., A. Rollett and D. L. Kaplan. 2015. Silk-elastin-like protein biomaterials for the controlled delivery of therapeutics. Expert Opin. Drug Deliv. 12: 779–791.

Hubbell, J. A. 1995. Biomaterials in tissue engineering. Nat. Biotechnol. 13: 565–576.

Huisgen, R. 1963. 1, 3-dipolar cycloadditions. Past and future. Angew. Chem. Internat. Ed. English 2: 565–598.

Hutmacher, D. W. 2000. Scaffolds in tissue engineering bone and cartilage. Biomaterials 21: 2529–2543.

Islam, M. M., V. Cèpla, C. He, J. Edin, T. Rakickas, K. Kobuch et al. 2015. Functional fabrication of recombinant human collagen–phosphorylcholine hydrogels for regenerative medicine applications. Acta Biomater. 12: 70–80.

Jeon, W. B., B. H. Park, S. K. Choi, K. M. Lee and J. K. Park. 2012. Functional enhancement of neuronal cell behaviors and differentiation by elastin-mimetic recombinant protein presenting Arg-Gly-Asp peptides. BMC Biotechnol. 12: 61.

Jia, L., Z. Duan, D. Fan, Y. Mi, J. Hui and L. Chang. 2013. Human-like collagen/nano-hydroxyapatite scaffolds for the culture of chondrocytes. Mater. Sci. Eng. 33: 727–734.

Kilic, C., A. Girotti, J. C. Rodriguez-Cabello and V. Hasirci. 2014. A collagen-based corneal stroma substitute with micro-designed architecture. Biomater. Sci. 2: 318–329.

Kimmerling, K. A., B. D. Furman, D. S. Mangiapani, M. A. Moverman, S. M. Sinclair, J. Huebner et al. 2015. Sustained intra-articular delivery of IL-1Ra from a thermally-responsive elastin-like polypeptide as a therapy for post-traumatic arthritis. Eur. Cells Mater. 29: 124–140.

Ko, M. S. and M. P. Marinkovich. 2010. Role of dermal-epidermal basement membrane zone in skin, cancer, and developmental disorders. Dermatol. Clin. 28: 1–16.

Kolb, H. C., M. Finn and K. B. Sharpless. 2001. Click chemistry: diverse chemical function from a few good reactions. Angew. Chem. Int. Ed. 40: 2004–2021.

Kopeček, J. 2003. Smart and genetically engineered biomaterials and drug delivery systems. Eur. J. Pharm. Sci. 20: 1–16.

Lampe, K. J., A. L. Antaris and S. C. Heilshorn. 2013. Design of three-dimensional engineered protein hydrogels for tailored control of neurite growth. Acta biomater. 9: 5590–5599.

Lewicka, M., O. Hermanson and A. U. Rising. 2012. Recombinant spider silk matrices for neural stem cell cultures. Biomaterials 33: 7712–7717.

Li, X., K. Wu, M. Edman, K. Schenke-Layland, M. MacVeigh-Aloni, S. Janga et al. 2010. Increased expression of cathepsins and obesity-induced proinflammatory cytokines in lacrimal glands of male NOD mouse. Invest. Ophthalmol. Vis. Sci. 51: 5019–5029.

Liu, K., A. Tedeschi, K. K. Park and Z. He. 2011. Neuronal intrinsic mechanisms of axon regeneration. Annu. Rev. Neurosci. 34: 131–152.

Liu, W., K. Merrett, M. Griffith, P. Fagerholm, S. Dravida, B. Heyne et al. 2008. Recombinant human collagen for tissue engineered corneal substitutes. Biomaterials 29: 1147–1158.

Liu, Y., L. Gan, D. J. Carlsson, P. Fagerholm, N. Lagali, M. A. Watsky et al. 2006. A simple, cross-linked collagen tissue substitute for corneal implantation. Invest. Ophthalmol. Vis. Sci. 47: 1869–1875.

Liu, Z., A. J. Huang and S. C. Pflugfelder. 1999. Evaluation of corneal thickness and topography in normal eyes using the Orbscan corneal topography system. Br. J. Ophthalmol. 83: 774–778.

Macaya, D. and M. Spector. 2012. Injectable hydrogel materials for spinal cord regeneration: a review. Biomed. Mater. 7: 012001.

MacEwan, S. R. and A. Chilkoti. 2014a. Applications of elastin-like polypeptides in drug delivery. J. Control. Release 190: 314–330.

MacEwan, S. R. and A. Chilkoti. 2014b. Controlled apoptosis by a thermally toggled nanoscale amplifier of cellular uptake. Nano Lett. 14: 2058–2064.

Machula, H., B. Ensley and R. Kellar. 2014. Electrospun tropoelastin for delivery of therapeutic adipose-derived stem cells to full-thickness dermal wounds. Adv. Wound Care 3: 367–375.

Mackay, J. A. and A. Chilkoti. 2008. Temperature sensitive peptides: engineering hyperthermia-directed therapeutics. Int. J. Hyperthermia 24: 483–495.

Martinez-Osorio, H., M. Juárez-Campo, Y. Diebold, A. Girotti, M. Alonso, F. J. Arias et al. 2009. Genetically engineered elastin-like polymer as a substratum to culture cells from the ocular surface. Curr. Eye Res. 34: 48–56.

Massodi, I., S. Moktan, A. Rawat, G. L. Bidwell and D. Raucher. 2010. Inhibition of ovarian cancer cell proliferation by a cell cycle inhibitory peptide fused to a thermally responsive polypeptide carrier. Inter. J. Cancer 126: 533–544.

Matsumoto, R., R. Hara, T. Andou, M. Mie and E. Kobatake. 2014. Targeting of EGF-displayed protein nanoparticles with anticancer drugs. J. Biomed. Mater. Res. B: Appl. Biomater. 102: 1792–1798.

McDaniel, J. R., D. J. Callahan and A. Chilkoti. 2010. Drug delivery to solid tumors by elastin-like polypeptides. Adv. Drug Deliv. Rev. 62: 1456–1467.

McGann, C. L., E. A. Levenson and K. L. Kiick. 2013. Resilin-based hybrid hydrogels for cardiovascular tissue engineering. Macromol. Chem. Phys. 214: 203–213.

McKenna, K. A., K. W. Gregory, R. C. Sarao, C. L. Maslen, R. W. Glanville and M. T. Hinds. 2012. Structural and cellular characterization of electrospun recombinant human tropoelastin biomaterials. J. Biomater. Appl. 27: 219–230.

McLaughlin, C. R., R. Osborne, A. Hyatt, M. A. Watsky, E. V. Dare, B. B. Jarrold et al. 2009. Tissue engineered models for *in vitro* studies. Fundamentals of Tissue Engineering and Regenerative Medicine. Springer 1: 759–772.

Meilander, N. J., H. J. Lee and R. V. Bellamkonda. 2004. Biomaterials to promote tissue regeneration. pp. 445–447. *In*: Kutz, M. (ed.). Standard Handbook of Biomedical Engineering and Design, Second Edition, Vol. 1. McGraw-Hill, New York.

Mithieux, S. M., S. G. Wise and A. S. Weiss. 2013. Tropoelastin—a multifaceted naturally smart material. Adv. Drug Deliv. Rev. 65: 421–428.

Moisenovich, M. M., O. Pustovalova, J. Shackelford, T. V. Vasiljeva, T. V. Druzhinina, Y. A. Kamenchuk et al. 2012. Tissue regeneration *in vivo* within recombinant spidroin 1 scaffolds. Biomaterials 33: 3887–3898.

Mottaghitalab, F., H. Hosseinkhani, M. A. Shokrgozar, C. Mao, M. Yang and M. Farokhi. 2015. Silk as a potential candidate for bone tissue engineering. J. Control. Release 215: 112–128.

Mutsaers, S. E., J. E. Bishop, G. McGrouther and G. J. Laurent. 1997. Mechanisms of tissue repair: from wound healing to fibrosis. Int. J. Biochem. Cell Biol. 29: 5–17.

Myllyharju, J. and K. I. Kivirikko. 2004. Collagens, modifying enzymes and their mutations in humans, flies and worms. Trends Genet. 20: 33–43.

Nakayama, Y., S. Nishi, H. Ueda-Ishibashi and T. Matsuda. 2003. Fabrication of microporous elastomeric film-covered stents and acute-phase performances. J. Biomed. Mater. Res. A 64: 52–61.

Newman, A. P. 1998. Articular cartilage repair. Am. J. Sports Med. 26: 309–324.

Nichol, J. W. and A. Khademhosseini. 2009. Modular tissue engineering: engineering biological tissues from the bottom up. Soft Matter. 5: 1312–1319.

Numata, K., M. R. Reagan, R. H. Goldstein, M. Rosenblatt and D. L. Kaplan. 2011. Spider silk-based gene carriers for tumor cell-specific delivery. Bioconjugate Chemistry 22: 1605–1610.

Numata, K., A. J. Mieszawska-Czajkowska, L. A. Kvenvold and D. L. Kaplan. 2012. Silk-based nanocomplexes with tumor-homing peptides for tumor-specific gene delivery. Macromol. Biosci. 12: 75–82.

Nyström, A., D. Velati, V. R. Mittapalli, A. Fritsch, J. S. Kern and L. Bruckner-Tuderman. 2013. Collagen VII plays a dual role in wound healing. J. Clin. Invest. 123: 3498–3509.

Olthoff, C. M., J. S. Schouten, B. W. van de Borne and C. A. Webers. 2005. Noncompliance with ocular hypotensive treatment in patients with glaucoma or ocular hypertension: an evidence-based review. Ophthalmol. 112: 953–961.

Panda, A., M. Vanathi, A. Kumar, Y. Dash and S. Priya. 2007. Corneal graft rejection. Surv. Ophthalmol. 52: 375–396.

Parmar, P. A., L. W. Chow, J. P. St-Pierre, C. M. Horejs, Y. Y. Peng, J. A. Werkmeister et al. 2015. Collagen-mimetic peptide-modifiable hydrogels for articular cartilage regeneration. Biomaterials 54: 213–225.

Pascolini, D. and S. P. Mariotti. 2011. Global estimates of visual impairment: 2010. Br. J. Ophthalmol. 96: 614–618.

Pereira, R. F., C. C. Barrias, P. L. Granja and P. J. Bartolo. 2013. Advanced biofabrication strategies for skin regeneration and repair. Nanomedicine 8: 603–621.

Polo-Corrales, L., M. Latorre-Esteves and J. E. Ramirez-Vick. 2014. Scaffold design for bone regeneration. J. Nanosci. Nanotechnol. 14: 15–56.

Price, R., A. Poursaid and H. Ghandehari. 2014. Controlled release from recombinant polymers. J. Control. Release 190: 304–313.

Price, R., A. Poursaid, J. Cappello and H. Ghandehari. 2015. *In vivo* evaluation of matrix metalloproteinase responsive silk–elastinlike protein polymers for cancer gene therapy. J. Control. Release 213: 96–102.

Pulkkinen, H. J., V. Tiitu, P. Valonen, J. S. Jurvelin, L. Rieppo, J. Töyräs et al. 2013. Repair of osteochondral defects with recombinant human type II collagen gel and autologous chondrocytes in rabbit. Osteoarthr. Cartil. 21: 481–490.

Qiu, W., Y. Huang, W. Teng, C. M. Cohn, J. Cappello and X. Wu. 2010. Complete recombinant silk-elastinlike protein-based tissue scaffold. Biomacromolecules 11: 3219–3227.

Radtke, C., C. Allmeling, K. H. Waldmann, K. Reimers, K. Thies, H. C. Schenk et al. 2011. Spider silk constructs enhance axonal regeneration and remyelination in long nerve defects in sheep. PLoS ONE 6: e16990.

Raj, P. A., M. Johnsson, M. J. Levine and G. H. Nancollas. 1992. Salivary statherin. Dependence on sequence, charge, hydrogen bonding potency, and helical conformation for adsorption to hydroxyapatite and inhibition of mineralization. J. Biol. Chem. 267: 5968–5976.

Ratcliffe, A. 2000. Tissue engineering of vascular grafts. Matrix Biol. 19: 353–357.

Raucher, D. and J. S. Ryu. 2015. Cell-penetrating peptides: strategies for anticancer treatment. Trends Mol. Med. 21: 560–570.

Rnjak, J., S. G. Wise, S. M. Mithieux and A. S. Weiss. 2011. Severe burn injuries and the role of elastin in the design of dermal substitutes. Tissue Eng. Pt. B: Rev. 17: 81–91.

Rnjak-Kovacina, J., S. G. Wise, Z. Li, P. K. Maitz, C. J. Young, Y. Wang et al. 2012. Electrospun synthetic human elastin: collagen composite scaffolds for dermal tissue engineering. Acta Biomater. 8: 3714–3722.

Rodríguez-Cabello, J. C., A. Girotti, A. Ribeiro and F. J. Arias. 2012. Synthesis of genetically engineered protein polymers (recombinamers) as an example of advanced self-assembled smart materials. pp. 17–38. *In*: Navarro, M. and J. A. Planell (eds.). Nanotechnology in Regenerative Medicine. Methods in Molecular Biology. Springer.

Rodriguez-Cabello, J. C., F. J. Arias, M. A. Rodrigo and A. Girotti. 2015. Elastin-like polypeptides in drug delivery. Adv. Drug Deliv. Rev. 97: 85–100.

Rogers, S. L., P. C. Letourneau, B. A. Peterson, L. T. Furcht and J. B. McCarthy. 1987. Selective interaction of peripheral and central nervous system cells with two distinct cell-binding domains of fibronectin. J. Cell Biol. 105: 1435–1442.

Romano, N. H., K. J. Lampe, H. Xu, M. M. Ferreira and S. C. Heilshorn. 2015. Microfluidic gradients reveal enhanced neurite outgrowth but impaired guidance within 3D matrices with high integrin ligand densities. Small 11: 722–730.

Romano, N. H., C. M. Madl and S. C. Heilshorn. 2015. Matrix RGD ligand density and L1CAM-mediated Schwann cell interactions synergistically enhance neurite outgrowth. Acta Biomater. 11: 48–57.

Ruszczak, Z. 2003. Effect of collagen matrices on dermal wound healing. Adv. Drug Deliv. Rev. 55: 1595–1611.

Ryu, J. S. and D. Raucher. 2014. Anti-tumor efficacy of a therapeutic peptide based on thermo-responsive elastin-like polypeptide in combination with gemcitabine. Cancer Lett. 348: 177–184.

Ryu, J. S. and D. Raucher. 2015. Elastin-like polypeptide for improved drug delivery for anticancer therapy: preclinical studies and future applications. Expert Opin. Drug Del. 12: 653–667.

Sedaghati, T. and A. M. Seifalian. 2015. Nanotechnology and bio-functionalisation for peripheral nerve regeneration. Neural Regen. Res. 10: 1191–1194.

Sengupta, D. and S. C. Heilshorn. 2010. Protein-engineered biomaterials: highly tunable tissue engineering scaffolds. Tissue Eng. Pt. B: Rev. 16: 285–293.

Shah, M., M. C. Edman, S. R. Janga, P. Shi, J. Dhandhukia, S. Liu et al. 2013. A rapamycin-binding protein polymer nanoparticle shows potent therapeutic activity in suppressing autoimmune dacryoadenitis in a mouse model of Sjögren's syndrome. J. Control. Release 171: 269–279.

Shi, P., J. A. Gustafson and J. A. MacKay. 2014. Genetically engineered nanocarriers for drug delivery. Int. J. Nanomed. 9: 1617–1626.

Shilo, S., S. Roth, T. Amzel, T. Harel-Adar, E. Tamir, F. Grynspan et al. 2013. Cutaneous wound healing after treatment with plant-derived human recombinant collagen flowable gel. Tissue Eng. A 19: 1519–1526.

Shukla, P., M. Kumar and G. Keshava. 2008. Mycotic keratitis: an overview of diagnosis and therapy. Mycoses 51: 183–199.

Singh, A. K., G. K. Srivastava, L. Martín, M. Alonso and J. C. Pastor. 2014. Bioactive substrates for human retinal pigment epithelial cell growth from elastin-like recombinamers. J. Biomed. Mater. Res. A 102: 639–646.

Sofia, S., M. B. McCarthy, G. Gronowicz and D. L. Kaplan. 2001. Functionalized silk-based biomaterials for bone formation. J. Biomed. Mater. Res. 54: 139–148.

Son, Y. J. and W. J. Thompson. 1995. Schwann cell processes guide regeneration of peripheral axons. Neuron 14: 125–132.

Sreekumar, P. G., R. Kannan, M. Kitamura, C. Spee, E. Barron, S. J. Ryan et al. 2010. alphaB crystallin is apically secreted within exosomes by polarized human retinal pigment epithelium and provides neuroprotection to adjacent cells. PLoS One 5: e12578.

Srivastava, G. K., L. Martín, A. K. Singh, I. Fernandez-Bueno, M. J. Gayoso, M. T. Garcia-Gutierrez et al. 2011. Elastin-like recombinamers as substrates for retinal pigment epithelial cell growth. J. Biomed. Mater. Res. A 97: 243–250.

Sun, G., P. Y. Hsueh, S. M. Janib, S. Hamm-Alvarez and J. A. MacKay. 2011. Design and cellular internalization of genetically engineered polypeptide nanoparticles displaying adenovirus knob domain. J. Control. Release 155: 218–226.

Tan, D. T., J. K. Dart, E. J. Holland and S. Kinoshita. 2012. Corneal transplantation. Lancet 379: 1749–1761.

Tejeda-Montes, E., K. H. Smith, E. Rebollo, R. Gómez, M. Alonso, J. C. Rodriguez-Cabello et al. 2014. Bioactive membranes for bone regeneration applications: effect of physical and biomolecular signals on mesenchymal stem cell behavior. Acta Biomater. 10: 134–141.

Urry, D. W. 2007. What sustains life?: consilient mechanisms for protein-based machines and materials. Springer-Verlag, New York, NY, USA.

Vacanti, J. 2010. Tissue engineering and regenerative medicine: from first principles to state of the art. J. Pediatr. Surg. 45: 291–294.

van der Veen, V. C., M. B. van der Wal, M. C. van Leeuwen, M. M. Ulrich and E. Middelkoop. 2010. Biological background of dermal substitutes. Burns 36: 305–321.

Vedrenne, N., B. Coulomb, A. Danigo, F. Bonté and A. Desmoulière. 2012. The complex dialogue between (myo) fibroblasts and the extracellular matrix during skin repair processes and ageing. Pathol. Biol. 60: 20–27.

Vepari, C. and D. L. Kaplan. 2007. Silk as a biomaterial. Prog. Polym. Sci. 32: 991–1007.

Wakitani, S., T. Kimura, A. Hirooka, T. Ochi, M. Yoneda, N. Yasui et al. 1989. Repair of rabbit articular surfaces with allograft chondrocytes embedded in collagen gel. J. Bone Joint. Surg. Br. 71: 74–80.

Walker, L. R., J. S. Ryu, E. Perkins, L. R. McNally and D. Raucher. 2014. Fusion of cell-penetrating peptides to thermally responsive biopolymer improves tumor accumulation of p21 peptide in a mouse model of pancreatic cancer. Drug Des. Dev. Ther. 8: 1649–1658.

Wang, H. M., Y. T. Chou, Z. H. Wen, Z. R. Wang, C. H. Chen and M. L. Ho. 2013. Novel biodegradable porous scaffold applied to skin regeneration. PloS One 8: e56330.

Wang, W., J. Despanie, P. Shi, M. C. Edman, Y. A. Lin, H. Cui et al. 2014a. Lacritin-mediated regeneration of the corneal epithelia by protein polymer nanoparticles. J. Mater. Chem. B 2: 8131–8141.

Wang, W., P. G. Sreekumar, V. Valluripalli, P. Shi, J. Wang, Y. A. Lin et al. 2014b. Protein polymer nanoparticles engineered as chaperones protect against apoptosis in human retinal pigment epithelial cells. J. Control. Release 191: 4–14.

Wang, W., A. Jashnani, S. R. Aluri, J. A. Gustafson, P. Y. Hsueh, F. Yarber et al. 2015. A thermo-responsive protein treatment for dry eyes. J. Control. Release 199: 156–167.

Wang, X., P. Ghasri, M. Amir, B. Hwang, Y. Hou, M. Khilili et al. 2013. Topical application of recombinant type VII collagen incorporates into the dermal–epidermal junction and promotes wound closure. Mol. Ther. 21: 1335–1344.

Wang, Y., S. M. Mithieux, Y. Kong, X. Q. Wang, C. Chong, A. Fathi et al. 2015. Tropoelastin incorporation into a dermal regeneration template promotes wound angiogenesis. Adv. Healthc. Mater. 4: 577–584.

Weimer, T., H. J. Metzner and S. Schulte. 2013. Recombinant albumin fusion proteins. pp. 163–178. *In*: Schmidt, S. R. (ed.). Fusion Protein Technologies for Biopharmaceuticals: Applications and Challenges John Wiley & Sons, Inc.

Werkmeister, J. A. and J. A. Ramshaw. 2012. Recombinant protein scaffolds for tissue engineering. Biomed. Mater. 7: 012002.

Whitcher, J. P., M. Srinivasan and M. P. Upadhyay. 2002. Prevention of corneal ulceration in the developing world. Int. Ophthalmol. Clin. 42: 71–77.

White, J. D., S. Wang, A. S. Weiss and D. L. Kaplan. 2015. Silk–tropoelastin protein films for nerve guidance. Acta Biomater. 14: 1–10.

WHO, W. H. O. 2006. Neurological disorders: public health challenges. World Health Organization.

Wise, S. G. and A. S. Weiss. 2009. Tropoelastin. Int. J. Biochem. Cell Biol. 41: 494–497.

Włodarczyk-Biegun, M. K., M. W. Werten, F. A. de Wolf, J. J. van den Beucken, S. C. Leeuwenburgh, M. Kamperman et al. 2014. Genetically engineered silk–collagen-like copolymer for biomedical applications: Production, characterization and evaluation of cellular response. Acta Biomater. 10: 3620–3629.

Woodley, D. T., X. Wang, M. Amir, B. Hwang, J. Remington, Y. Hou et al. 2013. Intravenously injected recombinant human type VII collagen homes to skin wounds and restores skin integrity of dystrophic epidermolysis bullosa. J. Invest. Dermatol. 133: 1910–1913.

Wysocki, A. B. 1999. Skin anatomy, physiology, and pathophysiology. Nursing Clin. N. Am. 34: 777–797.

Xia, X. X., Q. Xu, X. Hu, G. Qin and D. L. Kaplan. 2011. Tunable self-assembly of genetically engineered silk–elastin-like protein polymers. Biomacromolecules 12: 3844–3850.

Xia, X. X., M. Wang, Y. Lin, Q. Xu and D. L. Kaplan. 2014. Hydrophobic drug-triggered self-assembly of nanoparticles from silk-elastin-like protein polymers for drug delivery. Biomacromolecules 15: 908–914.

Yang, S., K. F. Leong, Z. Du and C. K. Chua. 2001. The design of scaffolds for use in tissue engineering. Part I. Traditional factors. Tissue Eng. 7: 679–689.

Yildirimer, L., N. T. Thanh and A. M. Seifalian. 2012. Skin regeneration scaffolds: a multimodal bottom-up approach. Trends Biotechnol. 30: 638–648.

Zgheib, C., J. Xu and K. W. Liechty. 2014. Targeting inflammatory cytokines and extracellular matrix composition to promote wound regeneration. Adv. Wound Care 3: 344–355.

9

Cellulose Nanofibers for Biomedical Applications

Marité Cardenas and *Anna J. Svagan**

Introduction

The creation of materials exploiting molecules from renewable resources and green processing routes in order to minimize contamination of the environment with toxic solvents and starting components, is an important step towards a sustainable society, and sustainable development is critical in all technological fields including biomedical engineering. In this context, the polysaccharides are an important family of molecules, as they can be derived from numerous natural sources including plants, bacteria, insects, animals, and also from by-products/waste-materials obtained from agricultural or fishery activities. Also, polysaccharides are biodegradable and can be broken down by common microorganisms found on land or in water. In nature, polysaccharides can be composed of one type of repeating unit (homopolysaccharides; starch and cellulose) or two or more types of repeating monomer (heteropolysaccharides; pectin, alginate). But despite using only a few basic building blocks, many unique and complex molecular structures with specific features and functions are assembled giving rise to a plethora of diverse carbohydrates. Some of the polysaccharides are classified as polyelectrolytes, and these are either negatively or positively charged. The intrinsic properties of such ionic polysaccharides are used in material science to produce stimuli-responsive materials where external stimuli (pH, ionic strength, and temperature) trigger,

Malmö University, Department of Biomedical Science and Biofilm Research Center for Biointerfaces Health and Society, 20506 Malmö, Sweden.
* Corresponding author: anna.hanner@sund.ku.dk

for example, a mechanical response in the material or a swelling mechanism that can be exploited in drug delivery. In addition to conventional polysaccharides, advanced genetic engineering also opens up the possibility for new, innovative, and structurally designed macromolecules with specific chemical and physical properties, allowing for better material structure-property control. Natural polysaccharides are typically biocompatible, possibly bioadhesive, and generally recognized as safe (GRAS) and, in conclusion, they are attractive materials to use in biomedical applications.

One potentially interesting polysaccharide candidate in the biomedical context is cellulose, in the form of nanofibers. Traditionally, cellulose has already been used for a long time in formulations in the pharmaceutical industry in the form of microcrystalline cellulose (MCC) or a salt form or modified cellulose type (for example, Hydroxypropyl Methylcellulose). However, in comparison, cellulose in the form of cellulose nanofibers is still a relatively new concept. Cellulose is the most abundant polysaccharide polymer in the biosphere, and its versatility has recently been explored in several biomedical applications. However, this area is still much in its infancy. Thanks to its native molecular arrangement several unique properties are naturally obtained when it is utilized in the form of cellulose nanofiber, properties that cannot be found when cellulose is present/processed into another solid-state form (e.g., MCC, macro-scopic fibers, or salt form). Such properties include mechanical properties, barrier properties, and surface chemistry, to mention a few. Also, from a chemical point of view, the presence of many hydroxyl groups on the cellulose surface allows for further surface modification. Thanks to these properties and also the biocompatibility, cellulose materials hold great promise in a wide variety of biotechnological and biomedical applications. The aim of the present chapter is to provide an overview of the unique features of CNF and how these have been exploited in biomedical application to date and also highlight the many possibilities of using CNF in future biomedical applications.

The Structure of Cellulose Nanofibers

Cellulose is a linear polymer consisting of repeating cellobiose units, that is two anhydroglucose units connected via a β-1,4glycosidic bond as depicted (A) in Fig. 1. In nature, several such polymer chains are further assembled in parallel, forming semicrystalline microfibrils that are held together via van der Waals and inter- and intramolecular hydrogen bonds, see Fig. 1D. The hydrogen bonds are responsible for stability of the cellulose polymer, that is, it is has no melting point (it degrades prior to melting) and is not easy to dissolve in aqueous solvents (it cannot be dissolved in water) (Eichhorn et al. 2010). Recently, Lindman et al. (2012) hypothesized that the insolubility characteristics of cellulose is due to its largely overseen amphiphilicity and hydrophobic molecular interactions. This hypothesis for cellulose insolubility is based on fundamental polymer physicochemical principles and also on well-known inconsistencies in cellullose dissolution behavior.

The microfibrils are assembled into larger macroscopic fibres, such as those found in wood, Fig. 1D. Depending on the botanical source, the size of the microfibrils will vary—in wood the typical size is ca 4 nm. This corresponds to 36 cellulose chains (Endler and Persson 2011), see Fig. 1. In these microfibrils, the cellulose is typically

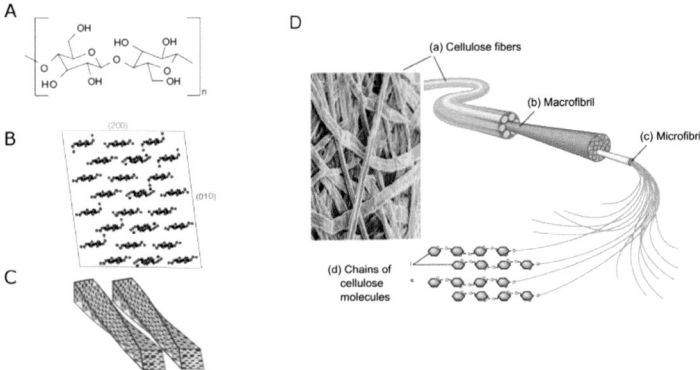

Fig. 1: In (A) the cellobiose unit is presented. A proposed model of the chain packing arrangements of spruce microfibrils. (B) the rectangular shape (24 cellulose chains) overall dimension 3.2 × 3.1 nm. In (C) two adjacent twisted microfibrils are presented. (D) The hierarchical structure of pulp fibers. The images in (B) and (C) are adapted from reference Fernandes et al. (2011). (D) is adapted from ref. (http://nutrition. jbpub.com/resources/chemistryreview9.cfm, 2016).

present in the cellulose-I crystal form, which is a combination of two allomorphs, the cellulose Iα and Iβ form—the ratio between these allomorphs again depending on the botanical origin. The native cellulose-I crystal form is not the most thermodynamically stable polymorph, and therefore upon recrystallization the more stable cellulose-II type will form. The microfibrils contain both crystalline and less ordered regions. However, the exact structure of the microfibril is still under debate. In a recent study by Fernandes (Fernandes et al. 2011), the structure of microfibrils in spruce were examined using a range of spectroscopic methods and small-angle neutron and wide-angle X-ray scatterings. From the experimental data, a microfibril model was proposed containing about 24 chains, with a possibly twisted structure (see (C) in Fig. 1) and with less ordered regions increasing towards the surfaces of the microfibril. More ordered regions were expected within the microfibrils. Previous studies have also suggested less ordered regions occur in segments along the length of the microfibrils (Battista and Smith 1962). A rectangular packing model was also suggested by Fernandes et al. (2011) for spruce microfibrils, consisting of both hydrophobic and hydrophilic surfaces, see B in Fig. 1.

Cellulose nanofibers (CNF), also denoted as microfibrillated cellulose (abbreviated MFC) or nanofibrillated cellulose (abbreviated NFC), can be derived by disintegrating the cell wall of cellulosic fibers. CNF can be individual microfibrils or bundles of microfibrils. The available botanical source of fiber are many such as wood, hemp, flax and cotton, and also non-plant sourced such as those produced by bacteria (gram-negative bacteria *Acetobacter xylinum* or *Gluconacetobacter xylinum*). To obtain CNF from wood pulp, typically a mechanical treatment step is combined with a chemical treatment step, for example, carbomethylation, hydrolysis, or enzymatic treatment (Mølgaard et al. 2014a; Pääkkö et al. 2007). The produced CNF is typically available as a suspension in water, and this is because upon drying re-dispersion is problematic, and thus the water enables the further easy use of CNF. Apart from cellulose, and depending on the botanical origin of the starting material, the CNF may also contain some lignin, hemicellulose, and pectin. CNF derived from wood pulp typically contains both hemicellulose and lignin. Bacterial Cellulose, on the other hand, is already in a pure form, that is, devoid of hemicellulose, lignin, and pectin. Also unlike CNF, which involves disintegrated of macroscopic pulp-fibers in the case of wood, the bacteria directly produce slender fibers with nano-size diameters and thus the fabrication is not connected with harsh chemical usage. The structure of BC and a scheme of the cellulose production by the bacteria are shown in Fig. 2—the interwoven extra-cellular cellulose ribbons (Brown et al. 1976) are clearly shown in (B).

CNF typically have a high aspect ratio (length/diameter) with diameters as small as that of the native microfibrils (~ 4 nm in diameter, botanical origin: wood) and lengths up to several micrometers. The surface chemistry of CNF is also quite unique. It is rich in reactive hydroxyl groups and, as a consequence, functionalization of the CNF surface has received increasing interest amongst CNF researchers in order to further improve the compatibility between CNF and different polymeric matrices but also in the development of smart or functional materials based on CNF.

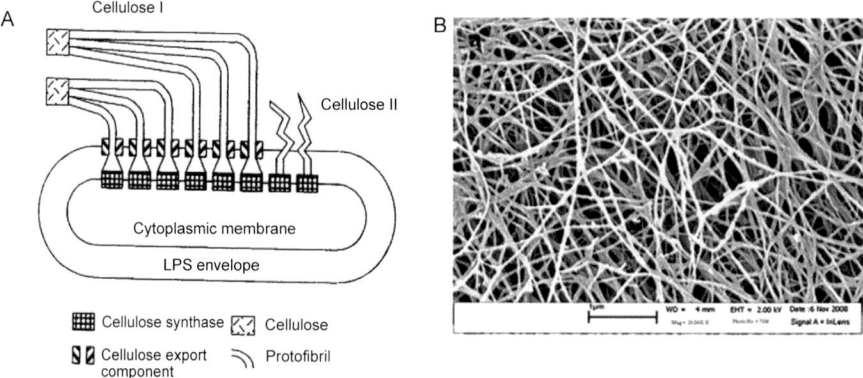

Fig. 2: The production of cellulose microfibrils by *A. Xylinium* (A). An interconnected network of cellulose ribbons (bacterial cellulose, BC) can be produced by bacteria (B). The image (A) is adapted from Chawla et al. (2009) and (B) is adapted from Szot et al. (2011).

Properties of CNF and CNF Based Materials

There are several unique properties with CNF that has made it interesting in biomedical applications, such as its extra-ordinary mechanical properties, good biocompatibility, low toxicity, and excellent barrier properties. The aim of this sub-chapter is to give a deeper understanding of these properties and in the next sub-chapter on "Biomedical Applications", we will show how some of these properties have been exploited in different biomedical applications.

Mechanical and rheological properties

The first interesting feature with CNF is the outstanding mechanical properties, which makes it attractive in applications where mechanical stability is important, for example, scaffolds. By breaking down the macroscopic cellulose fibers into tiny cellulose nanofibers and thereby decreasing the amount of amorphous material present, advantageous mechanical properties are gained. This is because the resulting cellulose nanofibers will be of high crystallinity and the high stiffness of the cellulose crystal ensures a strong reinforcement in nanocomposite materials (Eichhorn et al. 2010; Yamanaka et al. 1989). The advantage of using cellulose nanofibers over conventional fibers has been studied extensively and is also supported using micromechanical models, for example, the Halpin-Tsai model (Affdl and Kardo 1976). Several different techniques and theoretical approaches, for example, X-ray diffraction, atomic force microscopy, Raman Spectroscopy, inelastic X-ray scattering, have been used in the past to determine the crystal modulus of cellulose and the values reported have typically been in the range 100–160 GPa (Nishino et al. 1995; Sturcova et al. 2005). The Young's modulus of cellulose is quite high compared to other materials such as steel (E = 200 GPa) in particular if the density of cellulose is taken into account, for example, the so-called specific density (= modulus/density). Steel has a specific modulus of 36 GPa Mg^{-1} m^3 whereas crystalline cellulose has a value of 92 GPa Mg^{-1} m^3.

A mechanical advantage of using cellulose nanofibers is that they typically have a high aspect ratio (aspect ratio = length/width). This aspect is desirable as this enables a critical length for stress transfer from the matrix to the reinforcing phase—nanofibers with aspect ratios larger than 50 are said to have an efficient reinforcements' effect (Eichhorn et al. 2010).

Another interesting feature is the mechanical strength of CNF. In a recent study by Saito et al. (2013), the mechanical strength of individual cellulose nanofibers were evaluated. Their results showed a mean strength of wood cellulose nanofibrils of 1.6–3 GPa, the exact value depending on the method used to determine the nanofibril width. These values are comparable to those of multiwalled carbon nanotubes and ultrastrong para-aramid fibers (Kevlar).

To obtain efficient reinforcement properties, a homogenous dispersion of the CNF in the matrix material is of immense importance. As a consequence, water is typically the preferred processing medium, mainly due to the high-stability of CNF in water. However, CNF can also be dispersed in dimethylformamide, dimethyl sulfoxide, or N-methyl pyrrolidine (van den Ber 2007; Vie 2007). Adaptation to non-aqueous processing conditions, that is, in organic solvents, can also be achieved by utilizing surfactants adsorbed to the CNF surface or chemical modification of the CNF surface. When prepared from aqueous suspension, CNF typically forms a percolating network upon drying, which is held together via strong hydrogen-bonding. This network is responsible for the extraordinary strong mechanical reinforcement (Svagan et al. 2007, 2008). To retain the network and achieve a homogenous CNF dispersion, films of CNF can also be immersed in a polymer solution or monomer solution for further polymerization (Yano et al. 2005). However, a homogenous dispersion of CNF within polymeric matrices is not always possible. The nanofiber packing, nanocellulose network formation, and also the porosity of nanocellulose films, strongly depend on factors such as the type of nanocellulose (Fukuzumi et al. 2011) and the conditions and/or the dispersion media used during manufacturing (Henriksson 2008).

Cellulose nanofiber dispersions in, for example, water display unique rheology properties, and the CNF structure-morphology-rheology relationships has been studied in great detail in the past (Li et al. 2015). The rheological properties depend on parameters such as chemical composition, crystallinity, length, and aspect ratio of the CNF. For CNF suspensions, the entangled cellulose nanofibers network of the slender and long CNF in water gives rise to a rigid solid-like viscoelastic behavior, even at the low concentration of 0.25 wt% (Li et al. 2015). The properties can be further changed by, for example, decreasing the aspect ratio of the CNF. CNF suspensions could potentially be used as a rheological modifier in, for example, pharmaceutical applications.

Barrier properties

If a densely packed arrangement of nanofibers can be achieved then this could potentially be used to reduce permeability of small molecules (e.g., incorporated drugs), which represents another interesting property of CNF (Fukuzumi et al. 2011; Kolakovic et al. 2013). It was recently demonstrated that the neat CNF based film exhibits excellent oxygen barrier properties at low relative humidity. Aulin et al. (2010) reported an oxygen barrier coefficient of 0.0006 mL μm m^{-2} day^{-1} kPa^{-1} at 0% RH. Similar values were reported by Fukuzumi (2011). This value is 2 to 3 orders of magnitude lower that ethylene vinyl alcohol (EVOH) at 0% RH (Lange and Wyse 2003), which is a petro-chemically derived material typically used in high oxygen barrier applications. Low oxygen permeability coefficients are interesting in the context of improving the oxidative stability of potential oxygen sensitive molecules, for example, drug molecules, present in the materials. The high oxygen barrier properties are due to, amongst other factors, the high crystallinity of the CNF, and strong hydrogen bonding between nanofibers, which makes it more difficult for molecules to penetrate the CNF network. Also, small pores, low porosity, and pores that are not interconnected throughout the thickness of the material are important factors (Fukuzumi et al. 2011). However, polar molecules such as water act as plasticizers and disrupt these hydrogen bonds, which leads to inferior barrier properties—above 70% RH a rapid decrease in the barrier properties is observed (Aulin et al. 2010). Thus, CNF based films need to be protected from moisture, for example, by coating the surface with hydrophobic material.

Amphiphilic properties

Another interesting feature with cellulose nanofibers, and also cellulose nanocrystals, is that they display amphiphilic properties. This property is believed to be a consequence of the molecular arrangement of the cellulose molecules in the microfibril structure, giving raise to both hydrophilic and hydrophobic faces, see (B) and (C) in Fig. 1 (Mazeau and Wyszomirsk 2012). Recent studies have also shown their potential uses in Pickering stabilization producing very stable oil-in-water emulsion (Kalashnikova et al. 2012) by stabilizing the oil/water interphase. The resulting emulsions were quite stable and could withstand repeated centrifugation steps. The amphiphilic properties could also be used to stabilize small amphiphilic drug molecules or nanoparticles or can be used in a surfactant-free synthesis of nanocellulose reinforced capsules (Mølgaard et al. 2014a).

Toxicity of CNF

Given the great potential for using CNF as substrate in regenerative medicine and tissue engineering there have been various studies investigating whether such cellulose-based materials are biocompatible. As a consequence, the issue of cytotoxicity and other side-effects of CNF have been raised. Indeed, the answer to this question is rather complex and depends on factors such as surface charge, topography, surface chemistry, and the physical form, for example, film, suspension, or particles. The answer will also depend on the types of cells used in the toxicology assay and the specific approach used to testing cytotoxicity. For example, whether the nanocellulose particles have been pre-exposed to biological media or not can definitely have an impact on how the behave in the body (see the discussions regarding protein corona on nanoparticles and for example the review by (Nel et al. 2009)). Recent studies by Colic et al. (2015) suggested that unmodified CNF (diameters 10 to 70 nm, length of a few microns) at concentrations up to 1 mg mL^{-1} are cytocompatible according to the present ISO criteria (ISO10993-, 2009), with non-inflammatory and non-immunogenic properties. Also higher concentrations (250 µg mL^{-1} to 1 mg mL^{-1}) were reported to be tolerogenic to the immune system, which makes them suitable for use in implantable biomaterials. Jorfi and Foster (2015) have provided an excellent summary of the most recent toxicology report for CNF. The findings presented in their review show that studies performed up to date give little evidence of serious toxic effects of CNF on the cellular, genetic level, and *in vivo* animal experiments. Still, future investigations are needed to fully establish the genotoxicity and cytotoxicity of CNF *in vitro* and *in vivo*.

Biomedical Application

Wound healing

Since the 1980's, the so-called bacterial cellulose (BC) has shown promising properties for treatment of for example skin wounds (Czaja et al. 2006). Healing of wounds typically involves providing a moist environment, which is desired as it is proven that this gives a better and faster wound healing. Therefore, wound dressing is of key importance when treating wounds, especially those arising from burns and that involve ulcers. The extreme hydration capacity of BC (~ 99 wt% is water) makes this material a good candidate for wound dressing. In Fig. 3A, a hydrated sheet of BC is shown and in Fig. 3B the topical application of BC on the skin of a burn patient is illustrated. Studies have shown that BC is biocompatible, with good cell attachment and proliferation *in vitro* and enhanced tissue generation *in vivo* (Bäckdahl et al. 2006). In addition, the mechanical properties and highly porous structure of the BC mimic the extracellular matrix of the human skin. Helenius et al. implanted BC subcutaneously in rats for 1, 4, and 12 weeks, and their studies showed no sign of inflammations around the implants, also fibroblasts penetrated the BC network enabling a good integration and no chronical inflammatory response was observed (Bäckdahl et al. 2006; Helenius et al. 2006). In another study by Fu et al. (2013), large area full-thickness skin defects were made on mice, and wounds treated with BC demonstrated better tissue regeneration and faster and better healing effect of

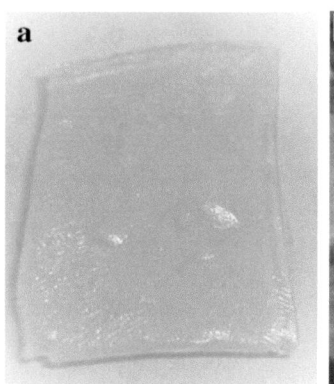
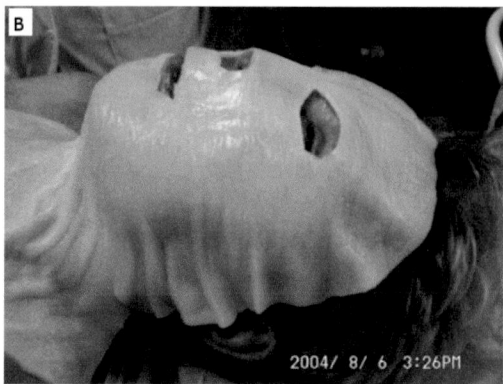

Fig. 3: A sheet of bacterial cellulose (A). Bacterial cellulose applied to a patient (B). (A) and (B) is used with permission from Pinto et al. (2009) and Czaja et al. (2007), respectively.

the epithelial tissue and lower inflammatory response when compared to results obtained for the control group. However, the important drawbacks of BC, is its poor antimicrobial activity and also that it is hard to rehydrate the material (once it has been dried). These features can, however, be addressed by modification of the BC. For example by incorporating hydrolyzed gelatin peptides and/or hydroxypropyl methylcellulose for improved rehydration properties (Chen et al. 2013) and chemical grafting of antimicrobial compounds for better antimicrobial activity, see section 4.3.

Today there are several companies that commercialize BC for wound healing; Biofill®, Bioprocess®, and XCell® (Czaja et al. 2007; Petersen and Gatenholm 2011). XCell® is produced by US based Xylos Corporation, which is a biomedical device company that develops cellulose-based wound-care products. Another example of is Epiprotect®, a wound care product which has antimicrobial properties and that mimics the collagen network, gives high biocompatibility, and full functionality as a synthetic epithelium and is now under use to treat burns, pressure ulcers, and diabetic ulcers (http://www.s2m.se/).

Tissue engineering

In tissue engineering, methods extracted from cell biology, biochemistry, engineering, and material science are combined to produce biomaterials with improved biological functions. Specifically, tissue engineering seeks at repairing or replacing tissues such as bone, cartilage, skin, and muscle. A critical parameter to take into account is biocompatibility. High porosity and fibril network structures are typical characteristics needed to create favorable interactions between the biomaterial and the cells in the body. Moreover, biomaterials that can tolerate high mechanical strains are very important for bone and cartilage tissue engineering for example.

Therefore, nanocellulose seems to be an ideal candidate in this respect, for a recent review see Jorfi et al. (2015). In particular, nanocellulose dispersions can be used as bioink in three dimensional (3D) printing with the aim to produce biomaterials with micrometer precision (Derb 2012). Bioinks need to be viscous enough to keep its shape during printing and must have cross-linking abilities to retain the wished 3D form after printing. These characteristics can be achieved using various types of cellulose including nanofibrils and bacterial cellulose. Here we will focus on some examples in which cellulose has been used to produce tissue like biomaterials. In the first example, CNF has been used in mixtures with other biopolymers. In the second and third examples, biomaterials made of only CNF or bacterial cellulose have been used (Mertaniemi et al. 2016 and Andrade et al. 2010).

The group of Prof. Gatenholm in Sweden has developed several approaches using various types of cellulose in tissue engineering (Markstedt et al. 2015). For example, Markstedt et al. (2015) prepared various bioinks for 3D printing based on formulations based on cellulose nanofibrils (CNF) and alginate. The bioinks were prepared by mixing concentrated CNF dispersions and alginate solutions at for example 90:10 CNF:alginate in weight percent (the total dry weight was 2.5%). The viscosity of the CNF/alginate mixtures was first measured to determine the optimal ratio for best printability. As expected, CNF has a high viscosity at low shear rates and then it shows a shear thinning behavior. The viscosity is in general lowered with alginate addition (Fig. 4A). Alginate solutions in the absence of CNF, on the other hand, presented overall lower viscosity. Cross-linking was performed on the CNF/alginate mixtures after printing by adding 90 mM aqueous solution of $CaCl_2$ (this was then called Ink9010 for the bioink prepared using 90:10 CNF:alginate. Ink fidelity (the ability to line width upon printing) was quite poor for alginate dispersions lacking CNF but it was considerably improved by addition of CNF (Fig. 4B). Moreover, the mechanical stability of the printed grids was quite poor for alginate and NCF inks: The grid shape was only retained upon using mixtures of NCF and alginate. This example clearly illustrates the main challenge in 3D printing: how low viscosity solutions reduce the printing resolution and how high viscosity solutions cannot often be gelled. The authors then proceeded to optimize the bioink formulation by changing the ratio of alginate and CNF. They found that Ink8020 (that is 80:20 alginate:CNF weight ratio with total dry weight of 2%) was the best bioink in terms of rheological properties, compression, and shape deformation. Ink8020 showed good gelling and crosslinking ability, showing little tendency of shape deformation.

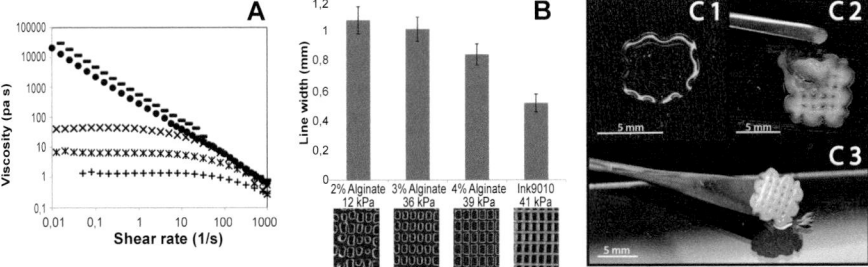

Fig. 4: Production of bioinks for 3D printing based on mixtures of alginate and nano cellulose fibrils (NCF). Viscosity measurements of 2.5% CNF (-), Ink 9010 (Ÿ) and alginate solutions at increasing concentration 4 (x), 3 (*) and 2 (+) wt% (A). Ink fidelity measurements for alginate solutions at increasing concentration and the CNF-alginate Ink9010 (B). The grid shape upon applying mechanical force is quite poor for inks based on 3% alginate (C1) and 2.5% CNF (C2). However, the grid shape remained for printed and cross-linked mixtures of alginate and CNF (Ink9010). Reproduced from Markstedt et al. (2015).

The authors then proceeded to demonstrate that the CNF/alginate based bioink could be used to make 3D constructs that mimic human nasoseptal chondrocytes (hNC). hND are cells found in human cartilage connective tissue, and basically are responsible for the cartilage matrix structure. The authors engineered small grids (Fig. 5A) using Ink8020 that showed remarkable mechanical properties after squeezing with a tweezer (Fig. 5B) and release (Fig. 5C). These grids were then used to make a 3D printed version of a human ear (Fig. 5D–F). 3D grids based on bioink Ink8020 were then used to test the bioink biocompatibility towards hND. The authors found good

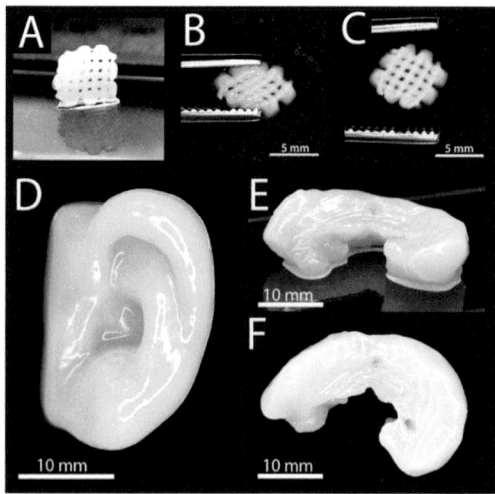

Fig. 5: The CNF/alginate based bioink was used to print small 3D grids (A) that upon cross-linking with CaCl$_2$ retained their shape after mechanical stress (B-C). These grids were used to make 3D human ears. Reproduced from Marksted et al. (2015).

cell viability after 1 and 7 days of culture growth. Moreover, this type of constructs allows the further study of how cells behave in 3D, which so far has not been possible, and thus better mimic the behavior in the body.

In the second example, cellulose nanofibers were used to engineer threads for biomedical applications. Mertaniemi et al. (2016) used CNF hydrogels to make thin threads (0.1–0.2 mm in diameter) using a 3D printer, see Fig. 6. Upon printing and after immersion in ethanol, the threads were cross-linked using glutaraldehyde and zinc nitrate, and cured for 30 min at 130°C. The cross-linking step was necessary to produce ductile threads in both the dry and wet state, the latter being the relevant state for biomedical applications. Indeed, these threads embedded in water were able to retain up to 40% of the dry-state tensile strength of CNF, resulting in a wet strength in the range of strongest human tendons (Woo and Levin 1998).

The threads were then exposed to a culture of human adipose stem primary cells (hASC) and the cells retained viability and remained attached even after one week of exposure. hASC cells have demonstrated very similar phenotypic and functional characteristics to that of bone marrow-derived mesenchymal stem cell, and therefore are very interesting for using in stem cell therapies. The main challenge in stem cell

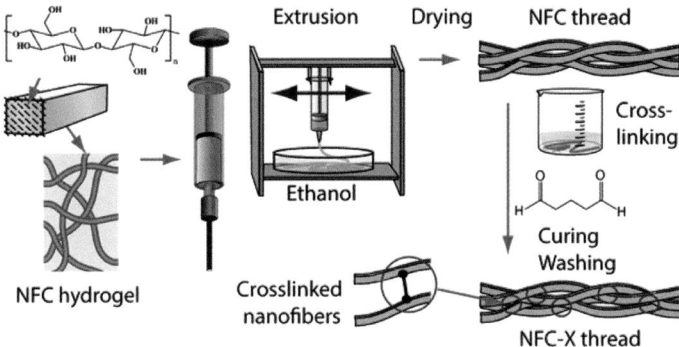

Fig. 6: Schematics for 3D printing of biocompatible threads based on CNF hydrogels and crosslinking with glutaraldehyde (CNF-X). Reproduced from Mertaniemi et al. (2016).

therapy is to increase cell retention rate in the injured area. The hASC coated CNF based threads could be then used as effective stem cell carriers. Therefore, the authors used the hASC coated CNF based threads to penetrate pig tissue (muscle, fat, and skin). The threads were mechanically robust enough to pass through such tissues. Moreover, the authors demonstrate that in using this approach, the cells hASC cells remain attached to CNF-based threads after suturing in an *ex vivo* wound model, and that they maintained their metabolic activity. These exciting results make possible a new generation of highly reproducible, zoonosis free, functionalized nanobiomaterials for biomedical applications.

In the third example, the tissue like network of bacterial cellulose (see section 4.1) has been used for blood vessel replacement. This is a very important field in biomedicine, as vascular problems often arise in patients suffering from cardiovascular diseases—the leading cause of mortality in westernized societies. There are several studies covering this approach (Andrade et al. 2010; Esguerra et al. 2010; Klemm et al. 2001; Malm et al. 2012; Schumann et al. 2008). In order to further the biocompatibility and effectiveness for vascular grafts, improved cellular adhesion to cellulose is needed. This is very important when treating implantation of blood vessels since there is a great loss of endothelial cells after surgery (Bos et al. 1998). Andrade et al. (2010) functionalized a chimeric protein that contains a cellulose-binding module and an adhesion protein on the surface of BC. The authors attempted coating by simple physisorption of the proteins and peptides to BC for 12 h at 4°C and rinse with PBS buffer. By coating BC with these adhesion peptides, enhanced adhesion to human microvascular endothelial cells (HMEC-1) was achieved therefore improving the biocompatibility and performance of BC: The incubation time for endothelial cell adsorption to BC was shorter than in the absence of adhesion peptides and furthermore it stimulated angiogenesis (i.e., the formation of new blood vessels).

Antimicrobial films

Antimicrobial compounds are nowadays widely used and are an integrated part of industrialized societies, for example, they are used to prevent the host of bacteria and viruses in wounds, water, food, household items, cosmetics, paints, and medical supplies. For instance, in 2006, the market for biocides in the EU amounted to €10–11 billion with a growth of 4–5% per annum for the previous 15 years and predicted to continue expanding ("Pesticide Action Network"). The increasing use of antimicrobial compounds is in part due to their extensive use that often occurs at concentrations too low to kill bacteria. Furthermore, there is also evidence that the use or misuse of antimicrobial compounds is leading to the increased occurrence of bacteria that are resistant to both biocides (disinfectants, antiseptics, and preservatives) and antibiotics (agents that act against infections) (Fortunati et al. 2014). Addressing biocide resistance and the subsequent risk of antibiotic resistance is a complex problem that requires the concerted action of people, policymakers, scientist, and industry. It is clear that the development of novel and more effective biocides and biocidal coatings (in different applications such as wound dressings and wood or food preservation, biocides need to be incorporated in coatings) will aid in this direction. Indeed, the need to develop novel biocides is not only driven by this reason. European regulations such as the Biocidal Product Regulation (BPR, Regulation (EU) 528/2012) state the need to replace toxic biocides. Therefore, there has been lately several research groups studying and developing antimicrobial coatings based on cellulose.

As described in section 3, the broad range of properties (e.g., biodegradability, easy to be chemically and physically modified, mechanical stress, and biocompatibility) makes cellulose an ideal candidate for a range of applications including packaging and in biomedical applications. The ability to modify cellulose surface properties has been exploited recently to produce cellulose surfaces with antimicrobial properties. There are two types of modifications that can be used to prepare cellulose-based materials with antimicrobial properties. In one hand, nano-composites can be produced based on cellulose and the antimicrobial compound. For example, nano-composites were recently produced from poly(lactic acid) (PLA), cellulose nanocrystals modified with acid phosphate ester of ethoxylatednonylphenol (s-CNC), and silver nanoparticles (Fortunati et al. 2014). Silver nanoparticles are known to have antimicrobial properties against Gram-positive and Gram-negative bacteria (Dallas et al. 2011). Currently, however, there are concerns about the cytotoxicity of silver nanoparticles (de Lima et al. 2012). Despite these concerns, silver nanoparticles are approved by the Food and Drug Administration as a food additive in bottled water and no safety concerns were concluded by the European Food Safety Authority (EFSA) when the migration of silver ion does not exceed the group specific migration limit of 0.05 mgAg kg^{-1} food (Anadón et al. 2011). On the other hand, the surface of cellulose nanofibers and nanocrystals can be functionalized with antimicrobial compounds. Some examples include the surface functionalization of cellulose nanocrystals with, for example, nontoxic rosin acids and benzylpenicillin (Saini et al. 2015; Saini et al. 2016).

Let's first discuss the production of nanocomposites with antimicrobial properties. This is an approach that has so far been commercialized by several companies. For example, Smith Nephew has developed a series of antimicrobial dressings for the management of wound infection and chronic wounds and burns (http://www.smith-nephew.com/key-products/advanced-wound-management/dressing-types/antimicrobial-dressings/). Most of these products are based on nanocomposites between cellulose and, for example, silver nanoparticles. A recently published study discussed the formation of antimicrobial films by solvent casting using PLA, s-CNC, and Ag nanoparticles (Fortunati et al. 2014). Briefly, chloroform solutions of PLA, s-CNC, and silver nanoparticles were mixed under stirring before being casted onto glass Petri dishes (Fig. 7A). This simple procedure gave homogeneous particle dispersion in the polymer matrix (Fig. 7B) that did not affect the transparency of PLA. Interestingly, a synergistic effect on the barrier properties to oxygen and water (approximately 50% improvement) was observed when both s-CNC and silver nanoparticles were present. If PLA was mixed only with silver nanoparticles or s-CNC, a reduction of the barrier properties by approximately 40–45% was observed instead. This suggests that the silver nanoparticles act as linkers of s-CNC fibers further strengthening the film structure. A synergistic effect was also observed in regards with antimicrobial activity. Moreover, the migration values for silver ions were well below the limits by EFSA although these values were above the limits for biocomposites containing 1 wt% Ag and upon treatment with ethanol based solutions.

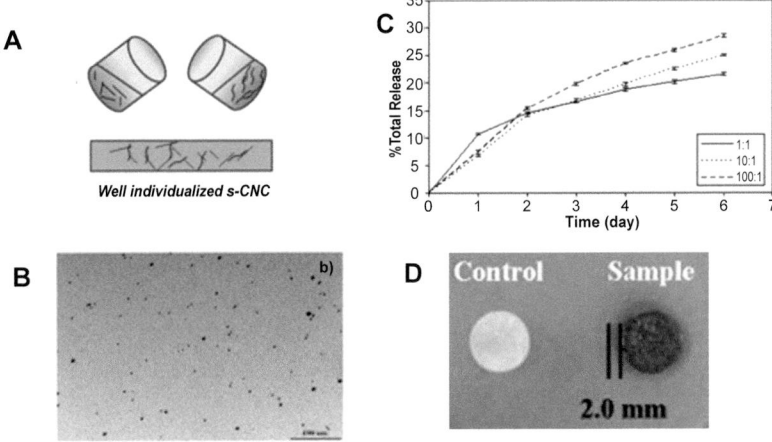

Fig. 7: Preparation on antimicrobial cellulose films via by mixing PLA with cellulose nanofibers using the solvent cast method in the presence of Ag nanoparticle (A). Reproduced from ref. (Fortunati et al. 2014) Ag nanoparticles are evenly distributed in the film and penetrate the pores of the film (B). Reproduced from (Fortunati et al. 2014). For antimicrobial BC films (no PLA present), the Ag release rate decreases with the ratio of AgNO3 to NaBH4 during impregnation (C). Reproduced from ref. (Maneerung et al. 2008). The antimicrobial capacity of these films is confirmed using the disc diffusion method for *E. coli* (D).Reproduced from ref. (Maneerung et al. 2008).

Bacterial cellulose has also been used mixed with Ag nanoparticles to produce antimicrobial wound dressings. Maneerung et al. used BC pellicles that are produced on the surface of the liquid culture medium, and impregnated them in $AgNO_3$ solutions (Maneerung et al. 2008). The films were then let to stand for 1 h and then washed with ethanol. Rinsing with ethanol ensures the removal of excess Ag nanoparticles. The silver-ion saturated films were then reduced using $NaBH_4$ and finally rinsed with water and dried. This produced thin pellicles showing the characteristic cellulose nanofibers (Fig. 2) and a very large surface are that can hold large amounts of water. Ag nanoparticles readily integrated into these pores and remained bound electrostatically to the polar group of cellulose (He et al. 2003). The films prepared using a higher molar ratio of $NaBH_4$ to $AgNO_3$ during the impregnation step showed smaller particle sizes and slower Ag ion release rate (Fig. 7C). Since the nanoparticles were prepared within the BC film, the nanoparticles were probably found deeper within the film the higher $NaBH_4$:$AgNO_3$ molar ratio. Finally, the films showed great antimicrobial activity against Gram-positive and Gram-negative strains using the disc diffusion method (Fig. 7D) among other approaches. In the disc diffusion method, a sterilized disc shape piece of the antimicrobial film and placed on a bacterium culture agar plate for 24 h at 37°C. If the film presents antimicrobial activities, the bacteria that surrounds the film will die and the radii around which dead bacteria is found will depend on the diffusion of antimicrobial compounds from the film. This method is used in comparative purposes by measuring such radii in comparison to a control (for instance the BC that did not have any Ag nanoparticles). This clearly demonstrates the potential of using cellulose for antimicrobial purposes by including Ag nanoparticles during the film preparation or via simple impregnation.

The second modification type that can produce antimicrobial films is based on the chemical modification of cellulose. The simple introduction of cationic charges in cellulose pulp via chemical reaction with 2,3 epoxypropyltrimethylammonium chloride and its subsequent fibrillation to nanofibers allowed to form fibers with antimicrobial properties (Saini et al. 2016). Similarly, 3-aminopropyltrimethoxysilane was used to induce cationic charges in BC with the purpose of producing antimicrobial materials (Fernandes et al. 2013). More advanced modifications can be introduced via surface functionalization of cellulose fibers. For example, Saine et al. (2016) prepared microfibrillated cellulose films grafted with penicillin (Fig. 8). First a microcellulose pellicle (Fig. 8i) was produced using a handsheet former and standard protocols. Then, the film was dipped for 10 seconds at room temperature into a sodium penicillin solution at pH 4 in acetic acid. The film was then cured at 150°C under flowing air to covalently graft the penicillin on the surface of the films via esterification. Finally, an extraction of excess penicillin was performed in ethanol for at least 12 hours. Alternatively, penicillin was grafted in the cellulose suspension prior to formation of cellulose pellicles (Fig. 8ii). This type of chemical grafting ensures that non-leaching

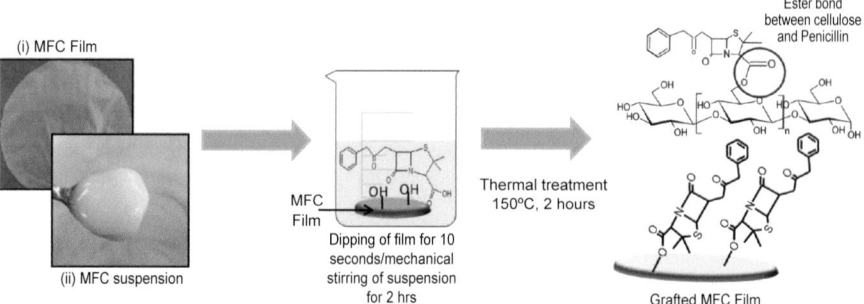

Fig. 8: Penicillin was grafted on microfibrillated cellulose (CNF) using esterification. Two approaches were used for incorporation of penicillin: (i) after CNF film formation or (ii) in the CNF suspension prior to film formation. Used with permission from Saini et al. (2015).

pellicles are produced. This is of extreme importance when it comes to the production of resistant bacterial strains, as it is precisely the leaking of antibiotics below the total inhibitory concentration that creates resistance in bacteria. Interestingly, the degree of grafting was higher when done directly on the film than when done on cellulose suspension prior to film formation.

Smart protective coatings

Another interesting biomedical application for cellulose-based products is that of targeted delivery at the human gut. Humans lack enzymes to degrade cellulose. However, there is a wide range of anaerobic bacterial present in the human gut that is able to ferment cellulose. Therefore, the possibility of targeted release at the gut can be achieved via the use of coatings made of cellulose. Inclusion of active compounds in cellulose matrices that resist the harsh conditions during the passage on the stomach (pH could be as low as 1.5 for up to 2 h) should in principle be able to release the active compound via the fermentation (or enzymatic degradation) of the cellulose-based matrix by the gut bacteria. This concept has been explored in 2014 by Mølgaard et al. (2014a) who produced a coating based on the layer by layer technology based on poly(galacturonic acid) and cationic nanofibrillated cellulose, see Fig. 9. In this method, a surface is immersed in a cationic polymer. This leads to adsorption of the polymer on the surface. Excess polymer is removed by rinsing with water. Then the surface is immersed in an anionic polymer solution that leads to further adsorption onto the surface due to electrostatic interactions. The surface is then rinsed with water to remove excess negative polymer. Then one layer by layer step has been completed and the process can be repeated until the desired film thickness is produced. Figure 9 shows that this method is able to produce thick films that are dense and resistant to acid treatment. Moreover, the film is partially degraded by pectinase and thus this work demonstrates the potential of pectin-cellulose composites for targeted delivery to the human gut. Another important property of these coatings is their good barrier properties against oxygen, which could allow for encapsulation of, for instance, anaerobic bacteria as an alternative for fecal transplant. Fecal transplant is a method that raises ethical questions, in which stool from a healthy donor is transferred into the gastrointestinal tract for the purpose of treating recurrent C. difficile colitis, among other diseases (Gough et al. 2011).

Conclusions and Future Perspectives

The intrinsic properties of cellulose nanofibers offer great potential for its use in biomedical applications. More specifically, such properties include biocompatibility, nanofiber network formation, high hydration capability, controllable porosity, tailorable rheological properties, lack of toxicity, high specific surface area and unique surface chemistry, excellent mechanical properties, barrier properties, and biodegradability. On January the 14th 2016, a search in the web of science for "cellulose" and "biomedical" give 933 articles since 1997. For "cellulose" and "tissue engineering" 712 articles are found since 1997. In both cases the growth is exponential. In this chapter, we have

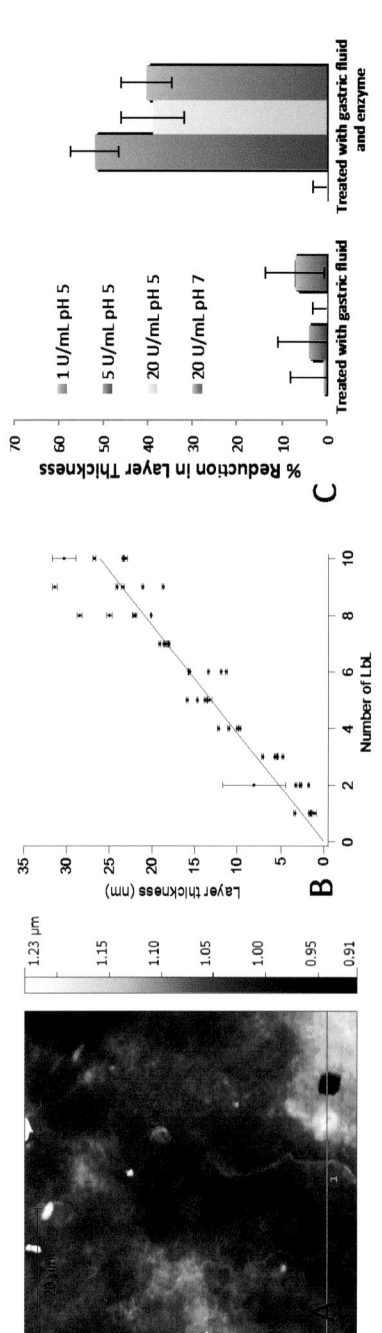

Fig. 9: Film formed using poly(galacturonic acid) and cationic nanofibrillated cellulose following the layer by layer approach. Atomic force microscopy shows a dense and uniform film is formed upon the deposition of 8 LbL (A). The growth upon number of LbL deposited on the surface is linear as measured by spectroscopic ellipsometry (B). The film thickness is not affected by treatment with gastric fluid mimics but it is partially destroyed when subjected to gastric fluid mimics that contain pectinase, a bacterial enzyme present in human gut that is able to degrade poly(galacturonic acid). Adapted with permission (Molgaard et al. 2014b).

presented an overview of the cellulose properties and also selected a couple of very interesting examples of the current state of research on nanocellulose based materials for biomedical applications. Undoubtedly, the use of cellulose in biomedicine will grow and many biotech companies are currently developing and commercializing products based on cellulose nanofibers. A recent report from Markets and Markets (2015) shows that the nanocellulose market was of $ 250 million in 2014 and it was then estimated to grow by 19% from 2014 to 2016 where the main players for this market are biotech companies (e.g., Novozymes) and electronic companies.

There is no doubt that nanocellulose fibers and bacterial cellulose are promising candidates for a wide range of biomedical applications, from simple wound dressings to tissue engineering scaffolds. However, to further revolution this specific field, more *in vivo* studies are needed to understand the interactions between cells and nanocellulose—this will provide further understanding of how the nanocellulose should be modified to enhance positive interactions, avoiding toxic effects.

References

Affdl, J. C. H. and J. L. Kardos. 1976. The Halpin-Tsai equations: a review. Polymer Engineering & Science 16(5): 344–352. doi: 10.1002/pen.760160512.

Anadón, A., M.-L. Binderup, W. Bursch, L. Castle, R. Crebelli, K.-H. Engel et al. 2011. Scientific opinion on the safety evaluation of the substance, silver zeolite A (silver zinc sodium ammonium alumino silicate), silver content 2–5%, for use in food contact materials. EFSA J. 9(2): 4034–4041.

Andrade, F. K., R. Costa, L. Domingues, R. Soares and M. Gama. 2010. Improving bacterial cellulose for blood vessel replacement: Functionalization with a chimeric protein containing a cellulose-binding module and an adhesion peptide. Acta Biomaterialia 6(10): 4034–4041. doi: http://dx.doi.org/10.1016/j.actbio.2010.04.023.

Aulin, C., M. Gallstedt and T. Lindstrom. 2010. Oxygen and oil barrier properties of microfibrillated cellulose films and coatings. Cellulose 17(3): 559–574. doi: 10.1007/s10570-009-9393-y.

Battista, O. A. and P. A. Smith. 1962. Microcrystalline Cellulose. Industrial & Engineering Chemistry 54(9): 20–29. doi: 10.1021/ie50633a003.

Bos, G. W., A. A. Poot, T. Beugeling, W. G. van Aken and J. Feijen. 1998. Small-diameter vascular graft prostheses: current status. Archives of Physiology and Biochemistry 106(2): 100–115. doi: 10.1076/apab.106.2.100.4384.

Bäckdahl, H., G. Helenius, A. Bodin, U. Nannmark, B. R. Johansson, B. Risberg et al. 2006. Mechanical properties of bacterial cellulose and interactions with smooth muscle cells. Biomaterials 27(9): 2141–2149. doi: http://dx.doi.org/10.1016/j.biomaterials.2005.10.026.

Brown, R. M., J. H. Willison and C. L. Richardson. 1976. Cellulose biosynthesis in Acetobacter xylinum: visualization of the site of synthesis and direct measurement of the *in vivo* process. Proc. Natl. Acad. Sci. 73(12): 4565–4569.

Chawla, P. R., I. B. Bajaj, S. A. Survase and R. S. Singhal. 2009. Microbial cellulose: fermentative production and applications. Food Technology and Biotechnology 47(2): 107–124.

Chen, H. H., S. B. Lin, C. P. Hsu and L. C. Chen. 2013. Modifying bacterial cellulose with gelatin peptides for improved rehydration. Cellulose 20(4): 1967–1977. doi: 10.1007/s10570-013-9931-5.

Colic, M., D. Mihajlovic, A. Mathew, N. Naseri and V. Kokol. 2015. Cytocompatibility and immunomodulatory properties of wood based nanofibrillated cellulose. Cellulose 22(1): 763–778. doi: 10.1007/s10570-014-0524-8.

Czaja, W., A. Krystynowicz, S. Bielecki and R. M. Brown, Jr. 2006. Microbial cellulose—the natural power to heal wounds. Biomaterials 27(2): 145–151. doi: http://dx.doi.org/10.1016/j.biomaterials.2005.07.035.

Czaja, W. K., D. J. Young, M. Kawecki and R. M. Brown. 2007. The future prospects of microbial cellulose in biomedical applications. Biomacromolecules 8(1): 1–12. doi: 10.1021/bm060620d.

Dallas, P., V. K. Sharma and R. Zboril. 2011. Silver polymeric nanocomposites as advanced antimicrobial agents: Classification, synthetic paths, applications, and perspectives. Advances in Colloid and Interface Science 166(1–2): 119–135. doi: http://dx.doi.org/10.1016/j.cis.2011.05.008.

de Lima, R., A. B. Seabra and N. Durán. 2012. Silver nanoparticles: a brief review of cytotoxicity and genotoxicity of chemically and biogenically synthesized nanoparticles. Journal of Applied Toxicology 32(11): 867–879. doi: 10.1002/jat.2780.

Derby, B. 2012. Printing and prototyping of tissues and scaffolds. Science 338(6109): 921–926. doi: 10.1126/science.1226340.

Eichhorn, S. J., A. Dufresne, M. Aranguren, N. E. Marcovich, J. R. Capadona, S. J. Rowan et al. 2010. Review: current international research into cellulose nanofibres and nanocomposites. Journal of Materials Science 45(1): 1–33. doi: 10.1007/s10853-009-3874-0.

Endler, A. and S. Persson. 2011. Cellulose Synthases and Synthesis in Arabidopsis. Molecular Plant (Oxford University Press/USA) 4(2): 199–211. doi: 10.1093/mp/ssq079.

Esguerra, M., H. Fink, M. W. Laschke, A. Jeppsson, D. Delbro, P. Gatenholm et al. 2010. Intravital fluorescent microscopic evaluation of bacterial cellulose as scaffold for vascular grafts. Journal of Biomedical Materials Research Part A, 93A(1): 140–149. doi: 10.1002/jbm.a.32516.

Fernandes, A. N., L. H. Thomas, C. M. Altaner, P. Callow, V. T. Forsyth, D. C. Apperley et al. 2011. Nanostructure of cellulose microfibrils in spruce wood. Proceedings of the National Academy of Sciences 108(47): E1195–E1203. doi: 10.1073/pnas.1108942108.

Fernandes, S. C. M., P. Sadocco, A. Alonso-Varona, T. Palomares, A. Eceiza, A. J. D. Silvestre et al. 2013. Bioinspired antimicrobial and biocompatible bacterial cellulose membranes obtained by surface functionalization with aminoalkyl groups. ACS Applied Materials & Interfaces 5(8): 3290–3297. doi: 10.1021/am400338n.

Fortunati, E., S. Rinaldi, M. Peltzer, N. Bloise, L. Visai, I. Armentano et al. 2014. Nano-biocomposite films with modified cellulose nanocrystals and synthesized silver nanoparticles. Carbohydrate Polymers 101: 1122–1133. doi: http://dx.doi.org/10.1016/j.carbpol.2013.10.055.

Fu, L. N., P. Zhou, S. M. Zhang and G. Yang. 2013. Evaluation of bacterial nanocellulose-based uniform wound dressing for large area skin transplantation. Materials Science & Engineering C-Materials for Biological Applications 33(5): 2995–3000. doi: 10.1016/j.msec.2013.03.026.

Fukuzumi, H., T. Saito, S. Iwamoto, Y. Kumamoto, T. Ohdaira, R. Suzuki et al. 2011. Pore size determination of TEMPO-oxidized cellulose nanofibril films by positron annihilation lifetime spectroscopy. Biomacromolecules 12(11): 4057–4062. doi: 10.1021/bm201079n.

Gough, E., H. Shaikh and A. R. Manges. 2011. Systematic review of intestinal microbiota transplantation (fecal bacteriotherapy) for recurrent Clostridium difficile infection. Clinical Infectious Diseases 53(10): 994–1002. doi: 10.1093/cid/cir632.

He, J., T. Kunitake and A. Nakao. 2003. Facile *in situ* synthesis of noble metal nanoparticles in porous cellulose fibers. Chemistry of Materials 15(23): 4401–4406. doi: 10.1021/cm034720r.

Helenius, G., H. Bäckdahl, A. Bodin, U. Nannmark, P. Gatenholm and B. Risberg. 2006. *In vivo* biocompatibility of bacterial cellulose. Journal of Biomedical Materials Research Part A 76A(2): 431–438. doi: 10.1002/jbm.a.30570.

Henriksson, M., L. A. Berglund, P. Isaksson, T. Lindstrom and T. Nishino. 2008. Cellulose nanopaper structures of high toughness. Biomacromolecules 9(6): 1579–1585. doi: 10.1021/bm800038n. http://nutrition.jbpub.com/resources/chemistryreview9.cfm. (2016). http://nutrition.jbpub.com/resources/chemistryreview9.cfm.

ISO10993-5. 2009. Biological evaluation of medical devices. Part 5. Test for *in vitro* cytotoxicity.

Jorfi, M. and E. J. Foster. 2015. Recent advances in nanocellulose for biomedical applications. Journal of Applied Polymer Science 132(14): n/a-n/a. doi: 10.1002/app.41719.

Kalashnikova, I., H. Bizot, B. Cathala and I. Capron. 2012. Modulation of cellulose nanocrystals amphiphilic properties to stabilize oil/water interface. Biomacromolecules 13(1): 267–275. doi: 10.1021/bm201599j.

Klemm, D., D. Schumann, U. Udhardt and S. Marsch. 2001. Bacterial synthesized cellulose—artificial blood vessels for microsurgery. Progress in Polymer Science 26(9): 1561–1603. doi: http://dx.doi.org/10.1016/S0079-6700(01)00021-1.

Kolakovic, R., L. Peltonen, A. Laukkanen, M. Hellman, P. Laaksonen, M. B. Linder et al. 2013. Evaluation of drug interactions with nanofibrillar cellulose. European Journal of Pharmaceutics and Biopharmaceutics 85(3): 1238–1244. doi: 10.1016/j.ejpb.2013.05.015.

Lange, J. and Y. Wyser. 2003. Recent innovations in barrier technologies for plastic packaging—a review. Packaging Technology and Science 16(4): 149–158. doi: 10.1002/pts.621.

Li, M.-C., Q. Wu, K. Song, S. Lee, Y. Qing and Y. Wu. 2015. Cellulose nanoparticles: structure–morphology–rheology relationships. ACS Sustainable Chemistry & Engineering 3(5): 821–832. doi: 10.1021/acssuschemeng.5b00144.

Malm, C. J., B. Risberg, A. Bodin, H. Bäckdahl, B. R. Johansson, P. Gatenholm et al. 2012. Scand. Cardiovasc. J. 46: 57–62.

Maneerung, T., S. Tokura and R. Rujiravanit. 2008. Impregnation of silver nanoparticles into bacterial cellulose for antimicrobial wound dressing. Carbohydrate Polymers 72(1): 43–51. doi: http://dx.doi.org/10.1016/j.carbpol.2007.07.025.

Markets, M. 2015. Nanocellulose market by type, application, and geography, Regional trends and forecast to 2019 by Markets and Markets Report code CH 3320.

Markstedt, K., A. Mantas, I. Tournier, H. Martínez Ávila, D. Hägg and P. Gatenholm. 2015. 3D Bioprinting human chondrocytes with nanocellulose–alginate bioink for cartilage tissue engineering applications. Biomacromolecules 16(5): 1489–1496. doi: 10.1021/acs.biomac.5b00188.

Mazeau, K. and M. Wyszomirski. 2012. Modelling of Congo red adsorption on the hydrophobic surface of cellulose using molecular dynamics. Cellulose 19(5): 1495–1506. doi: 10.1007/s10570-012-9757-6.

Medronho, B., A. Romano, M. G. Miguel, L. Stigsson and B. Lindman. 2012. Rationalizing cellulose (in) solubility: reviewing basic physicochemical aspects and role of hydrophobic interactions. Cellulose 19(3): 581–587. doi: 10.1007/s10570-011-9644-6.

Mertaniemi, H., C. Escobedo-Lucea, A. Sanz-Garcia, C. Gandía, A. Mäkitie, J. Partanen et al. 2016. Human stem cell decorated nanocellulose threads for biomedical applications. Biomaterials 82: 208–220. doi: http://dx.doi.org/10.1016/j.biomaterials.2015.12.020.

Mølgaard, S. L., M. Henriksson, M. Cárdenas and A. J. Svagan. 2014a. Cellulose-nanofiber/polygalacturonic acid coatings with high oxygen barrier and targeted release properties. Carbohydrate Polymers 114(0): 179–182. doi: http://dx.doi.org/10.1016/j.carbpol.2014.08.011.

Mølgaard, S. L., M. Henriksson, M. Cárdenas and A. J. Svagan. 2014b. Cellulose-nanofiber/polygalacturonic acid coatings with high oxygen barrier and targeted release properties. Carbohydrate Polymers 114: 179–182. doi: http://dx.doi.org/10.1016/j.carbpol.2014.08.011.

Nel, A. E., L. Madler, D. Velegol, T. Xia, E. M. V. Hoek, P. Somasundaran et al. 2009. Understanding biophysicochemical interactions at the nano-bio interface. Nat. Mater. 8(7): 543–557.

Nishino, T., K. Takano and K. Nakamae. 1995. Elastic-modulus of the crystalline regions of cellulose polymorphs. Journal of Polymer Science Part B-Polymer Physics 33(11): 1647–1651. doi: 10.1002/polb.1995.090331110.

Pesticide Action Network. from http://www.pan-europe.info/campaigns/biocides.

Petersen, N. and P. Gatenholm. 2011. Bacterial cellulose-based materials and medical devices: current state and perspectives. Applied Microbiology and Biotechnology 91(5): 1277–1286. doi: 10.1007/s00253-011-3432-y.

Pääkkö, M., M. Ankerfors, H. Kosonen, A. Nykänen, S. Ahola, M. Österberg et al. 2007. Enzymatic hydrolysis combined with mechanical shearing and high-pressure homogenization for nanoscale cellulose fibrils and strong gels. Biomacromolecules 8(6): 1934–1941. doi: 10.1021/bm061215p.

Pinto, R. J. B., P. Marques, C. P. Neto, T. Trindade, S. Daina and P. Sadocco. 2009. Antibacterial activity of nanocomposites of silver and bacterial or vegetable cellulosic fibers. Acta Biomaterialia 5(6): 2279–2289. doi: 10.1016/j.actbio.2009.02.003.

Saini, S., N. Belgacem, J. Mendes, G. Elegir and J. Bras. 2015. Contact antimicrobial surface obtained by chemical grafting of microfibrillated cellulose in aqueous solution limiting antibiotic release. ACS Applied Materials & Interfaces 7(32): 18076–18085. doi: 10.1021/acsami.5b04938.

Saini, S., Ç. Yücel Falco, M. N. Belgacem and J. Bras. 2016. Surface cationized cellulose nanofibrils for the production of contact active antimicrobial surfaces. Carbohydrate Polymers 135: 239–247. doi: http://dx.doi.org/10.1016/j.carbpol.2015.09.002.

Saito, T., R. Kuramae, J. Wohlert, L. A. Berglund and A. Isogai. 2013. An ultrastrong nanofibrillar biomaterial: the strength of single cellulose nanofibrils revealed via sonication-induced fragmentation. Biomacromolecules 14(1): 248–253. doi: 10.1021/bm301674e.

Schumann, D. A., J. Wippermann, D. O. Klemm, F. Kramer, D. Koth, H. Kosmehl et al. 2008. Artificial vascular implants from bacterial cellulose: preliminary results of small arterial substitutes. Cellulose 16(5): 877–885. doi: 10.1007/s10570-008-9264-y.

Sturcova, A., G. R. Davies and S. J. Eichhorn. 2005. Elastic modulus and stress-transfer properties of tunicate cellulose whiskers. Biomacromolecules 6(2): 1055–1061. doi: 10.1021/bm049291k.

Svagan, A. J., M. A. S. A. Samir and L. A. Berglund. 2007. Biomimetic polysaccharide nanocomposites of high cellulose content and high toughness. Biomacromolecules 8(8): 2556–2563. doi: 10.1021/bm0703160.

Svagan, A. J., M. A. S. A. Samir and L. A. Berglund. 2008. Biomimetic foams of high mechanical performance based on nanostructured cell walls reinforced by native cellulose nanofibrils. Advanced Materials 20(7): 1263–1269. doi: 10.1002/adma.200701215.

Szot, C. S., C. F. Buchanan, P. Gatenholm, M. N. Rylander and J. W. Freeman. 2011. Investigation of cancer cell behavior on nanofibrous scaffolds. Materials Science and Engineering: C 31(1): 37–42. doi: http://dx.doi.org/10.1016/j.msec.2009.12.005.

van den Berg, O., J. R. Capadona and C. Weder. 2007. Preparation of homogeneous dispersions of tunicate cellulose whiskers in organic solvents. Biomacromolecules 8(4): 1353–1357. doi: 10.1021/bm061104q.

Viet, D., S. Beck-Candanedo and D. Gray. 2007. Dispersion of cellulose nanocrystals in polar organic solvents. Cellulose 14(2): 109–113. doi: 10.1007/s10570-006-9093-9.

Woo, S. Y. and R. E. Levine. 1998. Ligament, tendon and fascia. pp. 59–65. *In*: Black, J. and G. Hastings (eds.). Handbook of Biomaterial Properties. Springer, US.

Yamanaka, S., K. Watanabe, N. Kitamura, M. Iguchi, S. Mitsuhashi, Y. Nishi et al. 1989. The structure and mechanical properties of sheets prepared from bacterial cellulose. Journal of Materials Science 24(9): 3141–3145. doi: 10.1007/bf01139032.

Yano, H., J. Sugiyama, A. N. Nakagaito, M. Nogi, T. Matsuura, M. Hikita et al. 2005. Optically transparent composites reinforced with networks of bacterial nanofibers. Advanced Materials 17(2): 153–155. doi: 10.1002/adma.200400597.

10

Modelling and Simulation of Biological Systems in Medical Applications

S. Balaji

Introduction

A model basically represents a system or an object under study, or may be an idea which might represent the system. Simulation actually represents the operation of the model which mimics the system as a whole. A model can be treated as an alternative way to realize the system which might be impractical or too expensive to perform in real for the studies. From this model, the system can be built and simulated to study its operation and behaviour. This is the primary reason for an extensive use of simulation in every scientific research in studying a system for its behaviour in different circumstances (Durairaj et al. 2012; Miller et al. 2012). Modelling and simulation mainly focuses on collecting information about the system under study and building a computational model of that system, which helps in analysing the system. Analysis can easily be done once we have built the model and its dependencies across different elements without actually building the whole system and thus the real system can be studied through simulation by taking all the parameters into consideration (Durairaj et al. 2012). Systems biology, as a field of study, is the computational and

Jain University, Centre for Emerging Technologies, Jain Global Campus, Jain University, 45th KM, NH 209, Kanakapura Road, Kanakapura Taluk, Ramanagara Dist., Karnataka-562112, India.
E-mail: drsbalaji@gmail.com

mathematical modelling of complex biological systems and studying the interactions among the components of biological systems. Modelling and Simulation studies are common in all areas of systems biology including simulation of neurons, cells, tissues, biochemical reactions, gene regulatory networks, and so on.

A complex system consists of interconnected processes or networks. These inter-related components must be considered while modelling since they play a major role when we consider the system as a whole. These networks or interconnected smaller parts produce large data and computing is the only option to analyse such huge data (Miller et al. 2012). The goal is to create a model of the real system and collect all the responses from the system over a period of time. The collected data is used to simulate the system for different inputs and to study the behaviour with varied parameters. The functional aspects of any system are basically represented by models and the interconnections among several subsystems. The simulation software converts this model into a feasible computational model which helps in studying the functional and non-functional system properties. Modelling and simulation involves getting information about behaviour and properties of the system under study without actually building it in real life. For instance, to determine which type of car design would be suitable for a particular road can be inferred just by simulating the car design process. Useful insights about different decisions in the design could be gleaned without actually building the car. The terms "modelling" and "simulation" are often used interchangeably. In general, modelling and simulation refer to using models, including emulators, prototypes, and simulators, either statically or over time, to develop data as a basis for making managerial or technical decisions.

Modelling and simulation have been extensively used in engineering for virtual realization of the systems under study. Engineering management is equipped with large number of tools to accomplish modelling and simulation. By using modelling and simulation, we are able to produce high quality products and also able to decrease the development cost, since much of the trials can be done virtually. It has to be noted that modelling and simulation have emerged as pure applications without being any cross application interface. Hence, the modelling and simulation find their application in fields where real testing proves to be costly.

Mathematical modelling plays a very important role in understanding the complexity involved in biological systems. Mathematical formulations make it easy to clearly understand the dynamics of any system. This has proved to be a success in simulating complex biological processes like biochemical pathways, cell signalling pathways, etc. A mathematical model is very useful in studying gene expression or behaviour of complex systems because it helps in generalization of a system in a mathematical way. Figure 1 depicts typical modelling and simulation study. In general, modelling and simulation of a system depends on the way we develop new mathematical representations. The main step is to find a mathematical representation for each component or sub-system and their inter-relationships. Since any biological system consists of a complex network of entities which interact among themselves to perform various vital biological processes, there is a huge demand for computing power to model and simulate such systems.

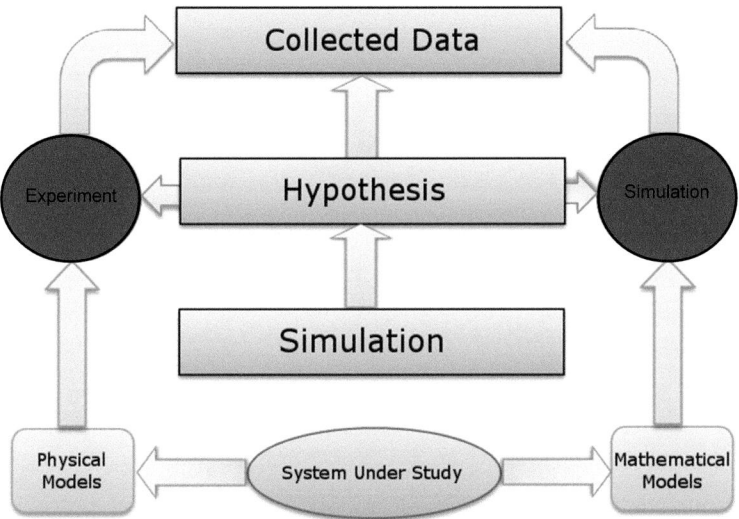

Fig. 1: Modelling and Simulation.

Biological Systems

Numerous specific functions in the human body are carried out by independent systems which facilitate the human body to work as a system. For example, if we consider the digestive system, it mainly consists of connected organs which help in movement of food, digestion, and excretion. Similarly, the circulatory system consists of veins, heart, capillaries which help in blood movement and transport of food and oxygen to all cells in the body. The immune system plays a role in protecting the body against various invasions by micro-organisms. The immune system consists of bone marrow, lymphocytes, lymph nodes, etc.

The nervous system is responsible for various control and coordination aspects of the body. This includes the brain, nervous system, spinal cord, etc. The nervous system is responsible for generating any action or reactions for an event and also the control of voluntary organs in the human body. If we consider the human body muscular system, it has around 650 muscles which help in the movement, blood flow, food movement in the digestive system and so on. Skeletal muscle is connected to the body and helps in the body movement. Similarly, muscles in different areas of the human body have different roles to play. The male reproductive system includes the penis and testis while the female reproductive system includes the vagina, uterus, and ovaries.

Oxygen is taken into the respiratory system and carbon-di-oxide is expelled out. The respiratory system consists of trachea, lungs, and diaphragm. The waste generated in the human body is removed by excretory system which consists of bladder, kidneys, and ureters. The urine produced by the kidneys travels to ureters and then to the bladder and exits through the urethra. The skin is considered to be the largest organ in the human body. The skin basically protects the body from the outer temperature variations and also micro-organisms. It helps in eliminating body waste and also temperature control of body through sweating.

Computer modelling and simulation have changed the way medicine is practised and taught. The fundamental idea behind modelling is to first build a system which is the virtual copy of the real system. Once it is built, it is easy to observe the system parameters by exerting the model through simulations and tweak the design to improve the system performance. Finally, one can test the design using the real system (Pavlick et al. 2011) to validate the system design. The issues which have to be considered during simulations are:

- Providing appropriate user interface.
- Determining the complexity of simulation.
- Coverage of all inputs.
- Evaluating the hardware requirements.

In modelling, it is important to consider the modelling scheme which covers all the important properties of the system under study and also carefully examine all the inputs and outputs (Zeng and Chen 2011). Since all the processes do not normally affect the behaviour of a system, we select the important processes that have a major impact on the system. The modelling process typically involves the following steps (Monroe and Hoffman 2006; Zhu 2007):

1. Familiarize with the system to be modelled.
2. Identify important variables that are volatile over time.
3. Detect interconnections among key variables.
4. Investigate how to measure and collect data.
5. Finalize selection of model and its architecture.
6. Build a model by stipulating all parameters. Operate the model and measure the behaviour.
7. Compare measurements with the model concepts. If the model is getting improved return to Stage 6; otherwise return to Stages 3, 4, and 5.
8. Perform sensitivity analysis to study the effect of variation in one independent variable on other dependent variables. Return to Stage 6 and 7, if required.
9. Study how to control policy and other initial conditions' impact.
10. Using these criteria, decide the choice that affects the policy trade off.

Use of these steps in modelling and simulation of biological systems is an involved process since biological systems are complex and are interconnected with many important physiological and pathological roles. A biological system may be seen as a complex adaptive system where each individual component is connected through various feedback and feed forward loops (Monroe and Hoffman 2006). The non-linear relationships between these factors can be interchanged among the components of the biological systems that render the study of biology at a molecular and cellular level which is nearly impossible (Zhu 2007).

Modelling and Simulation

Scientific domains such as engineering, social sciences, and economics generally use modelling and simulation. Healthcare experts examine the disease mechanisms and design pharmaceutical agents using modelling techniques. In production sector and logistics, modelling and simulation methods are used for development in choice making, competence, and quality. A real system is modelled to understand the behaviour. After observing the system, we test it by varying the system parameters using simulations. This allows testing various scenarios, and the performance results of the simulated system can help in devising different approaches for effective and well-organized system operation. The results of simulation indicate the quality of model itself and gives the insight in to the real system. A model is used to highlight the absence of parts of a system and to forecast the influence of planned outages without interfering with the regular working of the system. Medical applications such as learning disease and physiological procedures, forecasting and investigating human performance, and directing system assessments in difficult, high-risk healthcare situations are the important applications of modelling and simulation.

Social simulation relates mathematical frameworks to investigate matters in social sciences. The matters include problems in psychology, structural behaviour, sociology, political science, finances, anthropology, topography, manufacturing, archaeology, morphology, etc. These simulations target to close the gap between expressive approaches used in social sciences and formal approaches used in hard sciences.

Computational experiments of biological systems have been discussed in An et al. (2010). The physical laws that govern all the processes of the organisms, the way molecules interact to perform complex functions of the brain and other whole organs are strictly to be obeyed while performing these experiments. The coded information related to a living organism is very different from that related to the matter which is decaying (An et al. 2010). The computational biology's task is to find those differences. This process has been barely started. Also, many researchers are trying computational tools that have been utilized effectively in different fields to understand biological systems. The modelling of mathematical and statistical networks is an essential step towards uncovering the behaviour of biological networks and the organizational principles. Without doubt, there is a need for new mathematical tools to address these challenges. The main effort presently is to use standard tools especially from applied mathematics that have proved successful for solving many problems in other disciplines. These new areas of mathematics contribute very powerful tools to solve practical problems.

Stochastic simulations for parameter sweep applications

The stochastic modelling and optimization are important parts in the field of systems biology in terms of atomic level and the natural framework originating from both within the cell (intrinsic) and outside the cell in interaction with the environment (extrinsic). Parameter sweep applications can be used to explore the large spaces generated by the variables and parameters and help in the study of the dynamics of a system. The stochastic simulation traces the evolution of variables that change stochastically, that is, randomly with certain probabilities. The recreation of the stochastic approach depicts how each framework is connected to another framework which gives an insight of how handling of arrangements of different biochemical responses for every species that is stochastically ready. In the stochastic demonstration setting, the Parameter Sweep Applications (PSAs) approach helps to investigate the huge spaces that are being created by framework's various variables and parameters (Mosca et al. 2009). The researchers demonstrate a matrix based variant of multi-volume stochastic test system, tau-DPP, which tests the quality of PSAs that has been done to indicate the basic variables, bottlenecks, and versatility over the information being shared for natural displaying and reproductions (Jiang and Luo 2010).

Non-linear biological phenomena using Bayesian method

The dynamics of a biological system can be captured by non-linear ODEs (Ordinary Differential Equations). Bayesian method is used to study a system by considering only that part of data which has dependency on other system functions. An S-system is a set of non-linear ODEs which is derived from mass action law and is widely used as an effective model for various biological systems (Mansouri et al. 2012). The main challenge is to model the biological systems by considering various model parameters using the Bayesian approach (Mansouri et al. 2012) where the states and parameters estimation of biological events are modelled using S-systems. The non-linear states and the estimation of various parameters have been very challenging for the biological systems. Nevertheless, it is the key approach for finding the quantitative and qualitative information of the dynamic and structured models of the biological systems. To estimate the model parameters of Cad System in *E. Coli* (CSEC), a Particle Filter (PF) is used which is non-linear. Gaussian noise is the statistical noise that affects any data set in a Gaussian distribution. Most of these non-linear systems and non-Gaussian noise observations are practically untraceable in terms of the closed-form expressions of the posterior distribution of the states. To overcome these shortfalls, non-parametric particle filtering is becoming more popular. The simulation analysis done by evaluating models using Root Mean Square Error (RMSE) shows that the Bayesian algorithm efficiently measures the different parameters of unknown models and provides accurate estimation of states.

Global methodology for simulating medical systems

Various variables are given as inputs to the gadgets used to numerically represent the patients, which yield an arrangement of mathematical statements that shows how the variables are allied (Ch et al. 2014). Numerous procedures are followed to build the frameworks for the human system simulations, which have specific targets in breaking down the execution and administration of all the framework parts. A patient or device can be mathematically represented by using a number of variables. These variables represent input, output, and set of equations which describe interactions among themselves. Using these variables, one can use a global method for analysing the human system. This helps in understanding human organism control and also to analyse the results of the clinical trials.

Modelling and Simulation in Medical Applications

Modelling and simulation techniques are used extensively for various medical applications including drug discovery, gene regulatory networks, medical implantations, nanoparticle applications, tissue simulation, and so on. The rest of this section briefly addresses some of these applications.

Drug discovery

Drug discovery is concerned with discovering new drugs and studying their possible adverse effects on the biological system(s) without actually inducing the drugs into the humans. The most important research and development in pharma bioinformatics is in automating and speeding drug discovery process. The drug discovery process is shown in Fig. 2 (Bergeron 2002; Partl et al. 2014; Evangelidis and Xie 2014; Xie et al. 2012; Tobinick 2009) and depicts the set of events that starts with 5000 drug molecules and completes with one product that comes to the market. Any technology that reduces the research process has potential to save the industry billions of dollars. Modelling and simulation accelerate the drug discovery research. A better study of metabolism of a disease can suggest which molecule will be most effective for treatment and which one causes toxic reactions in the patient (Bergeron 2002; Partl et al. 2014; Evangelidis and Xie 2014; Xie et al. 2012; Tobinick 2009). Modelling protein structure and differentiating it with important drugs can potentially serve as an effective screener for candidate drugs.

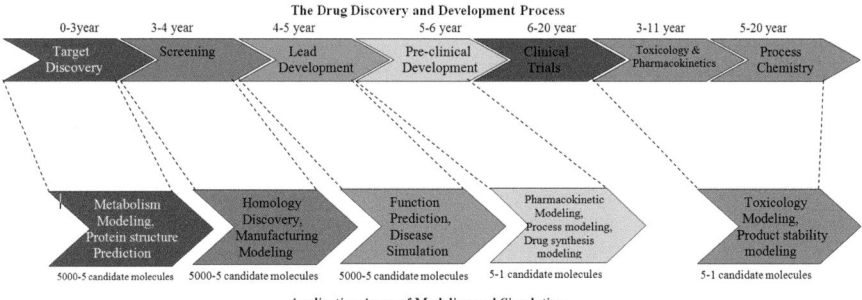

Fig. 2: Drug Discovery and Development Process.

Another major research area in drug discovery is the virtual screening for drug discovery. Virtual screening basically screens many proteins in the data set and finds the matching ligand in less time. In cell signalling, also known as signal transduction, an external stimulus brings about response by triggering a chain of molecular events within the cell. Understanding of this signalling process helps in discovering new drugs since the molecular interactions can be found using this. Finding out protein ligand affinity is one of the most important processes in drug discovery.

Virtual screening for drug discovery

The process of finding out protein-ligand affinity is an important research area in bioinformatics. It is a computational technique used in drug discovery to search libraries of small molecules in order to identify those structures which are most likely to bind to a drug target, typically a protein receptor or enzyme. The basic goal of the virtual screening is the reduction of the enormous virtual chemical space of small organic molecules, to synthesize and/or screen against a specific target protein, to a manageable number of the compound that inhibits the highest chance to lead to a drug candidate. Additionally, the 3-D space is usually larger than what it appears to be; this brings about more particulate estimations requiring huge computing resources. Docking is one of the methods in virtual screening. This process involves finding the location where the ligand can be introduced and it is a computationally intensive task. In docking, researchers investigate studies related to bonding a ligand to specific protein (Hu et al. 2008; Smith et al. 2011; Erwin and Davidson 2010). In rigid body docking techniques, one utilizes either a solitary adaptation or multi conformer libraries to consider ligand adaptability. In these methods, the little particles are docked using shape complementarity or cooperation site coordinating calculations (for instance, ADAM, DOCK, FRED, FTDock, LIGIN, SANDOCK, and YUCCA). In coordinating calculations, a pharmacophore speaking to the protein is at first created and used to direct the docking. A starting ligand adaptation is created and a ligand pharmacophore is obtained from this compliance.

The process of binding a ligand to a protein includes and relies on two components: (i) a method to explore the conformational space of the ligand and/or the protein target and (ii) a Scoring Function (SF) to evaluate the proposed binding modes referred to as poses. An SF should first assign the best score to the 'correct pose' (that is, the native pose observed in crystal structures), thus 'guiding' the conformational sampling algorithm. The prediction of the accurate binding mode is very crucial which forms the first step since it is the major part of docking process. In the second phase, poor binders or non-binders are identified and active compounds are assigned with higher scores. This second aspect is critical in lead optimization and in Virtual Screening (VS), where potential hits are to be extracted from large libraries. In fact, some programs use multiple SFs, such as a crude SF to direct the docking and a more refined SF for scoring the final poses. Figure 3 shows the time taken to dock protein to the ligand (Zhang et al. 2013) using single core and multi core computers. The current drug discovery procedure is centred on discrete targets and streamlined measures. Certain improvement exercises result in less demanding procedures with critical drawbacks. The single-target methodology disregards the fact that numerous medications have different objectives without a focus on the viability. The single target based approach likewise restricts the capacity of scientists to distinguish creative targets and/or components of activity by constraining druggable space (Kirshner et al. 2013; Nilmeier et al. 2013) to perceived targets and modalities.

Choosing the right molecule as a drug within the large set of chemical database is a computationally challenging task. It is known that a typical pharmaceutical compound collection contains ~ 1 million compounds. The common practices in computer-aided docking employed in pharmaceutical companies are still dominated

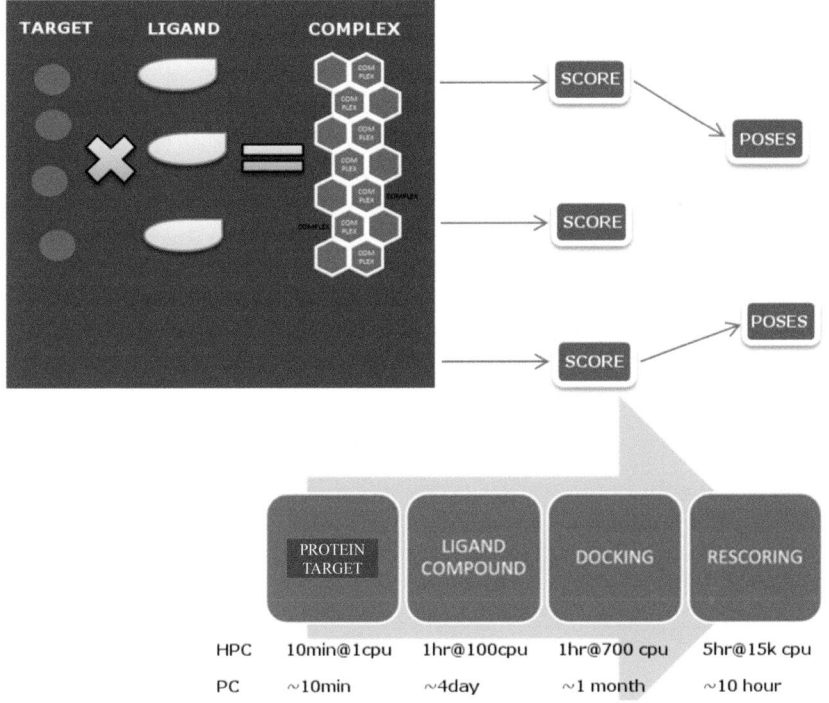

Fig. 3: Protein-Ligand Docking Time (Single Core vs. Multicore).

by personal computers and midsize clusters with hundreds of CPU cores. This limited computational resource can cap the database size that can be screened in practice.

It has been documented that for a typical data set, the time scales of a target of ~ 4000 atoms and ~ 40000 ligands running through the pipeline of drug design process, if done on a single CPU, takes ~ 10 minutes to prepare the protein target, ~ 4 days to prepare the ligands, ~1 month to dock the ligands into the target, and ~ 10 years to re-score the top 20 docking poses of all ligands. Supercomputers, although mature and popular in the field of molecular simulations and modelling, are seldom used in the in-silica drug design process since they are very expensive to use. Applying High Performance Computing (HPC) towards drug design could be a game-changing strategy for pharmaceutical companies.

Regulatory and signalling in protein interaction

High throughput study of proteins and functions along with microarray technology have paved the way for better understanding of regulatory networks and signalling in protein interactions. Proteomics is the large-scale study of proteins, particularly their structures and functions. There is currently no satisfactory method to construct an integrated cellular network that combines the gene regulatory network and the signalling regulatory pathway. Proteomics is the large-scale study of proteins, particularly their structures and functions, which provides unprecedented views of cellular components in the biological systems. However, the challenge for current researchers lies in how to interpret these large-scale data sets and extract true information to understand biological systems more thoroughly.

Signalling networks can be mathematically represented using different types of formalisms. A more sophisticated and principled way consists of writing rules describing the interactions among the different proteins that are then instantiated into biochemical reactions. Gene regulatory networks are responsible for the control of gene expression and, therefore, have direct impact on virtually all processes in the cell. Given the large set of possible interactions, the construction of regulatory networks is far from trivial and our knowledge is still very limited. No single mathematical formalism currently seems capable of simulating the phenotype of a cell taking signalling, gene regulation, and metabolic systems into account. With the advent of high-throughput experimental data, network reconstruction is moving towards an integration of all kinds of biological molecules based on different types of 'omics' data. There are undoubtedly many challenges, modelling approaches that leverage these data, as well as improved parameter optimisation algorithms and high-performance computing (Goncalves et al. 2013).

Gene regulatory networks

A Generic Regulatory Network (GRN) is a combination of different regulators that communicate with each other and with other particles within the cell that control the level of gene expression in mRNA and in proteins. The combination within the cells can be either direct or indirect. Overall, the molecules of mRNA make an explicit set of proteins. Certain proteins also act as enzymes which help in breakdown of food molecules. If protein is structural, it will accumulate at the membranes of the cell or inside the cell so as to provide detailed properties of the cell structure (Haseong and Gelenbe 2012; Yong et al. 2011; Shih 2004). Modelling and simulation of gene regulatory networks helps in identifying gene patterns and gene expressions. There are some proteins that provide assistance to trigger other genes. In the organisms that are unicellular, the controlling networks of the cell responds to the surrounding that enhances the cell at a particular time for existence in the environment. For example, the yeast cell in the solution containing sugar triggers the genes within the yeast cell to use an enzyme to prepare alcohol from the sugar solution. Thus, the yeast cell multiplies its energy and makes a living within the solution and assists in making wine, which in the normal situation (Carro et al. 2010). Bayesian model averaging is applied in gene regulatory networks to build large scale gene regulatory systems. Gene regulatory memories try to find out information about frameworks that have been inherited.

Reconstruction of large-scale GRNs

A GRN gives enormous information regarding the interaction of different molecules in a biological system (Haseong and Gelenbe 2012). Here, the main challenge is to build a large scale gene regulatory system. Also, the procedure includes a lot of information that might require a legitimate incorporation system such as Bayesian model averaging which rests on finding out a criterion.

The GRN plays a pivotal role in discovering different biological problems, where it can recognize the transcription factors of specific disease marker genes (Carro et al. 2010) and is utilized to find out the information in the developmental processes that influence in improving some disease conditions (Erwin and Davidson 2010). With this, various scientific and measurable systems have been acquainted with different quality administrative systems which induce connections among qualities. Probabilistic models have been used for computer system performance analysis (Gelenbe 1973) and to find gene regulatory networks (Gelenbe 2007). Recently, various studies have been done to find different methods that have been assessed in a competition called DREAM (Dialogue for Reverse Engineering Assessments and Methods) (Erwin and Davidson 2010).

Gene-regulatory memories

The progress made in gene-regulatory memory circuits (Zhang and Li 2009; Nido et al. 2012; Ferreira and Vendramini 2010) has made a breakthrough in finding out the information that has been stored and has enabled new natural science applications. The computer models and simulations give quantitative examination and finding of the practices and components of the frameworks that has been inherited. The non-linear movement clubbed with various substance reactions in quality authoritative memory frameworks which use compound reaction scientific explanations are demonstrated. The reactions are mapped in the process of electrical-similar models. The researchers address the most important problem related to showing framework model parameters, that is, by adding to a multiplication driven Bayesian structure for recognizing various parameters. To make sure the trustworthy identification of some of the crucial system properties, the researchers have proposed a two-stage structure that defends parameter unmistakable confirmation philosophy. Initial step collects bi-strength; the next step is adjusts towards recognizing dynamic properties of framework while keeping up the perceived bi-security.

Human physiology simulation

Human physiology refers to the study of how tissues and organs of a normal human being function mechanically, physically and in terms of biochemical functions (Viceconti 2011; Huertas and Ceccaroni 2013; Kulhanek et al. 2014; Das et al. 2013; Rubenfeld et al. 2005; Esteban et al. 2002; Esteban et al. 2008). The primary focus is at the level of human organs. It contains various systems like digestive, reproductive, nervous, musculoskeletal, circulatory, and respiratory systems. The virtual physiological human vision for collaborative modelling and simulation discusses about the framework phases which can be used to understand human physiology and pathology. Many tools exist to simulate human physiology.

Collaborative modelling and simulation

The Virtual Physiological Human (VPH) (Viceconti 2011; Martins and de Araujo 2001) is an intercontinental research initiative. Different framework phases and technologies of human physiology are discussed in VPH. The term integrative shows the essential limitations of the reductionist methodology, trying to capture the appearances due to complete collaboration between space-time measures, organ schemes. The early results of the VPH creativity claim that the VPH is the first and primary attempt to progress to collective modelling and simulation.

Simulation environment for heterogeneous physiology models

Many tools exist for the simulation of models that signify the human physiology (Huertas and Ceccaroni 2013; Martins and de Araujo 2001). These models and simulation tools are established in specific languages and models are interoperable with other models developed in the same or similar languages. A new tool is being developed to offer a common structure of simulation for models developed in different programming languages. This simulation environment is directed at bio-researchers and medical students, and establishes a framework to support the opinion and analysis of physiological appliances. The tool has been validated using models of the physiology of a chronic disease, namely, the chronic obstructive pulmonary disease. Eight deterministic models and one probabilistic model which are related to the respiratory chain have been considered and are represented in different languages.

Medical implantations

Medical implants are devices or tissues which can be placed inside the body. These implants are basically used to monitor body functions or in some cases provide support to organs and tissues. In some cases, these can also be used to deliver medications. These implants can be permanently placed in the body or can be removed when the intended purpose is met (Gamini and Shastry 2009; Merli et al. 2011; Freeman et al. 2010; Latsios et al. 2010; Chaufour et al. 1998; Grube et al. 2005). Medical implantations, when modelled and simulated, reveal a lot of information about how the device responds to the inner body parts. Active medical implantable devices can be artificially or surgically introduced into the human body to study the internal changes and behaviours. Medically implantable devices vary a lot in complexity and application. Examples include thermometers which gauge the temperature and send the data. Also, many advanced devices or computers help in testing and prosthesis. The design guidelines for the wireless biomedical telemetry system such as Radio Frequency (RF) can be used to detect the values in monitoring the physiological system.

Planar multi-turn loop antenna for wireless bio-medical telemetry

The radio frequency telemetry system detects the system values in monitoring physiological variables of independent medical diagnostic systems. This is required to meet isolated, separated chip sensors that are coupled to externally monitored devices (Gamini and Shastry 2009; Werber et al. 2006; Balanis 2005). The wireless blood pressure monitoring devices are pressure sensitive Micro Electro Mechanical Systems (MEMS) capacitor coupled with chip inductors to make passive sensor devices or loop antenna that function as the receptors of external observation devices. The external loop antenna is inductively controlled with the implanted chip inductive sensor. The limitation of the size of the implanted sensor controls the working of the system. The research carried out impacts changing the values of planar multi-turn circle devices. In this, sensitivity of the antenna is matched with the required frequency in the range that has been improved using tuneable antenna identical networks.

Miniature antenna for implantable wireless communication

The techniques used for designing, understanding, and finding the implanted radiators for telemetry applications are discussed in Merli et al. (2011). The analysis lets us use the free space of antenna topology for reduced calculation time. Consequently, antenna inserted in a body phantom is designed to account for all important electronic devices, power supply, and insulation of bio-computable system to realize complete implantable system. The simulation showed the gain in the two required frequency ranges between 2.4–2.5 GHz (Merli et al. 2011; Panescu 2008; Medical Implanted Communication System (MICS) 2009; Dissanayake et al. 2009). Three antennas are identified to improve performance of the system.

Wireless medical implant

The medicinal supplements are the tools that are prepared to replace the fractured biological frameworks. These are embedded to interact with other devices external to the body (Ma et al. 2012; Morari et al. 1999; Yang 2006; McCaffrey 2008). This research deals with the new Wireless Medicinal Insert (WMI) fake pancreas. There are complexities and subjects related to artificial pancreas frameworks. It is important to achieve low power consumption in a medical implant device for a virtual patient to measure control designs and communicate in the background without consuming much power.

Nanoparticles for biological applications

Nanoparticles are materials with overall dimensions in the nano scale, that is, under 100 nm (An et al. 2010; Ogomi et al. 2006; Ouyang et al. 2012; Zhang and Tam 2003; Hodzic et al. 2007; Yan et al. 2006; Kunii and Levenspiel 1991; Jung and Gidaspow 2002; Jaraiz et al. 1992; Ouyang et al. 2011; Tran et al. 2000; Otsuka et al. 2002). In recent years, these materials have emerged as important players in modern medicine, with clinical applications ranging from contrast agents in imaging to carriers for drug and drug delivery into tumors. Indeed, there are some instances where nanoparticles enable analyses and therapies that simply cannot be performed otherwise. Nano particles have advantages over today's therapies because they can be engineered to have certain properties or to behave in a certain way. These properties are selectivity, size, shape, and biocompatibility. Such properties allow for nanoparticles to affect the human body differently than traditional therapies. Nano particles are being used to increase image contrast of ultrasound and MRI technology. They are used in ultrasound to increase the acoustic reflectivity, ultimately leading to an increase in brightness and creation of a clearer image. Nano particles also help increase the image quality of MRI technology. However, nanoparticles also bring with them unique environmental and societal challenges, particularly with regard to toxicity. Here are some of the instances of applications of nanoparticles in biological applications and the need for modelling and simulation of such systems.

Nano particle targeted drug delivery

Nano medicine is a promising application of nano technology in medicine, which can drastically improve drug delivery efficiency through targeted delivery. However, characterization of the nanoparticle targeted delivery process within the vascular environment is very challenging due to the small scale of nanoparticles and the complexity *in vivo* vascular system. To understand such complicated systems, various computational models are developed to help reveal the nano particle targeted delivery process and design of nano particles for optimal delivery (Moffat 2015). The modelling approaches span from continuum vascular flow, particle Brownian adhesion dynamics, to molecular level ligand-receptor binding. Computer simulation is envisioned to be able to optimize drug carrier design and predict drug delivery efficiency for patient specific vascular environment. Mathematical modelling of targeted drug delivery systems provides quantitative description of the drug transportation in biological systems. Therefore, it can be utilized to evaluate efficiency of drug delivery and to estimate dose response. It is a very time consuming and challenging task for researchers to predict behaviour of various nano carriers in the physiological environment. Owing to the limitation of experiments, computational work would be a crucial tool for engineering shape and size of these nano carriers.

Nano informatics

The medical applications of information systems sciences (i.e., informatics) have gained prominence as essential sciences in nano biotechnology research, and have become particularly suitable in generating the appropriate research design frameworks. While these two concepts rely on computational and DNA analyses as well as protein sequencing, nano informatics specifically relates to the characterization of particles with applications in nano biotechnology using strategies in computational and analytical chemistry. The exponential generation of nano scale data have also enabled multi band interdisciplinary research to harness skills in creating new nano particles with relevant biomedical applications. Computational chemistry has helped in the design, modelling, and simulation of nano materials, nano particles, metallic nano particles, nano spheres, nano capsules, and quantum dots. These nano sized particles are currently being used as carriers for early diagnosis in nano medicine.

In modelling and simulation, the application of molecular dynamics requires an accurate characterization of the physico chemical properties of the nano system, in order to obtain accurate results about the structural dynamics at the atomic level. It is expected that most of the computer-related techniques in nano biotechnology and nano informatics would accelerate discoveries specific for biomedical treatments in a bottom-up approach (Liu et al. 2012).

Neuro prosthesis

The device that supplies or provides input and output to the nervous system is called neuro prosthesis (de Castro and Timmis 2002; Jerne 1974; Kohonen 1989). For many years the studies have been mainly focused on neuro prosthesis as a different way to escape the shortcomings of the neural system caused by the diseases. The neural prosthesis is a chain of different devices that provides assistance to sensory and motor modality which is damaged due to an injury or a disease. The cochlear transplants are an example of the devices being used. This provides assistance in performing the functions of ear drums while analysing the frequency during simulation of the cochlea. A microphone used in the device collects the sound and processes the signal and is transferred to the transplanted unit that simulates the acoustic nerve through an electrode array which are micro in size. Now, with the replacement and expansion of the injured senses, these implements aim to recover the disabilities of the organs (Zhang et al. 2014; Chun et al. 2014). The advancements in neuro prosthesis include the brain controlled prosthetic hand which learns the brain signals and controls the prosthetic hand. This process consumes much energy since stimulators are not energy efficient.

Brain control prosthetic hand

Recently biosensors and the brain-computer interface have seen a lot of advancements. This involves electromechanical tools other than computer (Zhang et al. 2014; Wolpaw et al. 2002; Allison et al. 2012; Zhang et al. 2011). This has led to the emergence of a new domain called brain control technology. The brain control technology involves brain signal detection, intelligent control, and man-system cooperation model. The neural prosthesis system was run by Brain Computer Interface (BCI) which was first constructed and integrated with EEG detector system, BCI analyses recognition and prosthesis control system. An Intelligent Mind Control Prosthetic Hand (IMCP Hand) was discovered with integrated multipoint tactile and sensor prosthetic space and 3-D acceleration sensor fusion. This improves the condition of people with upper limb disability.

Low power retinal prosthesis with charge balance

The safe working of stimulators is a very important issue in neural stimulation (Chun et al. 2014; Butterwick et al. 2007; McCreery et al. 1990; Merrill et al. 2005) for electrical performance. This has a direct relation with zero-net charge transfer and also heat generated in the tissue. The CMOS process increases the charge balancing capability and also lowers power consumption. The charge balance accuracy is achieved by creating the dynamic current mirror at the output of a stimulator. Low power consumption was achieved by using bias current, sharing with key bias blocks.

Spiking neural networks

Spiking Neural Networks (SNNs) is one of the neural network models, which also uses the concept of time in the model. It is called spiking because the neuron states are spiked or pushed by the triggers from the synaptic ends. Among the neural network models, the spiking neural network model comes in third generation that improves the level of practicality in the neural simulation. Additionally, the state of neuronal and synaptic timing concepts has been integrated into the SNN working model. The main aim here is to avoid the SNNs' neurons to reach the circulation cycle but fire when it is membrane prospective. When the neuron fires, a signal is generated which reaches the other neurons and as a result it either ups or lowers the capabilities in relation to the signal (Soleimani et al. 2012; Valova et al. 2005; Seth and Pandy 2007; Cisi and Kohn 2008; Schouten et al. 2008; Doya 2000). It is very difficult to simulate large scale neural networks.

Large scale simulation of SNNs on fast system C simulator

Spiking neural networks have attracted widespread attention in the artificial neural network community. Pulse coupled neural networks are important components processed by the brain. Several models are presented for spiking neural networks (Soleimani et al. 2012; Hodgkin and Huxley 1952; Gerstner and Kistler 2002; Izhikevich 2003; Renaud et al. 2007; Wijekoon and Dudek 2008) to replicate the behaviour of the networks. Detailed models such as the Hodgkin Huxley model, imitate research data to accuracy, but find it difficult to simulate large networks. Simplified frameworks are popular for large network dynamic studies of neural information coding, network dynamics, and memory. Integrate and Fire (IF) model is far from describing accurate data for real neurons. This research work focuses on various frameworks developed by Izhikevich which balances the mathematical efficiency of IF models of biological adaptability of Hodgkin-Huxley type frameworks (Soleimani et al. 2012). Neurons work in parallel for a large scale simulation. Mathematical environments are required for running large number of concurrent equations in massively parallel organization. Different digital and software implementations of spiking networks are reported in the literature.

Spinnaker is one approach for building specific neural system simulation. Other examples are BlueBrain, IFAT4G, BRAINSCALEs, and Neurogrid. These approaches are challenging in the field because they are expensive and require new operating system and software environment and their usage is limited to the research groups. Recent developments in high performance, low cost GPU (Soleimani et al. 2012) created new research opportunities to facilitate mathematical and computational resources to perform high speed simulations. A GPU consists of a number of processors framed as a grid working in parallel; this structure is suitable for small tasks in parallel. This assembly seems very suitable for neural network simulation where there area large number of neurons, each of them performing a basic operation.

System C procedures can cut design cycles permitting designers to optimize the ever narrowing time to market challenges. A key contributing factor to t h e success of System C is its capability to afford instruments for fast simulation as the RTL abstraction level language. A simplified cortical network is illustrated in Fig. 4. In this figure, the neurons are indicated by the label Nj and the presynaptic connections (Xi) of a neuron are represented as small circles with the weight Wi. The synaptic weight computation formula for each neuron is also shown in Fig. 4.

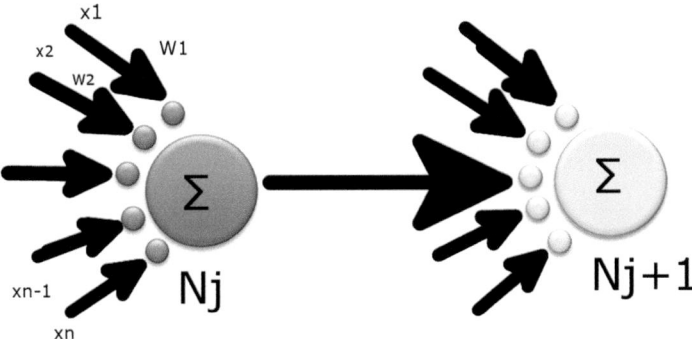

Fig. 4: A Simplified Illustration of the Cortical Networks.

The SNN (Soleimani et al. 2012) is based on four component neurons for spike processing, axons and dendrites for spike input and output communication and synapses for learning and storage. Figure 5 shows the overall simulation and design flow of the method. Simulation of SNN is one of the most challenging computational tasks because of its numerical complexity and simulation time.

Modelling weakly connected networks

The spiking neural systems are the systems built on the naturally stimulated models of the neurons of computation as they take the accurate timing of the spiking events into account. These are more suited to find out the dynamic aspects of the broadcasting of the neuron signals. These neurons' basic units for the processing form the main part of nervous system and then interact with one another with electrochemical pulses. Cortical neurons, analogue neurons, and spiking neurons are various types of neurons. Spiking neurons are used to process the data through the impulses of the nerves thus releasing into the axons, the spikes of electrical fissures. It later sends the signal to other cells that release the chemical affluences which later are attached to the neuron membrane as a receiver of chemical substances. These spiking neural structures of the human are mainly influenced by the neural models of the computation as they take accurate timing of the spiking signals and thus are very useful to find the features on

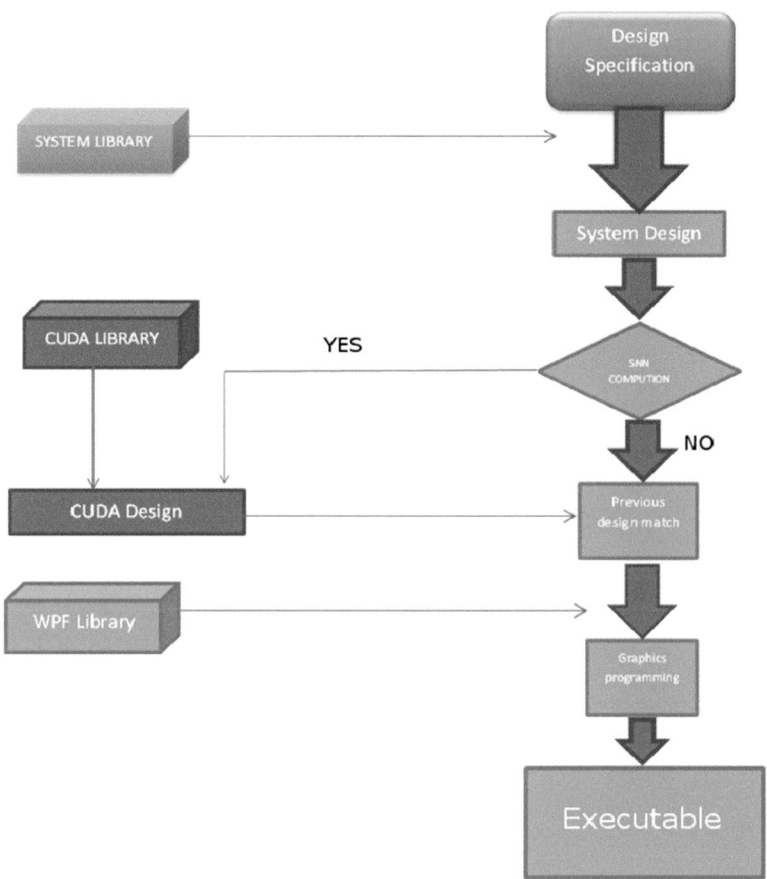

Fig. 5: GPU Simulation Flow Diagram.

the transmission of the signals of the neurons. These schemes gain attention as they are better defined than any neuron models which are simple by nature. They are also very close to the models that show the neurons and other elements synchronizing with the removal of assembled structure of neurons; this helps to serve the brain as a coding for feature binding and division into different shapes of outlines (Valova et al. 2005; Bialek et al. 1999; Gestner and Kistler 2002; Abbott and Dayan 2001).

Tissue simulation

Tissue simulation involves simulation of tissues to reveal various biochemical interactions. It focuses on various tissue properties like elasticity, specific absorption, etc. Also, the simulation can be applied to check stress and strain on a tissue and to study how it gets deformed or how it changes with the application of pressure. The tissue simulation is complicated because of its non-linear nature of response. The tissue has a sneak response which is dependent on time (Chanthasopeephan 2007).

Further, tissues are of extreme varieties including the walls of arteries, bone cartilages and organs, tissues of the skin, etc. The material characteristics of many tissues are not yet understood and, hence, several simulation experiments (Wang et al. 2006) are being conducted. There is a need for quicker algorithms to simulate surgical methods. Many sophisticated tools are available for bone surgery. Attempts are being made to the study the tissue deformation without actually cutting in surgery (Perrin et al. 2009; Terzopoulos et al. 1987; Meier et al. 2005; McInerney et al. 1996).

Modelling and simulation of tissue based CT images

Building of the surgical simulators needs better and quicker algorithms to calculate in real-time how the tissues are warped and the precise properties of these tissues. Development of sophisticated tools for organizing bone surgery is under-way. A simulation tool is developed for planning of treatment for bone surgery based on the Computerised Tomography (CT) data. The major ligaments were simulated using tension by connecting attachment point to the bone surface. Here, the main objective is to build a simulating device that plans the bone surgical diagnosis which is done on the data collected through CT scan of the patient. The surgery in this simulation will need a precise representation of the gentle tissues and the bones. In the model, all the joints are categorized as the interaction sides that allow the comparative building. The accurate ligaments are replicated by joining to apply the pressure that binds the constituents that compares the assembled ligament surfaces. The muscles are then categorized as the viscoelastic materials that are non-directional in nature (Wang et al. 2006; Woo et al. 2006; Pyburn and Goswami 2004; Jiang 2007).

Modelling soft-tissue deformation for surgical simulation

The soft tissue present in the human body gets deformed when it is cut before surgery. The study in (Chanthasopeephan et al. 2007) focuses on how the soft tissues get deformed during cutting. This can be used to show as simulated surgical trainings. The study is done for the soft tissues to cut with a blade while observing the forces involved whenever cut and the blade movement for different speeds of the cutting and angles of cutting. The deformation resistance is a property of Local Effective Modulus (LEM). The deformation resistance is calculated using the experimental data. During the distortion stage there is a need for closely observing formerly cracked extension of the tissue (Wang et al. 2006; Daigo et al. 2003; Mendoza and Laugier 2003; Cotin et al. 1999; Hirota et al. 1999). Living tissue usually exhibits non-linear deformation which might be considered for simulation.

Drug delivery

The drug delivery is a method, design, or skill for transporting the compound of medicine into body as and when needed. It involves the location targeting (where the medicine is needed to be delivered). The drug delivery is often viewed as the formulation of drug's chemical compounds. It also has to incorporate the amount of dosage (Park et al. 2009). These are basically used to modify the drug release profile and absorption. The most common ways of delivering drugs include non-invasive peroral (mouth), skin or through inhalation. Current focus in this domain is on targeted delivery. In the targeted delivery the drug is active only on the specified location or target (Fournier-Bidoz et al. 2004). An important drug delivery method is antibody mediated drug delivery system which uses antibodies and sticks to the receptors (sick cells). Nano robots can also be used to deliver the drugs, which is a unique application for drug delivery. The simulation and modelling of drug delivery helps in understanding the effects of drug without actually inducing (Singh et al. 2008; Nir et al. 2003; Cevc et al. 1996; Prausnitz et al. 2004) drugs into human body.

Antibody-mediated Drug Delivery Systems (ADDS)

The ADDS are emerging as the most promising solution to heal and diagnose various cancers. It uses antibodies that increase in large number and stick to the receptors which are sick cells known as antigens where it communicates. The Molecular Communication (MC) is used to transfer the data to core part of the atom and supports in constructing ADDS. The point-to-point response for ADDS from infusion of medicine into cells to ingestion of medicine from the cells is numerically calculated on account of the cell geometry that counter these performing agents. The accuracy attained for this MC model is agreed upon in the limited module restorations (COMSOL) (Park et al. 2009; Akyildiz et al. 2008; Berezhkovskii and Skvortsov 2013; Boswell et al. 2010; Brenner 1967).

Pt/Au hybrid self-actuating nano-robot for drug delivery

A model is being developed to examine and construct micro nano-sized robots (Chen et al. 2015; Smagilov et al. 2002; Paxton et al. 2004). The primary objective is to bring out unique applications of nano robots in drug delivery system, medical, health care, environmental monitoring, and so on. The initial step for reducing the self-impelled items is brought by white sides bunch (Zhang et al. 2013), which has the ability to change the artificially induced strength from hydrogen peroxide in its space. The nano rod made up of bimetal platinum (Pt) and gold (Au) is introduced by Tom Mallouk (Paxton et al. 2004; Fournier-Bidoz et al. 2004). The usage of nano rod has led to self-impetus hydrogen peroxide fuel. Besides that, there is a nano robot being developed in the University of Toronto (Fournier-Bidoz et al. 2004). In later stages, the researchers plan to produce self-fuelled colloidal miniaturized scale engines joining synergistic and attractive top structures, and show their execution for control, for example, transferring, transportation, conveyance, and sorting of small scale objects on microfluidic chips. Anderson and other analysts drive the nano robots with the outside field including attractive (Vickrey and Garcia-Ramirez 1980; Watarai et al. 2004), electric (Delgado 2001), warm (Derjaguin et al. 1987; Zhang and Briggs 1999; Piazza 2004) and fixation fields (Lin and Prieve 1983; Ebel et al. 1988; Keh and Wei 2000). Bao et al. (2013) present a novel reactant versatile small scale/nano robot made just of platinum that acknowledges nano meter headway in hydrogen peroxide arrangement.

Drug side effects detection

All drugs come with some side effects. Some of the common drug side effects include allergy, itching or development of rashes. Other side effects include nausea, constipation, and diarrhoea. In the case of cancer treatment, the side effects include hair loss, skin mutations (Valafar and Valafar 1999). Simulating drug side effects helps in analysing the side effects without causing them in reality. Drug side effects or opposing medicine reactions have become a major communal health alarm. It is one of the leading causes of disappointment in the process of drug growth and of drug removal once they have reached the market. Initial in silica forecast of potential side-effects in the drug detection process and getting early in to the clinical stages is of great importance to improve the long drug detection process and to deliver new, effective and harmless therapies for patients (Wada and Ward 1995; Rowland and Tozer 1989; Sheiner et al. 1979; Schwilden 1981; Alvis et al. 1985).

Open loop control of multiple drug effects in anaesthesia

Present open-loop computer-controlled infusion pumps do not clearly govern the temporary contrary side effects of circulatory drugs through anaesthesia. Researchers used ideal control values to produce a single-input multiple production controller that adjusts attentions at the site of required drug effect while correcting excessive side-effect drug attentions. The price function integrates framework based forecasts of upcoming effect-site concentrations, and the ability of the anaesthesiologist to anticipate future surgical proceedings. The regulator was evaluated and then associated with other control approaches through computer simulation of a physiologically based pharmacokinetic framework for the circulatory drug alfentanil. Multiple-effect control offers an analytic method to limit the overshoot in opposing side-effect concentrations at the significance of growing the time to attain the preferred drug outcome (Wada and Ward 1995; Valafar and Valafar 1999; Halford 1943; Mancia et al. 1984; Jacobs and Reves 1993).

Prediction of a patient's response to a specific drug treatment

A recent research uses the features of Artificial Neural Networks (ANNs) in forecasting the reaction of patient's pain from a particular disease or illness to a particular drug (Lori et al. 1994; Rodgers et al. 1990; Ajay 1990). As a case study, researcher illustrates that ANNs can be used to forecast sickle cell anaemia patients' reaction to hydroxyl urea behaviour. Hydroxyl urea is an orally transported medicine that partially eases the indications of sickle cell anaemia. Further research using neural networks is required to identify those patients who will not benefit adequately from hydroxyl urea risking its harmful side effects. The skilled artificial neural networks were capable of forecasting the potential reaction of a patient to hydroxyl urea with 86% with as high as 100% accuracy depending on the meaning of a positive reaction. This forecast was attained by preparation of the network with the 23 parameters. Also, it was possible to reduce the 23 input dimensional spaces into only 8 by manipulating the choice of variables (Valafar and Valafar 1999).

Predicting protein function

To allocate the biological and biochemical characteristics of the proteins, the bioinformaticians use the method of protein function prediction. These proteins are the ones that are ill-researched based on the genomic data sequence. The estimations are often data driven computational process. The data for these come from the nucleic acid series and gene expressions. Text mining of various materials also form the domain of structure of a protein and the interaction between the proteins (Yang et al. 2015; Gonzalez-Alvarez et al. 2015). The modelling and simulation helps in predicting protein functions which include protein similarity analysis and finding patterns in the protein sequence (Kramer 2003; Kola and Landis 2004; Fishman and Porter 2005; Barabasi and Oltvai 2004).

Protein sequence similarity analysis

An important task in the area of bioinformatics is to compare protein sequences and to derive some results out of it. This comparison also helps in prediction and classification of protein structure and function. A new distance based protein similarity analysis is done in this study which uses a new encoding method of protein sequence. The protein sequence is first represented in the 1-D space. The phylogenic tree can be constructed and used for similarity analysis. The proposed model is more accurate when compared to existing models like Su's model, Zhang's model, Yao's model (Yang et al. 2015; Shi and Niu 2007; Cheung and Jia 2013).

Finding patterns in protein sequences

The mass of any living being is primarily made up of proteins. These proteins are further dissociated or decomposed into many molecules like amino-acids and carry out various biological functions. All the body reactions are controlled by the participation of proteins. This is the reason protein studies are very important in bioinformatics. The identification of patterns in the protein sequence reveals a lot of information about functions and expressions. For performance evaluation, protein sequences are obtained from the database and fed to the bioinformatics computing system. The performance was far better compared to the existing pattern finding technique (Gonzalez-Alvarez et al. 2015; Fogel et al. 2008; Crooks et al. 2004).

Stochastic model of protease-ligand reactions

The protein tertiary structure prediction is a very computationally intensive task. We can use two methods to predict the structure; one is using X-ray crystallography and the other is using Nuclear Magnetic Resonance (NMR). Both are actually very expensive and time consuming processes. Some proteins are basically resistant to crystallization. Many techniques exist to solve this problem but all are inaccurate and also time consuming. The main objective of the research is to build a model which is reliable and time efficient in protein prediction. A stochastic simulation model is used that validates rate constant prediction which will be used for refinement of structure determination (Anderson et al. 2005; Crooks et al. 2004).

Metabolic pathways visualization

New methods are needed for analysis at a higher level of the sequenced genomes. To identify the metabolic pathway there is a need for data to be collected on gene expression and regulation (Bourqui et al. 2006). The discovery of the pathways provides aid to improve the genome annotations which are being discovered continuously. The analysis of the genome on the metabolic pathway level requires different methods for showing the pathways which are required (Rojdestvenski and Cottam 2002). Metabolic pathways can be simulated by using virtual reality and 3D structures of pathways. VRML software helps in realising 3D abstracts of metabolic pathways. Metabolic networks can be visualised using constraint planar graph drawing algorithm (Siegel et al. 2013; Miyamoto et al. 2000; Ross et al. 2004).

Visualizing metabolic networks in VRML

Successful data collection and visualization should satisfy conflicting requirements: unification of diverse data formats, support for serendipity research, support of hierarchical structures, algorithmizability, vast information density, Internet-readiness, etc. The traditional 2D representations of metabolic pathways lack compactness and information density. Virtual Reality (VR) has made significant progress in engineering, architectural design, entertainment, and communication. Evident advantages of using VR for scientific visualization are subconscious orientation, compromise between overview and detail, memorizing search results, and customization. Researchers experiment with the possibility of using immersive abstract 3D visualizations of metabolic networks. They present the trial Metabolic Network Visualizer (MNV) software, which produces graphical representation of a metabolic network as a Virtual Reality Modelling Language (VRML) world. The entities in the metabolic network are identified as "compartment", "species", "reaction," and "transporter". The properties of the above objects are described using a simple scripting language (Rojdestvenski and Cottam 2002; Jin et al. 2013; Yeoh et al. 2002).

Metabolic network visualization

A metabolic network is a set of interconnected metabolic pathways (sub networks). Until recently, metabolic studies were dedicated to a single pathway, but current researches now consider the entire network. Existing visualization tools cannot be used to undertake these global studies since they have been designed to probe metabolic pathways. For the purpose of making it feasible, work in (Bourqui et al. 2006) presents a graph drawing algorithm for the whole metabolic network. Collaboration with biologists led the researchers to introduce drawing constraints which take into account the decomposition of the network into metabolic pathways as well as biochemical textbook drawing conventions. These constraints give raise to numerous graph drawing problems which are solved by first recursively decomposing the network then applying suitable graph drawing algorithms. Finally, authors present an application that illustrates the advantage of this representation when visualizing groups of reactions which span several metabolic pathways (Bourqui et al. 2006; Bruchova et al. 2004; Haouas et al. 2010; Lamb et al. 2006).

GPU-Powered Simulation in Medical Applications

The experiments carried out in biological systems involve lengthy, slow processes. They require the use of various tools and equipment during the experiments in addition to involving laboratory specialists to carry out the experiments. For many years the studies carried out in molecular biology have been motivated to find out the protein structure. The proteins used for the experiments are isolated and are purified. The clear form of protein is then imaged for analysis. The various steps during the process involve many unsuccessful iterations because many researchers mainly focus on the data to be extracted over the different experimental methods followed. While studying the structure of a protein, the main alternate experiment used in bioinformatics is wet lab method. In this, many computational techniques are used. The protein structure determined is used to estimate different problems faced while creating a molecular model of structured protein and to discover the extrinsic factors that affect the protein structure (Lamb et al. 2006; Lamb 2007).

GPU-powered simulation methodologies

The last few years, very important research is being carried out in the area of biological systems with a focus on the cross-fertilization to find the experimental results to tackle the complexities of the biological systems. For a given computational model of the complex system of biology, it is possible to define the structural properties to estimate the systems normal behaviour and its response in abnormal conditions. Computer algorithms are used to find the changes that are equivalent to changes in biological systems starting from the initial model conditions to the target system behaviour. The results then rely upon many repeated iterations. Costs of obtaining the concrete results depend on the computational needs. Use of General-Purpose Graphics Processing Unit (GPGPU) is a promising cost-cutting technology (Dematte and Prandi 2009; Besozzi et al. 2013). Although Graphics Processing Unit (GPU) has the computational speed advantages, GPU programming requires non-conventional talent as GPU programming is drastically different from CPU programming. Biological systems simulation requires ever increasing computational power and GPGPU computing has the potential to face this challenge. Numerous attempts are being made in using simple GPUs to study biological systems (Dematte and Prandi 2009; Besozzi et al. 2013; Smalley et al. 2010).

GPU-powered simulation methodologies for biological systems

In the last decade, the interdisciplinary research focused on the computation methods that yield high throughput and high performance. This resulted in developing unique methods that simplified the complex nature of the biological systems. For example, in the formalization of the complex biological frameworks, it is possible to find the evolving structural properties with appropriate methods to find the way systems behave in normal as well as in abnormal conditions (Besozzi et al. 2013; Ashburn and Thor 2004; McArt et al. 2013).

GPU accelerated program for gene expression connectivity mapping

Modern studies carried out on cancer use very large data and many highly advanced statistical methods. Collectively, they bring in heavy computational burden during the analysis stage. The connectivity mapping is a progressive approach in the field of bioinformatics in finding the treatment and the drug resolving methods on the basis of the analysis done on different gene expressions. It requires more than two hours for sscMap technique, a Java application that runs on a normal CPU to carry out the connectivity mapping of a single gene expression. The cudaMap developed by using CUDA C/C++ language has computational power of the NVIDIA GPUs that reduces the processing time of the connectivity mapping technique (McArt et al. 2013; Iorio et al. 2013).

Mapping single nucleotide polymorphisms using GPUs

The genotyping study used in Single Nucleotide Polymorphism (SNP) is highly exposed to misplacement errors in the chromosomal position of SNP. The SNP mapping data along with the array of the SNPs provide accuracy without any need for additional information. Further, mapped data that are linked to a given genome needs to be updated to a given build whenever a new build is available. This requires remapping of SNPs to get a more updated SNP chromosomal position. To map SNPs on a genome, the GPU tool G-SNPM is effectively used (Manconi et al. 2014; Smalley et al. 2010; Zhang and Gant 2009).

Fast short read sequence aligner using GPUs

With the advancement of Next-Generation DNA Sequencing (NGS) technologies, there has been a dramatic increase in the DNA sequencing reads to over 600 gigabases due to high throughput of the NGS machines. This exponentially increases the demand for computational power. The GPGPU provides the computational speed using the parallel stream processors within the cores of GPUs and provides cost as well as energy efficient computing power. The BarraCUDA, a GPGPU sequence alignment software improves the speed of sequencing using the tools that are specifically developed for DNA sequence analysis (Klus et al. 2012; Zhang and Gant 2008).

Multilevel modelling and quantitative analysis of bone remodelling

Paoletti et al. (2012) focus on remodelling of bone with numerous scales of breadth that ranges between inter-and-intra cell ranking (RANK/RANKL) signals providing tissue dynamics to build several levels of modelling structure. Various crucial findings carried out by Paoletti et al. (2012) suggest that there is a clear indication of the multi-scale properties of bone structuring and the connection between the ranking signals and density in the bone both in healthy and in the diseased conditions. The recent studies done by Paoletti et al. (2012) specifies the circulating levels of OPG and RANKL which have relations that are contrary to bone turnover and Bone Mineral Density (BMD) that aid in the growth of osteoporosis in thalassemic patients and also help the women in postmenopausal stage. The dimensional algebra and the shape calculus are used to regulate the stochastic cell agents that are used for remodelling the bone constantly. The efficiency of these multilevel process and ranking signals as a result provides the method to find out the need for the continuous alteration and also to improve the defects in the bone structure. The research done by Paoletti et al. (2012) also contributes to the complex computational modelling with multi-level methods that connect the formal languages and agent-based simulation tools (Paoletti et al. 2012; Zhang and Gant 2009; McArt and Zhang 2011).

Parallelizing epistasis detection in GWAS

The genotyping technologies with high-throughput in the SNP-arrays bring in the quicker collection of up to millions of genetic markers of a person. Finding the epistasis for 2-SNP interactions in the studies carried out by Genome-Wide Associations (GWA) is crucial but also consumes a lot of time as it requires computations to be carried out statistically for the pair of measured markers. The computational methodologies developed show that epistasis is a setback for longer runs. Gonzalez-Dominguz et al. (2015) demonstrate how the task has to be carried out to speed up by using a combination of fine as well as coarse-grained parallelism on different computing systems. The first architecture mentions about Field-Programmable Gate Array (FPGA) which is reconfigurable hardware while the second architecture utilizes the many GPUs that are connected to the same host. Gonzalez-Dominguz et al. (2015) demonstrate that both the system architectures have the ability to accelerate four orders-of-magnitude as compared to the sequential implementation. This results in reducing the run times for finding out the epistasis to few minutes for reasonable sized datasets to a few hours for large-scale datasets (Gonzalez-Domınguez et al. 2015; Schatz et al. 2007; Park et al. 2012).

Multi-GPU hitting set algorithm for GRNs inference

Gene regulatory network research requires extensive computational power. The large number of genes involved in the study results in high dimensionality and selection of a restricted amount of samples making estimation to find out the gene dependencies difficult. Apart from the estimation problem, another issue is the computational complexity of the inference methods for GRN. Carastan-Santos et al. (2015) focus on avoiding the performance bottlenecks of a method based on the signal disruption in gene dependencies.

The difficulty is that the Hitting Set Problem (HSP) is NP-Hard. Several applications are needed to find the estimate or accurate solution to the problem. One of these applications uses a GPU based algorithm that obtains accurate solution to the HSP. The studies carried out by Carastan-Santos et al. (2015) augments the HSP algorithm to deal with the input set that contains many variables, almost thousands in number, by introducing new methods in the data structure and categorizing the arrangement that permit the effective discarding of non-solution candidates of HSP. The experiment done by Carastan-Santos et al. (2015) on a multi-core cluster of CPUs and GPUs demonstrates that the usage of sorting scheme brings increased speed of up to 3.5 in times compared to the CPU implementation. A single GPU achieves 4.7 times of speed up in comparison with CPU implementation with multi-thread. Also, in GPU clusters with 8 GPUs speed up achieved is 6.6 times. Combination of all methods results in a speed up of up to about 60 times (Carastan Santos et al. 2015; Mitsis and Marmarelis 2002; Mitsis et al. 2002).

GPU-Based alignment of protein interaction networks

Network alignment is important to understand the Protein to Protein Interactions (PPIs) in humans and it functions through model organisms. Sub-graph isomorphism problem is complex and requires a lot of time to align the Protein Interaction Networks (PINs). The parallel computing technology provides a solution to the challenges faced in aligning large scale networks via serial computing. Researchers have developed an algorithm known as HGA—Hungarian Greedy Algorithm for PIN alignment (Xie et al. 2015). They suggest that an HGA along with the two adjacent neighbours (HGA-2N) are instrumental in accelerating the GPU. Various experiments show that HGA-2N can discover the alignments that are adjacent to the one created by HGA in reduced computation time. HGA-2N improves the parallel outline in GPU computation and storage mode thus improving the overall computation. With this, the estimations are done on 25 common gene ontology terms with reference to the human protein that are found in the database, which is found to be about 42.8%. Additionally, a new method of rebuilding phylogenetic trees is used that demonstrates the identical relationships amid the five herpes viruses that are attained by using alternative methods (Xie et al. 2015; Mitsis et al. 2004; Chrysos et al. 2014).

Interactive visualization of large deformations and variability

The large image distortions are a challenge in visualizing and analysing the spatial images common in the field of biology and in medicine. Simple linear interruption in the tangent space of the group introduces the artifacts that are anatomical in structure which hampers the application of directed shape analysis techniques. Hermann et al. (2016) and Wenfeng et al. (2010) use the concept of stationary velocity field that helps interactive non-direct image interruption and possible hypothesis for high quality translation of the large distortions. They devise an effective image restoration method using a GPU. This not only improves the quality of current imagining methods but also opens up a ground for innovative communicating systems for shape ensemble analyses.

Evaluation on the dataset demonstrates that the introduced method has the capability to do well in visual quality while keeping the interactive frame rates (Hermann et al. 2016; Kostoglou et al. 2012).

Conclusions

Modelling and simulation play an important role in modern research whether it is pure or applied sciences, social sciences, economics, or management. The inherent advantages of modelling and simulation make them to be a tool of choice to study biological systems especially in medical applications. The complexity of biological systems, sub-systems, sub-sub-systems, etc. and interactions among them demand huge computing resources to simulate them. In the study of biological systems, typically a model of the system is built which is then transformed in to a computational model. The computational model is exerted for various inputs to observe the model to arrive at the functional and behavioural properties of the system under study. Advancements in heterogeneous parallel processing have helped in handling the complexities of simulating biological systems by utilizing the cost and energy efficient multi-core CPU and many-core GPU processing power.

Use of modelling and simulation in medical applications such as drug discovery, gene regulatory networks, human physiology simulation, medical implantations, nano-particles for biological applications, neuro prosthesis, spiking neural networks simulation, tissue simulation, drug delivery, drug side effects detection, predicting protein function, and metabolic pathways visualization have been briefly discussed. The current research focus is on the use of heterogeneous parallel processing to speed up the simulation of biological systems in medical applications. Few case studies that exploit the power of GPUs have then been dealt with. Apart from the heterogeneous parallel architectures, development of libraries, frameworks, and tools that help in developing efficient parallel programs for bioinformatics applications will be the next major agenda for the researchers.

Acknowledgements

The author thankfully acknowledges his colleague Rashmi K.S. for the review of the manuscript and the suggestions made. He also acknowledges the research scholars Abhishek K., Aditya Pai H., and Sreenivasa N. for the help provided by them in preparing this manuscript.

References

Abbott, L. F. and P. Dayan. 2001. Theoretical Neuroscience: Computational and Mathematical Modeling of Neural Systems. MIT Press, Cambridge, MA, USA.

Ajay, M. 1990. A unified framework for using neural networks to build QSARs. J. Med. Chem. 36(23): 3565–3571.

Akyildiz, Ian F., Fernando Brunetti and Cristina Blazquez. 2008. Nanonetworks: a new communication paradigm at molecular level. Comput. Netw. J. 52(12): 2260–2279.

Allison, B. Z., C. Brunner, V. Kaiser, G. R. Muller-Putz, C. Neuper and G. Pfurtschellar. 2012. Toward a hybrid brain-computer interface based on imagined movement and visual attention. Journal of Neural Engineering, 7(2): 1–9.

Alvis, J. M., J. G. Reves, A. V. Govier, P. G. Menkhaus, C. E. Henling, J. A. Spain et al. 1985. Computer-assisted continuous infusion of the intravenous analgesic fentanyl during general anesthesia-An interactive system. IEEE Transaction on Biomedical Engineering Vol. BME-32: 323–329.

An, H., Q. Liu, Q. Ji and B. Jin. 2010. DNA binding and aggregation by carbon nanoparticles. Biochemical and Biophysical Research Communications 393: 571–576.

Anderson, Paul, Douglas Raiford, Deacon Sweeney, Travis Doom and Michael Raymer. 2005. Stochastic model of protease-ligand reactions. Fifth IEEE Symposium on Bioinformatics and Bioengineering (BIBE), pp. 306–310.

Ashburn, T. T. and K. B. Thor. 2004. Drug repositioning: identifying and developing new uses for existing drugs. Nat. Rev. Drug Discovery, pp. 673–683.

Balanis, Constantine A. 2005. Antenna Theory Analysis and Design, 3rd Ed. Wiley-Interscience, New Jersey.

Bao, J. J., M. Nakajima, Z. Yang and T. Fukuda. 2013. Self-actuating asymmetric platinum catalytic mobile nanorobot. IEEE Transaction on Robotics 30(1): 33–39.

Barabasi, A. L. and Z. N. Oltvai. 2004. Network biology: understanding the cell's functional organization. Nat. Rev. Genet. 5: 101–113.

Berezhkovskii, A. M. and A. T. Skvortsov. 2013. Aris-taylor dispersion with drift and diffusion of particles on the tube wall. J. Chem. Phys. 139(8): 84–101.

Bergeron, Bryan. 2002. Bioinformatics Computing. Upper Saddle River, NJ, Prentice Hall PTR.

Besozzi, Daniela, Giulio Caravagna, Marco Nobile, Dario Pescini, Paolo Cazzaniga and Alessandro Re. 2013. GPU-powered simulation methodologies for biological systems. Italian Workshop on Artificial Life and Evolutionary Computation, EPTCS 130: 87–91.

Bialek, W., F. Rieke, R. van Steveninck and D. Warland. 1999. Spikes: Exploring the neural code (computational neuroscience).

Boswell, C. A., D. B. Tesar, K. Mukhyala, F. P. Theil, P. J. Fielder and L. A. Khawli. 2010. Effects of charge on antibody tissue distribution and pharmacokinetics. Bioconjugate Chem. 21(12): 2153–2163.

Bourqui, Romain, David Auber, V. Lacroix and F. Jourdan. 2006. Metabolic network visualization using constraint planar graph drawing algorithm. Tenth International Conference on Information Visualization, IEEE, pp. 489–496.

Brenner, H. 1967. Coupling between the translational and rotational Brownian motions of rigid particles of arbitrary shape II. General theory. J. Colloid Interface Sci. 23(3): 407–436.

Bruchova, H., M. Kalinova and R. Brdicka. 2004. Array-based analysis of gene expression in childhood acute lymphoblastic leukemia. Leuk. Res. 28(1): 1–7.

Butterwick, A., A. Vankov, P. Huie, Y. Freyvert and D. Palanker. 2007. Tissue damage by pulsed electrical stimulation. IEEE Trans. Biomed. Eng. 54(12): 2261–2267.

Carastan Santos, Danilo, R. Yokoingawa De Camargo, D. Correa Martins, Siang Wun Song, L. C. Silva Rozante and F. Ferreira Borelli. 2015. A multi-GPU hitting set algorithm for GRNs inference. 15th IEEE/ACM International Symposium on Cluster, Cloud and Grid Computing, pp. 313–322.

Carro, M. S., W. K. Lim, M. J. Alvarez, R. J. Bollo, X. Zhao, E. Y. Snyder et al. 2010. The transcriptional network for mesenchymal transformation of brain tumours. Nature 463(7279): 318–325.

Cevc, G., G. Blume, A. Schätzlein, D. Gebauer and A. Paul. 1996. The skin: a pathway for systemic treatment with patches and lipid-based agent carriers. Adv. Drug Del. Rev. 18(3): 349–378.

Ch. El-Gemayel, F. Jumel, N. Abouchi, J. Constantin and D. Zaouk. 2014. A global methodology for modelling and simulating medical systems. 16th International Conference on e-Health Networking, Applications and Services (Healthcom), IEEE, pp. 466–471, October, 2014.

Chanthasopeephan, Teeranoot, Jaydev P. Desai and Alan C. W. Lau. 2007. Modelling soft-tissue deformation prior to cutting for surgical simulation: finite element analysis and study of cutting parameters. IEEE Transactions on Biomedical Engineering 54(3): 349–359.

Chaufour, X., G. White, B. Hambly, W. Yu, J. May, J. Harris et al. 1998. Evaluation of the risks of using an oversized balloon catheter in the human infrarenal abdominal aorta. Eur. J. Vasc. Endovasc. Surg. 16(2): 142–147.

Chen, Kai, Tao Chen, Huicong Liu and Zhan Yang. 2015. A Pt/Au hybrid self-actuating nanorobot towards to durg delivery system. Proceedings of the 10th IEEE International Conference on Nano/Micro Engineered and Molecular Systems (IEEE-NEMS 2015), pp. 286–289, Xi'an, China, April, 2015.

Cheung, Y. M. and H. Jia. 2013. Categorical-and-numerical-attribute data clustering based on a unified similarity metric without knowing cluster. Pattern Recognition, 46(8): 2228–2238.

Chrysos, G., E. Sotiriades, C. Rousopoulos, K. Pramataris, I. Papaefstathiou, A. Dollas et al. 2014. Reconfiguring the bioinformatics computational spectrum: challenges and opportunities of FPGA-based bioinformatics. IEEE Design and Test Magazine 31(1): 62–73.

Chun, Hosung, Yuanyuan Yang and Torsten Lehmann. 2014. Safety ensuring retinal prosthesis with precise charge balance and low power consumption. IEEE Transactions on Biomedical Circuits and Systems 8(1): 108–118.

Cisi, R. R. L. and A. F. Kohn. 2008. Simulation system of spinal cord motor nuclei and associated nerves and muscles, in a web-based architecture. J. Comp. Neurosci. 25: 520–542.

Cotin, S., H. Delingette and N. Ayache. 1999. Real-time elastic deformations of soft tissue for surgery simulation. IEEE Trans. Vis. Comput. Graphics 5(1): 62–73.

Crooks, G. E., G. Hon, J. M. Chandonia and S. E. Brenner. 2004. WebLogo: a sequence logo generator. Genome Res. 14: 1188–1190.

Daigo, Y., Y. Masanori, O. Homa, Y. Yasunori and T. Kanji. 2003. A comparison between electrocautery and scalpel plus scissor in breast conserving surgery. Oncol. Rep. 10: 1729–1732.

Das, Anup, Prathyush P. Menon, Jonathan G. Hardman and Declan G. Bates. 2013. Optimization of mechanical ventilator settings for pulmonary disease states. IEEE Transactions on Biomedical Engineering 60(6): 1599–1607.

de Castro, L. N. and J. Timmis. 2002. Artificial Immune Systems: A New Computational Intelligence Approach. Springer-Verlag, Berlin, Germany.

Delgado, Angel V. 2001. Electrokinetic phenomena and their experimental determination: an overview. pp. 1–54. *In*: Delgado, R. V. (ed.). Interfacial Electrokinetics and Electrophoresis. Dekker, CRC Press, New York.

Dematte, Lorenzo and Davide Prandi. 2009. GPU computing for systems biology. Briefing in Bioinformatics 2(3): 323–333, 20 November 2009.

Derjaguin, B. V., N. V. Churev and V. M. Muller. 1987. Surface Forces (Engl. transl.). Consultants Bureau, Edition 1, New York.

Doya, K. 2000. Complementary roles of the basal ganglia and cerebellum in learning and motor control. Curr. Opin. Neurobiology 10: 732–739.

Dissanayake, T., K. P. Esselle and M. R. Yuce. 2009. Dielectric loaded impedance matching for wide band implanted antennas. IEEE Trans. Microwave Theory Tech. 57(10): 2480–2487.

Durairaj, R. B., P. Shanker and M. Sivasankar. 2012. Nano robots in bio medical application. International Conference on Advances in Engineering, Science and Management, IEEE, pp. 67–72, 30–31 March, 2012.

Ebel, J. P., J. L. Anderson and D. C. Prieve. 1988. Diffusiophoresis of latex particles in electrolyte gradients. Langmuir 4: 396–406.

Erwin, D. and E. Davidson. 2010. The evolution of hierarchical gene regulatory networks. Nature Reviews Genetics 10(2): 141–148.

Esteban, A., A. Anzueto, F. Frutos, I. Alia, L. Brochard, T. E. Stewart et al. 2002. Characteristics and outcomes in adult patients receiving mechanical ventilation: A 28-day international study. J. Amer. Med. Assoc. 287: 345–355.

Esteban, A., N. D. Ferguson, M. O. Meade, F. Frutos-Vivar, C. Apezteguia, L. Brochard et al. 2008. Evolution of mechanical ventilation in response to clinical research. Am. J. Resp. Crit. Care 177: 170–177.

Evangelidis, Thomas and Lei Xie. 2014. An integrated workflow for proteome-wide off-target identification and polypharmacology drug design. Tsinghua Science and Technology 19(3): 275–284.

Ferreira, R. and J. C. G. Vendramini. 2010. FPGA-accelerated attractor computation of scale free gene regulatory networks. International Conference on Field Programmable Logic and Applications (FPL), IEEE, pp. 550–555.

Fishman, M. C. and J. A. Porter. 2005. Pharmaceuticals: a new grammar for drug discovery. Nature 437: 491–493.

Fogel, G. B., V. W. Porto, G. Varga, E. R. Dow, A. M. Crave, D. M. Powers et al. 2008. Evolutionary computation for discovery of composite transcription factor binding sites. Nucleic Acids Res. 36(21): 1–14.

Fournier-Bidoz, S., A. C. Arsenault, I. Manners and G. A. Ozin. 2004. Synthetic self-propelled nanorobots. Chem. Commun. 4: 441–443.

Freeman, J. W., P. B. Snowhill and J. L. Nosher. 2010. A link between stent radial forces and vascular wall remodeling: the discovery of an optimal stent radial force for minimal vessel restenosis. Connect. Tissue Res. 51(4): 314–326.

Gamini, D. S. and P. N. Shastry. 2009. Development of implantable spiral chip radiator and external receptor for wireless blood pressure monitoring system. IEEE MTT-S International Microwave Symposium Digest, pp. 1681–1684, 7–12 June, 2009.

Gamini, D. S. and P. N. Shastry. 2009. EuMC: design guidelines for a planar multi-turn loop antenna for wireless bio-medical telemetry system. Microwave Conference, EuMC, IEEE, pp. 649–652, October, 2009.

Gelenbe, E. 1973. A unified approach to the evaluation of a class of replacement algorithms. IEEE Transaction on Computers C22(6): 611–618.

Gelenbe, E. 2007. Steady-state solution of probabilistic gene regulatory networks. Phys. Rev. 76(3): p. 031903.

Gerstner, W. and W. M. Kistler. 2002. Spiking Neuron Models: Single Neurons, Populations, Plasticity, First Edition. Cambridge University Press.

Gonçalves, Emanuel, Joachim Bucher, Anke Ryll, Jens Niklas, Klaus Mauch, Steffen Klamt et al. 2013. Bridging the layers: towards integration of signal transduction, regulation and metabolism into mathematical models. Molecular BioSystems 9: 1576–1583.

Gonzalez-Alvarez, David L., Miguel A. Vega-Rodrıguez and Alvaro Rubio-Largo. 2015. Finding patterns in protein sequences by using a hybrid multiobjective teaching learning based optimization algorithm. IEEE/ACM Transactions on Computational Biology and Bioinformatics 12(3): 656–666, May/June, 2015.

Gonzalez-Domınguez, J. L. Wienbrandt, J. C. Kassens, D. Ellinghaus, M. Schimmler and B. Schmidt. 2015. Parallelizing epistasis detection in GWAS on FPGA and GPU-accelerated computing systems. IEEE/ACM Transactions on Computational Biology and Bioinformatics 12(5): 982–994.

Grube, E., J. C. Laborde, B. Zickmann, U. Gerckens, T. Felderhoff, B. Sauren et al. 2005. First report on a human percutaneous transluminal implantation of a self-expanding valve prosthesis for interventional treatment of aortic valve stenosis. Catheter. Cardiovasc. Intervention 66(4): 465–469.

Halford, F. J. 1943. A critique of intravenous anaesthesia in war surgery. Anaesthesiology 4: 57–59.

Haouas, H., S. Haouas, G. Uzan and A. Hafsia. 2010. Identification of new markers discriminating between myeloid and lymphoid acute leukemia. Haematology 15(4): 193–203.

Haseong Kim and Erol Gelenbe. 2012. Reconstruction of large-scale gene regulatory networks using Bayesian model averaging. IEEE Transactions on Nanobioscience 11(3): 202–207, September, 2012.

Hermann, Max, A. C. Schunke, T. Schultz and R. Klein. 2016. Accurate interactive visualization of large deformations and variability in biomedical image ensembles. IEEE Transactions on Visualization and Computer Graphics 22(1): 708–717, January, 2016.

Hirota, K., A. Tanaka and T. Kaneko. 1999. Representation of force in cutting operation. Proc. IEEE Virtual Reality Conf., pp. 77.

Hodgkin, L. and A. F. Huxley. 1952. A quantitative description of membrane current and its application to conduction and excitation in nerve. Journal of Physiology 117(4): 500–544.

Hodzic, V., V. Hodzic and R. W. Newcomb. 2007. Modeling of the electrical conductivity of the DNA. IEEE Trans. on Circuit and Systems 54(11): 2360–2364.

Hu, Gibson, Ying Guo and Rongxin Li. 2008. A self-organizing nano particle simulator and its applications. Adaptive Hardware System (AHS), IEEE, pp. 451–458, 22–25, June, 2008.

Huertas, Mercedes and Luigi Ceccaroni. 2013. A simulation and integration environment for heterogeneous physiology-models. e-Health Networking, Applications & Services (Healthcom), IEEE, pp. 228–232, October, 2013.

Iorio, F., T. Rittman, H. Ge, M. Menden and J. Saez-Rodriguez. 2013. Transcriptional data: a new gateway to drug repositioning? Drug Discover Today, pp. 350–357.

Izhikevich, E. M. 2003. Simple model of spiking neurons. IEEE Transactions on Neural Networks 14(6): 1569–1572.

Jacobs, I. R. and J. G. Reves. 1993. Effect site equilibration time is a determinant of induction dose requirement. Anesth. Analg. 76: 14.

Jaraiz, E., S. Kimura and O. Levenspiel. 1992. Vibrating beds of fine particles: estimation of inter particle forces from expansion and pressure drop experiments. Powder Technology 72: 23–30.

Jerne, N. K. 1974. Towards a network theory of the immune system. Ann. Immunol. (Inst. Pasteur), pp. 373–389.

Jiang, Haibo. 2007. Static and dynamic mechanics analysis on the artificial hip joints with different interface designs by finite element method. Journal of Bionic Engineering, 4(2): 123–131.

Jiang, Haibo and Yong Luo. 2010. Biological modelling and simulations of human lower limb joint system. International Conference on Computational and Information Sciences, IEEE, pp. 81–84, Chengdu, December, 2010.

Jin, W., K. Wu, Y.-Z. Li, W.-T. Yang, B. Zou, F. Zhang et al. 2013. AML1-ETO targets and suppresses cathepsin G, a serine protease, which is able to degrade AML1-ETO int (8; 21) acute myeloid leukemia. Oncogene 32(15): 1978–1987.

Jung, J. and D. Gidaspow. 2002. Fluidization of nano-size particles. Journal of Nano particle Research 4: 483–497.

Keh, H. J. and Y. K. Wei. 2000. Diffusiophoresis in a concentrated suspension of colloidal spheres in nonelectrolyte gradients. Colloid Polym. Sci. 278: 539–546.

Kirshner, D. A., J. P. Nilmeier and F. C. Lightstone. 2013. Catalytic site identification–a web server to identify catalytic site structural matches throughout PDB. Nucleic Acids Res. 41: 256–265.

Klus, Petr, S. Lam, D. Lyberg, MS. Cheung, G. Pullan, I. McFarlane et al. 2012. BarraCUDA—a fast short read sequence aligner using graphics processing units. BMC Research Notes, 13 January, 2012.

Kohonen, T. 1989. Self-Organization and Associative Memory. Springer-Verlag, 3rd Edition, New York, USA.

Kola, I. and J. Landis. 2004. Can the pharmaceutical industry reduce attrition rates? Nature Reviews Drug Discovery 3: 711–716.

Kostoglou, K., G. D. Mitsis, K. P. Michmizos, P. Stathis, D. Sakas and K. S. Nikita. 2012. Prediction of the Parkinsonian subthalamic nucleus spike activity from local field potentials using nonlinear dynamic models. 12th International Conference on Bioinformatics & Bioengineering (BIBE 2012), pp. 298–302, 11–13 November, 2012.

Kramer, T. 2003. Side effects and therapeutic effects. Medscape General Medicine 5: 28.

Kulhanek, T., M. Matejak, J. Silar and J. Kofranek. 2014. Parameter estimation of complex mathematical models of human physiology using remote simulation distributed in scientific cloud. Journal of Biomedical and Health Informatics (BHI), IEEE-EMBS Internal conference, pp. 712–715.

Kunii, D. and O. Levenspiel. 1991. Fluidization Engineering, Second Edition. Butterworth-Heinemann, Boston.

Lamb, J., E. D. Crawford, D. Peck, J. W. Modell, I. C. Blat, M. J. Wrobel et al. 2006. The connectivity map: using gene-expression signatures to connect small molecules, genes, and disease. Science 1929–1935.

Lamb, J. 2007. The connectivity map: a new tool for biomedical research. Nat. Rev Cancer, 7(1): 54–60.

Latsios, G., U. Gerckens, L. Buellesfeld, R. Mueller, D. John, S. Yuecel et al. 2010. Device landing zone calcification, assessed by MSCT, as a predictive factor for pacemaker implantation after TAVI. Catheter. Cardiovascular Intervention 76(3): 431–439.

Lin, M. M. and D. C. Prieve. 1983. Electromigration of latex induced by a diffusion potential. J. Colloid Interface Sci. 95: 327–339.

Liu, Yaling, Samar Shah and Jifu Tan. 2012. Computational modeling of nanoparticle targeted drug delivery. American Scientific Publishers, Reviews in Nanoscience and Nanotechnology 1: 66–83.

Lori, F., A. Malykh, A. Cara, D. Sun, J. N. Weinstein, J. Lisziewicz et al. 1994. Hydroxyl urea as an inhibitor of human immunodeficiency virus-type I replication. Science 266: 801–805.

Ma, Di, Sumei Sun, Ho Chin Keong, Daniel Mok, Chee Kong Chui and Stephen Kin Yong Chang. 2012. Wireless medical implant: a case study on artificial pancreas. International Conference on Communication (ICC), pp. 6096–6100, June, 2012.

Mancia, G., G. Grassi, G. Bertinieri, A. Ferrari and A. Zanchetti. 1984. Arterial baroreceptor control of blood pressure in man. J. Auton. Nervous System 11(2): 115–124.

Manconi, Andrea, A. Orro, E. Manca, G. Armano and L. Milanesi. 2014. A tool for mapping single nucleotide polymorphisms using graphics processing units. BMC Bioinformatics 15(1): 1.

Mansouri, Majidi, Hazem Nounou, M. N. Nounou and A. A. Datta. 2012. Modelling of nonlinear biological phenomena modelled by S-systems using Bayesian Method. EMBS International Conference on Biomedical Engineering and Sciences, IEEE, pp. 305–310, Langkawi, December, 2012.

Martins, W. and I. Z. De Araújo. 2001. Soft control of human physiological signals by reinforcement learning. International Joint Conference on Neural Networks (IJCNN) 4: 2501–2505, July, 2001.

McArt, D. G. and S. D. Zhang. 2011. Identification of candidate small-molecule therapeutics to cancer by gene-signature perturbation in connectivity mapping. PLoS ONE: e16382.

McArt, D. G., P. Bankhead, P. D. Dunne, M. Salto-Tellez, P. Hamilton and S. D. Zhang. 2013. cudaMap: a GPU accelerated program for gene expression connectivity mapping. BMC Bioinformatics 14(1): 1.

McCaffrey, C., O. Chevalerias, C. O. Mathuna and K. Twomey. 2008. Swallowable-capsule technology. IEEE Pervasive Computing 7(1): 23–29.

McCreery, D., W. Agnew, T. Yuen and L. Bullara. 1990. Charge density and charge per phase as cofactors in neural injury induced by electrical stimulation. IEEE Trans. Biomed. Eng. 37(10): 996–1001.

McInerney, T. and D. Terzopoulos. 1996. Deformable models in medical image analysis: a survey. Medical Image Analysis 1(2): 91–108.

Medical Implanted Communication System (MICS), FCC Std. CFR, Part 95, 2009.

Meier, U., O. Lopez, C. Monseratt, M. C. Juan and M. Alcaniz. 2005. Real-time deformable models for surgery simulation: a survey. Computer Methods and Programs in Biomedicine 77(3): 183–197.

Mendoza, C. and C. Laugier. 2003. Simulating soft tissue cutting using finite element methods. The IEEE International Conference on Robotics and Automation, 1: 1109–1114, Taipei, Taiwan, 14–19 September, 2003.

Merli, Francesco, Léandre Bolomey, Jean-François Zürcher, Giancarlo Corradini, Eric Meurville and Anja K. Skrivervik. 2011. Design, realization and measurements of a miniature antenna for implantable wireless communication systems. IEEE Transactions on Antennas and Propagation, pp. 3544–3555, October, 2011.

Merrill, D. R., M. Bikson and J. G. Jefferys. 2005. Electrical stimulation of excitable tissue: design of efficacious and safe protocols. J. Neurosci. Methods 141(2): 171–198.

Miller III, B. R., T. Dwight McGee, Jr., Jason M. Swails, Nadine Homeyer, Holger Gohlke and Adrian E. Roitberg. 2012. MMPBSA.py: an efficient program for end-state free energy calculations. Journal of Chemical Theory and Computation 8(9): 3314−3321.

Mitsis, G. D. and V. Z. Marmarelis. 2002. Modeling of nonlinear physiological systems with fast and slow dynamics. I. Methodology. Ann. Biomed. Eng. 30(2): 272–281.

Mitsis, G. D., R. Zhang, B. D. Levine and V. Z. Marmarelis. 2002. Modeling of nonlinear physiological systems with fast and slow dynamics. II. Application to cerebral autoregulation. Ann. Biomed. Eng. 30(4): 555–565.

Mitsis, G. D., M. J. Poulin, P. A. Robbins and V. Z. Marmarelis. 2004. Nonlinear modeling of the dynamic effects of arterial pressure and CO_2 variations on cerebral blood flow in healthy humans. IEEE Transactions on Biomedical Engineering 51(11): 1932–1943.

Miyamoto, T., I. L. Weissman and K. Akashi. 2000. AML1/ETO-expressing non leukemic stem cells in acute myelogenous leukaemia with 8; 21 chromosomal translocation. Proc. Natl. Acad. Sci. 97(13): 7521–7526.

Moffat, Stanley. 2015. Convergence of Nanoinformatics Nanobiotechnology and Bioinformatics. MOJ Proteomics Bioinform 2(6): 00068.

Monroe, D. M. and M. Hoffman. 2006. What does it take to make the perfect clot? Arteriosclerosis Thrombosis and Vascular Biology 26(1): 2463–2469.

Morari, M., J. H. Lee and C. E. Garcia. 1999. Model predictive control. Computers and Chemical Engineering 23(4/5): 667–682.

Mosca, Ettore, Ivan Merelli, Luciano Milanesi, P. Cazzaniga, D. Pescini and G. Mauri. 2009. Stochastic simulations on a grid framework for parameter sweep applications in biological models. International Workshop on High Performance Computational Systems Biology, IEEE, pp. 33–42, October, 2009.

Nido, G. S., J. M. Williams and L. Benuskova. 2012. Bistable properties of a memory-related gene regulatory network. International Joint Conference on Neural Networks (IJCNN), pp. 1–6, 2012.

Nilmeier, J. P., D. A. Kirshner, S. E. Wong and F. C. Lightstone. 2013. Rapid catalytic template searching as an enzyme function prediction procedure. PLoS ONE 8: 1–17.

Nir, Y., A. Paz, E. Sabo and I. Potasman. 2003. Fear of injections in young adults: prevalence and associations. Amer. J. Tropical Med. Hygiene 68(3): 341–344.

O'Regan, B. and M. Grätzel. 1991. A low-cost, high efficiency solar cell based on dyesensitized colloidal $TiO2$ films. Nature 353: 737–740.

Ogomi, S. Sakaguchi, T. Katoh, T. Kado, Y. Yamaguchi, M. Kono and S. Hayase. 2006. Dye sensitized solar cells with high photo-energy conversion-control of nano-particle surfaces. IEEE 4th World Conference on Photovoltaic Energy Conversion, pp. 167–170, May, 2006.

Otsuka, Yoichi, Hea-Yeon Lee, Jian-Hua Gu, Jeong-O Lee, Kuang-Hwa Yoo and Hidekazu Tanaka et al. 2002. Influence of humidity on the electrical conductivity of synthesized DNA film on nanogap electrode. Japanese Journal of Applied Physics 41: 891–894.

Ouyang, M., Y. M. Ho, Wen. Li and Ka Wai Won. 2011. Fabrication and manipulation of fluorescent carbon nanoparticles for biosensing applications. IEEE Int. Conference on Nano/Micro Engineered and Molecular Systems (IEEE-NEMS 2011), pp. 893–896, 20–23 February, 2011.

Ouyang, Mengxing, Wen J. Li, Ka Wai Wong and Wing Keung Liu. 2012. Investigation of electrical properties of DNA-attached carbon nano-particles for biological applications. IEEE International Conference on Nano/Micro Engineered Molecular Systems (NEMS), pp. 429–432, Kyoto, Japan, March, 2012.

Panescu, D. 2008. Emerging technologies: wireless communication systems for implantable medical devices. IEEE Eng. Med. Biol. Mag. 27(2): 96–101.

Paoletti, Nicola, P. Lio, E. Merelli and M. Viceconti. 2012. Multilevel computational modelling and quantitative analysis of bone remodelling. IEEE/ACM Transactions on Computational Biology and Bioinformatics 9(5): 1366–1378, 5 April, 2012.

Park, S., S. Y. Shin and K. B. Hwang. 2012. CFMDS: CUDA-based fast multidimensional scaling for genome-scale data. BMC Bioinformatics 13(17): 1.

Park, Yongjin, S. Shackney and Russell Schwartz. 2009. Network-based inference of cancer progression from microarray data. IEEE/ACM Trans. Comput. Biol. Bioinform. 6(2): 200–12, April–June, 2009.

Partl, Christian, Alexander Lex, M. Streit, H. Strobelt, A. M. Wassermann, H. Pfister et al. 2014. ConTour: data-driven exploration of multi-relational datasets for drug discovery. IEEE Transactions on Visualization and Computer Graphics 20(12): 1883–1892, December, 2014.

Pavlick, R. A., S. Sengupta, T. McFadden, H. Zhang and A. Sen. 2011. A polymerization-powered motor. Angewandte Chemie International Edition 50: 9374–9377.

Paxton, W. F., K. C. Kistler, C. C. Olmeda, A. Sen, St. S. K. Angelo, Y. Y. Cao et al. 2004. Catalytic nanomotor: autonomous movement of striped nanorods. J. Am. Chem. Soc. 126(41): 13424–13431.

Perrin, D. P., N. V. Vasilyev, P. Novotny, J. Stoll, R. D. Howe, P. E. Dupont et al. 2009. Image guided surgical interventions. Current Problems in Surgery 46(9): 730–766.

Piazza, R. 2004. Thermal forces: colloids in temperature gradient. J. Phys. Condens. Matter 16: S4195–S4211.

Prausnitz, M. R., S. Mitragotri and R. Langer. 2004. Current status and future potential of transdermal drug delivery. Nature Rev. Drug Discovery 3(2): 115–124.

Pyburn, E. and T. Goswami. 2004. Finite element analysis of gemoral components paper III-hip joint. Materials and Design 25(8): 705–713.

Renaud, S., J. Tomas, Y. Bornat, A. Daouzli and S. Saighi. 2007. Neuromimetic ICs with analog cores: an alternative for simulating spiking neural networks. ISCAS'07: IEEE International Symposium on Circuits and Systems, May 2007, pp. 3355–3358.

Rodgers, G. P., G. J. Dover, C. T. Noguchi, A. N. Schechter and A. W. Nienhuis. 1990. Hematologic responses of patients with sickle cell disease to treatment with hydroxyurea. New Engl. J. Med. 322(15): 1037–1045.

Rojdestvenski, Igor and M. Cottam. 2002. Visualizing metabolic networks in VRML. Sixth International Conference on Information Visualization, IEEE, pp. 175–180.

Ross, M. E., R. Mahfouz, M. Onciu, H. Liu, X. Zhou, G. Song et al. 2004. Gene expression profiling of paediatric acute myelogenous leukaemia. Blood 104(12): 3679–3687.

Rowland, M. and T. N. Tozer. 1989. Clinical Phamcokinetics: Concepts and Applications, 2nd Ed. Lea and Febiger, Philadelphia.

Rubenfeld, G. D., E. Caldwell, E. Peabody, J. Weaver, D. P. Martin, M. Neff et al. 2005. Incidence and outcomes of acute lung injury. New Engl. J. Med. 353: 1685–1693.

Schatz M., C. Trapnell, A. Delcher and A. Varshney. 2007. High-throughput sequence alignment using graphics processing units. BMC Bioinformatics 8(1): 474.

Schouten, A. C., E. de Vlugt, J. B. van Hilten and F. C. van der Helm. 2008. Quantifying proprioceptive reflex during position control of the human arm. IEEE Transaction on Biomedical Engineering 55(1): 311–321.

Schwilden, H. 1981. A general method for calculating the dosage scheme in linear pharmacokinetics. Eur. Journal of Clinical Pharmacology 20: 379–386.

Seth, A. and M. G. Pandy. 2007. A neuromusculoskeletal tracking method for estimating individual muscle forces in human movement. J. Biomech. 40: 356–366.

Sheiner, L. B., D. R. Stanski, S. Vozeh, R. D. Miller and J. Ham. 1979. Simultaneous modeling of pharmacokinetics and pharmacodynamics: application to d-tubocurarine. Clin. Phamcol. Therapy 25: 358–371.

Shi, F., Q. Chen and X. Niu. 2007. Functional similarity analysing of protein sequences with empirical mode decomposition. Proceedings of 4th International Conference on Fuzzy System Knowledge Discovery 2: 766–770.

Shih, K. C., R. M. Chen, R. M. Hu, F. M. Liu, H. K. Chen and J. J. P. Tsai. 2004. Prediction of gene regulatory networks using differential expression of cDNA microarray data. Sixth International Multimedia Software Engineering, IEEE, pp. 378–385, December, 2004.

Siegel, R., D. Naishadham and A. Jemal. 2013. Cancer statistics. CA. Cancer J. Clin. 63(1): 11–30.

Singh, R., S. Singh and J. W. Lillard. 2008. Past, present, and future technologies for oral delivery of therapeutic proteins. J. Pharm. Sci. 97(7): 2497–2523.

Smagilov. R. F., A. Schwartz, N. Bowden and G. M. Whitesides. 2002. Autonomous movement and self-assembly. Angew. Chem., Int. Ed. 41: 652–654.

Smalley, J. L., T. W. Gant and S. D. Zhang. 2010. Application of connectivity mapping in predictive toxicology based on gene-expression similarity. Toxicology 268(3): 143–146.

Smith, R. D., J. B. Dunbar, P. M. U. Ung, E. X. Esposito, C. Y. Yang, S. M. Wang. 2011. Combined evaluation across all submitted scoring functions. J. Chem. Inf. Model. 51: 2115−2131.

Soleimani, Hamid, Arash Ahmadi, Mohammad Bavandpour, A. Ali Amirsoleimani and Mark Zwolinski. 2012. A large scale digital simulation of spiking neural networks (SNN) on Fast System C Simulator. 14th International Conference on modelling and Simulation, IEEE, pp. 25–30.

Terzopoulos, Demetri, John Platt, Alan Barr and Kurt Fleischer. 1987. Elastically deformable models. Computer Graphics 21(4): 2005–2014.

Tobinick, E. L. 2009. The value of drug repositioning in the current pharmaceutical market. Drug News Perspective 22(2): 119–125.

Tran, P., B. Alavi and G. Gruner. 2000. Charge transport along the x-DNA double helix. Phys. Rev. Lett. 85(7): 1564–1967.

Valafar, Homayoun and F. Valafar. 1999. Prediction of a patient's response to a specific drug treatment using artificial neural networks. International Joint Conference on Neural Networks (IJCNN), IEEE 5: 3694–3697.

Valova, Iren, Natacha Gueorguieva and George Georgiev. 2005. Modeling weakly connected networks of neural oscillators with spiking neurons. IEEE Conference on Systems, Man and Cybernatics 1: 810–815, 10–12 October, 2005.

Viceconti, Marco. 2011. Collaborative modelling and Simulation: the virtual physiological human vision. Enabling Technologies: Infrastructure for Collaborative Enterprises, IEEE, pp. 229–234, June, 2011.

Vickrey, T. M. and J. A. Garcia-Ramirez. 1980. Magnetic field-flow fractionation: theoretical basis. Sep. Sci. Technol. 15: 1297–1304.

Wada, D. Russell and Denham S. Ward. 1995. Open loop control of multiple drug effects in anesthesia. IEEE Transactions on Biomedical Engineering 42(7): 666–677, July, 1995.

Wang, Monan, Lining Sun, Zhijiang Du and Zhiheng Jia. 2006. Model and simulation research of tissue based CT images. Proceedings of the IEEE International Conference on Mechatronics and Automation, pp. 1387–1391, Luoyang, China, 25–28 June, 2006.

Watarai, H., M. Suwa and Y. Iiguni. 2004. Migration analysis of micro-particles in liquids using microscopically designed external fields. Anal. Bioanal. Chem. 20(3): 423–434.

Wenfeng, S., W. Daming, X. Weimin, Z. Xin and Y. Shizhong. 2010. Parallelized computation for computer simulation of electrocardiograms using personal computers with multi-core CPU and general-purpose GPU. Computer Methods and Programs in Biomedicine 100(1): 87–96.

Werber, D., A. Schwentner and E. M. Biebl. 2006. Investigation of RF transmission properties of human tissues. Adv. Radio Sci. 4: 357–360.

Wijekoon, J. H. B. and P. Dudek. 2008. Special issue: Compact silicon neuron circuit with spiking and bursting behaviour. Neural Networks 21(2-3): 524–534.

Wolpaw, J. R., N. Birbaumer, D. J. McFarland, G. Pfurtschellar and T. M. Vaughan. 2002. Brain-computer interfaces for communication and control. Clin. Neurophysiol. 113(6): 767–791.

Woo, S. L., S. D. Abramowitch, R. Kilger and R. Liang. 2006. Biomechanics of knee ligaments: injury, healing, and repair. Journal of Biomechanics 39: 1–20.

Xie, Jiang, Zhonghua Zhou, Jin Ma, Chaojuan Xiang, Qing Nie and Wu Zhang. 2015. Graphics processing unit-based alignment of protein interaction networks. IET Syst. Biol. 9(4): 120–127.

Xie, L., S. L. Kinnings and P. E. Bourne. 2012. Novel computational approaches to polypharmacology as a means to define responses to individual drugs. Annu. Rev. Pharmacol. Toxicology 52: 361–379.

Yan, A., B. W. Lau, B. S. Weissman, I. Külaots, N. Y. Yang, A.B. Kane et al. 2006. Biocompatible, hydrophilic, supramolecular carbon nanoparticles for cell delivery. Adv. Mater. 18: 2373–2378.

Yang, G. Z. 2006. Body Sensor Networks. Springer-Verlag. London Limited, Springer London.

Yang, Lina, Yuan Yan Tang, Yang Lu and Huiwu Luo. 2015. A fractal dimension and wavelet transform based method for protein sequence similarity analysis. IEEE/ACM Transactions on Computational Biology and Bioinformatics 12(2): 348–359, March/April, 2015.

Yeoh, E.-J., M. E. Ross, S. A. Shurtleff, W. K. Williams, D. Patel, R. Mahfouz et al. 2002. Classification, subtype discovery, and prediction of outcome in pediatric acute lymphoblastic leukemia by gene expression profiling. Cancer Cell 1(2): 133–143.

Yong, Wang, H. Katsuhisa and Chen Luonan. 2011. An integrated gene regulatory network inference pipeline. 30th Chinese Control Conference, IEEE, pp. 6593–6598, July, 2011.

Zeng, T. and Luonan Chen. Identifying temporal trace of biological process during phase transition. International Conference on Systems Biology (ISB), IEEE, pp. 368–373, 2–4 September, 2011.

Zhang, Dan, Yijun Wang, Alexander Maye, Andreas K. Engel, Xiaorong Gao and B. Hong. 2011. A Brain-computer interface based on multi-modal attention. 3rd International IEEE/EMBS Conference on Neural Engineering, pp. 133–139.

Zhang, K. J. and M. E. Briggs. 1999. Optical measurement of the Soret coefficient and the diffusion coefficient of liquid mixtures. Solid State Physics: Proceedings of the D. A. E. Solid State Physics Symposium, J. Chem. Phys. 104(17): 6881–6892.

Zhang, M. and T. J. Tam. 2003. DNA electrical properties and potential nano-applications. Third International Conference on Nanotechnology 2: 512–515.

Zhang, S. D. and T. Gant. 2008. A simple and robust method for connecting small molecule drugs using gene-expression signatures. BMC Bioinformatics 9(1): 258–259.

Zhang, S. D. and T. Gant. 2009. sscMap: an extensible Java application for connecting small-molecule drugs using gene-expression signatures. BMC Bioinformatics 10(1): 1.

Zhang, X., S. E. Wong and F. C. Lightstone. 2013. Message passing interface and multithreading hybrid for parallel molecular docking of large databases on petascale high performance computing machines. J. Comput. Chem. 34: 915−927.

Zhang, Xiaodong, Rui Li and Yaonan Li. 2014. Research on brain control prosthetic hand. The 11th International Conference on Ubiquitous Robots and Ambient Intelligence, IEEE, pp. 554–557, Malaysia, 12–15 November, 2014.

Zhang, Yong and Peng Li. 2009. Gene-regulatory memories: electrical-equivalent modelling, simulation and parameter identification. IEEE/ACM International Conference on Computer-Aided Design Digest of Technical Papers, pp. 491–496, November, 2009.

Zhu, D. 2007. Mathematical modelling of blood coagulation cascade: kinetics of intrinsic and extrinsic pathways in normal and deficient conditions. Blood Coagul Fibrinolysis, pp. 637–46, 18 October, 2007.

11

High-Order Perturbation Theory Models of Drug-Target Interactomes for Proteins Expressed on Networks of Hippocampus Brain Region of Alzheimer Disease Patients

Francisco J. Romero-Durán,[1,2] *Edgar Lopez-Castro,*[3]
Xerardo García-Mera[1] *and Humberto González-Díaz*[4,5,]*

Abstract

Predicting drug-target protein interactions networks (interactomes) in the proteome of specific regions of the brain of Alzheimer Disease (AD) patients may be relevant in the development of treatments for this neurodegenerative

[1] Department of Organic Chemistry, Faculty of Pharmacy, University of Santiago de Compostela (USC), 15782, Santiago de Compostela.
[2] IMQ Zorrotzaurre Clinic, 48014, Bilbao, Spain.
[3] Department of Pharmacology, Faculty of Science and Technology, University of Basque Country (UPV/EHU), 48940, Leioa, Spain.
[4] Department of Organic Chemistry II, Faculty of Science and Technology, University of Basque Country (UPV/EHU), 48940, Leioa, Spain.
[5] IKERBASQUE, Basque Foundation for Science, 48011, Bilbao, Spain.
* Corresponding author: humberto.gonzalezdiaz@ehu.es

disease. However, many computational models are unable to take into consideration the effects, over the interaction of new compounds, of changes (perturbations) on the experimental conditions of assay with respect to a lead compound of reference including changes of molecular or cellular target, specie of the organism of assay, protocol of assay, etc. In this chapter, we report the following results. We start it proposing the first Higher Order Perturbation Theory (HOPT) model of Quantitative Structure-Binding Relationships (PT-QSBR) for a drug-protein interactome. HOPT-QSBR model predicts the interaction of a new drug with different proteins starting from the experimental binding of a drug of reference and adding higher order (n >= 2) corrections in the form of perturbation operators. The tests included the evaluation of different equations with linear, quadratic, and higher-order operators. Next, we carry out a crossover analysis of proteins expressed on the proteome of the Hippocampus of AD patients vs. compounds downloaded from the database ChEMBL. The linear HOPT-QSBR model showed the best results for the dataset studied. This model predicted correctly 70,000 perturbations or variations in experimental data with specificity, sensitivity, and accuracy of 85–90% in training and validation series.

Introduction

The use of Chemoinformatics to predict the binding targets for drug lead compounds in Alzheimer Disease (AD) research may help to develop treatments for this neurodegenerative disease (Dominguez et al. 2015; Liu et al. 2014; Valasani et al. 2014; Roos et al. 2014; Prado-Prado et al. 2012; Nastase and Boyd 2012; Cosconati et al. 2012; Barman and Prabhakar 2012; Speck-Planche et al. 2012; Garcia et al. 2011; Sopkova-de Oliveira Santos et al. 2010; Vijayan et al. 2009; Zaheer-ul et al. 2008; Karsai et al. 2005). The output property of a Quantitative Structure-Binding Relationships (QSBR) model is a parameter of drug affinity or binding to a protein target. We can use different types of molecular descriptors (Jewison et al. 2014) of the chemical structure for a given molecule M_i as inputs of data analysis techniques. As a result, we can obtain Chemoinformatics models able to predict drug—protein interactions (Gonzalez-Diaz 2008). These Chemoinformatics models are useful to predict the biological activity of one compound based on the molecular descriptors Di. In classic Chemoinformatics models, the molecules studied are low molecular weight compounds. In the particular case of a binding interaction, we can use the term QSBR (Zhang et al. 2006). In QSBR models, one measure of drug-target binding plays the role of biological activity. The constant K_{ij} of binding of the drug i-th to the j-th protein is a common parameter of drug binding in these studies. We can define a classic form of a linear QSBR model as follow:

$$K_i = \sum_{i=1}^{imax} a_i \cdot D_i + e_0 \qquad (1)$$

Unfortunately, classic QSBR models based on this equation can predict only the interaction of one drug with a single target out of multiple proteins in one proteome.

In fact, classic QSBR models reported until now predict the interaction of drugs with only one single protein target in a proteome. Consequently, classic QSBR models are unable to predict drug-target interactomes (networks of interactions for a large set of drugs and all the multiple proteins in one proteome). For instance, Hansch et al. (Hansch et al. 1977a; Hansch et al. 1977b) have published two of the first papers in QSBR studies. One was about anti-malarial and dihydrofolate reductase inhibition by quinazolines and diaminopyrimidines and the other on chymotrypsin-ligand interactions. In 1979, Hansch published other paper of high relevance to QSBR studies of the interaction of ligands with enzymes. In 1985, Hansch and McClarin et al. developed a QSBR model for the binding of a set of substituted benzene sulfonamides to the human enzyme carbonic anhydrase (the drug target). They used Hammett sigma electronic substituent constant, octanol/water partition coefficient (P), and substituent indicator variables (I_1 and I_2) to predict drug-target binding constants (K). The equation of this model is the following.

$$\log K = 1.55 \cdot \sigma + 0.64 \cdot \log P - 2.0711 \cdot I_1 - 3.2812 \cdot I_2 + 6.94 \tag{2}$$

In 1990, Compadre et al. developed a QSBR model for the Michaelis-Menten constants (K_m) for the papain hydrolysis of benzoylglycine esters. The inputs of the model are related to field inductive parameter (F), Van der Waals distance (Z), and hydrophobic constant (π) of substituent with different restrains (see details on the original reference). The equation of this model is the following.

$$\log\left(\frac{1}{K_m}\right) = 8.13 \cdot F + 0.33 \cdot Z + 1.27 \cdot \pi + 1.95 \tag{3}$$

However, more recently Chou (Chou and Shen 2010, 2008; Chou and Shen 2007; Chou and Shen 2006a; Chou and Shen 2006b; Chou and Cai 2006; Chou 2005), Cai (Cai and Chou 2005a, 2005b; Cai et al. 2003), Marrero-Ponce (Marrero-Ponce et al. 2005), Agüero-Chapin (Aguero-Chapin et al. 2011; Aguero-Chapin et al. 2009; Aguero-Chapin et al. 2008; Aguero-Chapin et al. 2006), González-Díaz (Gonzalez-Diaz et al. 2011; González-Díaz et al. 2007; Munteanu et al. 2009; Rodriguez-Soca et al. 2010; Gonzalez-Diaz et al. 2008), and other authors have extended Chemoinformatics—like modeling to proteins and proteome research; developing predictive models that take into consideration different proteins. Recently, some authors have assembled large drug-target interactomes (drug-target network) (Yildirim et al. 2007). In addition, our group has reported some predictive models of drug-target interactomes based on descriptors of molecular structure of both drugs and proteins (Prado-Prado et al. 2012; Prado-Prado et al. 2011; Gonzalez-Diaz et al. 2011; Gonzalez-Diaz et al. 2011; Vina et al. 2009). This field of research is evolving very fast in the development of computational target profiling and network pharmacology methods able to identify the most probable target of a query molecule (Cereto-Massague et al. 2015; Antolin and Mestres 2015; Anighoro et al. 2015; Fang 2015; Tang and Aittokallio 2014; Reutlinger et al. 2014; Perez-Nueno et al. 2014).

However, many of them are still unable to account for changes on the conditions of assay with respect to a drug of reference. We refer here to changes (perturbations) on the molecular or cellular target, experimental measure, specie of the organism of assay, protocol of assay, etc. More recently, we have developed models of drug interactomes that account for many of these factors (Casanola-Martin et al. 2015; Gonzalez-Diaz et al. 2014; Tenorio-Borroto et al. 2013). In some of our more recent works, we reported predictive models for multi-target interactomes of neuroprotective drugs (Alonso et al. 2013; Romero Duran et al. 2014; Luan et al. 2013). Nevertheless, these models are not strictly speaking QSBR models and do not account for multiple perturbations with respect to different assays of references in one specific human tissue. In closing, on-target and also multi-target QSBR are still an active field of research.

AlzPlatform (www.cbligand.org/AD/) developed by Liu et al. (2014) is one of the more advanced computational platforms useful to manage target profiling and polypharmacology data in AD research. The platform has assembled various AD-related chemogenomics data records, including 928 genes and 320 proteins related to AD, 194 AD drugs approved or in clinical trials, and 405,188 chemicals associated with 1,023,137 records of reported bioactivities from 38,284 corresponding bioassays and 10,050 references. In this work, we report a new model with similar objective but inspired on different methodology and datasets. We start the work with a review of the state of art on this area. Next, we propose the first QSBR-Perturbation Theory (PT-QSBR) model for the drug-protein interactome of one human proteome. The interactome studied here contain compounds downloaded from the database ChEMBL and protein of the proteome of the Hippocampus of Alzheimer Disease (AD) patients. In this chapter, we report the following results. Firstly, we performed a review and discussion about the theoretical basis and past applications of QSBR analysis. Next, we developed a new QSBR-Perturbation Theory (PT-QSBR) model for prediction of a drug interactome (set of drug-target interactions) for proteins present in the proteome of Hippocampus region of the brain of Alzheimer's disease (AD) patients. Previous drug interactome networks have been constructed by other authors (Yildirim et al. 2007). The PT-QSBR model can predict the probability of interaction for a large number of drugs reported in CheMBLwith targets expressed by the human brain of AD patients. We carry out different tests in order to seek a good model. The tests included the evaluation of different equations with linear, quadratic, and higher-order free-energy operators. Lastly, we applied our model in theoretical-experimental studies presented as a proof-of-concept. This last part included the organic synthesis, pharmacological assay, and prediction of unmeasured results for series of compounds similar to Rasagiline (compound of reference) with potential neuroprotection effect.

Cheminformatics Models for Drug-Protein Interactions in Neurodegenerative Diseases

The discovery of new drugs for the treatment of neurodegenerative diseases is an important goal of medicinal chemistry (Allegri and Guekht 2012; Park 2012; Morris et al. 2012; Trushina and McMurray 2007). Despite the serious scientific efforts these disorders continue to threaten the viability of our health systems in the near future (Pisani et al. 2015). To illustrate this point, in the entire world more than 44 million people are estimated to be living with dementia (Wang et al. 2014). This figure is expected to rise to 135 million by 2050. In 2010 the global societal economic cost of dementia exceeded $600 billion USD, over 1% of global GDP. These costs are estimated to rise over the next few decades, particularly in middle- and low-income countries (Prince and Albanese 2014). Probably the most universal of them, Alzheimer´s disease (AD), (Salmon and Watts 2000) is a serious and degenerative disorder that causes a gradual loss of neurons. In spite of the efforts realized by the big pharmaceutical companies of the world, the origin of this pathology is still not very clear and the molecular mechanisms of the neuronal degeneration have not been totally understood yet (Martin 2012).

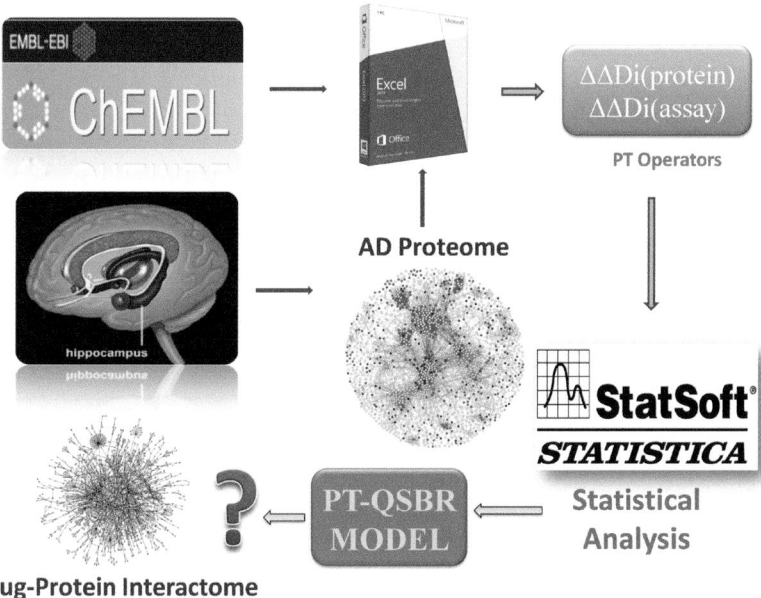

Fig. 1: Workflow for development of the PT-QSBR model for drug-target interactome of AD hippocampus proteome.

The previous picture, and the disappointing results in the major part of clinical trials, makes interesting the prediction of drug and drug targets candidates with mathematical and computational techniques (Howells et al. 2012; Nurisso et al. 2012). In fact, theoretical models in general are indispensable for the analysis of Big Data sets coming from Crystallography, Omics, or Clinical Research towards drug and target discovery (Zhang and Brusic 2014; Zheng et al. 2014; Sahin et al. 2014). In order to develop such computational models, we need to use modeling techniques to process chemical information from public databases. These databases have accumulated immense sets of experimental results of pharmacological trials for many compounds. This includes data from a large number of chemical libraries, target proteins, and Interactomes (Nantasenamat and Prachayasittikul 2015). For instance, CHEMBL (Heikamp and Bajorath 2011; Gaulton et al. 2012) is one of the biggest with more than 11,420,000 activity data for more than 1,295,500 compounds, and

9,844 targets. This huge amount of information offers a fertile field for the application of computational techniques (Gaulton et al. 2012; Mok and Brenk 2011). Another example is The Small Molecule Pathway Database (SMPDB) (Jewison et al. 2014), with data about human metabolism, drug action, drug metabolism, physiological activity, and metabolic disease pathways for more than 600 pathways. The capacity of production of new data is so high that in some cases a single group report in one work really important amounts of data. For instance, Liu et al. (2014) reported a large library with 533 drug relevant targets of 179,807 active ligands. The analysis of all this data is very complex due to three features of the chemical and pharmacological information present: (1) multi-targeting, (2) multi-output, and/or (3) multi-scaling. Multi-targeting complication emerges due to the existence of multi-target compounds (Hu and Bajorath 2010; Erhan et al. 2006; Namasivayam et al. 2013), which led to the formation of complex networks of drug-target and/or target-target interactions (Yildirim et al. 2007; Csermely et al. 2013).

Multi-output feature refers to the necessity of prediction of different experimental parameters to characterize the biological activity of drugs versus different targets under different assay conditions. Multi-scaling refers to the different structural levels of the organization of matter that input variables have to describe. It includes molecular structure (drugs), macromolecular structure (molecular targets), cellular (cellular line targets), and organisms that express the target. In these models we have a high number of assays carried out in very different conditions (c_q) for the same or different targets, which may be molecular or not. The non-structural information here refers to different assay conditions (c_q) like time, concentrations, temperature, cellular targets, tissues, organisms, etc. (Vergara-Galicia et al. 2014; Tenorio-Borroto et al. 2014; Gonzalez-Diaz et al. 2014).

Neuroprotection and Neuroinformatics

Neuroprotection and Neuroprotectants

Neuroprotection is any therapeutic intervention that prevents or delays damage to nonneuronal or neuronal cells of CNS after an acute or chronic degenerative injury, interfering with one or more of the pathophysiological steps that leads to neuronal dysfunction or death. Neuroprotectant is an agent which shows neuroprotective properties. Sometimes the term neuroprotective, originally an adjective, is used like a substantive. Over 500 products with neuroprotective effects, that can be grouped into 80 categories, are under investigation at various stages (Jain 2011). Some examples of these groups of drugs and neuroprotective interventions are: free radical scavengers (antioxidants), anti-excitotoxic agents like glutamate antagonists, antidepressants, antiepileptics, apoptosis inhibitors, anti-inflammatory agents, neurotrophic factors, metal ion chelators, ion channel modulators, or gene therapy (Morales-Camilo et al. 2014). However, human clinical trials of these compounds h ave been mostly disappointing and only a few of them has been used in clinical practice. By now, only a few examples of neuroprotectants are available in everyday clinical practice and their neuroprotective potential remains controversial and not well understood yet.

More important SNC drugs targets in ChEMBL database

The public database ChEMBL report a large number of results of assays of organic compounds against different protein targets expressed on nervous systems (NS) of distinct organisms. Many of these targets may play an important role in the mechanism of action of NS active compounds, including relevant neuroprotective compounds for neurodegenerative diseases, as is reflected in scientific literature and showed in next paragraphs. In Table 1, we depicted the names, organism of expression, and number of compounds assayed (n_j) for many of these targets.

Table 1: ChEMBL dataset for promising neuroprotective targets.

CHEMBL ID	Target Proteins [a]	UniProt	TT[b]	Org.[c]	n_j^d
1293232	Survival motor neuron (SMN) protein	Q16637	SP	*Hsa*	33607
249	NK1R	P25103	SP	*Hsa*	3607
4777	NPYR1	P25929	SP	*Hsa*	2151
1951	MAO-A	P21397	SP	*Hsa*	2751
2815	Trk-A NGFR	P04629	SP	*Hsa*	1995
2327	NK2R	P21452	SP	*Hsa*	1922
2039	MAO-B	P27338	SP	*Hsa*	1897
4296	Sodium channel protein type IX α subunit	Q15858	SP	*Hsa*	1824
4898	Neurotrophic tyrosine kinase R2 (NTKR2)	Q16620	SP	*Hsa*	1702
4018	NPYR2	P49146	SP	*Hsa*	1682
3048	NOS, brain	P29476	SP	*Rno*	1565
1907596	Neuronal AChR; α4/β2	P12390	PC	*Rno*	1533
4561	NPYR5	Q15761	SP	*Hsa*	1291
3358	MAO-A	P21396	SP	*Rno*	1280
2993	MAO-B	P19643	SP	*Rno*	1268
4980	Neuronal AChR protein α-7 subunit	Q05941	SP	*Rno*	1262
5608	NT-3 GFR	Q16288	SP	*Hsa*	1208
3568	NOS, brain	P29475	SP	*Hsa*	1142
1907589	Neuronal AChR; α4/β2	P17787	PC	*Hsa*	1142
2492	Neuronal AChR protein α-7 subunit	P36544	SP	*Hsa*	872
4027	NK1R	P14600	SP	*Rno*	789
5122	Discoidin domain-containing R2	Q16832	SP	*Hsa*	688

Table 1: contd....

Table 1: contd.

CHEMBL ID	Target Proteins [a]	UniProt	TT[b]	Org.[c]	n_j^d
4429	NK3R	P29371	SP	*Hsa*	675
1907594	Neuronal AChR; α3/β4	P30926	PC	*Hsa*	673
3942	NK1R	P30547	SP	*Cpo*	640
1293293	Neuropeptides B/W R1	P48145	SP	*Hsa*	530
2097170	A1 Amyloidβ A4 precursor	Q02410	PPI	*Hsa*	449
4123	NeurotensinR1	P30989	SP	*Hsa*	432
2094110	Neuronal AChR	Q9JLB5	PCG	*Rno*	390
5072	Ephrin type-B R1	P54762	SP	*Hsa*	327
4554	NK2R	P16610	SP	*Rno*	302
2096621	Nitric oxide sythases; iNOS & nNOS	P29475	SG	*Hsa*	286
5192	Botulinum neurotoxin type A	P10845	SP	*Cbo*	268
2647	NK2R	Q64077	SP	*Cpo*	265
1907593	Neuronal AChR; α3/β4	P04757	PC	*Rno*	257
3636	Neuromedin B receptor	P28336	SP	*Hsa*	210
1882	Neuronal AChR protein α-4 subunit	P43681	SP	*Hsa*	202
307	Neuronal AChR protein α-4 subunit	P09483	SP	*Rno*	200
3433	NK2R	P79218	SP	*Ocu*	192
1907595	Neuronal AChR; α4/β4	P09483	PC	*Rno*	181
1907587	Neuronal AChR; α3/β2	P04757	PC	*Rno*	169
2721	Excitatory amino acid transporter 3	P43005	SP	*Hsa*	165
3068	Neuronal AChR subunit α-3	P32297	SP	*Hsa*	160
2111405	NOS (endothelial and brain)	P29475	SG	*Hsa*	156
4921	Urotensin II receptor	P49684	SP	*Rno*	143
5344	Botulinum neurotoxin type A	A5HZZ9	SP	*Cbo*	140
5368	Amiloride-sensitive cation channel 3	Q9UHC3	SP	*Hsa*	131
5174	Neuropilin-1	O14786	SP	*Hsa*	129
4877	NPYR4	P50391	SP	*Hsa*	129
3802	NPYR5	O70342	SP	*Mmu*	126
3154	NK 3 receptor	P16177	SP	*Rno*	126
1907590	Neuronal AChR; α2/β4	P12389	PC	*Rno*	126
2221348	Voltage-gated potassium channel, KQT	O43526	PC	*Hsa*	122

Table 1: contd....

Table 1: contd....

CHEMBL ID	Target Proteins [a]	UniProt	TT[b]	Org.[c]	n_j^d
2304405	NK2R	P51144	SP	*Mau*	122
5497	Neuropeptide S receptor	Q8BZP8	SP	*Mmu*	117
1907592	Neuronal AChR; α2/β2	P12389	PC	*Rno*	112
2514	NeurotensinR2	O95665	SP	*Hsa*	104
2007627	Botulinum neurotoxin type F	P30996	SP	*Cbo*	97
5951	Neuropeptide FF R1	Q9GZQ6	SP	*Hsa*	94
5952	Neuropeptide FF R2	Q9Y5X5	SP	*Hsa*	94
5158	Sodium channel protein type X α subunit	Q6QIY3	SP	*Mmu*	81
1907591	Neuronal AChR; α4/β4	P43681	PC	*Hsa*	80
5852	Pyroglutamylated RF-amide peptide receptor	Q96P65	SP	*Hsa*	77
2476	Voltage-gated potassium channel subunit Kv7.2	O43526	SP	*Hsa*	73
1795111	BDNF/NT-3 GFR	Q63604	SP	*Rno*	71
2109234	Neuronal AChR; α3/β2	P17787	PC	*Hsa*	69
1783	Vascular endothelial growth factor A	P15692	SP	*Hsa*	66
2548	NPYR5	Q63634	SP	*Rno*	66
3309	NPYR2	Q9ERC0	SP	*Rno*	62
4017	Sodium channel protein type X α subunit	Q62968	SP	*Rno*	61
3799	NK 3 receptor	P30098	SP	*Cpo*	59
5850	Mas-related G-protein coupled RX1	Q96LB2	SP	*Hsa*	57
3461	Neuronal AChR protein α-10 subunit	Q9JLB5	SP	*Rno*	53
1075108	Solute carrier family 12 member 5	Q63633	SP	*Rno*	53
3027	NeurotensinR1	P20789	SP	*Rno*	51
3425	Neuropeptide FFR2	Q9EQD2	SP	*Rno*	48
5295	Kinesin heavy chain isoform 5A	Q12840	SP	*Hsa*	45
3074	Tyrosine-protein kinase SRC	P05480	SP	*Mmu*	44
2109238	Neuronal AChR; α9/α10	Q9UGM1	PC	*Hsa*	43
2111384	Nicotinic AChR α3/βX	Q05901	PCG	*Hsa*	41
1938219	Neuropeptides B/W R1	P49681	SP	*Mmu*	41

Table 1: contd....

Table 1: contd.

CHEMBL ID	Target Proteins [a]	UniProt	TT[b]	Org.[c]	$n_j{}^d$
3818	Neuronal AChR subunit α-3	P04757	SP	*Rno*	38
2073673	Solute carrier family 22 member 3	O75751	SP	*Hsa*	37
3570	NeurotensinR1	O88319	SP	*Mmu*	32
6159	Ubiquitincarboxyl-terminal hydrolaseisozyme L1	P09936	SP	*Hsa*	30
4719	NOS, brain	Q9Z0J4	SP	*Mmu*	28
4762	Low affinity p75NTR	P08138	SP	*Hsa*	24
2109230	Neuronal AChR; α2/β4	Q15822	PC	*Hsa*	22
3091	Neurotensin receptor 3	Q99523	SP	*Hsa*	22
4747	Neuronal AChR subunit α-6	P43143	SP	*Rno*	22
2813	NK2R	P30549	SP	*Mmu*	21
3365	Neuronal AChR protein α-7 subunit	P49582	SP	*Mmu*	21
2221346	Neuronal AChRs; α-3/β-4, α-5, β-2	P17787	PCG	*Hsa*	15
2109233	Neuronal AChR; α3/α6/β2/β3	P32297	PC	*Hsa*	15
1615384	Solute carrier family 12 member 5	Q9H2X9	SP	*Hsa*	15
2111438	NeurotensinR	O95665	PF	*Hsa*	13
2585	Neuronal AChR protein α-9 subunit	P43144	SP	*Rno*	13
2584	Neuronal AChR protein α-2 subunit	P12389	SP	*Rno*	13

[a]Target proteins: R = Receptor, NKR = Neurokinin Receptor or Tachykinin receptor 1 (TACR1), NPYR = Neuropeptide Y Receptor, AchR = AChR, MAO = Monoamine Oxidase, NOS = Nitric Oxide Synthase, NTR = Neurotrophin Receptor, NGFR = Nerve growth factors receptor. [b]TT = Target types: SP = Single Protein, PC = Protein Complex, ND = No Data, PCG = Protein complex group, CL = Cell line, PPI = Protein-Protein Interaction, SG = Selectivity Group, PF = Protein Family. [c]Animal species: Hsa = *Homo sapiens*, Rno = *Rattusnorvegicus*, Mmu = *Musmusculus*, Cpo = *Caviaporcellus*, Cbo = *Clostridium botulinum*, Ocu = *Oryctolaguscuniculus*, Mau = *Mesocricetusauratus*. [d]Number of compounds assayed against target and reported in ChEMBL until 05/2014.

According to this, the Survival Motor Neuron (SMN) protein is one of the more promising targets with > 30000 compounds assayed. SMN is involved in spinal muscular atrophy which are a group of neuromuscular disorders characterized by degeneration of the anterior horn cells of the spinal cord. The clinical severity is dependent on the levels of functional Survival Motor Neuron (SMN) protein (Sen et al. 2013). There is increasing evidence indicating a key regulatory anti-apoptotic role for the SMN protein in modulating cell survival that is important in motor neuron survival (Zhou et al. 2014). Another work revealed the involvement of SMN protein in naloxone protection and oxidative stress-related neurotoxicity (Hsu et al. 2014).

And more importantly, it has been showed recently that SMN up-regulation slows locomotor deficit onset and motor neuron loss in a mouse model of amyotrophic lateral sclerosis (Matos et al. 2014).

NK1R is another important target according to the number of assays in ChEMBL (n_j = 3607). It is a Substance P receptor abundantly distributed in the basal ganglia. Substance P has a pro-inflammatory role and has been implicated in the pathogenesis of PD, given it that can initiate neurogenic inflammation. Treatment of NK1 receptor was demonstrated to provide neuroprotection through the inhibition of an apoptotic pathway in dopaminergic neurons (Juarez-Jimenez et al. 2014; Mao et al. 2013).

Also important as target according to the number of assays of compounds in ChEMBL (n_j = 1995) is the Tyrosine Kinase A Nerve Grow Factor Receptor (Trk-A NGFR). It is a receptor involved in the development and the maturation of the central and peripheral nervous systems (Klein et al. 1991). Jang (Jang et al. 2009) showed that the tricyclic antidepressant amitriptyline interacts with Trk-A NGFR. Inhibition of TrkA abolished the neuroprotective effect of amitriptyline without affecting its antidepressant activity.

Human Neuropeptide Y2 receptor (NPYR2) is a small peptide that inhibits glutamatergic neurotransmission. The NPYergic system has potential relevance in neuroprotection against excitotoxicity by acting on hyperexcitability, neuronal death or brain repair, and also proves to be a good target for the treatment of pharmaco-resistant forms of temporal lobe epilepsy (Coelho-Cerqueira et al. 2014).

NOS Brain, a nitric oxide producing enzyme, is implicated in oxidative stress, and several isoforms are elevated in Alzheimer's disease. This increased expression of NOS isoforms in astrocytes and neurons contributes to the synthesis of peroxynitrite, which leads to generation of nitrotyrosine. Nitrotyrosine was detected in neurons, astrocytes, and blood vessels in Alzheimer Disease cases. Physiological concentrations of NO also elicit anti-apoptotic effects against various neurotoxic conditions and brain insults through multiple mechanisms (Bonaiuto et al. 2013; Vishnu Nayak et al. 2013).

Heteromeric nicotinic acetylcholine receptors (AchR) with α4β2 subunits are a family of ACh-gated ion channels. They appear to mediate the essential features of nicotine-addiction, and have important roles in other neurological diseases like epilepsies. Significant loss of α4β2 AChR may contribute to the cognitive deficits in Alzheimer's disease (Hung et al. 2013). In addition, nicotinic acetylcholine receptor (nAChR) drugs could have clinical potential for Parkinson's disease (Xi et al. 2013).

Alpha-7 subunit of the Neuronal AChR protein is expressed on cholinergic projection neurons, and target regions have been implicated in neuroprotection against beta-amyloid toxicity, possibly through influences on beta-amyloid accumulation and oligomerization (Yang et al. 2013).

Another interesting example is the receptor of growth factor Neurotrophin-3 (NT-3 GFR). Several lines of evidence have suggested a possible involvement of neurotrophic factors in the pathogenesis of neurodegenerative disease. NT-3 prevents the degeneration of noradrenergic neurons of the locus coeruleus in a lesion model that resembles the pattern of cell loss found in Alzheimer's dementia (Ferino et al. 2013).

Monoamine oxidase A (MAO-A) in the brain have also been implicated in the etiology of Alzheimer's disease. Elevated levels of this enzyme have been linked to increases in neurotoxic metabolites and neuron loss. However, paradoxically, its activity was found significantly decreased by 17% in Alzheimer patients versus normal subjects in the prefrontal cortex. The changes in MAO A occur very early in Alzheimer's disease and remain relatively constant as the disease progresses (Matos et al. 2013).

MAO-B inhibitors are unique in that they exert protective effects on both vascular and neuronal tissue (Gao et al. 2013). The properties of propargyl-based inhibitors of MAO-B in preclinical experiments have drawn attention to their neuroprotective effect in neurodegenerative diseases, and have raised the question of the MAO-B implication in the generation of free radicals (Pisani et al. 2013). A series of novel multi-target neuroprotective drugs has been developed exploiting their ability against MAO-B receptors (Salgin-Goksen et al. 2013; Tripathi et al. 2013).

Classic Cheminformatics models in Neuropharmacology

In the last few years, several Cheminformatics approaches resembling our work on the prediction of different drugs in this area have been published. These models are useful to predict different series of compounds active against diverse nervous systems targets implicated in neurodegenerative diseases. A subset of them that have attracted special attention are MAO, AChE, and BACE1 inhibitors. In the following paragraphs we show briefly some relevant theoretical models published on this area.

Prediction of MAO inhibitors

Santana et al. (2006) developed a model to correctly classify 1406 active/non-active MAO-A inhibitors compounds with > 90% of accuracy. Later, Santana et al. (2008), reported an interesting model for the prediction of both MAO-A and MAO-B inhibitors using the same methodology employing coumarine derivatives. Molina et al. 2012 carried out a review about Cheminformatics models for the prediction of the MAO-A inhibitors. Pisani et al. (2015) uses Gaussian field-based three dimensional (3D) Quantitative structure-activity relationship (QSAR) and docking with 67 2H-chromen-2-one derivatives to obtain inhibition data on rat MAO-B. Morales-Camilo et al. (2014) synthesized and evaluated *in vitro* a series of chalcones and aurones, and the structural requirements for their activity were characterized with the aid of 3D-QSAR and docking studies. Pettersson (Pettersson et al. 2013) synthesized a series of 4-phenylpiperidines and piperazines and reported QSAR models of binding affinities to the dopamine D2 receptor and MAO-A enzyme. Fresqui et al. (2013) obtained a satisfactory QSAR model of thirty-four amphetamines against the enzyme MAO-A through three latent variables extracted for a set of initial thirty-eight molecular descriptors. Vilar et al. (2012) synthesized and assayed and studied different classes of MAO-A and MAO-B inhibition. Helguera et al. (2013) built QSAR models from a dataset of heterocyclic compounds which could be used to predict the inhibitory activity and selectivity toward human MAO. Prado-Prado et al. (2012) developed 3D multi-target QSAR models using the 3D MI-DRAGON technique. They used the MARCH-INSIDE and DRAGON software to calculate 3D structural parameters for a set of US FDA approved drugs and their targets to predict the complex network made up of all drug-target interactions. Molina et al. (2012) provided a review and new tools prediction of MAO-A inhibitors was validated through a new series of oxoisoaporphine derivatives.

Prediction of β-secretase inhibitors

Beta-secretase 1 is implicated in the pathway that induces formation of amyloid beta and its inhibition has been investigated as a promising therapeutic approach in the treatment of AD. Hossain et al. (2014) uses 3D QSAR modeling approaches to identify structural requirements for a potential BACE inhibitor employing 980 structurally diverse compounds. Chakraborty et al. (2014) incorporates receptor flexibility to identify potential compounds and identifies 24 highly potent novel BACE1 inhibitors. Huang et al. (2013) elaborated a 3D-QSAR model and designed 30 new molecules with high BACE 1 inhibitory activity. Cruz and Castilho (2014) designed aminoimidazoles, aminohydantoins, and aminopyridines derivatives that inhibit BACE-1. Nastese and Boyd (2012) used available structural data on protein-inhibitor complexes in the Protein Data Bank, and found a remarkable relationship with two simple descriptors in a QSAR model of known BACE 1 inhibitors. Ginman et al. (2013) synthesized diverse compounds based on cyclic amidine and guanidine cores with the goal of finding BACE-1 inhibitors. Liu et al. (2012) explores the mechanism of inhibition through the use of 46 X-ray crystallographic BACE-1/inhibitor complexes to derive quantitative structure-activity relationship (QSAR) models. Niño et al. (2012) revised QSAR studies using method of Artificial Neural Network (ANN) in order to understand the essential structural requirement for binding with receptor for β and γ-secretase inhibitors.

Prediction of AChE inhibitors

Acetylcholinesterase is an enzyme that catalyzes the hydrolysis of the acetylcholine neuro transmitter thereby terminating neurotransmission in the synaptic cleft of neuromuscular junctions or cholinergic brain synapses. The inhibition of this relevant enzyme is an important therapeutic target in clinical entities like myasthenia gravis or Alzheimer's disease. Shaikh et al. (2014) published a concise update about the study of inhibitors of the acetylcholinesterase from a neuroinformatics perspective. Natural and traditional inhibitors as well as novel inhibitors have been covered. Additionally they review the current clinical benefit of this molecule. Bautista-Aguilera et al. (2014) used a 3D-QSAR study to define 3D-pharmacophores for inhibition of MAO A/B, acetylcholinesterase (AChE), and butyrylcholinesterase enzymes with donepezil-pyridyl hybrids. They found a donepezil-pyridyl that is a potent, moderately selective human AChE and selective irreversible MAO B. In another methodologically similar study from the same group (Bautista-Aguilera et al. 2014), they found a donepezil-indolyl hybrid like a promising drug for potential treatment of AD. Gholivand et al. (2014) synthesized new phosphoramidate derivatives. Molecular docking and QSAR were used to understand the relationship between molecular structural features and anti-ChE activity, and to predict the affinity of phosphoramidopiperidinecarboxamides to ChE receptors. Korabecny et al. (2014) generated a novel series of 7-methoxytacrine donepezil-like compounds and tested it for their ability to inhibit several acetylcholinesterases, and butyrylcholinesterases. QSAR studies were performed to rationalize studies from *in vitro* interesting candidates. Islam et al. (2013) made molecular docking of conventional AchE inhibitors and, quercetin, a plant flavonoid, on the active site of AchE. Next, they added different functional groups to quercetin to perform QSAR analysis. From this approach, they predicted the superiority of the natural compound quercetin over the conventional drugs as AchE inhibitor. Abuhamdah et al. (2013) examined 85 AChE inhibitors implementing genetic algorithm-based QSAR modeling to discriminate optimal combination of pharmacophoric models and 2D physicochemical descriptors. They identified twenty-four low micromolar AChE inhibitors. Correa-Basurto et al. (2014) used a set of N-aryl-monosubstituted derivatives with inhibitory activity toward both acetylcholinesterase and butyrylcholinesterase for QSAR studies employing docking data. They included clinical approved acetylcholinesterase inhibitors to contrast their results and concluded that the complex formed between ChEs and the best N-aryl compound could be a valuable inhibitor.

Multi-target cheminformatics models for neuropharmacology

Our group also has been working on the development of new computational models for predicting multiple targets of drugs in relationship with neurotoxicity/neuroprotective effects from multiplexing assay outcomes reported in CHEMBL. We have reported three different models in this field. The three models can give different outcomes for > 30 experimental measures in > 400 different experimental protocols, related to > 150 molecular and cellular targets present in 11 different organisms (including human). The three methods showed excellent values of accuracy, specificity, and sensitivity in both training and validation series. These models should predict different probabilities if we change the organisms (c_1), the biological assays (c_2), the molecular/cellular target (c_3), or the standard experimental parameter measured (c_4), for the same compound. The statistical parameters used to select the best models are: Number of cases used to train the model (N), Canonical Regression Coefficient (Rc), Chi-square (χ^2), and p-level. The probability cut-off for this LDA model is $^i p_1(c_q) > 0.5 => L_{ij}(c_q) = 1$. It means that the drug d_i predicted by the model with probability > 0.5 are expected to give a positive outcome in the qth assays carry out under the given set of conditions c_q.

TM-moments multi-target models for neuroprotective effects

In a previous paper (Luan et al. 2013), we developed the first multitarget-QSAR model for multiplexing assays of neurotoxicity/neuroprotective effects of drugs. We used the method TOPS-MODE (http://scorpio.biophysics.ismb.lon.ac.uk/scorpio.html) to calculate the structural parameters of drugs. The best model classified correctly 4,393 out of 4,915 total cases. This model used the spectral moments μ_k of order k^{th} of the bond adjacency matrix ($^1\mathbf{B}$); calculated with the TM approach. The TM-spectral moment model is able to classify correctly 83-82% of 4915 cases in total. Apparently, the TM-moments model shows better values of these parameters, but we have to take into account the differences in the complexity of the datasets used to train and validate these models. The equation of this model is the following:

$$S_{ij}\left(c_q\right) = -7.01 \cdot 10^{-4} \cdot p\left(c_j\right) \cdot \mu_5^i - 7.84 \cdot 10^{-4} \cdot \Delta\mu_5^i\left(s\right) - 2.93 \cdot 10^{-4} \cdot \Delta\mu_5^i\left(a\right)$$
$$+ 1.16 \cdot 10^{-4} \cdot \Delta\mu_5^i\left(o\right) + 2.84 \cdot 10^{-4} \cdot \Delta\mu_5^i\left(t\right) + 4.198684 \tag{4}$$
$$N = 3683 \quad R_c = 0.7 \quad p < 0.005$$

MI-moments multi-target models for neuroprotective effects

In another work (Alonso et al. 2013), we introduce the first multiplexing QSAR model for neurotoxicity/neuroprotective effects of drugs based on the MARCH-INSIDE (MI) method to calculate the stochastic spectral moments (structural descriptors) of all compounds. This second model, utilized as input the π_k^i values of the Markov matrix ($^1\mathbf{\Pi}$) of atom-atom electron delocalization calculated with the software MI. In the TM method, we weighted the edges of the molecular graph with standard distances of chemical bonds whereas the MI algorithm employs atom standard electronegativities to weight the nodes of molecular graph. The MI-spectral moment model is able to classify correctly 89–92% of 3598 cases. The equation of the second model is:

$$S_{ij}\left(c_q\right) = 1.139556 - 0.403994 \cdot p\left(c_j\right) \cdot \pi_5^i + 0.199322 \cdot \Delta\pi_5^i\left(s_x\right) + 0.434889 \cdot \Delta\pi_5^i\left(a_u\right)$$
$$- 0.020189 \cdot \Delta\pi_5^i\left(o_t\right) - 0.001660 \cdot \Delta\pi_1^i\left(t_e\right) \tag{5}$$
$$N = 2661 \quad R_c = 0.72 \quad \chi^2 = 1913.007 \quad p < 0.005$$

MI-entropy multi-target models for neuroprotective effects

In the third work, we introduce the first multitarget QSAR model based again on the method MI. We found a model that classified correctly 2,955 out of 3,548 total cases in the training and validation series. Then, we made a multi-target complex network where the links (Lij) represent the interactions between the drug (di) and the target (Olsson et al. 2008) characterized by different experimental measures obtained in pharmacological assays under diverse boundary conditions of (cj). Notably, the MI-entropy model is able to classify correctly 89–92% of 8309 cases. Consequently, the statistics for this last model refer to a dataset with more than twice the number of cases present in previous models. The best ALMA-entropy model found in this work was:

$$S_{ij}\left(c_q\right) = 1.1396 - 0.4039 \cdot p(c_1) \cdot \theta_1^i + 0.1993 \cdot \Delta\theta_1^i\left(s_x\right) + 0.4349 \cdot \Delta\theta_1^i\left(a_u\right)$$
$$- 0.0202 \cdot \Delta\theta_1^i\left(o_t\right) - 0.0017 \cdot \Delta\theta_1^i\left(t_e\right) \tag{6}$$
$$N = 2661 \quad R_c = 0.72 \quad \chi^2 = 1913.007 \quad p < 0.005$$

Methods

Drug-receptor affinity, that is, the tendency of a drug molecule to bind to one or more receptors due to the collective influence of multiple molecular forces, plays an important role in pharmacology. Consequently, prediction of drug affinity as a dissociation constant (reciprocal of the equilibrium constant) is extraordinarily valuable. Quantification of the changes in the system due to perturbations (e.g., to a change in drug structure, concentration, or temperature) may yield important information in this sense. As we mentioned above Gonzalez-Díaz et al. introduced a general-purpose extra-thermodynamic perturbation theory or model for multiple-boundary Chemoinformatics problems (Gonzalez-Diaz et al. 2011a,b; Gonzalez-Diaz et al. 2013; Gonzalez-Diaz et al. 2014a,b,c).

Let us consider that we know the values in the state of reference $f(\varepsilon_{ij})_{ref}$ of a function (f) for the parameter ε_{ij} that characterizes the efficiency of transformation of the ith molecule (M_i) by bio-molecular process. We also have to consider that the process is determined by a set of boundary conditions $c_j = (c_0, c_1, c_2, \ldots c_n)$. In addition, we know the values of these boundary conditions for the state of reference or initial $^{ref}c_j = (c_0, c_1, c_2, \ldots c_n)_{ref}$ and for a new state of the system $^{new}c_j = (c_0, c_1, c_2, \ldots c_n)_{new}$. Lastly, we know the values $D_k(M_j)$ of the molecular descriptors D_k of type k for each molecule M_i at the state of reference and in the new state (after the process). Therefore, to predict the change $\Delta f(\varepsilon_{ij})$ we have to predict only $f(\varepsilon_{ij})_{new}$. We can predict the new values $f(\varepsilon_{ij})_{new}$ based on the values of $f(\varepsilon_{ij})_{ref}$ of reference, the change on the molecular descriptors $\Delta D_k(M_j)$, and the changes in the boundary conditions. In this work, we developed the first Higher Order QSBR-Perturbation Theory (HOPT-QSBR) model to predict activity of organic compounds upon different proteins located in the hippocampus brain region having great possibilities of being implicated in AD. In so doing, we extended the idea behind Hansch's analysis to search the first HOPT-QSBR models with applications to Neuropharmacology. In a previous work, we developed a linear PT-QSBR model. It lets the door open to generalization of this model. We can use higher order exponents (n >= 2) for the Box-Jenkins Operators used on this PT-QSBR equation. We created the acronym HOPT-QSBR by contraction of these terms. The general equation of the HOPT-QSBR model introduced here by the first time is:

$$f(\varepsilon_{ij})_{new} = a_0 \cdot f(\varepsilon_{qr})_{ref} + \sum_{n=1}^{n\,max} \sum_{k=0}^{k\,max} b_{nk} \cdot O_{nk} + \sum_{n=1}^{n\,max} \sum_{k=0}^{k\,max} \sum_{j=1}^{4} c_{nkj} \cdot O_{nkj} + e_0 \qquad (7)$$

We can decompose the HOPT equation into perturbation terms according to the order n. In the particular case when we add to the perturbation model only the terms with n = 1 we obtain the linear perturbation model LPT-QSBR. In the case when we add also the quadratic terms, we obtain the QPT-QSBR version of LPT-QSPR model. When, n > 2, we are in the presence of HOPT-QSBR model for higher orders.

$$f(\varepsilon_{ij})_{new} = a_0 \cdot f(\varepsilon_{qr})_{ref} + \sum_{k=0}^{k\,max} b_{1k} \cdot O_1 + \sum_{k=0}^{k\,max} \sum_{j=1}^{4} b_{1kj} \cdot O_{1kj} + \sum_{k=0}^{k\,max} c_{2k} \cdot O_{2k}$$

$$+ \sum_{k=0}^{k\,max} \sum_{j=1}^{4} c_{2kj} \cdot O_{2kj} + \sum_{n=1}^{n\,max} \sum_{k=0}^{k\,max} \sum_{j=1}^{4} d_{nkj} \cdot O_{n>2} + e_0 \qquad (8)$$

$$f(\varepsilon_{ij})_{new} = a_0 \cdot f(\varepsilon_{qr})_{ref} + \sum_{k=0}^{k\,max}\sum_{j=1}^{4} b_{nkj} \cdot \left[\left(\Delta D_{kj}\right)_{new} - \left(\Delta D_{kj}\right)_{ref}\right] + e_0$$

$$+ \sum_{k=0}^{k\,max}\sum_{j=1}^{4} c_{nkj} \cdot \left[\left(\Delta D_{kj}\right)_{new} - \left(\Delta D_{kj}\right)_{ref}\right]^2 + \sum_{n=1}^{n\,max}\sum_{k=0}^{k\,max}\sum_{j=1}^{4} d_{nkj} \cdot O_{n>2} + e_0 \tag{9}$$

$$f(\varepsilon_{ij})_{new} = a_0 \cdot f(\varepsilon_{qr})_{ref} + \sum_{k=0}^{k\,max}\sum_{j=1}^{4} b_{nkj} \cdot \left[\left(\Delta D_{kj}\right)_{new} - \left(\Delta D_{kj}\right)_{ref}\right]$$

$$+ \sum_{k=0}^{k\,max}\sum_{j=1}^{4} c_{nkj} \cdot \left[\left(\Delta D_{kj}\right)_{new} - \left(\Delta D_{kj}\right)_{ref}\right]^2 + d_n \cdot O(n>2) + e_0 \tag{10}$$

The operators of the type $O_{nk} = [(D_{kj})_{new} - (D_{kj})_{ref}]^n$ only account for perturbations on molecular structure. However, the operators with the form $O_{nkj} = [(\Delta D_{kj})_{new} - (\Delta D_{kj})_{ref}]^n$ account for perturbations on molecular structure of the compounds and on the boundary conditions of the assay (c_j). In this work, we also developed the first HOPT-QSBR model of order $n \leq 5$. We carried out the study with the previous dataset downloaded from ChEMBL. In so doing, we explored the terms of order $n = 1, 2, 3, 4,$ and 5, automatically in the software STATISTICA with the option Polynomial LDA. Following that, we wrote down the general equation of the HOPT model for all terms of order $n = 1, 2,$ and 3 letting higher terms on compact notation for the sake of simplicity.

$$f(\varepsilon_{ij})_{new} = a_0 \cdot f(\varepsilon_{qr})_{ref} + \sum_{k=0}^{k\,max}\sum_{j=1}^{4} b_{1k} \cdot \left[\left(D_{kj}\right)_{new} - \left(D_{kj}\right)_{ref}\right] + \sum_{k=0}^{k\,max}\sum_{j=1}^{4} b_{1kj} \cdot \left[\left(\Delta D_{kj}\right)_{new} - \left(\Delta D_{kj}\right)_{ref}\right]$$

$$+ \sum_{k=0}^{k\,max}\sum_{j=1}^{4} b_{2k} \cdot \left[\left(D_{kj}\right)_{new} - \left(D_{kj}\right)_{ref}\right]^2 + \sum_{k=0}^{k\,max}\sum_{j=1}^{4} c_{2kj} \cdot \left[\left(\Delta D_{kj}\right)_{new} - \left(\Delta D_{kj}\right)_{ref}\right]^2 \tag{11}$$

$$+ \sum_{k=0}^{k\,max}\sum_{j=1}^{4} b_{3k} \cdot \left[\left(D_{kj}\right)_{new} - \left(D_{kj}\right)_{ref}\right]^3 + \sum_{k=0}^{k\,max}\sum_{j=1}^{4} c_{3kj} \cdot \left[\left(\Delta D_{kj}\right)_{new} - \left(\Delta D_{kj}\right)_{ref}\right]^3$$

$$+ \sum_{n=1}^{n\,max}\sum_{k=0}^{k\,max} d_{nk} \cdot O_{n>3} + \sum_{n=1}^{n\,max}\sum_{k=0}^{k\,max}\sum_{j=1}^{4} d_{nkj} \cdot O_{n>3} + e_0$$

As a proof-of-concept test, we studied a large dataset of drugs downloaded from ChEMBL. The dataset contains (see materials and methods) the outcomes of a large number of experimental pharmacological assays. The results are for assays of binding of drugs to different proteins expressed by the Central Nervous System (CNS) tissues. The model presupposes that the changes in drug binding occur due to perturbations on the input boundary conditions c_j. The boundary conditions considered in this work are $c_1 =$ molecular target selected, $c_2 =$ type of assay. We do not consider, by the moment, changes in other boundary conditions like $c_3 =$ organisms of assay, $c_4 =$ different experimental parameters, $c_5 =$ brain cortex area, etc. We focused on those proteins that express highly in a specific area of the brain (Hippocampus). This interest takes into account the involvement of these area in pathological processes linked to diseases like AD. We do not consider either changes in $c_3 =$ organisms of assay or in $c_4 =$ pharmacological experimental parameters. Our dataset contains only values of drug binding constant for humans ($\varepsilon_{ij} = K_{ij}$). In fact, we focused only on a drug binding pseudo-constant ($\varepsilon_{ij} = {}^*K_{ij}$) defined by us to quantify the probability of binding of a drug highly expressed on hippocampus. In this work, we also developed the first PT-QSBR model of order 2 as a generalization of the Hansch's model derived from the previous dataset. In this sense, this extra-thermodynamic model may be annotated as a Quadratic PT-QSBR (QPT-QSBR). In so doing, explored the terms of order n = 1 and 2 automatically with the software STATISTICA using the option Polynomial LDA. The best QPT-QSBR model found here with LDA was:

$$S\left({}^*K_{ij}\right)_{new} = -3.49867 \cdot f\left(\varepsilon_{ij}\right)_{ref} - 4.17669 \cdot \Delta LogP - 0.16334 \cdot \Delta PSA$$
$$+ 0.18587 \cdot \Delta\Delta LogP_{protein} + 0.0151 \cdot \Delta\Delta PSA_{protein} + 4.08016 \cdot \Delta\Delta LogP_{assay} \quad (12)$$
$$+ 0.1525 \cdot \Delta\Delta PSA_{assay} + 0.00163 \cdot \left(\Delta LogP\right)^2 - 0.89129$$
$$N = 49312 \quad Rc = 0.76 \quad F = 13154.02 \quad p < 0.005$$

Notably, the model incorporated a quadratic term. The quadratic term presented the form $(\Delta LogP)^2 = [LogP(M_i)_{ref} - LogP(M_i)_{new}]^2$. This quadratic term is the analogue of Hansch quadratic term $LogP(M_i)^2$ for the LogP of a single molecule. Anyhow, the term is a perturbation or change in LogP due to changes in the structure of the new molecule with respect to the molecule of reference. In any case, the coefficient of the term in the equation is not a negative value as expected for a negative parabolic

Table 2: Results of PT-QSBR models developed in this work for drug-target interactome of proteins expressed in the proteome of the hippocampus of AD patients.

PT-QSBR Model	Data Sets[a]	Observed sets train (t)	Statistical Parameter[b]	Predicted Statistics	Predicted sets		
					n_j	$L_{ij} = 0$	$L_{ij} = 1$
Quadratic	$L_{ij} = 0$	0	Sp	90.9	53783	48870	4913
(n = 2)	$L_{ij} = 1$	1	Sn	77.7	21245	4736	16509
	Train	total	Ac	87.1			
	$L_{ij} = 0$	0	Sp	90.9	17927	16289	1638
	$L_{ij} = 1$	1	Sn	77.6	7045	1581	5464
	Validation	total	Ac	87.1			
High Order	$L_{ij} = 0$	0	Sp	90.9	53783	48879	4904
(2 < n ≤ 5)	$L_{ij} = 1$	1	Sn	77.7	21245	4739	16506
	Train	total	Ac	87.1			
	$L_{ij} = 0$	0	Sp	90.9	17927	16293	1634
	$L_{ij} = 1$	1	Sn	77.6	7045	1580	5465
	Validation	total	Ac	87.1			

[a]We used as input effects perturbation theory operators based on the values reported by ChEMBL: PSA = Polar Surface Area, LogP = Logarithm of n-Octanol/Water Partition coefficient, Nro = Number of Rotable Bonds, and Mw = Molecular weight. [b]The positive (1) and negative control cases (0) were assigned as follows $f({}^*K_{ij})_{new} = L_{ij} = 1$ (links in the interactome) => $z_{ij} > 0$ => $v_j > avg(v_j)$ otherwise $L_{ij} = 0$. [c]Sn = Sensitivity (%), Sp = Specificity (%), and Ac = Accuracy (%).

Hansch effect (Hansch et al. 1964). In addition, the introduction of quadratic term do not outperformed the linear model. In Table 2, we give the training, validation, and overall classification results obtained with this HOPT-QSBR model in terms of Sn = Sensitivity (%), Sp = Specificity (%), and Ac = Accuracy (%). The results obtained in the same range of other excellent multi-target models reported in the literature for other problems (Casanola-Martin et al. 2015; Tenorio-Borroto et al. 2014; Romero Duran et al. 2014; Luan et al. 2014; Kleandrova et al. 2014b; Kleandrova et al. 2014a; Gonzalez-Diaz et al. 2014; Gonzalez-Diaz et al. 2014; Luan et al. 2013; Speck-Planche 2012; Speck-Planche 2012; Molina Matos 2012; Speck-Planche et al. 2011, 2011).

According to the previous sections, the first input term is the value $f(^*K_{ij})_{ref}$. This is the scoring function (f) of the parameter of binding efficiency ($^*K_{ij}$) of the drug of reference to the protein defined in c_j = target (known solution). The function $f(^*K_{ij})_{ref} = 1$ if the molecule M_i interacts with the target in the boundary conditions c_j and $f(^*K_{ij})_{ref} = 0$ otherwise. We decided the strength of the interaction (efficiency of binding) with a cut-off or threshold value: $f(^*K_{ij})_{ref} = 1$ if $^*K_{ij} > 1000$. The parameter

Table 3: Probability of expression of proteins p(prot) in the proteome of the hippocampus of AD patients.

Gen	p(prot)	Protein	Gen	p(prot)	Protein
PIK3R1	1.000	PI3-kinase p110-delta/p85-alpha	TAP1	0.550	Methionine aminopeptidase 1
CHRNA3	1.000	Neuronal acetylcholine receptor; alpha3/beta2	INS	0.530	Vascular endothelial growth factor receptor 2
CSF1	1.000	Macrophage colony stimulating factor receptor	CASP3	0.470	Caspase-3
IGF1R	1.000	Insulin-like growth factor I receptor	PLAT	0.400	LDL-associated phospholipase A2
GSK3B	1.000	Glycogen synthase kinase-3 beta	FYN	0.380	Tyrosine-protein kinase FYN
CCNT1	1.000	CDK9/cyclin T1	VDR	0.370	Integrin alpha-IIb/beta-3
CCR5	1.000	C-C chemokine receptor type 5	RXRB	0.360	Retinoid X receptor beta
CASP6	1.000	Caspase-6	CHRNA7	0.300	Neuronal acetylcholine receptor protein alpha-7 subunit
BACE2	1.000	Beta secretase 2	INSR	0.270	Insulin receptor
NOS1	0.990	Nitric-oxide synthase, brain	NGFR	0.270	Low affinity neurotrophin receptor p75NTR
CHRNB4	0.990	Neuronal acetylcholine receptor; alpha4/beta4	FOS	0.240	Carbonic anhydrase II
GRIN2B	0.990	Glutamate NMDA receptor; GRIN1/GRIN2B	HTR2C	0.240	Serotonin 2c (5-HT2c) receptor

Table 3: contd....

Table 3: contd.

Gen	p(prot)	Protein	Gen	p(prot)	Protein
ENPP1	0.990	Ectonucleotide pyrophosphatase/ phosphodiesterase family member 1	C1R	0.230	Melanocortin receptor 1
CASP8	0.990	Caspase-8	CASP4	0.230	Caspase-4
IL1B	0.990	Caspase-1	NOS3	0.220	Nitric-oxide synthase, endothelial
ADRB1	0.990	Beta-1 adrenergic receptor	BIRC3	0.210	Baculoviral IAP repeat-containing protein 3
PLAU	0.980	Urokinase plasminogen activator surface receptor	CHRNA2	0.180	Neuronal acetylcholine receptor; alpha2/ beta4
PLG	0.980	Plasminogen	GRN	0.180	Cell division control protein 42 homolog
DRD4	0.980	Dopamine D4 receptor	CCR2	0.140	C-C chemokine receptor type 2
NR3C1	0.970	Glucocorticoid receptor	LPL	0.140	Alkaline phosphatase, tissue-nonspecific isozyme
CRP	0.970	ATP-binding cassette sub-family G member 2	CTSD	0.130	Cathepsin D
ALOX5	0.950	Arachidonate 5-lipoxygenase	FADD	0.130	Caspase-8
PRKAB2	0.940	AMP-activated protein kinase, alpha-1 subunit	NTRK1	0.110	Nerve growth factor receptor Trk-A
RXRA	0.930	Retinoid X receptor alpha	TNF	0.110	ADAM17
APP	0.920	Insulin-like growth factor I receptor	PTGS2	0.100	Cyclooxygenase-2
AKT2	0.910	Serine/threonine-protein kinase AKT2	FAS	0.070	Fatty acid synthase
CAV1	0.890	Voltage-gated L-type calcium channel alpha-1C subunit	CD36	0.070	Sphingosine 1-phosphate receptor Edg-1
CTSS	0.890	Cathepsin S	ADRA2A	0.060	Alpha-2a adrenergic receptor
ESR1	0.880	Estrogen receptor	PPARG	0.050	Peroxisome proliferator-activated receptor gamma
ESR2	0.870	Estrogen receptor beta	GSTP1	0.040	Glutathione S-transferase Pi
RXRG	0.850	Retinoid X receptor gamma	BDNF	0.040	Neurotrophic tyrosine kinase receptor type 2

Table 3: contd....

Table 3: contd.

Gen	p(prot)	Protein	Gen	p(prot)	Protein
TANK	0.840	Serine/threonine-protein kinase TBK1	CLU	0.030	Bcr/Abl fusion protein
TP53	0.840	Tumour suppressor p53/ oncoprotein Mdm2	CAV3	0.030	Voltage-gated T-type calcium channel alpha-1I subunit
LCK	0.830	Tyrosine-protein kinase LCK	FABP4	0.020	Fatty acid binding protein adipocyte
MMP3	0.810	Matrix metalloproteinase 3	BACE1	0.020	Beta-secretase 1
CHRNA4	0.800	Neuronal acetylcholine receptor; alpha4/beta2	TAP2	0.020	Methionine aminopeptidase 2
MME	0.790	Matrix metalloproteinase 12	SLK	0.020	Tyrosine-protein kinase FYN
NTRK2	0.790	Nerve growth factor receptor Trk-A	CHRNB2	0.010	Neuronal acetylcholine receptor; alpha4/beta2
BCL2	0.790	Bcl2-antagonist of cell death (BAD)	RFC1	0.010	Folate transporter 1
EIF2AK2	0.760	Interferon-induced, double-stranded RNA-activated protein kinase	BCR	0.010	Peroxisome proliferator-activated receptor alpha
MMP1	0.750	Matrix metalloproteinase 13	PARP1	0.000	Poly [ADP-ribose] polymerase-1
ACHE	0.730	Microtubule-associated protein tau	DAPK1	0.000	Death-associated protein kinase 1
PPARA	0.730	Peroxisome proliferator-activated receptor alpha	ALB	0.000	Cytochrome P450 3A4
CTSG	0.720	Granzyme B	GAPDH	0.000	Glyceraldehyde-3-phosphate dehydrogenase liver
SIRT1	0.720	NAD-dependent deacetylasesirtuin 1	GBA	0.000	Beta-glucocerebrosidase
SLC6A3	0.710	Dopamine transporter	HK2	0.000	Serine/threonine-protein kinase Chk2
ADRB2	0.600	Serotonin 1a (5-HT1a) receptor	PSAP	0.000	Phosphoribosyl pyrophosphate synthetase-associated protein 2
KCNJ11	0.570	Sulfonylurea receptor 2, Kir6.2	S100B	0.000	S-100 protein beta chain
REN	0.570	Apoptosis regulator Bcl-X	SNCA	0.000	Alpha-synuclein

[a]The equation p(prot) = 1 – p(Whelch) was introduced in this work to calculate the probability p(prot) of expression of a protein in the Hippocampus brain region of AD patients based on the probabilities p(Whelch).

$^{*}K_{ij}$ is a corrected constant of drug binding to the target protein introduced to in this work by first time. The definition of the parameter is $^{*}K_{ij} = p(error) \cdot p(prot) \cdot K_{ij}$. This value K_{ij} is the binding constant of the molecule M_i for the jth protein measured *in vitro* or *in vivo* but not in the Hippocampus brain region of AD patients (value reported in ChEMBL). The parameter p(error) measures the confidence of the value of K_{ij}. It does not measure the experimental error on the determination of K_{ij} but the probability of human error during the introduction of data on the dataset (data-collation error). This probability take the values p(error) = 1, 0.75, and 0.65 for the expert, intermediate, or auto-collation degrees of verification of the data point reported in ChEMBL. In Table 3, we show the values of probability of differential expression p(prot) of proteins in the Hippocampus brain region of AD patients.

The term p(prot) = 1 – p(Whelch) was introduced in this work to calculate the probability p(prot). The value p(prot) measure the probability of differential expression of the jth protein in the Hippocampus brain region of AD patients based on the probabilities p(Whelch). The p(Whelch) were determined experimentally by using a Welch's upper-tailed t-test from control to disease in six brain regions individually (including Hippocampus). A gene is significantly expressed for p(Whelch)-value < 0.05.

The other input terms are the following. The first, $\Delta PSA = PSA_{new} - PSA_{ref}$ is the perturbation term for the variation of Polar Surface Area (PSA) in the new molecule with respect to the molecule of reference. The other variational-perturbation terms are $\Delta\Delta LogP$ and $\Delta\Delta PSA$. These are at the same time typical terms of Perturbation Theory and Moving Average (MA) functions used in Box-Jenkin models in time series (Box and Jenkins 1970). These new types of terms account for both the deviation of the ClogP and PSA of all the new organic compounds with respect to compound of reference and with respect to all boundary conditions. For instance $\Delta\Delta PSA_{protein} = \Delta PSA_{ref} - \Delta PSA_{new} = [PSA(M_i)_{ref} - < PSA(M_i) >_{prot}] - [PSA(M_i)_{new} - < PSA(M_i) >_{new} >_{prot}]$. The quantities $< PSA(M_i)_{new} >_{prot}$ and $< PSA(M_i)_{ref} >_{prot}$ are the average values of PSA(Mi) for all molecules Mi assayed against the same protein than the new or reference compound. In the case, when the new and reference compound were assayed against the same protein $< PSA(M_i)_{new} >_{prot} = < PSA(M_i)_{ref} >_{prot}$.

The values of the terms of type $< PSA(M_i) >_{prot}$ have been calculated by us and tabulated for a large number of proteins. We must substitute the values of PSA(M$_i$) calculated for a new drug and the values of PSA(M$_i$) for known drugs of reference in the equation to predict $f(^{*}K_{ij})_{new}$. We also have to substitute the tabulated values of $< PSA(M_i) >_{prot}$ for different proteins. The situation is similar for the third term of the equation $\Delta\Delta LogP_{protein} = \Delta LogP_{ref} - \Delta LogP_{new} = [LogP(M_i)_{ref} - < LogP(M_i) >_{prot}] - [LogP(M_i)_{new} - < LogP(M_i)_{new} >_{prot}]$. The quantities $< LogP(M_i)_{new} >_{prot}$ and $< LogP(M_i)_{ref} >_{prot}$ are the average values of LogP(Mi) for all molecules Mi assayed against the same protein than the new or reference compound, respectively. In Table 4 we give some of these values of $< PSA(M_i) >_{prot}$ and $< LogP(M_i) >_{prot}$ for the proteins with the higher number of cases (n$_j$) in the dataset studied. For comparative purposes, we included the values of $< Mw(M_i) >_{prot}$; average value of molecular weight Mw for all compounds assayed against the same protein. The LogP values used here were calculated with the method ALogP for calculation of LogP values (see introduction).

Table 4: Values of $< D_k(M_i) >_{prot}$ for different molecular descriptor D_k = Mw, LogP, and PSA, for the proteins with the higher number of cases (n_j) in the dataset studied.

GEN	cases	$<D_k(M_i)>_{prot}$			GEN	cases	$<D_k(M_i)>_{prot}$		
symbol	n_j	MW	LogP	PSA	symbol	n_j	MW	LogP	PSA
INS	5562	404.33	2.90	107.02	GRIN2B	292	326.42	3.74	46.45
FOS	5137	340.84	0.59	137.47	PPARG	292	442.99	5.33	89.25
ADRB2	3352	389.31	3.95	57.26	CHRNA3	285	237.55	1.40	37.85
PLAT	2241	466.70	2.51	125.10	NOS1	266	233.62	0.97	95.45
MMP1	2071	464.41	2.50	132.15	MME	237	461.19	3.03	132.45
DRD4	2029	359.84	3.95	41.36	CHRNB4	223	237.66	1.29	37.51
FYN	1932	383.28	3.40	93.38	CCR5	210	540.21	4.38	61.15
SLC6A3	1753	334.48	3.88	36.94	ALB	202	411.85	4.07	79.28
HTR2C	1741	339.81	3.33	47.21	CCR2	186	478.16	5.11	83.39
LCK	1645	383.50	3.37	94.28	RXRA	174	400.54	6.74	53.24
SLK	1480	382.06	3.38	93.55	TAP2	153	284.22	3.27	82.41
GSK3B	1411	368.31	3.31	90.22	BCR	136	463.47	6.00	89.53
CSF1	993	371.01	3.26	91.57	PPARA	134	463.88	6.04	89.73
NR3C1	968	454.99	5.10	68.78	CASP3	131	516.89	1.61	186.56
BDNF	949	377.24	3.31	92.78	GBA	104	307.96	0.67	104.09
PRKAB2	936	376.94	3.31	92.88	RXRG	98	399.42	6.69	52.25
NTRK1	918	377.28	3.31	93.08	NOS3	97	217.04	1.05	76.46
NTRK2	918	377.28	3.31	93.08	RXRB	95	404.54	6.71	53.76
MMP3	915	465.63	2.62	127.05	TP53	92	534.77	5.04	81.56
PLAU	906	401.86	2.65	126.00	CCNT1	91	379.23	3.27	123.06
IGF1R	882	388.72	3.38	93.45	PIK3R1	66	503.69	0.85	146.87
APP	882	388.72	3.38	93.45	CTSG	49	558.08	2.07	154.20
C1R	870	585.87	4.75	91.56	BACE2	45	482.68	3.50	108.19
ADRA2A	833	354.92	3.28	55.93	FABP4	44	449.29	6.65	70.44
REN	832	573.55	5.74	132.12	CAV1	43	424.70	3.71	102.23
AKT2	813	374.29	3.22	94.23	TAP1	35	263.92	1.04	93.75
PLG	775	491.46	2.25	147.78	BIRC3	28	557.38	2.56	120.32
INSR	757	375.33	3.21	94.21	CASP8	20	448.65	1.72	155.84
HK2	711	378.50	3.31	93.86	FADD	20	448.65	1.72	155.84
CHRNA4	616	266.90	1.91	43.57	SNCA	19	297.60	3.65	75.38
CHRNB2	556	273.75	2.01	43.36	CASP6	17	459.87	1.55	165.77
TNF	544	443.64	2.12	116.00	CASP4	17	459.87	1.55	165.77
ESR1	514	418.82	5.85	62.45	KCNJ11	16	297.36	2.37	85.10

Table 4 contd....

Table 4 contd.

GEN	cases	$<D_k(M_i)>_{prot}$			GEN	cases	$<D_k(M_i)>_{prot}$		
symbol	n_j	MW	LogP	PSA	symbol	n_j	MW	LogP	PSA
CHRNA7	504	353.32	2.23	44.61	FAS	15	340.05	−1.48	148.26
CTSS	504	465.92	3.71	107.10	GSTP1	13	405.93	−1.72	167.38
BACE1	451	566.66	3.40	145.37	GAPDH	9	388.18	0.36	151.18
VDR	419	498.49	1.28	162.77	CHRNA2	8	224.99	1.40	37.86
ESR2	416	426.45	6.04	64.36	ACHE	8	376.67	3.99	56.67
PARP1	396	293.61	2.02	74.18	CD36	8	349.63	2.43	123.61
IL1B	328	489.87	1.58	148.16	ENPP1	8	536.12	−0.71	265.17
TANK	326	381.70	3.44	88.18	CLU	6	330.89	1.32	88.29
CTSD	316	657.47	3.54	153.69	LPL	6	246.97	1.92	60.63
ADRB1	294	411.20	2.93	97.11	PTGS2	5	351.89	4.07	72.25

Conclusions

We can develop linear and non-linear PT-QSBR models of drug-protein target interactome networks combining Hansch's chemoinformatic analysis with Perturbation Theory ideas. Multi-target PT-QSBR models are useful to classify drugs based on their constant of binding *in vitro* to many different proteins reported in ChEMBL and the experimental expression of these proteins in the Hippocampus region of the brain of AD patients. We can include quadratic (in analogy to Hansch's parabolic terms) or even higher-order terms in PT-QSBR models. However, the inclusion of these terms into the PT-QSBR models did not improved the accuracy of the model to fit the ChEMBL dataset studied. We can use the new PT-QSBR models to predict the interaction of new drugs with many different drug target proteins.

Acknowledgments

The authors acknowledge partial financial support from grants MINECO (CTQ2013-41229-P) and Xunta de Galicia (07CSA008203PR).

Supporting Information

Tables SM1−SM4 contain detailed results of the computational studies, available upon corresponding author's request at humberto.gonzalezdiaz@ehu.es.

References

Abuhamdah, S., M. Habash and M. O. Taha. 2013. Elaborate ligand-based modeling coupled with QSAR analysis and *in silico* screening reveal new potent acetylcholinesterase inhibitors. J. Comput. Aided Mol. Des. 27(12): 1075–92.

Aguero-Chapin, G., H. Gonzalez-Diaz, R. Molina, J. Varona-Santos, E. Uriarte and Y. Gonzalez-Diaz. 2006. Novel 2D maps and coupling numbers for protein sequences. The first QSAR study of polygalacturonases; isolation and prediction of a novel sequence from Psidium guajava L. FEBS Lett. 580(3): 723–30.

Aguero-Chapin, G., H. Gonzalez-Diaz, G. de la Riva, E. Rodriguez, A. Sanchez-Rodriguez, G. Podda et al. 2008. MMM-QSAR recognition of ribonucleases without alignment: comparison with an HMM model and isolation from Schizosaccharomyces pombe, prediction, and experimental assay of a new sequence. J. Chem. Inf. Model 48(2): 434–48.

Aguero-Chapin, G., J. Varona-Santos, G. A. de la Riva, A. Antunes, T. Gonzalez-Vlla, E. Uriarte et al. 2009. Alignment-free prediction of polygalacturonases with pseudofolding topological indices: experimental isolation from Coffea arabica and prediction of a new sequence. J. Proteome Res. 8(4): 2122–8.

Aguero-Chapin, G., G. Perez-Machado, R. Molina-Ruiz, Y. Perez-Castillo, A. Morales-Helguera, V. Vasconcelos et al. 2011. TI2BioP: Topological Indices to BioPolymers. Its practical use to unravel cryptic bacteriocin-like domains. Amino Acids 40(2): 431–42.

Allegri, R. F. and A. Guekht. 2012. Cerebrolysin improves symptoms and delays progression in patients with Alzheimer's disease and vascular dementia. In Drugs Today (Barc). United States: 2012 Prous Science, S.A.U. or its licensors.

Alonso, N., O. Caamano, F. J. Romero-Duran, F. Luan, M. N. Dias Soeiro Cordeiro, M. Yanez et al. 2013. Model for high-throughput screening of multi-target drugs in chemical neurosciences: synthesis, assay and theoretic study of rasagiline carbamates. ACS Chem. Neurosci. 4(10): 1393–1403.

Anighoro, A., D. Stumpfe, K. Heikamp, K. Beebe, L. M. Neckers, J. Bajorath et al. 2015. Computational polypharmacology analysis of the heat shock protein 90 interactome. J. Chem. Inf. Model. 55(3): 676–86.

Antolin, A. A. and J. Mestres. 2015. Distant polypharmacology among MLP chemical probes. ACS Chem. Biol. 10(2): 395–400.

Barman, A. and R. Prabhakar. 2012. Protonation states of the catalytic dyad of beta-secretase (BACE1) in the presence of chemically diverse inhibitors: a molecular docking study. J. Chem. Inf. Model. 52(5): 1275–87.

Bautista-Aguilera, O. M., G. Esteban, I. Bolea, K. Nikolic, D. Agbaba, I. Moraleda et al. 2014a. Design, synthesis, pharmacological evaluation, QSAR analysis, molecular modeling and ADMET of novel donepezil-indolyl hybrids as multipotent cholinesterase/monoamine oxidase inhibitors for the potential treatment of Alzheimer's disease. Eur. J. Med. Chem. 75: 82–95.

Bautista-Aguilera, O. M., G. Esteban, M. Chioua, K. Nikolic, D. Agbaba, I. Moraleda et al. 2014b. Multipotent cholinesterase/monoamine oxidase inhibitors for the treatment of Alzheimer's disease: design, synthesis, biochemical evaluation, ADMET, molecular modeling, and QSAR analysis of novel donepezil-pyridyl hybrids. Drug Des. Devel. Ther. 8: 1893–910.

Bonaiuto, E., A. Milelli, G. Cozza, V. Tumiatti, C. Marchetti, E. Agostinelli et al. 2013. Novel polyamine analogues: from substrates towards potential inhibitors of monoamine oxidases. Eur. J. Med. Chem. 70: 88–101.

Cai, Y. D., G. P. Zhou and K. C. Chou. 2003. Support vector machines for predicting membrane protein types by using functional domain composition. Biophys. J. 84(5): 3257–63.

Cai, Y. D. and K. C. Chou. 2005a. Predicting enzyme subclass by functional domain composition and pseudo amino acid composition. J. Proteome Res. 4(3): 967–71.

Cai, Y. D. and K. C. Chou. 2005b. Using functional domain composition to predict enzyme family classes. J. Proteome Res. 4(1): 109–11.

Casanola-Martin, G. M., H. Le-Thi-Thu, F. Perez-Gimenez, Y. Marrero-Ponce, C. Merino-Sanjuan, C. Abad et al. 2015. Multi-output model with Box-Jenkins operators of linear indices to predict multi-target inhibitors of ubiquitin-proteasome pathway. Mol. Divers. 19(2): 347–56.

Cereto-Massague, A., M. J. Ojeda, C. Valls, M. Mulero, G. Pujadas and S. Garcia-Vallve. 2015. Tools for *in silico* target fishing. Methods 71: 98–103.

Chakraborty, S., B. Ramachandran and S. Basu. 2014. Encompassing receptor flexibility in virtual screening using ensemble docking-based hybrid QSAR: discovery of novel phytochemicals for BACE1 inhibition. Mol. Biosyst. 10(10): 2684–92.

Chou, K. C. 2005. Prediction of G-protein-coupled receptor classes. J. Proteome Res. 4(4): 1413–8.

Chou, K. C. and H. B. Shen. 2006a. Predicting eukaryotic protein subcellular location by fusing optimized evidence-theoretic K-nearest neighbor classifiers. J. Proteome Res. 5: 1888–1897.

Chou, K. C. and H. B. Shen. 2006b. Large-scale predictions of Gram-negative bacterial protein subcellular locations. J. Proteome Res. 5: 3420–3428.

Chou, K. C. and Y. D. Cai. 2006. Predicting protein-protein interactions from sequences in a hybridization space. J. Proteome Res. 5(2): 316–22.

Chou, K. C. and H. B. Shen. 2007. Euk-mPLoc: a fusion classifier for large-scale eukaryotic protein subcellular location prediction by incorporating multiple sites. J. Proteome Res. 6: 1728–1734.

Chou, K. C. and H. B. Shen. 2008. Cell-PLoc: a package of Web servers for predicting subcellular localization of proteins in various organisms. Nat. Protoc. 3(2): 153–62.

Chou, K. C. and H. B. Shen. 2010. Plant-mPLoc: a top-down strategy to augment the power for predicting plant protein subcellular localization. PLoS ONE 5: e11335.

Coelho-Cerqueira, E., P. A. Netz, V. P. do Canto, A. C. Pinto and C. Follmer. 2014. Beyond topoisomerase inhibition: antitumor 1,4-naphthoquinones as potential inhibitors of human monoamine oxidase. Chem. Biol. Drug Des. 83(4): 401–10.

Compadre, C. M., C. Hansch, T. E. Klein and R. Langridge. 1990. The structure-activity relationship of the papain hydrolysis of N-benzoylglycine esters. Biochim. Biophys. Acta. 1038(2): 158–63.

Correa-Basurto, J., M. Bello, M. C. Rosales-Hernandez, M. Hernandez-Rodriguez, I. Nicolas-Vazquez, A. Rojo-Dominguez et al. 2014. QSAR, docking, dynamic simulation and quantum mechanics studies to explore the recognition properties of cholinesterase binding sites. Chem. Biol. Interact. 209: 1–13.

Cosconati, S., L. Marinelli, F. S. Di Leva, V. La Pietra, A. De Simone, F. Mancini et al. 2012. Protein flexibility in virtual screening: the BACE-1 case study. J. Chem. Inf. Model. 52(10): 2697–704.

Cruz, D. S. and M. S. Castilho. 2014. 2D QSAR studies on series of human beta-secretase (BACE-1) inhibitors. Med. Chem. 10(2): 162–73.

Csermely, P., T. Korcsmaros, H. J. Kiss, G. London and R. Nussinov. 2013. Structure and dynamics of molecular networks: A novel paradigm of drug discovery: a comprehensive review. Pharmacol. Ther. 138(3): 333–408.

Dominguez, J. L., F. Fernandez-Nieto, M. Castro, M. Catto, M. R. Paleo, S. Porto et al. 2015. Computer-aided structure-based design of multitarget leads for Alzheimer's disease. J. Chem. Inf. Model. 55(1): 135–48.

Erhan, D., J. L'Heureux P., S. Y. Yue and Y. Bengio. 2006. Collaborative filtering on a family of biological targets. J. Chem. Inf. Model. 46(2): 626–35.

Fang, Y. 2015. Combining label-free cell phenotypic profiling with computational approaches for novel drug discovery. Expert Opin. Drug Discov. 10(4): 331–43.

Ferino, G., E. Cadoni, M. J. Matos, E. Quezada, L. Santana et al. 2013. MAO inhibitory activity of 2-arylbenzofurans versus 3-arylcoumarins: synthesis, *in vitro* study, and docking calculations. ChemMedChem. 8(6): 956–66.

Fresqui, M. A., M. M. Ferreira and M. Trsic. 2013. The influence of R and S configurations of a series of amphetamine derivatives on quantitative structure-activity relationship models. Anal. Chim. Acta 759: 43–52.

Gao, L., J. S. Fang, X. Y. Bai, D. Zhou, Y. T. Wang, A. L. Liu et al. 2013. *In silico* target fishing for the potential targets and molecular mechanisms of baicalein as an antiparkinsonian agent: discovery of the protective effects on NMDA receptor-mediated neurotoxicity. Chem. Biol. Drug Des. 81(6): 675–87.

Garcia, I., Y. Fall, G. Gomez and H. Gonzalez-Diaz. 2011. First computational chemistry multi-target model for anti-Alzheimer, anti-parasitic, anti-fungi, and anti-bacterial activity of GSK-3 inhibitors *in vitro*, *in vivo*, and in different cellular lines. Mol. Divers. 15(2): 561–7.

Gaulton, A., L. J. Bellis, A. P. Bento, J. Chambers, M. Davies, A. Hersey et al. 2012. ChEMBL: a large-scale bioactivity database for drug discovery. Nucleic Acids Research 40(Database issue): D1100-7.

Gholivand, K., A. A. Ebrahimi Valmoozi and M. Bonsaii. 2014. Synthesis, biological evaluation, QSAR study and molecular docking of novel N-(4-amino carbonylpiperazinyl) (thio)phosphoramide derivatives as cholinesterase inhibitors. Pestic. Biochem. Physiol. 112: 40–50.

Ginman, T., J. Viklund, J. Malmstrom, J. Blid, R. Emond, R. Forsblom et al. 2013. Core refinement toward permeable beta-secretase (BACE-1) inhibitors with low hERG activity. J. Med. Chem. 56(11): 4181–205.

Gonzalez-Diaz, H., L. Saiz-Urra, R. Molina, L. Santana and E. Uriarte. 2007. A model for the recognition of protein kinases based on the entropy of 3D van der Waals interactions. J. Proteome Res. 6(2): 904–8.

Gonzalez-Diaz, H. 2008. Quantitative studies on Structure-Activity and Structure-Property Relationships (QSAR/QSPR). Curr. Top. Med. Chem. 8(18): 1554.

Gonzalez-Diaz, H., Y. Gonzalez-Diaz, L. Santana, F. M. Ubeira and E. Uriarte. 2008. Proteomics, networks and connectivity indices. Proteomics 8(4): 750–78.

Gonzalez-Diaz, H., F. Prado-Prado, X. Garcia-Mera, N. Alonso, P. Abeijon, O. Caamano et al. 2011a. MIND-BEST: web server for drugs and target discovery; design, synthesis, and assay of MAO-B inhibitors and theoretical-experimental study of G3PDH protein from Trichomonas gallinae. J. Proteome Res. 10(4): 1698–718.

Gonzalez-Diaz, H., F. Prado-Prado, E. Sobarzo-Sanchez, M. Haddad, S. Maurel Chevalley, A. Valentin et al. 2011b. NL MIND-BEST: a web server for ligands and proteins discovery—theoretic-experimental study of proteins of Giardia lamblia and new compounds active against Plasmodium falciparum. J. Theor. Biol. 276(1): 229–49.

Gonzalez-Diaz, H., S. Arrasate, A. Gomez-SanJuan, N. Sotomayor, E. Lete, L. Besada-Porto et al. 2013. General theory for multiple input-output perturbations in complex molecular systems. 1. Linear QSPR electronegativity models in physical, organic, and medicinal chemistry. Curr. Top. Med. Chem. 13(14): 1713–41.

Gonzalez-Diaz, H., S. Arrasate, A. G. Juan, N. Sotomayor, E. Lete, A. Speck-Planche et al. 2014a. Matrix trace operators: from spectral moments of molecular graphs and complex networks to perturbations in synthetic reactions, micelle nanoparticles, and drug ADME processes. Curr. Drug Metab. 15(4): 470–88.

Gonzalez-Diaz, H., D. M. Herrera-Ibata, A. Duardo-Sanchez, C. R. Munteanu, R. A. Orbegozo-Medina and A. Pazos. 2014b. ANN multiscale model of anti-HIV drugs activity vs. AIDS prevalence in the US at county level based on information indices of molecular graphs and social networks. J. Chem. Inf. Model. 54(3): 744–55.

Gonzalez-Diaz, H., L. G. Perez-Montoto and F. M. Ubeira. 2014c. Model for vaccine design by prediction of B-epitopes of IEDB given perturbations in peptide sequence, *in vivo* process, experimental techniques, and source or host organisms. J. Immunol. Res. 2014: 768515.

Hansch, C. and Steward, A. R. 1964. The use of substituent constants in the analysis of the structure-activity relationship in penicillin derivatives. J. Med. Chem. 7: 691–4.

Hansch, C., J. Y. Fukunaga and P. Y. Jow. 1977a. Quantitative structure-activity relationships of antimalarial and dihydrofolate reductase inhibition by quinazolines and 5-substituted benzyl-2,4-diaminopyrimidines. J. Med. Chem. 20(1): 96–102.

Hansch, C., C. Grieco, C. Silipo and A. Vittoria. 1977b. Quantitative structure-activity relationship of chymotrypsin-ligand interactions. J. Med. Chem. 20(11): 1420–35.

Hansch, C. 1979. The interaction of ligands with enzymes. A starting point in drug design. Farmaco [Sci.] 34(8): 729–42.

Heikamp, K. and J. Bajorath. 2011. Large-scale similarity search profiling of ChEMBL compound data sets. J. Chem. Inf. Model. 51(8): 1831–9.

Helguera, A. M., A. Perez-Garrido, A. Gaspar, J. Reis, F. Cagide, D. Vina et al. 2013. Combining QSAR classification models for predictive modeling of human monoamine oxidase inhibitors. Eur. J. Med. Chem. 59: 75–90.

Hossain, T., A. Mukherjee and A. Saha. 2014. Chemometric design to explore pharmacophore features of BACE inhibitors for controlling Alzheimer's disease. Mol Biosyst. 2015; 11(2): 549–57.

Howells, D. W., E. S. Sena, V. O'Collins and M. R. Macleod. 2012. Improving the efficiency of the development of drugs for stroke. Int. J. Stroke 7(5): 371–7.

Hsu, Y. Y., Y. J. Jong, Y. T. Lin, Y. T. Tseng, S. H. Hsu and Y. C. Lo. 2014. Nanomolar naloxone attenuates neurotoxicity induced by oxidative stress and survival motor neuron protein deficiency. Neurotox. Res. 25(3): 262–70. http://scorpio.biophysics.ismb.lon.ac.uk/scorpio.html.

Hu, Y. and J. Bajorath. 2010. Molecular scaffolds with high propensity to form multi-target activity cliffs. J. Chem. Inf. Model. 50(4): 500–10.

Huang, D., Y. Liu, B. Shi, Y. Li, G. Wang and G. Liang. 2013. Comprehensive 3D-QSAR and binding mode of BACE-1 inhibitors using R-group search and molecular docking. J. Mol. Graph Model. 45: 65–83.

Hung, M. S., Z. Xu, Y. Chen, E. Smith, J. H. Mao, D. Hsieh et al. 2013. Hematein, a casein kinase II inhibitor, inhibits lung cancer tumor growth in a murine xenograft model. Int. J. Oncol. 43(5): 1517–22.

Islam, M. R., A. Zaman, I. Jahan, R. Chakravorty and S. Chakraborty. 2013. *In silico* QSAR analysis of quercetin reveals its potential as therapeutic drug for Alzheimer's disease. J. Young Pharm. 5(4): 173–9.

Jain, Kewal K. 2011. The Handbook of Neuroprotection. Springer Science & Business Media. Basel, Switzerland.

Jang, S. W., X. Liu, C. B. Chan, D. Weinshenker, R. A. Hall, G. Xiao et al. 2009. Amitriptyline is a TrkA and TrkB receptor agonist that promotes TrkA/TrkB heterodimerization and has potent neurotrophic activity. Chem. Biol. 16(6): 644–56.

Jewison, T., Y. Su, F. M. Disfany, Y. Liang, C. Knox, A. Maciejewski et al. 2014. SMPDB 2.0: big improvements to the Small Molecule Pathway Database. Nucleic Acids Res. 42 (Database issue): D478–84.

Juarez-Jimenez, J., E. Mendes, C. Galdeano, C. Martins, D. B. Silva, J. Marco-Contelles et al. 2014. Exploring the structural basis of the selective inhibition of monoamine oxidase A by dicarbonitrile aminoheterocycles: role of Asn181 and Ile335 validated by spectroscopic and computational studies. Biochim. Biophys. Acta 2: 389–97.

Karsai, A., A. Nagy, A. Kengyel, Z. Martonfalvi, L. Grama, B. Penke et al. 2005. Effect of lysine-28 side-chain acetylation on the nanomechanical behavior of alzheimer amyloid beta 25–35 fibrils. J. Chem. Inf. Model. 45(6): 1641–6.

Kleandrova, V. V., F. Luan, H. Gonzalez-Diaz, J. M. Ruso, A. Melo, A. Speck-Planche et al. 2014a. Computational ecotoxicology: simultaneous prediction of ecotoxic effects of nanoparticles under different experimental conditions. Environ. Int. 73: 288–94.

Kleandrova, V. V., F. Luan, H. Gonzalez-Diaz, J. M. Ruso, A. Speck-Planche and M. N. Cordeiro. 2014b. Computational tool for risk assessment of nanomaterials: novel QSTR-perturbation model for simultaneous prediction of ecotoxicity and cytotoxicity of uncoated and coated nanoparticles under multiple experimental conditions. Environ. Sci. Technol. 48(24): 14686–94.

Klein, R., S. Q. Jing, V. Nanduri, E. O'Rourke and M. Barbacid. 1991. The trk proto-oncogene encodes a receptor for nerve growth factor. Cell 65(1): 189–97.

Korabecny, J., R. Dolezal, P. Cabelova, A. Horova, E. Hruba, J. Ricny et al. 2014. 7-MEOTA-donepezil like compounds as cholinesterase inhibitors: synthesis, pharmacological evaluation, molecular modeling and QSAR studies. Eur. J. Med. Chem. 82: 426–38.

Liu, H., L. Wang, M. Lv, R. Pei, P. Li, Z. Pei et al. 2014. AlzPlatform: an Alzheimer's disease domain-specific chemogenomics knowledgebase for polypharmacology and target identification research. J. Chem. Inf. Model. 54(4): 1050–60.

Liu, S., R. Fu, X. Cheng, S. P. Chen and L. H. Zhou. 2012. Exploring the binding of BACE-1 inhibitors using comparative binding energy analysis (COMBINE). BMC Struct. Biol. 12: 21.

Liu, X., Y. Xu, S. Li, Y. Wang, J. Peng, C. Luo et al. 2014. *In Silico* target fishing: addressing a "Big Data" problem by ligand-based similarity rankings with data fusion. J. Cheminform. 6: 33.

Luan, F., M. N. Cordeiro, N. Alonso, X. Garcia-Mera, O. Caamano, F. J. Romero-Duran et al. 2013. TOPS-MODE model of multiplexing neuroprotective effects of drugs and experimental-theoretic study of new 1,3-rasagiline derivatives potentially useful in neurodegenerative diseases. Bioorg. Med. Chem. 21(7): 1870–9.

Luan, F., V. V. Kleandrova, H. Gonzalez-Diaz, J. M. Ruso, A. Melo, A. Speck-Planche et al. 2014. Computer-aided nanotoxicology: assessing cytotoxicity of nanoparticles under diverse experimental conditions by using a novel QSTR-perturbation approach. Nanoscale 6(18): 10623–30.

Mandado, M., M. J. Gonzalez-Moa and R. A. Mosquera. 2007. Chemical graph theory and n-center electron delocalization indices: a study on polycyclic aromatic hydrocarbons. J. Comput. Chem. 28(10): 1625–33.

Mao, F., J. Chen, Q. Zhou, Z. Luo, L. Huang and X. Li. 2013. Novel tacrine-ebselen hybrids with improved cholinesterase inhibitory, hydrogen peroxide and peroxynitrite scavenging activity. Bioorg. Med. Chem. Lett. 23(24): 6737–42.

Marrero-Ponce, Y., R. Medina-Marrero, J. A. Castillo-Garit, V. Romero-Zaldivar, F. Torrens and E. A. Castro. 2005. Protein linear indices of the 'macromolecular pseudograph alpha-carbon atom adjacency matrix' in bioinformatics. Part 1: prediction of protein stability effects of a complete set of alanine substitutions in Arc repressor. Bioorg. Med. Chem. 13(8): 3003–15.

Martin, L. J. 2012. Biology of mitochondria in neurodegenerative diseases. *In*: Prog. Mol. Biol. Transl. Sci. Elsevier Inc., Netherlands.

Matos, M. J., S. Vilar, R. M. Gonzalez-Franco, E. Uriarte, L. Santana, C. Friedman, N. P. Tatonetti, D. Vina and J. A. Fontenla. 2013. Novel (coumarin-3-yl)carbamates as selective MAO-B inhibitors: synthesis, *in vitro* and *in vivo* assays, theoretical evaluation of ADME properties and docking study. Eur. J. Med. Chem. 63: 151–61.

Matos, M. J., P. Janeiro, R. M. Gonzalez Franco, S. Vilar, N. P. Tatonetti, L. Santana et al. 2014. Synthesis, pharmacological study and docking calculations of new benzo[f]coumarin derivatives as dual inhibitors of enzymatic systems involved in neurodegenerative diseases. Future Med. Chem. 6(4): 371–83.

Mok, N. Y. and R. Brenk. 2011. Mining the ChEMBL database: an efficient chemoinformatics workflow for assembling an ion channel-focused screening library. J. Chem. Inf. Model. 51(10): 2449–54.

Molina, E., E. Sobarzo-Sanchez, A. Speck-Planche, M. J. Matos, E. Uriarte, L. Santana et al. 2012. Monoamino Oxidase A: an interesting pharmacological target for the development of multi-target QSAR. Mini Rev. Med. Chem. 12(10): 947–58.

Morales-Camilo, N., C. O. Salas, C. Sanhueza, C. Espinosa-Bustos, S. Sepulveda-Boza, M. Reyes-Parada et al. 2014. Synthesis, biological evaluation, and molecular simulation of chalcones and aurones as selective MAO-B inhibitors. Chem. Biol. Drug Des. 23(10): 12458.

Morris, H. R., A. J. Waite, N. M. Williams, J. W. Neal and D. J. Blake. 2012. Recent advances in the genetics of the ALS-FTLD complex. Curr. Neurol. Neurosci. Rep. 12(3): 243–50.

Munteanu, C. R., J. M. Vazquez, J. Dorado, A. P. Sierra, A. Sanchez-Gonzalez, F. J. Prado-Prado et al. 2009. Complex network spectral moments for ATCUN motif DNA cleavage: first predictive study on proteins of human pathogen parasites. J. Proteome Res. 8(11): 5219–28.

Namasivayam, V., Y. Hu, J. Balfer and J. Bajorath. 2013. Classification of compounds with distinct or overlapping multi-target activities and diverse molecular mechanisms using emerging chemical patterns. J. Chem. Inf. Model 53 (6): 1272–81.

Nantasenamat, C. and V. Prachayasittikul. 2015. Maximizing computational tools for successful drug discovery. Expert Opin. Drug Discov., pp. 1–9.

Nastase, A. F. and D. B. Boyd. 2012. Simple structure-based approach for predicting the activity of inhibitors of beta-secretase (BACE1) associated with Alzheimer's disease. J. Chem. Inf. Model. 52(12): 3302–7.

Nino, H., J. E. Rodriguez-Borges, X. Garcia-Mera and F. Prado-Prado. 2012. Review of synthesis, assay, and prediction of beta and gamma-secretase inhibitors. Curr. Top. Med. Chem. 12(8): 828–44.

Nurisso, A., C. Simoes-Pires, S. Martel, D. Cressend, A. Guillot and P. A. Carrupt. 2012. How to increase the safety and efficacy of compounds against neurodegeneration? A multifunctional approach. Chimia (Aarau) 66(5): 286–90.

Olsson, Tjelvar S. G., Mark A. Williams, William R. Pitt and John E. Ladbury. 2008. The Thermodynamics of Protein-Ligand Interaction and Solvation: Insights for Ligand Design. J. Mol. Biol. 384(4): 1002–1017.

Park, N. H. 2012. Parkinson disease. JAAPA 25(5): 73–4.

Perez-Nueno, V. I., A. S. Karaboga, M. Souchet and D. W. Ritchie. 2014. GES polypharmacology fingerprints: a novel approach for drug repositioning. J. Chem. Inf. Model. 54(3): 720–34.

Pettersson, F., P. Svensson, S. Waters, N. Waters and C. Sonesson. 2013. Synthesis, pharmacological evaluation and QSAR modeling of mono-substituted 4-phenylpiperidines and 4-phenylpiperazines. Eur. J. Med. Chem. 62: 241–55.

Pisani, L., M. Barletta, R. Soto-Otero, O. Nicolotti, E. Mendez-Alvarez, M. Catto et al. 2013. Discovery, biological evaluation, and structure-activity and -selectivity relationships of 6'-substituted (E)-2-(benzofuran-3(2H)-ylidene)-N-methylacetamides, a novel class of potent and selective monoamine oxidase inhibitors. J. Med. Chem. 56(6): 2651–64.

Pisani, L., R. Farina, O. Nicolotti, D. Gadaleta, R. Soto-Otero, M. Catto et al. 2015. *In silico* design of novel 2H-chromen-2-one derivatives as potent and selective MAO-B inhibitors. Eur. J. Med. Chem. 89: 98–105.

Prado-Prado, F., X. Garcia-Mera, M. Escobar, E. Sobarzo-Sanchez, M. Yanez, P. Riera-Fernandez et al. 2011. 2D MI-DRAGON: a new predictor for protein-ligands interactions and theoretic-experimental studies of US FDA drug-target network, oxoisoaporphine inhibitors for MAO-A and human parasite proteins. Eur. J. Med. Chem. 46(12): 5838–51.

Prado-Prado, F., X. Garcia-Mera, M. Escobar, N. Alonso, O. Caamano, M. Yanez et al. 2012. 3D MI-DRAGON: new model for the reconstruction of US FDA drug-target network and theoretical-experimental studies of inhibitors of rasagiline derivatives for AChE. Curr. Top. Med. Chem. 12(16): 1843–65.

Reutlinger, M., T. Rodrigues, P. Schneider and G. Schneider. 2014. Multi-objective molecular *de novo* design by adaptive fragment prioritization. Angew. Chem. Int. Ed. Engl. 53(16): 4244–8.

Rodriguez-Soca, Y., C. R. Munteanu, J. Dorado, A. Pazos, F. J. Prado-Prado and H. Gonzalez-Diaz. 2010. Trypano-PPI: a web server for prediction of unique targets in trypanosome proteome by using electrostatic parameters of protein-protein interactions. J. Proteome Res. 9(2): 1182–90.

Romero Duran, F. J., N. Alonso, O. Caamano, X. Garcia-Mera, M. Yanez, F. J. Prado-Prado et al. 2014. Prediction of multi-target networks of neuroprotective compounds with entropy indices and synthesis, assay, and theoretical study of new asymmetric 1,2-rasagiline carbamates. Int. J. Mol. Sci. 15(9): 17035–64.

Roos, K., J. Viklund, J. Meuller, K. Kaspersson and M. Svensson. 2014. Potency prediction of beta-secretase (BACE-1) inhibitors using density functional methods. J. Chem. Inf. Model. 54(3): 818–25.

Sahin, M. E., T. Can and C. D. Son. 2014. GPCRsort-responding to the next generation sequencing data challenge: prediction of G protein-coupled receptor classes using only structural region lengths. OMICS 18(10): 636–44.

Salgin-Goksen, U., N. Gokhan-Kelekci, S. Yabanoglu-Ciftci, K. Yelekci and G. Ucar. 2013. Synthesis, molecular modeling, and *in vitro* screening of monoamine oxidase inhibitory activities of some novel hydrazone derivatives. J. Neural. Transm. 120(6): 883–91.

Salmon, S. A. and J. L. Watts. 2000. Minimum inhibitory concentration determinations for various antimicrobial agents against 1570 bacterial isolates from turkey poults. Avian Diseases 44(1): 85–98.

Santana, L., E. Uriarte, H. González-Díaz, G. Zagotto, R. Soto-Otero and E. Mendez-Alvarez. 2006. A QSAR model for *in silico* screening of MAO-A inhibitors. Prediction, synthesis, and biological assay of novel coumarins. J. Med. Chem. 49(3): 1149–56.

Santana, L., H. Gonzalez-Diaz, E. Quezada, E. Uriarte, M. Yanez, D. Vina et al. 2008. Quantitative structure-activity relationship and complex network approach to monoamine oxidase a and B inhibitors. J. Med. Chem. 51(21): 6740–51.

Sen, A., D. N. Dimlich, K. G. Guruharsha, M. W. Kankel, K. Hori, T. Yokokura et al. 2013. Genetic circuitry of Survival motor neuron, the gene underlying spinal muscular atrophy. Proc. Natl. Acad. Sci. USA 110(26): E2371–80.

Shaikh, S., A. Verma, S. Siddiqui, S. S. Ahmad, S. M. Rizvi, S. Shakil et al. 2014. Current acetylcholinesterase-inhibitors: a neuroinformatics perspective. CNS Neurol. Disord. Drug Targets 13(3): 391–401.

Sopkova-de Oliveira Santos, J., A. Lesnard, J. H. Agondanou, N. Dupont, A. M. Godard, S. Stiebing et al. 2010. Virtual screening discovery of new acetylcholinesterase inhibitors issued from CERMN chemical library. J. Chem. Inf. Model. 50(3): 422–8.

Speck-Planche, A., V. V. Kleandrova, F. Luan and M. N. Cordeiro. 2012a. Chemoinformatics in multi-target drug discovery for anti-cancer therapy: *in silico* design of potent and versatile anti-brain tumor agents. Anti-cancer Agents Med. Chem. 12(6): 678–85.

Speck-Planche, A., V. V. Kleandrova, F. Luan and M. N. Cordeiro. 2011b. Multi-target drug discovery in anti-cancer therapy: fragment-based approach toward the design of potent and versatile anti-prostate cancer agents. Bioorg. Med. Chem. 19(21): 6239–44.

Speck-Planche, A. and V. V. Kleandrova. 2012. *In silico* design of multi-target inhibitors for C-C chemokine receptors using substructural descriptors. Mol. Divers. 16(1): 183–91.

Speck-Planche, A., F. Luan and M. N. Cordeiro. 2012. Role of ligand-based drug design methodologies toward the discovery of new anti-alzheimer agents: futures perspectives in fragment-based ligand design. Curr. Med. Chem. 19(11): 1635–45.

Tang, J. and T. Aittokallio. 2014. Network pharmacology strategies toward multi-target anticancer therapies: from computational models to experimental design principles. Curr. Pharm. Des. 20(1): 23–36.

Tenorio-Borroto, E., X. Garcia-Mera, C. G. Penuelas-Rivas, J. C. Vasquez-Chagoyan, F. J. Prado-Prado, N. Castanedo et al. 2013. Entropy model for multiplex drug-target interaction endpoints of drug immunotoxicity. Curr. Top. Med. Chem. 13(14): 1636–49.

Tenorio-Borroto, E., F. R. Ramirez, A. Speck-Planche, M. N. Cordeiro, F. Luan and H. Gonzalez-Diaz. 2014. QSPR and flow cytometry analysis (QSPR-FCA): review and new findings on parallel study of multiple interactions of chemical compounds with immune cellular and molecular targets. Curr. Drug Metab. 15(4): 414–28.

Tripathi, R. K., O. Goshain and S. R. Ayyannan. 2013. Design, synthesis, *in vitro* MAO-B inhibitory evaluation, and computational studies of some 6-nitrobenzothiazole-derived semicarbazones. ChemMedChem. 8(3): 462–74.

Trushina, E. and C. T. McMurray. 2007. Oxidative stress and mitochondrial dysfunction in neurodegenerative diseases. Neuroscience 145: 1233–1248.

Valasani, K. R., J. R. Vangavaragu, V. W. Day and S. S. Yan. 2014. Structure based design, synthesis, pharmacophore modeling, virtual screening, and molecular docking studies for identification of novel cyclophilin D inhibitors. J. Chem. Inf. Model. 54(3): 902–12.

Vergara-Galicia, J., F. J. Prado-Prado and H. Gonzalez-Diaz. 2014. Galvez-Markov network transferability indices: review of classic theory and new model for perturbations in metabolic reactions. Curr. Drug Metab. 15(5): 557–64.

Vijayan, R. S., M. Prabu, N. M. Mascarenhas and N. Ghoshal. 2009. Hybrid structure-based virtual screening protocol for the identification of novel BACE1 inhibitors. J. Chem. Inf. Model. 49(3): 647–57.

Vilar, S., G. Ferino, E. Quezada, L. Santana and C. Friedman. 2012. Predicting monoamine oxidase inhibitory activity through ligand-based models. Curr. Top. Med. Chem. 12(20): 2258–74.

Vina, D., E. Uriarte, F. Orallo and H. Gonzalez-Diaz. 2009. Alignment-free prediction of a drug-target complex network based on parameters of drug connectivity and protein sequence of receptors. Mol. Pharm. 6(3): 825–35.

Vishnu Nayak, B., S. Ciftci-Yabanoglu, S. S. Jadav, M. Jagrat, B. N. Sinha, G. Ucar et al. 2013. Monoamine oxidase inhibitory activity of 3,5-biaryl-4,5-dihydro-1H-pyrazole-1-carboxylate derivatives. Eur. J. Med. Chem. 69: 762–7.

Wang, L., G. Esteban, M. Ojima, O. M. Bautista-Aguilera, T. Inokuchi, I. Moraleda et al. 2014. Donepezil + propargylamine + 8-hydroxyquinoline hybrids as new multifunctional metal-chelators, ChE and MAO inhibitors for the potential treatment of Alzheimer's disease. Eur. J. Med. Chem. 80: 543–61.

Xi, J., X. Zhu, Y. Feng, N. Huang, G. Luo, Y. Mao et al. 2013. Development of a novel class of tubulin inhibitors with promising anticancer activities. Mol. Cancer Res. 11(8): 856–64.

Yang, Y., J. Shen, X. Yu, G. Qin, M. Zhang, H. Shen et al. 2013. Identification of an inhibitory mechanism of luteolin on the insulin-like growth factor-1 ligand-receptor interaction. Chembiochem. 14(8): 929–33.

Yildirim, M. A., K. I. Goh, M. E. Cusick, A. L. Barabasi and M. Vidal. 2007. Drug-target network. Nature Biotechnology 25(10): 1119–26.

Zaheer-ul, H., R. Uddin, H. Yuan, P. A. Petukhov, M. I. Choudhary and J. D. Madura. 2008. Receptor-based modeling and 3D-QSAR for a quantitative production of the butyrylcholinesterase inhibitors based on genetic algorithm. J. Chem. Inf. Model. 48(5): 1092–103.

Zhang, P. and V. Brusic. 2014. Mathematical modeling for novel cancer drug discovery and development. Expert Opin. Drug Discov. 9(10): 1133–50.

Zhang, S., A. Golbraikh and A. Tropsha. 2006. Development of quantitative structure-binding affinity relationship models based on novel geometrical chemical descriptors of the protein-ligand interfaces. J. Med. Chem. 49: 2713–2724.

Zheng, H., J. Hou, M. D. Zimmerman, A. Wlodawer and W. Minor. 2014. The future of crystallography in drug discovery. Expert Opin. Drug Discov. 9(2): 125–37.

Zhou, C., D. Kang, Y. Xu, L. Zhang and X. Zha. 2014. Identification of novel selective lysine-specific demethylase 1 (LSD1) inhibitors using a pharmacophore-based virtual screening combined with docking. Chem. Biol. Drug Des. 23(10): 12461.

12

Structural Modeling for DNA and RNA Bindings to Breast Anticancer Drug Tamoxifen and Its Metabolites

H. A. Tajmir-Riahi,[1,*] *P. Bourassa*[2] and *T. J. Thomas*[3]

Abstract

In this chapter we have compared the structural models developed for the bindings of the breast antitumor drugs tamoxifen, 4-hydroxytamoxifen, and endoxifen with DNA and tRNA. Multiple spectroscopic methods and molecular modeling were used to characterize the drug binding sites, binding constant, and the effect of drug binding on DNA and tRNA stability and conformation. Structural analysis showed that tamoxifen and its metabolites bind DNA and tRNA *via* hydrophobic and hydrophilic interactions with tRNA forming more stable drug adducts than DNA and 4-hydroxytamoxifen forms stronger conjugate with polynucleotides. The negative free binding energy showed that drug complexation is spontaneous at room temperature.

[1] Department of Chemistry-Biochemistry and Physics, TR (Quebec), Canada G9A 5H7.
[2] Department of Chemistry-Biochemistry and Physics, University of Québec at Trois-Rivières, TR (Quebec) Canada G9A 5H7.
   E-mail: philippe.bourassa@gmail.com
[3] Department of Medicine, Rutgers Robert Wood Johnson Medical School and Rutgers Cancer Institute of New Jersey, New Brunswick, NJ 08901, USA.
   E-mail: thomastj@rwjms.rutgers.edu
* Corresponding author: tajmirri@uqtr.ca

Drug conjugation did not alter DNA and tRNA conformations, while major biopolymer aggregation occurred at high drug concentrations. The drug binding mode is correlated with the mechanism of action of antitumor activity of tamoxifen and its metabolites.

Introduction

Breast anticancer drug tamoxifen is a selective estrogen receptor modulator (SERMs), and is the most widely used breast cancer drug in pre- and post-menopausal women (Jordan 2006; Hughes-Davis et al. 2009; Sheen and Costantino 2008; Hayes 2009; Nabholtz and Gligorov 2006; Jordan 2008). Its target is the estrogen receptor α (ERα), the specific receptor of the female sex hormone, estradiol (Jordan 2003; Thomas et al. 2004). Estardiol is implicated in the origin and progression of breast cancer (Yue et al. 2013). The binding of estradiol with ERα-triggers a cascade of events, culminating in the transcription of estrogen-responsive genes, some of which contribute to the progression of breast tumor growth (O'Malley and Kumar 2009). Approximately 75% of breast tumors are the ERα-positive, and two-third of these tumors respond to tamoxifen and other SERMs (Rose-Innes et al. 2012). Tamoxifen exerts its action as a breast cancer drug/chemoprevention agent by antagonizing the action of estradiol, by its binding to the ligand binding domain of ERα and provoking a conformational state of the protein that is incapable of binding to the ERE (Ahn and Sheen 1997). However, tamoxifen is capable of triggering the effects of ERα in a tissue-specific manner in conjunction with coactivator proteins. Thus tamoxifen causes endometrial cancers in some patients (Bland et al. 2009).

Tamoxifen is metabolized in humans by the action of CYP2D6 and CYP3A4/5 enzymes, respectively, to 4-hydroxytamoxifen and N-desmethyltamoxifen (Jordan 2007; Lien et al. 1991; Furlanut et al. 2007). These metabolites are further converted to endoxifen (Scheme 1) by the action of CYP2D6 and CYP3A4/5 (Hoskins et al. 2009; Schroth et al. 2009; Bijil et al. 2009). 4-Hydroxytamoxifen and endoxifen are potent antiestrogens *in vitro* and have been used to understand the mechanism of action of tamoxifen using breast cancer cell culture models (Wu et al. 2009; Wiseman et al. 1993).

Tamoxifen is an antiestrogen and it acts on the ERα in target tissues. Approximately 75% of all breast tumors are ERα-positive; however, tamoxifen is effective in only two-third of this population. The female sex hormone, estradiol plays an important role in the induction and progression of breast cancer by its binding to the ERα and provoking a conformational state of the receptor for facile binding to coactivator proteins and recognition of the estrogen response element (ERE), that is present in the promoter/enhancer elements of estrogen-responsive genes (Thomas et al. 2004; Yue et al. 2013). In breast cancer, ERα binding to the ERE triggers a cascade of gene expression, leading to cell cycle regulation and cell proliferation.

Recent research has focused on the important role of RNA in transcriptional control and the mechanism of drug action. It has been known for a long time that tamoxifen and its metabolites form adducts with DNA, resulting in hepatic toxicity in rats and mice. Tamoxifen forms DNA adducts in the human colon after administration of a single therapeutic dose (Yue et al. 2013). A comparison of DNA

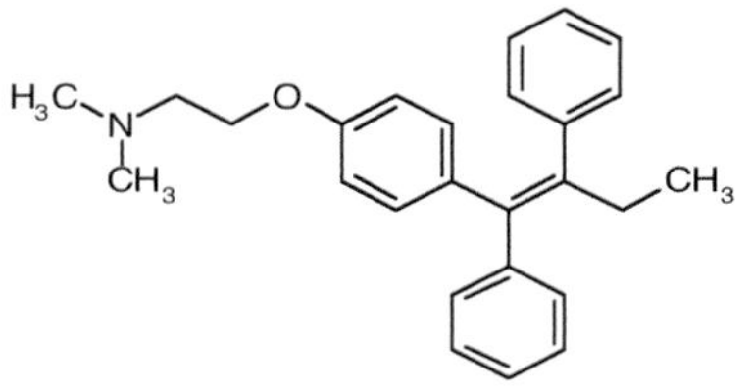

Tamoxifen

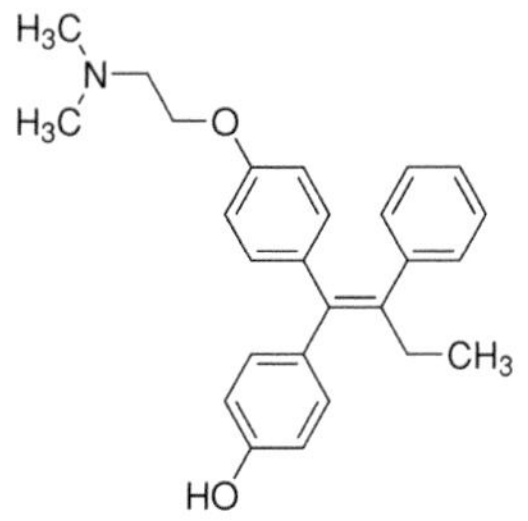

4-hydroxytamoxifen

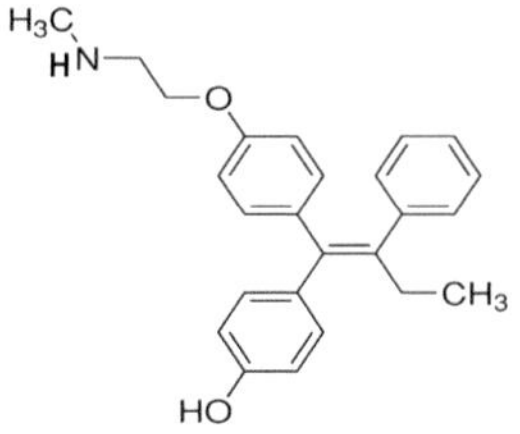

Endoxifen

Scheme 1: Chemical structures of tamoxifen, 4-hydroxytamoxifen and endoxifen.

adduct formation by tamoxifen and 4-hydroxytamoxifen *in vivo* has been reported (Randreath et al. 1994). We reported that tamoxifen and its metabolites, 4-hydroxy tamoxifen and endoxifen dock with DNA and tRNA as a first step in adduct formation (Bourassa et al. 2014a; Bourassa et al. 2014b). Therefore, considering the emerging role of RNA as a regulator of drug action and DNA as a target of antitumor drugs we compared the binding affinity of tamoxifen for DNA and tRNA using spectroscopic and molecular modeling approaches.

Analytical Methods

Molecular modeling

The docking studies were performed with ArgusLab 4.0.1 software (Mark A. Thompson, Planaria Software LLC, Seattle, Wa, http://www.arguslab.com). The structures of DNA and tRNA were obtained from the PDB (ID: 6TNA) (Privé et al. 1991; Sussman et al. 1978) and the three dimensional structure of drugs were generated from PM3 semi-empirical calculations using Chem3D Ultra 6.0. The docking runs were performed on the ArgusDock docking engine using high precision with a maximum of 150 candidate poses. The conformations were ranked using the Ascore scoring function, which estimates the free binding energy.

FTIR spectroscopy

Infrared spectra were recorded on a FTIR spectrometer (Impact 420 model), equipped with DTGS (deuterated triglycinesulfate) detector and KBr beam splitter, using AgBr windows. Spectra were collected after 2 h incubation of polymer with the DNA solution and measured. Interferograms were accumulated over the spectral range 4000–600 cm^{-1} with a nominal resolution of 2 cm^{-1} and a minimum of 100 scans. The difference spectra [(DNA solution + polymer) – (DNA solution)] were obtained, using a sharp band at 968 (DNA) as internal reference. This band, which is due to sugar C-C stretching vibrations, exhibits no spectral changes (shifting or intensity variations) upon polymer-polynucleotide complexation, and cancelled out upon spectral subtraction (Alex and Dupuis 1989).

CD spectroscopy

The CD spectra of DNA and its polymer adducts were recorded at pH 7.3 with a Jasco J-720 spectropolarimeter. For measurements in the Far-UV region (200–320 nm), a quartz cell with a path length of 0.01 cm was used. Six scans were accumulated at a scan speed of 50 nm per minute, with data being collected at every nm from 200 to 320 nm. Sample temperature was maintained at 25°C using a Neslab RTE-111 circulating water bath connected to the water-jacketed quartz cuvette. Spectra were corrected for buffer signal and conversion to the Mol CD ($\Delta\varepsilon$) was performed with the Jasco Standard Analysis software (Marty et al. 2009a; Marty et al. 2009b).

UV absorption spectroscopy

The absorption spectra were recorded on a Perkin Elmer Lambda 40 Spectrophotometer with a slit of 2 nm and scan speed of 240 nm min^{-1}. Quartz cuvettes of 1 cm were used. The absorbance assessments were performed at pH 7.3 by keeping the concentration of DNA constant (125 μM), while varying polymer contents (5 to 100 μM). The binding constants of polymer-DNA adducts were calculated as reported (Marty et al. 2009a; Connors 1987).

It is assumed that the interaction between the ligand L and the substrate S is 1:1; for this reason a single complex SL (1:1) is formed. It was also assumed that the sites (and all the binding sites) are independent and finally the Beer's law is followed by all species. A wavelength is selected at which the molar absorptivities ε_S (molar absorptivity of the substrate) and ε_{11} (molar absorptivity of the complex) are different. Then at total concentration S_t of the substrate, in the absence of ligand and the light path length is $b = 1$ cm, the solution absorbance is:

$$A_o = \varepsilon_S b S_t \tag{1}$$

In the presence of ligand at total concentration L_t, the absorbance of a solution containing the same total substrate concentration is:

$$A_L = \varepsilon_S b[S] + \varepsilon_L b[L] + \varepsilon_{11} b[SL] \tag{2}$$

(where [S] is the concentration of the uncomplexed substrate, [L] the concentration of the uncomplexed ligand and [SL] is the concentration of the complex) which, combined with the mass balance on S and L, gives:

$$A_L = \varepsilon_S b S_t + \varepsilon_L b L_t + \Delta\varepsilon_{11} b[SL] \tag{3}$$

where $\Delta\varepsilon_{11} = \varepsilon_{11} - \varepsilon_S - \varepsilon_L$ (ε_L molar absorptivity of the ligand). By measuring the solution absorbance against a reference containing ligand at the same total concentration L_t, the measured absorbance becomes:

$$A = \varepsilon_S b S_t + \Delta\varepsilon_{11} b[SL] \tag{4}$$

Combining equation (4) with the stability constant definition $K_{11} = [SL]/[S][L]$, gives:

$$\Delta A = K_{11}\Delta\varepsilon_{11} b[S][L] \tag{5}$$

where $\Delta A = A - A_o$. From the mass balance expression $S_t = [S] + [SL]$ we get $[S] = S_t/(1 + K_{11}[L])$, which is equation (5), giving equation (6) at the relationship between the observed absorbance change per centimeter and the system variables and parameters.

$$\frac{\Delta A}{b} = \frac{S_t K_{11} \Delta\varepsilon_{11}[L]}{1 + K_{11}[L]} \tag{6}$$

Equation (6) is the binding isotherm, which shows the hyperbolic dependence on free ligand concentration.

The double-reciprocal form of plotting the rectangular hyperbola $\frac{1}{y} = \frac{f}{d} \cdot \frac{1}{x} + \frac{e}{d}$, is based on the linearization of equation (6) according to the following equation:

$$\frac{b}{\Delta A} = \frac{1}{S_t K_{11}\Delta\varepsilon_{11}[L]} + \frac{1}{S_t\Delta\varepsilon_{11}} \tag{7}$$

Thus the double reciprocal plot of $1/\Delta A$ versus $1/[L]$ is linear and the binding constant can be estimated from the following equation:

$$K_{11} = \frac{intercept}{slope} \tag{8}$$

Fluorescence spectroscopy

Fluorimetric experiments were carried out on a Perkin-Elmer LS55 Spectrometer. Stock solution of drug (30 µM) in Tris-HCl (pH 7.4) was also prepared at 24 ± 1°C. DNA solutions (1 to 200 µM) were prepared from a stock solution by successive dilutions at 24 ± 1°C. Samples containing 0.06 ml of the drug solution and various DNA solutions were mixed to obtain final DNA concentrations ranging from 1 to 200 µM with constant drug content (30 µM). The fluorescence spectra were recorded at $\lambda_{ex} = 275$ nm and λ_{em} from 300 to 450 nm. The intensity of the band at 375 nm of tamoxifen and its metabolites (Engelke et al. 2001; Agudelo et al. 2013a) was used to calculate the binding constant (K), according to a previously reported method (Lakowics 2006).

Binding Analysis of Synthetic Polymer-DNA Adducts

Docking studies for drug adducts with DNA and tRNA

The docking results for drug bindings to DNA and tRNA are shown in Fig. 1 and Table 1. In drug-DNA adducts, tamoxifen was surrounded by C1, C2, T3, C4, T5, C18, C19, A20, G21, A22, and G23 with the free binding energy of –3.85 kcal/mol (Fig. 1A and Table 1). 4-hydroxytamoxifen was located in the vicinity of C4, T5, G6, G7, T8, G16, A17, C18, C19, and A20 with the free binding energy of –4.18 kcal/mol, while endoxifen was close to C4, T5, G6, G7, C18, and C19 with the free binding energy of –3.74 kcal/mol (Fig. 1A and Table 1). The binding energies (ΔG) show more stable complexes formed with 4-hydroxytamoxifen than tamoxifen and endoxifen.

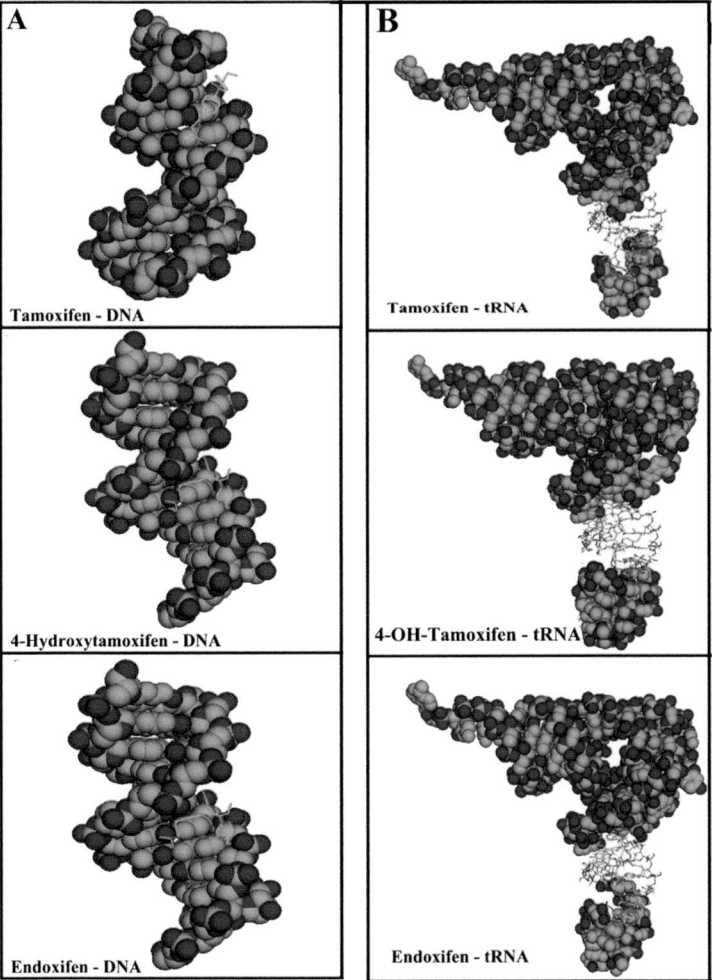

Fig. 1: Best docking positions for DNA (A) and tRNA (B) with tamoxifen, 4-hydroxytamoxifen and (C) endoxifen.

Table 1. Nucleobases involved in the interactions of tamoxifen and its metabolites with DNA and tRNA adducts with the free binding energies.

Complexes	Nucleobases involved in drug-DNA interaction	$\Delta G_{binding}$ (kcal/mol)
Tamoxifen - DNA	C1, C2, T3, C4, T5, C18, C19, A20, G21, A22, G23	−3.85
4-Hydroxytamoxifen - DNA	C4, T5, G6, G7, T8, G16, A17, C18, C19, A20	−4.18
Endoxifen - DNA	C4, T5, G6, G7, C18, C19	−3.74
Tamoxifen - tRNA	A29, A38, C25, C27, C28, C40, G26, G42, G43, U39, U41	−4.31
4-Hydroxytamoxifen - tRNA	A23, A29, A44, C25, C27, C28, C40, G24, G26 G42*, G43, G45, U41	−4.45
Endoxifen - tRNA	A23, A44, C25, C27, C28, C40, G26, G42*, G43, G45, U39, U41	−4.38

*Hydrogen bonding was observed with these nucleobases

In the drug-tRNA complexes, tamoxifen is surrounded by A29, A38, C25, C27, C28, C40, G26, G42, G43, U39, and U41 with the free binding energy of -4.31 kcal/mol, while 4-hydroxytamoxifen was located in the vicinity of A23, A29, A44, C25, C27, C28, C40, G24, G26, G42*, G43, G45, and U41 with the free binding energy of −4.45 kcal/mol (Fig. 1B and Table 1). Endoxifen was close to A23, A44, C25, C27, C28, C40, G26, G42*, G43, G45, U39, and U41 with the free binding energy of −4.38 kcal/mol (Fig. 6 and Table 2). The binding energies (ΔG) show more stable complexes formed with 4-hydroxytamoxifen than tamoxifen and endoxifen, which is consistent with those of drug-DNA adducts (Table 1). However, the presence of H-bonding network between G42* and drug OH group in 4-hydroxytamoxifen and endoxifen stabilizes drug-tRNA complexation (not present in drug-DNA adducts) (Table 1). It should be noted that most of the bound nucleobases are common in tamoxifen, 4-hydroxytamoxifen and endoxifen-DNA and tRNA complexes (Table 1).

Drug-DNA bindings by FTIR spectroscopy

Evidence for drug-base binding comes from the spectral changes observed for free DNA in-plane vibrational frequencies upon drug complexation (Ahmed Ouameur and Tajmir-Riahi 2004; Ahmed Ouameur et al. 2010; Andrushchenk et al. 2002; Dovbeshko et al. 2002; Froehlich et al. 2011a; Froehlich et al. 2011b; Froehlich et al. 2012; Froehlich et al. 2011c). At a low drug concentration of 0.125 mM, a minor intensity change was observed for the bands at 1710 (guanine) and at 1661 (thymine), in the difference spectra of drug-DNA adducts (Fig. 2A–C, diff., 0125 mM). The intensity variations of these vibrations were characterized by the presence of several weak positive and negative features at 1701–1695 (guanine), 1671–1657 (thymine), and 1610 cm^{-1} (adenine) in the difference spectra of tamoxifen-, 4-hydroxytamoxifen-, and endoxifen-DNA complexes (Fig. 2A–C, diff., 0.125 mM). The observed spectral changes are due to minor drug-DNA interaction at low drug concentration. As drug concentration increased to 0.5 mM, a major increase in intensity of base vibrations

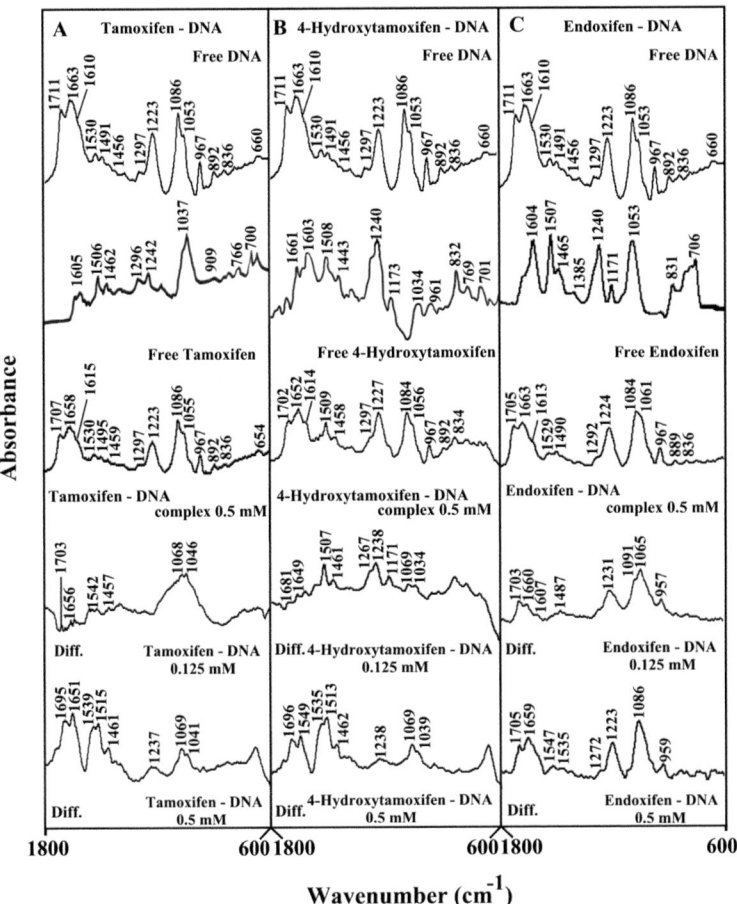

Fig. 2: FTIR spectra in the region of 1800–600 cm⁻¹ of hydrated films (pH 7.4) for free DNA (12.5 mM) and its complexes (A) for tamoxifen, (B) 4-hydroxytamoxifen, (C) endoxifen with difference spectra (diff.) (bottom two curves) obtained at different drug concentrations (indicated on the figure).

was observed, indicating continued drug interaction with DNA bases (Fig. 2A–C, diff., 0.5 mM). The major increase in intensity of DNA base vibrations comes from the strong positive features observed at 1703–1500 cm⁻¹ and major spectral shifting for guanine band at 1710 to 1707–1702 cm⁻¹, thymine band at 1663 to 1663–1652 cm⁻¹, and adenine band at 1610 to 1615–1613 cm⁻¹ (Fig. 2A–C, complex 0.5 mM). The observed spectral changes are due to strong drug-base binding *via* guanine and adenine N7 and thymine O2 atoms. Such spectral changes were observed for DNA vibrations upon several ligand-DNA complexes (Froehlich et al. 2011a; Froehlich et al. 2011b).

The drug-PO₂ interaction was evident from an increase in the intensity and shifting of the PO₂ antiymmetric band at 1223 and symmetric stretching at 1086 cm⁻¹, in the spectra of the drug-DNA complexes (Fig. 2A–C, complex 0.5 mM). The major intensity increase for the PO₂ bands at 1223 and 1086 cm⁻¹ are characterized by strong positive features around 1238–1223 and 1086–1070 cm⁻¹ in the difference spectra of drug-DNA complexes (Fig. 2A–C, diff. 0.5 mM). The observed positive features in the difference spectra of drug-DNA adducts are due to an increase in the intensity of the phosphate vibrational frequencies, upon drug-phosphate interaction (Fig. 2A–C diffs, 0.5 mM). Similar PO_2 spectral changes were observed in the spectra of several ligand-DNA adducts (Froehlich et al. 2011a; Froehlich et al. 2011b).

Drug-tRNA bindings by FTIR spectroscopy

There are several infrared spectroscopic evidence regarding drug binding to tRNA bases and the backbone phosphate group. Evidence for drug-base binding comes from the spectral changes observed for free tRNA in-plane vibrational frequencies upon drug complexation (Ahmed Ouameur et al. 2010; Froehlich et al. 2011c; N'soukpoé et al. 2009). At a low drug concentration of 0.125 mM, minor intensity changes were observed for the bands at 1698 (guanine) and at 1657 (uracil), in the difference spectra of drug-tRNA adducts (Fig. 3A–C, diff., 0125 mM). The intensity variations of these vibrations were characterized by the presence of several weak positive and negative features at 1700–1640 cm^{-1} for guanine and uracil vibrations in the difference spectra of tamoxifen-, 4-hydroxytamoxifen-, and endoxifen-tRNA complexes (Fig. 3A–C, diff., 0.125 mM). The observed spectral changes are due to minor drug-tRNA interaction at low drug concentration. As drug concentration increased to 0.5 mM, a major increase in intensity of base vibrations was observed, indicating of continued drug interaction with tRNA bases (Fig. 3A–C, diff., 0.5 mM). The major increase in intensity of tRNA base vibrations comes from the strong positive features observed at 1799–1500 cm^{-1} and major spectral shifting for guanine band at 1698 to 1679 (tamoxifen), 1679 (4-hydroxytamoxifen), and 1684 cm^{-1} (endoxifen), thymine band at 1657 to 1654 (tamoxifen), 1660 (4-hydroxtamoxifen) and 1656 cm^{-1} (endoxifen), adenine band at 1510 to 1610 (tamoxifen), 16011 (4-hydtoxytamoxifen), and 1607 cm^{-1} (endoxifen), upon drug complexation (Fig. 3A–C, complexes 0.5 mM). Strong positive features centered at 1690–1500 cm^{-1}, in the difference spectra of drug-tRNA complexes are also due to a major drug-base interaction (Fig. 3A–C, diff., 0.5 mM). The observed spectral changes are due to strong drug-base binding *via* guanine and adenine N7 and uracil O2 atoms. Similar spectral changes were observed for tRNA vibrations upon several ligand-tRNA complexation (Ahmed Ouameur et al. 2010; Froehlich et al. 2011c; N'soukpoé et al. 2009).

Evidence for drug-phosphate binding comes from major alterations of the phosphate vibrational frequencies. The drug-PO_2 leads to an increase in the intensity and shifting of the PO_2 antiymmetric band at 1237 and symmetric stretching at 1086 cm^{-1}, in the spectra of the drug-tRNA complexes (Fig. 3A–C, complex 0.5 mM). The major intensity increase for the PO_2 bands at 1237 and 1086 cm^{-1} are characterized by strong positive features around 1233–1220 cm^{-1} in the difference spectra of drug-DNA complexes (Fig. 3A–C, diff. 0.5 mM). The observed positive features in the difference spectra of drug-tRNA adducts are due to an increase in the intensity of the phosphate vibrational frequencies, upon drug-PO_2 interaction (Fig. 3A–C diffs., 0.5 mM). In addition, the phosphate symmetric vibration at 1086 cm^{-1} showed major shifting to lower frequencies at 1073 (tamoxifen), 1078 (4-hydroxytamoxifen), and

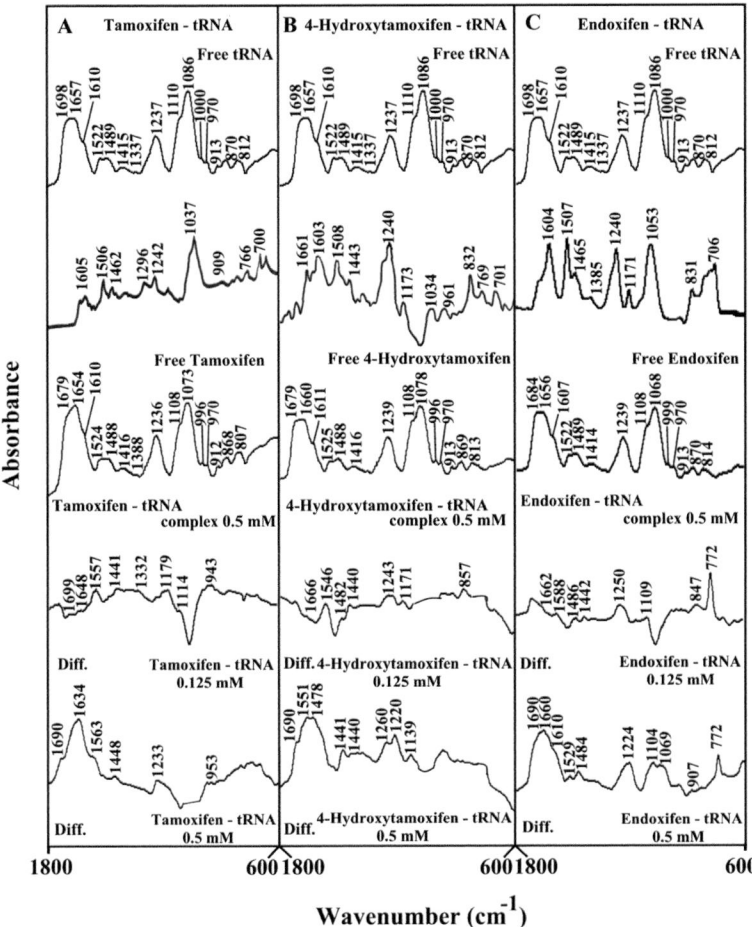

Fig. 3: FTIR spectra in the region of 1800–600 cm⁻¹ of hydrated films (pH 7.4) for free tRNA (12.5 mM) and its complexes (A) for tamoxifen, (B) 4-hydroxytamoxifen, (C) endoxifen with difference spectra (diff.) (bottom two curves) obtained at different drug concentrations (indicated on the figure).

1068 cm⁻¹ (endoxifen), upon drug–phosphate interaction (Fig. 3A–C complexes 0.5 mM). Similar PO_2 spectral changes were observed in the spectra of several ligand-tRNA adducts, where ligand-PO_2 interaction occurred (Ahmed Ouameur et al. 2010; Froehlich et al. 2011c; N'soukpoé et al. 2009).

DNA and tRNA conformations in drug-adducts

The CD spectrum of the free DNA had four major peaks: 210 (negative), 221 (positive), 246 (negative), and 278 nm (positive) (Fig. 4A). This result is consistent with CD spectra of double helical DNA in B conformation (Vorlickova 1995; Kypr and Vorlickova 2002). Upon drug interaction, no major shifting of the CD bands was observed at low drug concentration (0.125 to 0.25 mM), whereas, at higher polymer content (0.5 and 1 mM), a major increase in molar ellipticity of the band at 211 nm was observed, while the negativity of the band at 246 nm increased and the intensity of the band at 278 nm decreased in the spectra of tamoxifen, 4-hydroxytamoxifen, and endoxifen-DNA adducts (Fig. 4A). The loss of intensity of the CD band at 278 nm and the intensity variations of the band at 210, 221, and 246 nm in the spectra of drug-DNA complexes are due to DNA aggregation upon drug complexation and not due to DNA conformational changes (Fig. 4A). The CD results are also consistent with our infrared data on the drug-DNA complexes that showed no conformational changes for B-DNA with marker bands at 1710 (G), 1223 (PO_2), and 836 cm^{-1} (phosphodiester mode) (Fig. 2A).

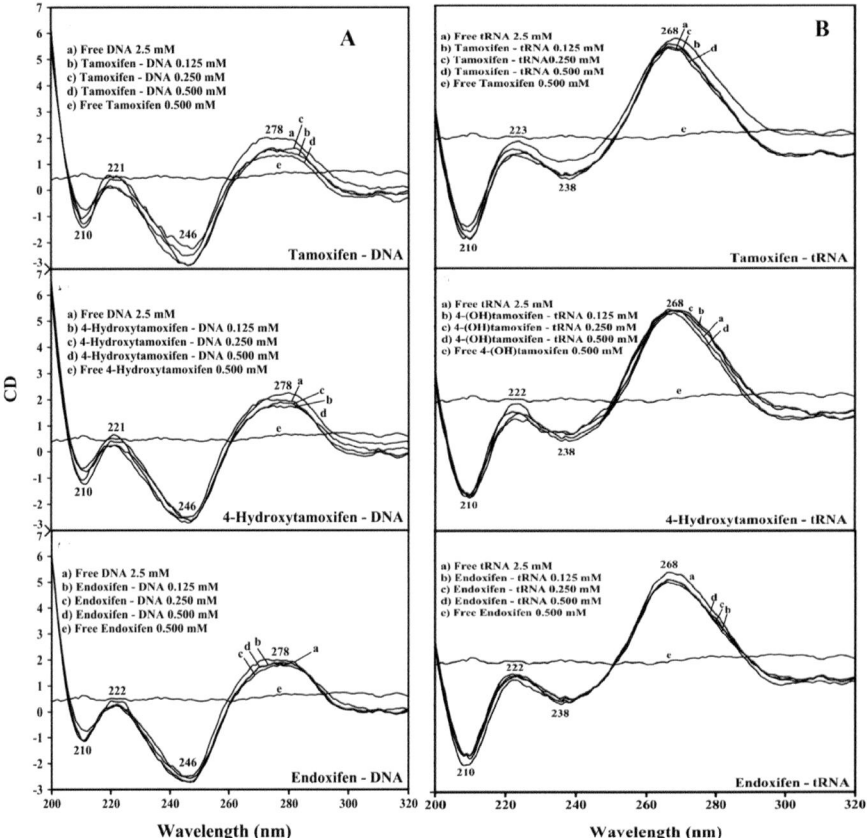

Fig. 4: CD spectra of free DNA (A) and free tRNA (B) at 2.5 mM and its complexes with tamoxifen, 4-hydroxytamoxifen, and endoxifen at different drug concentrations.

The CD spectrum of the free tRNA had four major peaks: 210 (negative), 223 (positive), 238 (negative), and 268 nm (positive) (Fig. 4B). This result is consistent with CD spectra RNA in A conformation (Vorlickova 1995; Kypr and Vorlickova 2002). Upon drug interaction, no major shifting of the CD bands was observed at low drug concentration (0.125 to 0.5 mM), whereas, at higher polymer content (0.5 mM), a major increase in molar ellipticity of the band at 210 nm was observed, while the negativity of the band at 238 nm increased and the intensity of the band at 268 nm decreased in the spectra of tamoxifen, 4-hydroxytamoxifen, and endoxifen-tRNA adducts (Fig. 4B). The loss of intensity of the CD band at 268 nm and the intensity variations of the band at 210, 223, and 238 nm in the spectra of drug-tRNA adducts are due to tRNA aggregation upon drug complexation and not due to tRNA conformational changes (Fig. 4B). The CD results are also consistent with our infrared data on the drug-tRNA complexes that showed no conformational changes for A-tRNA with marker bands at 1698 (G), 1237 (PO_2), and 812 cm^{-1} (phosphodiester mode) (Fig. 4 B). The shifting of the guanine bands at 1698 to lower frequency is due to drug interaction with guanine N7 site and not due to tRNA conformational transition, since the phosphodiester band at 810 cm^{-1} showed no major shifting in the spectra of the drug-tRNA complexes consistent with IR results discussed above (Fig. 3A).

Stability of drug-DNA and drug-tRNA complexes by fluorescence spectroscopy

Since DNA and RNA are weak fluorophore, the titrations of tamoxifen and its metabolites were done against different polynucleotide concentrations, using drug excitation at 280 nm and emission at 375 nm (Engelke et al. 2001; Agudelo et al. 2013a; Lakowicz 2006). The decrease of fluorescence intensity of tamoxifen and its metabolites has been monitored at 375 nm for drug-DNA and drug-tRNA systems (Figs. 5A and 5B). The plot of $F_0/(F_0 - F)$ vs. 1/[polynucleotides] is shown in Figs. 5A and 5B. Assuming that the observed changes in fluorescence come from the interaction between the drug and polynucleotides, the quenching constant can be taken as the binding constant of the complex formation. The overall binding constants were: $K_{tamox-DNA} = 3.5 (\pm 0.7) \times 10^4 M^{-1}$, $K_{4-hydroxytamox-DNA} = 4.3 (\pm 0.5) \times 10^4 M^{-1}$ and $K_{endox-DNA} = 2.8 (\pm 0.6) \times 10^4 M^{-1}$ and $K_{tamox-tRNA} = 5.2 (\pm 0.6) \times 10^4 M^{-1}$, $K_{4-hydroxytamox-tRNA} = 6.5 (\pm 0.5) \times 10^4 M^{-1}$ and $K_{endox-tRNA} = 1.3 (\pm 0.2) \times 10^4 M^{-1}$ (Fig. 5 A-B and Table 2), and suggesting that DNA and tRNA forms more stable complexes with 4-hydroxytamoxifen. More stable drug-tRNA adducts were formed due to the presence of several H-bonding contacts that are not present in drug-DNA complexes (Fig. 1). The results are consistent with the free binding energy from docking studies (Table 1).

The number of binding sites occupied by drug on DNA and tRNA (n) is found to be between 0.8 and 1.2 (Table 2).

The quenching coefficient constant Kq was calculated according to the Stern-Volmer equation (Lakowicz 2006):

$$F_0/F = 1 + k_Q t_0 [Q] = 1 + K_D [Q] \tag{9}$$

where F_0 and F are the fluorescence intensities in the absence and presence of quencher, [Q] is the quencher concentration and K_D is the Stern-Volmer quenching constant, which can be written as $K_D = k_Q t_0$; where k_Q is the bimolecular quenching rate constant and t_0 is the lifetime of the fluorophore in the absence of quencher ~ 2 ns for tamoxifen and its metabolites at neutral pH (Agudelo et al. 2013a). The quenching

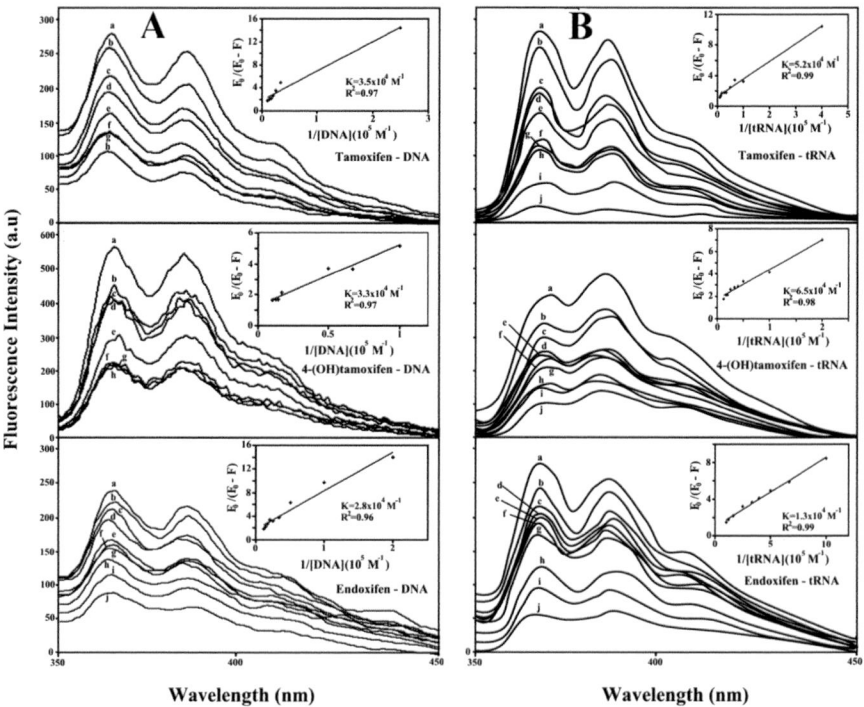

Fig. 5: Fluorescence emission spectra of drug-DNA (A) and drug-tRNA (B) in 10 mM Tris-HCl buffer pH 7.4 at 25°C for (A) tamoxifen–DNA: (a) free tamoxifen (20 M), (b-j) DNA at 4, 10, 20, 30 40, 50, 60, 70 and 100 μM 4-hydroxytamoxifen–DNA: (a) free 4-hydroxytamoxifen (20 μM), (b-j) DNA at 5, 10, 15, 20, 30, 60, 70, 80 and 100 μM endoxifen-DNA: (a): free endoxifen (20 μM); (b-j) DNA at 5, 10, 20, 30, 40, 50, 60, 70 and 90 μM. Inset: The plot of $F_0/(F_0-F)$ as a function of 1/DNA concentration. The binding constant K being the ratio of the intercept and the slope. Similar drug and tRNA concentrations were used for drug-tRNA systems (Fig. 5B).

coefficient constants (K_q) are about 10^{13} M^{-1}/s for these drug-DNA and drug-tRNA complexes (Table 2). Since these values are larger than the maximum collisional quenching constant $(2.0 \times 10^{10}$M^{-1}/s), we believe that static quenching is dominant in these drug-DNA complexes (Zhang et al. 2008).

We also compared the binding constants of drug-DNA and drug-tRNA complexes using fluorescence data and the model developed by McGhee and von Hippel 1974; Singhal and Rajeswari 2010; Tsodikov et al. 2001) for a non-linear non-cooperative ligand binding system. The results were analyzed using the following equation:

$$r/C_f = K(1-nr)[(1-nr)/1-(n-1)r]n-1 \qquad (10)$$

where r is the molar ratio of bound drug per DNA and C_f is the concentration of free drug given by $C_f = (C_t - C_b)$, where C_t is the total drug concentration and C_b is the concentration of bound drug, K the binding constant, and 'n' the number of binding sites occupied by the drug on the DNA molecule. The K values are comparable to those determined from the Stern-Volmer approach (Table 2).

Table 2. Binding parameters for drug-DNA and drug-tRNA complexes.

Complexes	K_{UV}	K_{fluo}	$K_{vonHippel}$	$K_q(M^{-1}s^{-1}) \times$	n
	$M^{-1} \times 10^4$	$M^{-1} \times 10^4$	$M^{-1} \times 10^4$	10^{13}	
Tamoxifen-DNA	2.8 ± 0.8	3.5 ± 0.7	1.5 ± 0.6	1.7 ± 0.5	0.90 ± 0.10
4-hydroxytamox-DNA	5.7 ± 0.6	4.3 ± 0.5	2.5 ± 0.7	2.1 ± 0.6	0.80 ± 0.10
Endoxifen-DNA	2.3 ± 0.4	2.8 ± 0.6	1.3 ± 0.4	1.4 ± 0.4	1 ± 0.10
Tamoxifen-tRNA	5.9 ± 1.9	5.2 ± 0.6	5.0 ± 1.4	2.6 ± 0.6	1 ± 0.10
4-hydroxytamox-tRNA	2.4 ± 0.5	6.5 ± 0.5	2.9 ± 1.5	3.2 ± 0.8	0.80 ± 0.10
Endoxifen-tRNA	4.9 ± 1	1.3 ± 0.2	1.7 ± 0.4	0.7 ± 0.2	1.2 ± 0.10

Stability of drug-DNA and drug-tRNA adducts by UV spectra

The drug-DNA and drug-tRNA binding constant were also determined by UV-Visible spectroscopy as reported (Marty et al. 2009a; Marty et al. 2009b; Connors 1987). An increase in drug concentration resulted in an increase in UV light absorption (Fig. 6). This is consistent with a reduction of base stacking interactions due to drug complexation (Figs. 6A-B). The double reciprocal plot of $1/(A-A_0)$ vs. $1/$(drug concentration) is linear and the binding constant (K) can be estimated from the ratio of the intercept to the slope (Figs. 6A-B). A_0 is the initial absorbance of free polynucleotides at 260 nm and A is the recorded absorbance of complex at different drug concentrations. The overall binding constants for drug-tRNA complexes are estimated to be $K_{tamox-DNA}$ = 2.8 ($\pm$ 0.8) x $10^4\,M^{-1}$, $K_{4-hydroxytamox-DNA}$ = 5.7 ($\pm$ 0.6) x $10^4\,M^{-1}$, $K_{endox-DNA}$ = 2.3 ($\pm$ 0.4) x $10^4\,M^{-1}$ and $K_{tamox-tRNA}$ = 5.9 ($\pm$ 1.9) x $10^4\,M^{-1}$, $K_{4-hydroxytamox-tRNA}$ = 2.4 ($\pm$ 0.5) x $10^4\,M^{-1}$ and $K_{endox-tRNA}$ = 4.9 ($\pm$ 1) x $10^4\,M^{-1}$ (Figs. 6A-B and Table 2). The binding constants estimated are mainly due to the drug-base binding and not related to the polymer-PO_2 interaction, which is largely ionic and can be dissociated easily in an aqueous solution. However, the overall binding constants calculated here for tamoxifen and its metabolites with DNA and tRNA are comparable with other drug-polynucleotides complexes (Agudelo et al. 2014; Agudelo et al. 2013b).

Summary and Key Points

In summary, this chapter provides important new information on the binding affinity of tamoxifen and two of its therapeutically important metabolites with DNA and tRNA: (1) The drug-polynucleotide interaction involves both hydrophilic and hydrophobic contacts. (2) Tamoxifen and its metabolites do not share similar binding sites on DNA and tRNA. (3) 4-hydroxytamoxifen forms more stable complex with DNA and tRNA than tamoxifen and endoxifen. (4) Several H-bonding contacts were observed in drug-tRNA adducts but not in drug-DNA complexes and this is the reason tRNA forms more stable drug conjugates than DNA. (5) At high drug concentrations, biopolymer aggregation is observed. (6) The information generated in this study can help to elucidate the mechanism of action of tamoxifen and its metabolites in cancer therapy.

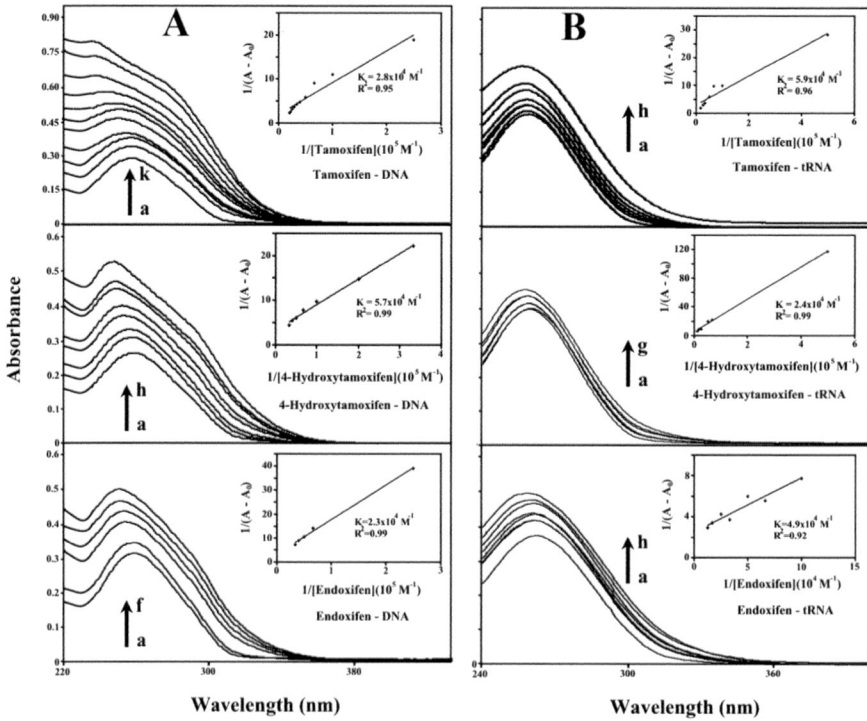

Fig. 6: UV-Visible spectra of drug-DNA (A) and drug-tRNA (B) in 10 mM Tris-HCl buffer pH 7.4 at 25 °C for (A) tamoxifen–DNA: (a) free DNA (50 µM), (b-h) tamoxifen at 4, 10 , 20, 30, 40, 45 and 50 µM 4-hydroxytamoxifen–DNA: (a) free DNA (50 µM), (b-g) 4-hydroxytamoxifen at 2, 5, 10, 20, 30 and 50 µM endoxifen-DNA: (a): free DNA (50 µM); (b-h) endoxifen at 4, 10, 20, 30, 40, 50 and 60 µM. Inset: The plot of $1/(A-A_0)$ as a function of 1/drug concentration. The binding constant K being the ratio of the intercept and the slope. Similar drug and tRNA concentrations were used for drug-tRNA systems (Fig. 6B).

Acknowledgments

This work was supported by grants from the Natural Sciences and Engineering Research Council of Canada (NSERC), and by the Foundation of the University of Medicine and Dentistry of New Jersey (Grant No. PC28-11).

Abbreviations: tamox, tamoxifen; 4-hydroxtamox, 4-hydroxytamoxifen; endox, endoxifen; FTIR, Fourier transform infrared spectroscopy; CD, circular dichroism.

References

Agudelo, D., S. Sanyakamdhorn, Sh. Nafisi and H. A. Tajmir-Riahi. 2013a. Transporting antitumor drug tamoxifen and its metabolites 4-hydroxytamoxifen and endoxifen by chitosan nanoparticles. PLOS ONE 8: 1–11, e60250.

Agudelo, D., P. Bourassa, M. Beauregard, G. Bérubé and H. A. Tajmir-Riahi. 2013b. tRNA binding to antitumor drug doxorubicin and its analogue. PLoS ONE 8(7): 1–8, e69248.

Agudelo, D., P. Bourassa, G. Bérubé and H. A. Tajmir-Riahi. 2014. Intercalation of antitumor drug doxorubicin and its analogue by DNA duplex: structural features and biological implications. Int. J. Biol. 66: 144–150.

Ahmed Ouameur, A. and H. A. Tajmir-Riahi. 2004. Structural analysis of DNA interactions with biogenic polyamines and cobalt (III) hexamine studied by Fourier transform infrared and capillary electrophoresis. J. Biol. Chem. 279: 42041–42054.

Ahmed Ouameur, A., P. Bourassa and H. A. Tajmir-Riahi. 2010. Probing tRNA interaction with biogenic polyamines. RNA 16: 1968–1979.

Ahn, M. R. and Y. Y. Sheen. 1997. Antiestrogen interaction with estrogen receptors and additional antiestrogen binding sites in human breast cancer MCF-7 cells. Arch. Pharm. Res. 20: 579–585.

Alex, S. and P. Dupuis. 1989. FTIR and Raman investigation of cadmium binding by DNA. Inorg. Chim. Acta 157: 271–281.

Andrushchenko, V. V., Z. Leonenko, H. van de Sande and H. Wieser. 2002. Vibrational CD (VCD) and atomic force microscopy (AMF) study of DNA interactions with Cr^{3+}: VCD and AFM evidence of DNA condensation. Biopolymers 61: 243–260.

Bijl, M. J., R. H. van Schaik, L. A. Lammers, A. Hofman, A. G. Vulto, E. V. Gelder et al. 2009. The CYP2D6*4 polymorphism affects breast cancer survival in tamoxifen users. Breast Cancer Res. Treat. 118: 125–130.

Bland, A. E., B. Calingaert, A. A. Secord, P. S. Lee, F. A. Valea, A. Berckuck et al. 2009. Relationship between tamoxifen use and high risk endometrial cancer histologic types. Gynecol. Oncol. 112: 150–154.

Bourassa, P., T. J. Thomas and H. A. Tajmir-Riahi. 2014a. Locating the binding sites of antitumor drug tamoxifen and its metabolites with DNA. J. Pharm. Biomed. Anal. 95: 193–199.

Bourassa, P., J. Bariyanga, T. J. Thomas and H. A. Tajmir-Riahi. 2014b. Breast anticancer drug tamoxifen and its metabolites bind tRNA at multiple sites. Int. J. Biol. Macromol. 72: 692–698.

Connors, K. 1987. Binding Constants: The Measurement of Molecular Complex Stability. John Wiley & Sons, New York.

Dovbeshko, G. I., V. I. Chegel, N. Y. Gridina, O. P. Repnytska, Y. M. Shirshov, V. P. Todor et al. 2002. Surface enhanced IR absorption of nucleic acids from tumor cells: FTIR reflectance study. Biopolymer (Biospectroscopy) 67: 470–486.

Engelke, M., P. Bojarski, R. Blob and H. Diehl. 2001. Tamoxifen perturbs lipid bilayer order and permeability: comparison of DSC, fluorescence anisotropy, Laurdan generalized polarization and carboxyfluoresceine leakage studies. Biophys. Chem. 90: 157–173.

Froehlich, E., J. S. Mandeville, C. M. Weinert, L. Kreplak and H. A. Tajmir-Riahi. 2011a. Bundling and aggregation of DNA by cationic dendrimers. Biomacromolecules 12: 511–517.

Froehlich, E., J. S. Mandeville, D. Arnold, L. Kreplak and H. A. Tajmir-Riahi. 2011b. PEG and mPEG-anthracene induce DNA condensation and particle formation. J. Phys. Chem. B115: 9873–9879.

Froehlich, E., J. S. Mandeville, L. Kreplak and H. A. Tajmir-Riahi. 2011c. Aggregation and particle formation of tRNA by dendrimers. Biomacromolecules 12: 2780–2787.

Froehlich, E., J. S. Mandeville, D. Arnold, L. Kreplak and H. A. Tajmir-Riahi. 2012. Effect of PEG and mPEG-anthracene on tRNA aggregation and particle formation. Biomacromolecules 13: 282–28.

Furlanut, M., L. Franceschi, E. Pasqual, S. Bacchetti, D. Poz, G. Giorda et al. 2007. Tamoxifen and its main metabolites serum and tissue concentrations in breast cancer women. Ther. Drug Monit. 29: 349–352.

Hayes, T. G. 2009. Pharmacologic treatment of male breast cancer. Expert Opin. Pharmacother. 10: 2499–2510.

Hoskins, J. M., L. A. Carey and H. L. McLeod. 2009. CYP2D6 and tamoxifen: DNA matters in breast cancer. Nat. Rev. Cancer 9: 576–586.

Hughes-Davies, L., C. Caldas and G. C. Wishart. 2009. Tamoxifen: the drug that came in from the cold. Br. J. Cancer 101: 875–878.

Jordan, V. C. 2003. Tamoxifen: a most unlikely pioneering medicine. Nat. Rev. Drug Discov. 3: 205–213.

Jordan, V. C. 2006. Tamoxifen (ICI46,474) as a targeted therapy to treat and prevent breast cancer. Br. J. Pharmacol. 147 Suppl. 1: S269–S276.

Jordan, V. C. 2007. New insights into the metabolism of tamoxifen and its role in the treatment and prevention of breast cancer. Steroids 72: 829–842.

Jordan, V. C. 2008. Tamoxifen: catalyst for the change to targeted therapy. Eur. J. Cancer 44: 30–38.

Kypr, J. and M. Vorlickova. 2002. Circular dichroism spectroscopy reveal invariant conformation of guanine runs in DNA. Biopolymers 67: 275–277.

Lakowicz, J. R. 2006. Principles of Fluorescence Spectroscopy, 3nd ed. Springer/Plenum, New York.

Lien, E. A., E. Solheim and P. M. Ueland. 1991. Distribution of tamoxifen and its metabolites in rat and human tissues during steady-state treatment. Cancer Res. 51: 4837–4844.

Marty, R., C. N. N' soukpoe-Kossi, D. Charbonneau, C. M. Wienert, L. Kreplak and H. A. Tajmir-Riahi. 2009a. Structural analysis of DNA complexation with cationic lipids. Nucl. Acids Res. 37: 749–757.

Marty, R., C. N. N' soukpoe-Kossi, D. Charbonneau, C. M. Weinert, L. Kreplak and H. A. Tajmir-Riahi. 2009b. Structural characterization of cationic lipid-tRNA complexes. Nucl. Acids Res. 37: 5197–5207.

McGhee, J. D. and P. H. von Hippel. 1974. Theoretical aspects of DNA-protein interactions: co-operative and non-co-operative binding of large ligands to a one dimensional homogeneous lattice. J. Mol. Biol. 25: 469–489.

Nabholtz, J. M. and J. Gligorov. 2006. The emerging role of aromatase inhibitors in the adjuvant management of breast cancer. Rev. Recent Clin. Trials 1: 237–249.

O'Malley, B. W. and R. Kumar. 2009. Nuclear receptor coregulators in cancer biology. Cancer Res. 69: 8217–8222.

Privé, G. G., K. Yanagi and R. E. Dickerson. 1991. Structure of the B-DNA decamer C- C-A-A-C-G-T-T-G-G and comparison with isomorphous decamers C-C-A-A-A-G-A-T-T-G-G and C-C-A-G-G-C-C-T-G-G. J. Mol. Biol. 217: 177–199.

Randerath, K., J. Bi, N. Mabon, P. Srir and B. Moorthy. 1994. Strong intensification of mouse hepatic tamoxifen DNA adduct formation by pretreatment with the sulfotransferase inhibitor and ubiquitous environmental pollutant pentachlorophenol. Carcinogenesis 15: 797–800.

Ross-Innes, C. S., R. Stark, A. E. Teschendorff, K. A. Holmes, H. R. Ali, S. F. Chin et al. 2012. Differential oestrogen receptor binding is associated with clinical outcome in breast cancer. Nature 481: 389–393.

Schroth, W., M. P. Goetz, U. Hamann, P. A. Fasching, M. Schmidt, S. Winter et al. 2009. Association between CYP2D6 polymorphisms and outcomes among women with early stage breast cancer treated with tamoxifen. JAMA 302: 1429–1436.

Sheen, Y. and J. P. Costantino. 2008. Tamoxifen chemoprevention treatment and time to first diagnosis of estrogen receptor-negative breast cancer. J. Natl. Cancer Inst. 100: 1448–1453.

Singhal, G. and M. R. Rajeswari. 2010. Molecular aspects of the interaction of Hoechst-33258 with GC-rich promoter region of c-met. DNA Cell Biol. 29: 91–100.

Soper, J. T. and L. Havrilesky. 2009. Relationship between tamoxifen use and high Risk endometrial cancer histologic types. Gynecol. Oncol. 112: 150–154.

Sussman, J. L., S. R. Holbrook, R. W. Warrant, G. M. Church and S.-H. Kim. 1978. Crystal structure of yeast phenylalanine transfer RNA: crystallographic refinement. J. Mol. Biol. 123: 607–630.

Thomas, T., M. A. Gallo and T. J. Thomas. 2004. Estrogen receptors as targets for drug development for breast cancer, osteoporosis and cardiovascular diseases. Curr. Cancer Drug Targets 4: 483–499.

Tsodikov, O. V., J. A. Holbrook, I. A. Shkel and M. T. Record, Jr. 2001. Analytic binding isotherms describing competitive interactions of protein ligand with specific and nonspecific sites on the same DNA oligomer. Biophys. J. 81: 1960–1969.

Vorlickova, M. 1995. Conformational transitions of alternating purin-pyrimidine DNAs in the perchlorate ethanol solutions. Biophys. J. 69: 2033–2043.

Wiseman, H., G. Pagang, C. Rice-Evan and B. Halliwell. 1993. Protective actions of tamoxifen and 4-hydroxytamoxifen against oxidative damage to human low-density lipoproteins: a mechanism accounting for the cardioprotective action of tamoxifen? Biochem. J. 292: 635–638.

Wu, X., J. R. Hawse, M. Subramaniam, P. M. Goetz, J. N. Ingle and T. C. Spelsherg. 2009. The tamoxifen metabolite, endoxifen, is a potent antiestrogen that targets estrogen receptor alpha for degradation in breast cancer cells. Cancer Res. 69: 1722–1727.

Yue, W., J. D. Yager, J. P. Wang, E. R. Jupe and R. J. Santen. 2013. Estrogen receptor-dependent and independent mechanisms of breast cancer carcinogenesis. Steroids 78: 161–170.

Zhang, G., Q. Que, J. Pan and J. Guo. 2008. Study of the interaction between icariin and human serum albumin by fluorescence spectroscopy. J. Mol. Struct. 881: 132–138.

13

Dynamic Analysis of Backbone-Hydrogen-Bond Propensity for Protein Binding and Drug Design

C. A. Menéndez, S. R. Accordino, J. A. Rodriguez Fris, D. C. Gerbino and *G. A. Appignanesi*[a]

Abstract

The three-dimensional shape of a protein recorded in the Protein Data Bank (PDB) provides valuable information regarding its structure and stability. However, such a static picture might be veiling relevant information regarding protein dynamics and function. In fact, backbone hydrogen bonds (BHBs), as main determinants of protein structure, constitute context-dependent non-covalent interactions. These interactions face different environments along the protein chain, particularly at protein binding sites which might present different hydration properties from that of other regions of the protein surface. Here we characterize the hydration and hydrophobicity of protein binding sites by molecular dynamics (MD) simulations, focusing particularly on their BHBs. We also carry out a time-averaged contact matrix study to reveal the existence of BHBs whose net persistence in time differs markedly from their corresponding PDB-reported state. Such interactions where the PDB fails

INQUISUR-UNS-CONICET and Departamento de Química, Universidad Nacional del Sur, Avenida Alem 1253, 8000-Bahía Blanca, Argentina.
[a] E-mail: appignan@criba.edu.ar

to predict their dynamical behavior will be termed as "chameleonic" BHBs (CBHBs), precisely to account for their tendency to change the structural prescription of the PDB for the opposite bonding propensity in solution. Additionally, such CBHBs are not found to be homogeneously distributed but to present a clear population enhancement at protein binding sites. We also relate them to local water exposure and analyze their behavior as ligand/drug targets. In fact, we find that when the apo protein forms its complex with its natural protein partner most of the CBHBs are quenched. A similar behavior is found when the apo protein binds a disruptive drug or ligand, albeit in a less optimal fashion in some cases. Thus, the dynamic analysis of hydrogen-bond propensity might lay the foundations for new tools of interest in protein binding-site prediction and in lead optimization for drug design.

Introduction

Backbone hydrogen bonds (BHBs) have been shown by Linus Pauling to constitute major determinants for protein structure, responsible for shaping their main secondary and tertiary structural motifs. In soluble proteins, such non-covalent interactions are stable provided water is significantly excluded from their local environment by amino acid side-chains. However, this requirement is not necessarily met all along the protein chain, particularly at protein binding sites (Qvist et al. 2008; Young et al. 2007; Wang et al. 2011; Friesner et al. 2006; Kulp et al. 2011; Fernández 2006; Fernández and Scott 2003; Accordino et al. 2012a,b; Sierra et al. 2013). Importantly, the hydration properties of binding sites have been suggested to play a main role in ligand-binding or in protein-protein association (Qvist et al. 2008; Young et al. 2007; Wang et al. 2011; Friesner et al. 2006; Kulp et al. 2011; Fernández 2006; Fernández and Scott 2003; Accordino et al. 2012a,b; Sierra et al. 2013; Accordino et al. 2013) since labile hydration-water molecules are expected to be displaced from the protein binding site (Qvist et al. 2008; Young et al. 2007; Wang et al. 2011; Friesner et al. 2006). Indeed, the replacement of so-called "unfavorable" water molecules by groups of the ligand complementary to the protein surface has been established as a principal driving force for binding (Qvist et al. 2008; Young et al. 2007; Wang et al. 2011; Friesner et al. 2006) and, as such, has been incorporated in computational structure-based strategies (Young et al. 2007; Wang et al. 2011; Friesner et al. 2006). Also, fragment clustering approaches (binding of small molecular probes) have been combined with exclusion maps dictated by the pattern of tightly-bond water molecules (Kulp et al. 2011) in order to detect protein binding sites.

In accord with this heterogeneous scenario for protein hydration, the existence of BHBs partially exposed to the solvent (incompletely wrapped BHBs or dehydrons) (Fernández 2006; Fernández and Scott 2003) have been established and their relevance for protein binding has been assessed (Fernández 2006; Fernández and Scott 2003; Accordino et al. 2012a,b; Sierra et al. 2013). This is so since soluble proteins tend to wrap or bury their intramolecular interactions (their BHBs) in order to be stable in water (Fernández 2006; Fernández and Scott 2003; Accordino et al. 2012a,b; Sierra et al. 2013; Accordino et al. 2013). Such protection is performed by surrounding the intramolecular interaction with hydrophobic residues which induce water removal

(Fernández 2006; Fernández and Scott 2003; Accordino et al. 2012a,b; Sierra et al. 2013). This stability requirement is not surprising since such BHB are expected to be very strong given the desolvation environment in which they are formed (with an "effective" dielectric constant much reduced as compared to that of bulk water) (Fernández 2006; Fernández and Scott 2003; Accordino et al. 2012a,b; Sierra et al. 2013). This strengthening of coulombic interactions in desolvation environments have been recognized in biophysics and have been regarded as central for the protein binding process (Fernández 2006; Fernández and Scott 2003; Accordino et al. 2012a,b; Sierra et al. 2013; Accordino et al. 2013). Indeed, O-Ring theories of protein binding (Bogan and Thorn 1998; Li and Liu 2009) propose that the structure of the binding hot spot, the reduced set of residues that mainly contribute to the binding free-energy change, comprises a central small subset of reactive residues surrounded by another subset of energetically less relevant residues whose function would be to occlude solvent in order to modulate the intramolecular interactions. This context-dependence of non-covalent interactions (like hydrogen bonds (HBs) and ionic interactions, which would be almost irrelevant in bulk water given solvation and screening) points to a revision of the so-called Gulliver principle used both in bioengineering and materials science: A strategy based on adding (weak) non-covalent interactions of equal or different nature, as if a giant were to be tied through many tiny ropes. However, for this strategy not to still remain conceptually "Lilliputian" it should be considered that the effects of these interactions are not necessarily simply additive, while the way they depend on the local environment should be properly understood. For instance, the glaring weakness of coulombic non-covalent interaction in bulk water might revert to a much stronger behavior in a nanoconfined environment where the local "effective dielectric" is diminished. This indiscriminate use of bulk-like intuition is common occurrence in contexts like material science, bioengineering, and drug design, so the scarcity of rational design elements and the overwhelming dominance of "trial and error" attempts (expensive and suboptimal) are not surprising.

In turn, the relevance of underwrapped intramolecular protein interactions, named as dehydrons (Fernández 2006; Fernández and Scott 2003), has been recognized. Such motifs, which are unshielded from water attack, have been shown to be sticky since they promote further removal of surrounding water (which otherwise would disrupt the intermolecular interaction) (Fernández 2006; Fernández and Scott 2003). Thus, dehydrons have been shown to be central for the protein-protein association phenomena upon which most biological functions rely (Fernández 2006; Fernández and Scott 2003). Such motif, which exhibits an enhanced dehydration propensity, represents a structural packing defect that is readily determined from PDB coordinates (Fernández 2006; Fernández and Scott 2003; Accordino et al. 2012a,b; Sierra et al. 2013; Accordino et al. 2013). Thus, this concept enabled a potent novel strategy for drug design (Fernández 2006; Fernández and Scott 2003; Accordino et al. 2012; Accordino et al. 2012b; Sierra et al. 2013) that simply relies on structural information (that is, on the structural characterization of the BHBs *already* present in the PDB of the apo protein). However, since proteins are inherently dynamical objects, the merely binary (formed/not formed) classification of non-covalent interactions provided by PDB structures might be veiling valuable information regarding protein interactions and function, as we shall show below. Specifically, we shall find that certain PDB

BHBs tend to be disrupted during the dynamics while other BHBs, completely absent from the PDB of the apo protein, display a significant dynamical persistence (Menéndez et al. 2015). We shall call such defects as "chameleonic" BHBs (CBHBs) since they change state from the PDB prescription to the opposite formation propensity in solution. We shall also show that these CBHBs are not homogeneously distributed along the protein chain but concentrate in binding regions. Additionally, we shall show that CBHBs are removed upon ligand binding, thus revealing their role as drug targets. These results imply that the dynamic analysis of BHB propensity might be easily translated into a novel drug-design concept.

Measure of Water Mobility Around Backbond Hydrogen Bonds

In order to determine the hydration properties of protein surfaces and, particularly, protein binding sites, we begin by studying protein hydration water mobility. We focused (Sierra et al. 2013) on the hydration layers of a set of complete (without missing residues) proteins without ligands (PDB IDs: 1AHO, 1AKI, 1B6D, 1BYI, 1CW6, 1d8v, 1DIV, 1DPT, 1DWU, 1EJG, 1GCN, 1GH5, 1IFB, 1L1I, 1M8L, 1N4I, 1TVM, 1UBI, 1UCS, 1UOY, 1VYC, 1WNJ, 2B4N, 2BZT, 2eyz, 2FDQ, 2GEQ, 2jqx, 2JQY, 2JU6, 2K0P, 2K4Q, 2KJG, 2KV4, 2KWD, 2KWL, 2L3V, 2L4V, 2L5R, 2L7W, 2LA1, 2LAO, 2LCU, 2LFN, 2LHC, 2LHS, 2LJM, 2LKB, 2LKY, 2LOL, 2LPK, 2PNE, 2PPP, 2QHE, 2QZW, 2RN2, 2RN4, 2ROG, 3A7L, 3IZP, 3N0K, 4GCR). These 62 PDBs were chosen at random, with an average residue number of 155 and standard deviation 151. The water molecules were modeled by the TIP3P model (Jorgensen et al. 1983; Mahoney and Jorgensen 2000) with the AMBER software versions 10 and 11 (Case et al. 2010), using periodic boundary conditions and a simulation box that extended more than 14 Å away from any protein atom. Therefore, we studied a total of 15,681 BHBs. We considered a BHB when the nitrogen bonded to the alpha carbon of a residue and the oxygen of the carbonyl bonded to the alpha carbon of another residue are less than 3.5 Å, and the (minimum) angle between O and H-N (H is the hydrogen bonded to the nitrogen) was greater than 140 degrees. The equilibration and molecular dynamics simulations were carried out according to the AMBER official tutorial (http://ambermd.org/tutorials/basic/tutorial1/section5.htm). We used a total production time of 4 ns, at 300 K, keeping the pressure at an average value of 1 atm, and a density around 1.0 kg/L.

In order to get an idea of the influence of the protein surface on water dynamics, we show in Fig. 1 the mean squared displacement, $MSD = \langle r^2(t) \rangle = \langle [r_i(t)-r_i(0)]^2 \rangle$, of water molecules close to the proteins studied, where $r_i(t)$ is the position of the oxygen of water molecule i at time t and $\langle \ldots \rangle$ is the average over all i water molecules. Based on previous results that indicate that only water molecules within the first peak of the water-protein radial distribution (or the surface density plot for model flat surfaces) exhibit a dynamics significantly different from that of the bulk (Bizzarri and Cannistraro 2002; Bizzarri et al. 2000; Malaspina et al. 2010; Accordino et al. 2012c; Kumar et al. 2006; Accordino et al. 2011) we have chosen to display the behavior of the molecules that are closer than 4 Å from the protein surface at the initial time. For comparison, we also include the case of water molecules initially far apart from the protein, with bulk-like behavior.

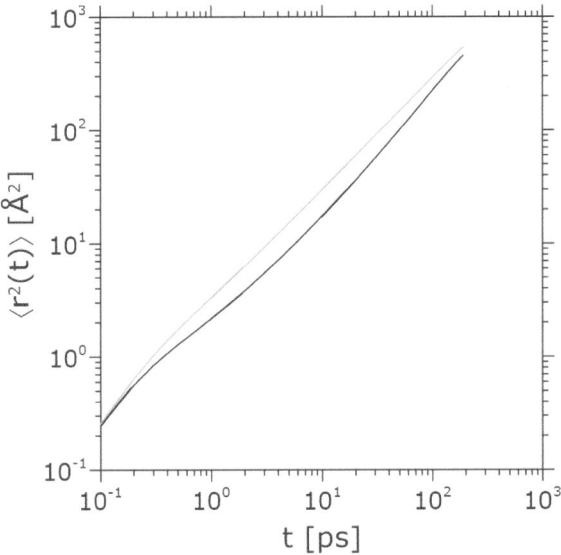

Fig. 1: Mean squared displacement plot for the water molecules close to the different proteins (water molecules whose minimum distance to the protein is lower than 4 Å, black curve) and for water molecules distant from the proteins (more than 14 Å, gray curve).

Direct inspection of Fig. 1 reveals that water dynamics close to the protein is slower than that of bulk dynamics. While the MSD curve for the molecules far from the protein surface displays, after around 0.3 ps, a behavior typical of bulk water, with a diffusive regime, the water molecules close to the protein evidence a slower, subdiffusive, regime and only tends to bulk behavior at large times (Sierra et al. 2013). This fact is consistent with previous results (Bizzarri and Cannistraro 2002; Bizzarri et al. 2000; Malaspina et al. 2010; Accordino et al. 2012c; Kumar et al. 2006) and also holds if one discriminates the parallel and perpendicular components of the MSD (Bizzarri and Cannistraro 2002; Bizzarri et al. 2000). Such sub-diffusive behavior of protein interfacial water implies certain reminiscence with the situation for supercooled water (Rodriguez Fris et al. 2007) and glass forming liquids (Debenedetti 1996; Appignanesi et al. 2006a; Rodriguez Fris et al. 2011). This behavior of the water molecules close to the protein speaks of the existence of a superficial regime at short times and distances and a bulk-like one which the molecules adopt when they get away from the protein surface. Thus, a calculation of the diffusion constant for the superficial water molecules (as obtained by the Einstein relation and which implies the extrapolation of the MSD at long times) would not be meaningful. To avoid this problem, we decided to adopt as a measure of water mobility the calculation of the MSD value at short times. We considered a timescale of $\varphi = 4$ ps (a timescale significantly larger than the end time of the ballistic regime in the MSD). As can be learnt from Fig. 1, at such timescale the superficial water molecules have moved on average one water-water distance, thus providing a reasonable measure of the local diffusivities.

On the basis of these results and to assess the mobility of the water molecules within the desolvation domains of BHBs, we calculated their MSD within a fixed time interval of length t = φ (Sierra et al. 2013). We applied this study to the hydration shell of the large set of proteins above-indicated. To get good statistics, for each of the 62 proteins we generated 400 different molecular-dynamics simulation runs of length t = φ (Sierra et al. 2013). Since we are interested on BHBs as main determinants of protein structure and protein binding, we calculated the mobility of the water molecules within the desolvation domain of each BHB of the different proteins studied. This desolvation domain was defined as the reunion of two intersecting spheres with radius 6 Å centered at the alpha carbons of the residues that form a BHB (Fernández 2006; Fernández and Scott 2003; Accordino et al. 2012a,b; Sierra et al. 2013; Accordino et al. 2013). Thus, most of the water molecules within this region are very close to the protein backbone and hence, are expected to present very low mobility values. The main result of this study was the finding that water molecules around BHBs located at protein binding sites are faster ($\langle r^2(\varphi) \rangle$ = 5 Å^2) as compared to that located away from binding sites ($\langle r^2(\varphi) \rangle$ = 3.5 Å^2) (Sierra et al. 2013). An example of such dewetting propensity of protein binding sites is represented by the p53 protein (PDB 2GEQ). The case was chosen given the practical relevance of p53, the tumor supresor (also called as the "genome guardian"), which is mutated in more than half of the cases of human cancer. From a 200 psMD simulation of p53 we found that the averaged mobility value (for a φ = 4 ps time interval) for the water molecules hydrating the desolvation domains of the BHBs located at the DNA recognition site is roughly $\langle r^2(\varphi) \rangle$ = 5 Å^2, significantly larger than the mean mobility value averaged over the water molecules within the desolvation domains of all the BHBs of the protein which gives $\langle r^2(\varphi) \rangle$ = 3.5 Å^2 (Sierra et al. 2013). These results show that the recognition site of p53 is indeed surrounded by labile water molecules that would be more easily displaced upon association with DNA. Given the large size of this binding site involving around 9 BHBs (we focused on the cluster of BHBs formed by (132, 270), (237, 271), (244, 239), (245, 237), (278, 274), (280, 276), (281, 277), (282, 279), and (284, 280), where we indicate both residues, by residue number, involved in the BHB), we can learn that this molecule presents a large patch of easily removable hydration water in its contact region, thus providing an expedient for DNA approaching and binding. This dehydration tendency is particularly relevant if we consider the neat electrostatic nature of this binding process. By promoting its local desolvation, this binding site quenches the local dielectric, thus triggering the electrostatic interaction between the positively charged arginines and the negatively charged backbone phosphates of the DNA. Another interesting observation (Sierra et al. 2013) we made was that the BHBs shaping the DNA recognition site are broken on average 15 percent of the simulation time, while the rest of the BHBs remain formed, on average, 97 percent of the time and none of them is broken more than 25 percent of the whole simulation time. In turn, one quarter of the BHBs of the binding site are broken more than such percentage and, indeed, 3 of them are broken more than 75 percent of the time. Such a lability of binding-site BHBs has also been observed by our group in the other binding cavity of p53 protein (Accordino et al. 2013).

The Y220C mutation (i.e., the replacement of tyrosine 220 by a cysteine) is one of the five major tumor suppressor p53 mutations. It creates a cavity in the surface of p53, at a region distal from the DNA recognition site, but that thermodynamically destabilizes the protein (which is already marginally stable), thus inactivating the protein and promoting disease. The possibility to find molecules that bind to such cavity and, therefore, re-establish the structure and thermodynamic stability (and hence the biological function of this molecule), becomes essential. In this context, our studies (Accordino et al. 2013) rationalized the oncogenic nature of the mutation by identifying the fact that it precisely destabilizes the structure by exposing protein backbone to the solvent and, thus, labilizing BHBs (in particular, one of them is significantly labilized and even broken: the BHB tyr220-thr155, which creates a dehydron). A molecule proposed by the group of AlanFersht (Boeckler et al. 2008; Wilcken et al. 2012a,b; Wang et al. 2012), named as PhiKan083, rescued the function of p53 inactivated by mutation Y220C. However, it did not recover the full stability since it left a flank of the cavity unguarded or solvent-accessible. Our computational results rationally re-engineered such molecule by adding a hydrophobic functional group in a specific region to stabilize such BHBs and increasing the affinity for p53.

The Fig. 2(a) shows the distribution of the number of water molecules (nW) within the desolvation domain of the BHB cys220-thr155 (this domain is built as a pair of spheres of radius 6 Å, centered at the alphacarbons of both residues involved in the BHB). The mean value of the distribution m and its standard deviation s are indicated in the caption. As expected, this BHB in the free protein 2J1X shows a higher water population than the same BHB in the protein 2VUK bonded to PhiKan083. In Fig. 2(b) we show the distribution of the cys220-thr155 N-O distance (dNO) during production runs. We show the results for the free protein molecule with the mutation Y220C (2J1X), the case for the complex with PhiKan083 (2VUK) and our modification of Phikan083 (2VUK molecule B), making the BHB even much more stable than PhiKan083 (lower m and s). In turn, Figs. 2(c), 2(d), and 2(e) exhibit the time evolution of dNO along a single production run. We can observe that the fluctuations are clearly more significant for the case of 2J1X. In fact, the BHB breaks (surpasses the BHB distance threshold of 3.5 Å) several times in the interval that goes from 500 ps to 1,000 ps. In the presence of the molecule PhiKan083 (2VUK), the dNO is a bit more stable during the whole simulation, fluctuating more smoothly around a mean value which is much lower than the BHB threshold value. This fact rationalizes the behavior of the small molecule which stabilizes the protein and raises its melting temperature, thus restoring function. It is also worth noting that the simulations show that the watermolecules approach the BHB cys220-thr155 from the side of the protein cavity not occupied by PhiKan083. Water molecules could penetrate the cavity from such a side and attack the intramolecular BHB. In fact, in Fig. 2(d) we can see that the dNO of such BHB indeed fluctuates and eventually slightly surmounts the BHB distance threshold. In Fig. 2(e) we have also included the case for our proposed modification of PhiKan083 (2VUK molecule B, in the inset of Fig. 2(e)), which indeed performs much better. Almost simultaneously, the experimental group of Alan Fersht continued working on this issue and published the discovery of a new molecule (Wilcken et al. 2012a,b), which precisely met the requirements of our work by occupying the indicated solvent-accessible region.

These results clearly denote the existence of a transference of constraints between regions of the protein chain with an enhanced dynamics and mobile hydration water molecules. This constitutes a very interesting piece of information since it anticipates the fact that the pattern of BHBs of the apo protein PDB might be hiding valuable

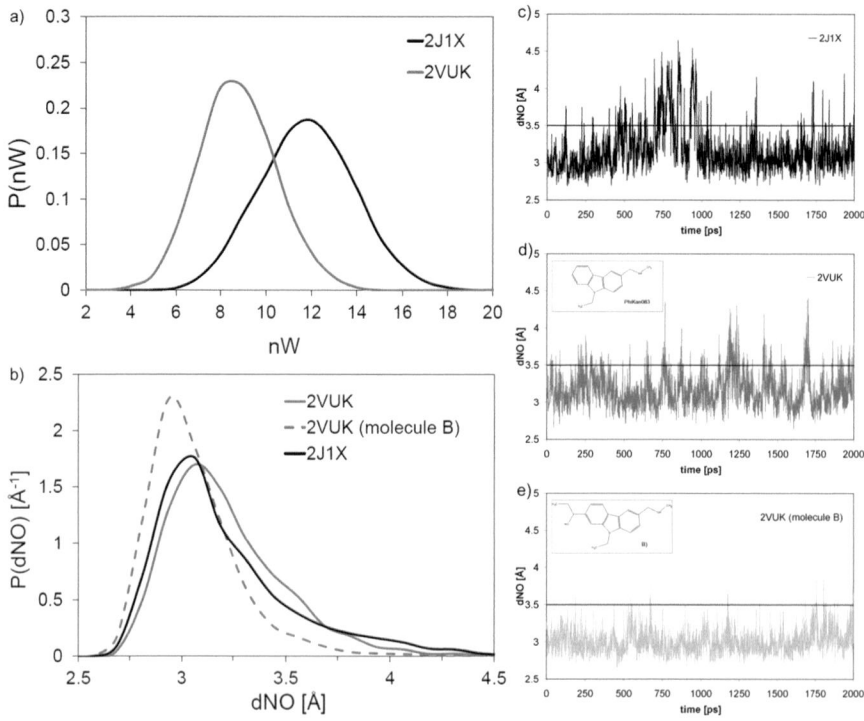

Fig. 2: (a) Distribution of the number of water molecules (nW) within the desolvation domain of the BHB cys220-thr155. 2VUK (T-p53C-Y220C-PhiKan083; m = 8.743 and s = 1.720) and 2J1X (T-p53C-Y220C; m = 11.819 and s = 2.111). (b) Distribution of the distance (dNO) between the N atom of the amide group and the O atom of the carbonyl. 2VUK (m = 3.150 and s = 0.288); 2J1X (m = 3.143 and s = 0.339) and 2VUK (molecule B) (m = 3.000 and s = 0.235). (c), (d), and (e) Time evolution of dNO for 2J1X, 2VUK, and 2VUK (molecule B).

information regarding protein dynamics and function and, thus, points to the relevance of performing a BHB dynamics propensity investigation.

Hydration Properties of Protein Binding Sites

Since the local mobility of hydration water is enhanced at protein binding sites, it is of interest to study in more detail protein hydration properties. To this end, as in the rest of this chapter, we shall focus on proteins involved in protein-protein interactions for which disruptive small molecules or drugs have been developed (Wells and McClendon 2007). Besides their main therapeutic relevance, these systems provide a more accurate means to determine the target protein binding site, since the small molecule/drug is significantly smaller than the partner protein they replace (Wells and McClendon 2007; Accordino et al. 2012b). This does not represent any loss in generality, since protein binding "hot spots" (the region that comprises the residues that mainly contribute to the binding free energy) are usually restricted to just a handful set of amino acids (Bogan and Thorn 1998; Wells and McClendon

2007; Accordino et al. 2012b). We shall study some successful cases (Wells and McClendon 2007): MDM2 (PDB: 1Z1M)/Nutlin-3 (PDB: 1RV1)/p53 (PDB: 1YCR) (Vassilev et al. 2004), IL-2 (PDB: 1M4C)/SP4206 (PDB: 1PY2)/IL-2 receptor alpha-chain (PDB: 1Z92) (Raimundo et al. 2004), BCL-XL (PDB: 1R2D)/ABT-73734 (PDB: 2YXJ)/BAD-derived peptide (amino acids: 100 to 126) (PDB: 2BZW) (Bruncko et al. 2007) and ZipA (PDB: 1F7W)/Compound 1 (PDB: 1Y2F)/FtsZ-derived peptide (PDB: 1F47) (amino acids: 367 to 383) (Rush et al. 2005). In each case the notation indicates first the target protein, then the disruptive drug and finally the partner protein, with the corresponding PDB entries for the apo protein, the drug-protein complex and the protein-protein complex. We have also chosen these cases for validation purposes (all 3D structures have been accurately determined and deposited in the PDB). However, our analysis is generally applicable to the broad realm of protein binding. To study the dynamical behavior of these systems were carried out MD simulations by means of AMBER simulation package 10 (Case et al. 2010), using TIP3P water and $T = 300$ K. For all apo proteins we performed production runs of 50 ns. For all other systems production runs were performed for 20 ns. To determine the binding site for each protein we used a simple geometrical method by finding BHBs in the target protein whose distance (measured form the N amide or the carbonyl O) to any heavy atom of their partner protein is less than 6 Å (Menéndez et al. 2015) in the PDB of the corresponding protein-protein complex (criterion 1). Another possibility (criterion 2), that yields a smaller size binding site, is to use the same geometrical criterion but with respect to the heavy atoms of the drug (small molecule) in the corresponding drug-protein complex PDB structure (Menéndez et al. 2015). We note that with these methods we determine the BHBs located within a certain interface or binding site. However, the protein might have other interacting/binding sites we are not considering here. For the four proteins studied, criterion 1 found that roughly 15 percent of the BHBs were located at binding sites, while criterion 2 reduced this percentage to half that value.

Water Vacating Probability Calculations for the Protein Hydration Layer

The nanoconfinement that arises upon the interaction of different assembling units, both in biological organization processes and in the supramolecular self-assembly of nanomaterials in a water environment, affects the thermodynamic properties of the hydration water which should be removed for the process to take place (Giovambattista et al. 2012). In realistic contexts, both chemistry and local geometry are expected to define the local hydrophobicity (Giovambattista et al. 2012). In fact, geometrically-induced surface dehydration (by means of water inaccessibly cavities) has been suggested to be central for the existence of reactive sites responsible for protein binding (Schulz et al. 2011) (this geometric effect might be responsible for the fact that the design of disruptive drugs has been much easier for enzyme receptors, with a pocket-like conformation, than for the much flatter typical protein binding sites). As already indicated, the replacement that a ligand performs of "unfavorable" hydration water molecules from the binding site has been established as a main driving force for binding (Qvist et al. 2008; Young et al. 2007; Wang et al. 2011; Friesner et al. 2006). In fact, this description has been shown to hold valid for a significant fraction of receptors of pharmaceutical interest (Young et al. 2007; Wang et al. 2011; Berne et al. 2009). Even in some cases, a portion of the receptor active site is so unfavorable for water molecules that it tends to remain practically dry (Young et al. 2007; Wang et al. 2011; Berne et al. 2009). Thus, the estimation of the free energy contribution involved in the displacement of quasilocalized (non-tightly-bonded) water molecules with unfavorable free energies in the receptor active site constitutes an issue of great interest in computational structure-based drug design (Young et al. 2007; Wang et al. 2011; Berne et al. 2009). Hence, it becomes relevant to develop a quantitative measure of hydrophobicity useful in determining such regions. Amongst the different structural, dynamical, and thermodynamical measures of hydrophobicity which have been proposed (Giovambattista et al. 2012; Giovambattista et al. 2008; Jamadagni et al. 2011), a very appealing one consists in the quantification of water density fluctuations (Raimundo et al. 2004). It has been demonstrated that superficial water density profiles do not represent a good measure of surface hydrophobicity. This can be expected in terms of the usual knowledge that water "abhors" vacuum and thus, water molecules tend to hydrate both polar and nonpolar surfaces and, thus, the density profiles normal to the surface plane display similar characteristics, with layering structure in both cases. However, at variance form hydrophilic surfaces where the water molecules are subject to significant attractive interactions, interactions are very weak at hydrophobic surfaces, which makes the hydrating water molecules display low residence times and be easily removed. Thus, such hydration layers display enhanced dynamics (Jamadagni et al. 2011), enhanced compressibility (Giovambattista et al. 2012; Giovambattista et al. 2008; Jamadagni et al. 2011), and enhanced density fluctuations (Jamadagni et al. 2011). In particular, the density fluctuations at differently functionalized self-assembled monolayers (SAMs) have been characterized demonstrating that hydrophobic-like surfaces do in fact present much larger density fluctuations than the ones displayed by hydrophilic-like surfaces, thus providing a good quantitative measure of hydrophobicity (Jamadagni et al. 2011). We have also studied (Alarcón et al. 2014) the role of curvature, determining that large holes in model hydrophobic systems display mild density fluctuations and even remain dry, a situation that has been experimentally found for certain protein pockets (Qvist et al. 2008). Additionally, we have studied water density fluctuations at graphitic-like surfaces determining a rather hydrophilic behavior, which we also found to be consistent with Potential of Mean Force calculations (Accordino et al. 2015). Normalized fluctuations of water number density, $\sigma^2/\langle N \rangle^2$, in small observation volumes (where N is the number of water molecules within such volume) are related to the free energy of formation of a cavity of such radius (Jamadagni et al. 2011). In fact, large water density fluctuations imply a high value of the water vacating probability in such an observation sphere (P ($N = 0$), which is calculated by computing the number of configurations the observational volume is empty of water molecules divided by the total number of configurations considered along the long MD runs performed). In small observation volumes $\mu = k_b T \ln[P(N = 0)]$, where μ is the free energy of formation of a cavity of such a small radius, k_b is Boltzmann constant and T is the absolute temperature (Jamadagni et al. 2011). Concurrently, a high value of water vacating probability at a given place indicates a favorable work of cavity creation at such place (Jamadagni et al. 2011) and, thus, a high hydrophobicity. We first calculated $P(N=0)$ at observation volumes centered at every heavy atom of the protein MDM2 for large simulation runs (50 ns) after equilibration, starting from the reported PDB structure. The protein MDM2 is interesting since it represents the natural regulator of the tumor supressor p53. A value of $P(N=0)$ close to unity implies that the atom is completely "dry" or desolvated (absence of a first hydration shell). If we focus on spheres centered at the heavy atoms of the protein surface we find that most of the surface is well hydrated (hydrophilic), while a patch of enhanced vacating probability (hydrophobic behavior) is observed at the p53 binding site. This result, compatible with studies of other proteins by the group of ShekharGarde (Jamadagni et al. 2011) supports the belief that ligands are expected to displace labile hydration water molecules from their protein binding site. However, since we are explicitly interested in the role of the BHB as protagonist of protein binding, we decided to calculate $P(N=0)$ at the amide (N atom) and carbonyl (O atom) moieties of each of the BHBs of the PDB.

Water Vacating Probability Around Backbone Hydrogen Bonds

As already indicated, the stability of non-covalent interactions like BHBs is expected to depend strongly on their local (hydration) environment (Fernández 2006; Fernández and Scott 2003; Accordino et al. 2012a,b; Sierra et al. 2013; Accordino et al. 2013). Thus, we next calculate the water vacating probability around the BHBs of the protein MDM2. The results of the calculations during simulation are displayed in Fig. 3(a), which depicts the behavior of $\langle P(N=0)\rangle$ for the complex MDM2-p53 and Fig. 3(b), for the apo form of protein MDM2. We simulated the apo form of the N-terminal domain of MDM2, MDM2^N, and a complex of MDM2^N with a peptide fragment taken from the transactivation domain of p53 (Uhrinova et al. 2005). The preponderance of red colors in Fig. 3(a) ($P(N=0)$ close to unity) speaks of the clear dehydration propensity of the BHBs of the MDM2 protein in complex with p53. This result implies that the above-mentioned predominance of hydrophilic regions ($P(N=0)$ close to zero) at the surface of the apo protein outside the binding site is given by well-hydrated side

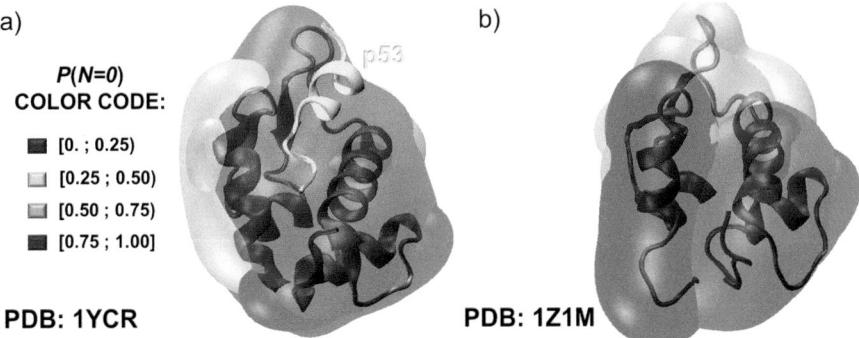

a)

$P(N=0)$
COLOR CODE:

■ [0. ; 0.25)
☐ [0.25 ; 0.50)
☐ [0.50 ; 0.75)
■ [0.75 ; 1.00]

PDB: 1YCR

b)

PDB: 1Z1M

Fig. 3: (a) Water vacating probability $P(N=0)$ for BHBs in the MDM2 protein in complex with p53. (b) Idem for the apo MDM2 protein.

chains that, in turn, protect the BHBs by promoting their drying. However, when we turn to Fig. 3(b), where we analyze the apo MDM2 protein, we can learn on the existence of a significant number of water-accessible BHBs (light-blue spheres) at the binding site. Thus, it is evident that the local environments of BHBs along the protein chain vary significantly, with predominance of buried or dry BHBs but also with binding-site BHBs which are (at least partially) water exposed. Thus, we expect binding regions to be more fluctuating and their BHBs to present a richer behavior with enhanced dynamics.

Dynamic Analysis of Backbone Hydrogen Bonds Propensity

In the last section we showed that BHBs, the main determinants of protein structure, might face different environments along the protein chain. Particularly, the situation at protein binding sites is very different from buried regions given the different local hydration/hydrophobicity conditions. The strength of non-covalent interactions is expected to change significantly their local environment and indeed, we have shown in a previous section (Sierra et al. 2013) (and also in other studies: Accordino et al. 2013) for one case study (the ADN recognition site of p53) that their dynamics and stability could be much altered at binding sites. Thus, now we build a time-averaged, or dynamic, BHB contact matrix (DBHB-CM) for the different proteins (Menéndez et al. 2015). This was done by calculating the fraction of time that each BHB is formed during long production runs. At each evaluation time, if a pair of residues i and j satisfy a hydrogen bonding criterion (N-O cutoff distance, $r < 3.5$ Å; N-H-O cutoff angle, $\theta > 140$ degrees (Menéndez et al. 2015), the corresponding $\{i,j\}$ matrix element becomes 1, while it is 0 otherwise. Then, we averaged the results for each matrix element at all evaluation times. Thus, the DBHB-CM contains values that range from 0 (never formed) to 1 (formed all the time) for the different matrix elements (for the sake of clarity, we discarded BHBs that were formed for less than 10 percent of the total run; this choice is arbitrary but the results do not depend on it). With this plot we can better learn on the correlation between BHB stability and water exposure. Thus, we calculated the mean value of the water vacating probability, $P(N = 0)$, for the BHBs whose average formation time was over 0.8 (very stable) and for the ones that were formed for a fraction of time less than 0.3 (the less persistent BHBs). Restricting the analysis for the BHBs located within the binding sites of the apo proteins (criterion 1, but similar results are obtained for criterion 2) we found that the very stable BHBs are practically dry ($\langle P(N = 0)\rangle = 0.9287$; $\sigma = 0.108$, where s is the standard deviation), while the less persistent ones are indeed water exposed ($\langle P(N = 0)\rangle = 0.3995$; with a larger σ-value of 0.228). These results can be seen in Fig. 4. Another interesting result is that the population of less persistent BHBs was greatly depleted when we considered the complexes of the target proteins with their partner proteins or with their corresponding disruptive molecules.

In Fig. 5(a) we show the DHBH-CM for the case of protein MDM2 in its apo form. We also show in Fig. 5(b) the PDB BHB Contact Matrix (PDB-BHB-CM) and in Fig. 5(c) we display the distance matrix (difference between the PDB-BHB-CM and the DHBH-CM).

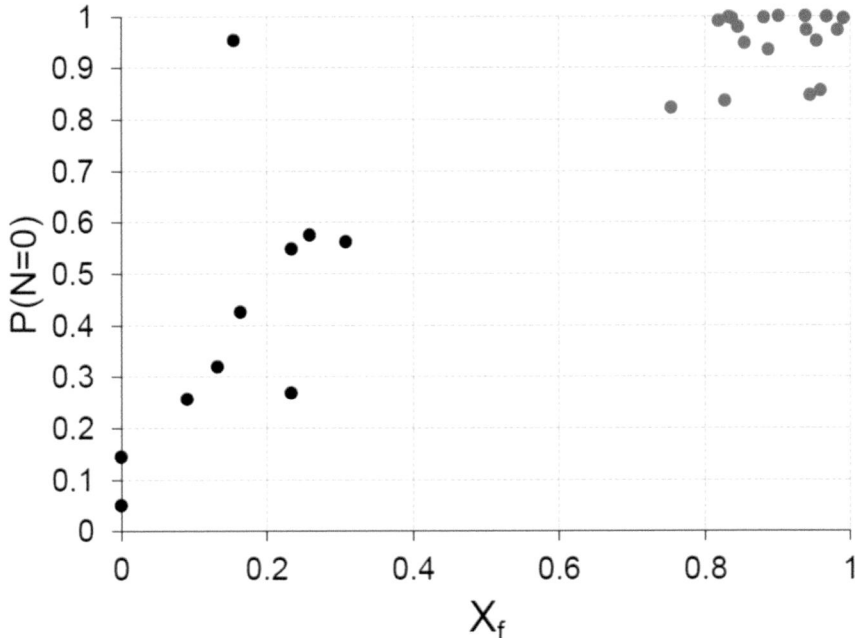

Fig. 4: Water vacating probability, $P(N=0)$, for the BHBs that were formed for a fraction of time, X_f, over 0.8 (very stable) and for the ones that were formed for X_f less than 0.3 (the less persistent BHBs).

To contrast the dynamical behavior of the protein with the information provided by the PDB structure we calculated, for each matrix element of the DBHB-CM, its distance, D, with respect to the corresponding matrix element of the PDB (PDB-BHB-CM, with values that are either strictly 1 or 0 if the BHB under consideration is formed or not in the PDB structure, respectively). In other words, for each BHB we calculated the difference between its formation propensity during the dynamics (its time-averaged state in the dynamics) and its corresponding state-value in the PDB structure. The resulting distance matrix (DM) is shown in Fig. 5(c) for the case of the protein MDM2 in its apo form, while in Fig. 6(a) we show the DM for MDM2 in complex MDM2-p53 calculated by comparing the DBHB-CM and the PDB-BHB-CM of the MDM2-p53 complex; we recall that we are studying MDM2^N and the complex of MDM2^N with a peptide fragment taken from the transactivation domain of p53 (Uhrinova et al. 2005). In turn, in Fig. 6(b) we present the case for the complex MDM2-Nutlin3.

The color intensity indicates the size of the distance, D: intense means large distance, while pale indicates low distance. If we focus on the case of the apo protein, we can learn that while most BHBs of the PDB are stable during the dynamics and thus yield a low D, there exist a significant number of BHBs that indeed display large D. Such BHBs represent either interactions that are present in the PDB but that disappear during the dynamics or interactions that are absent in the PDB but that are persistently formed during the dynamics. Such BHBs that "change color" (roughly from black/dark to white/pale or *vice versa*) between their PDB-BHB-CM (the matrix corresponding to the PDB) and the DBHB-CM (the matrix for the dynamics), will be

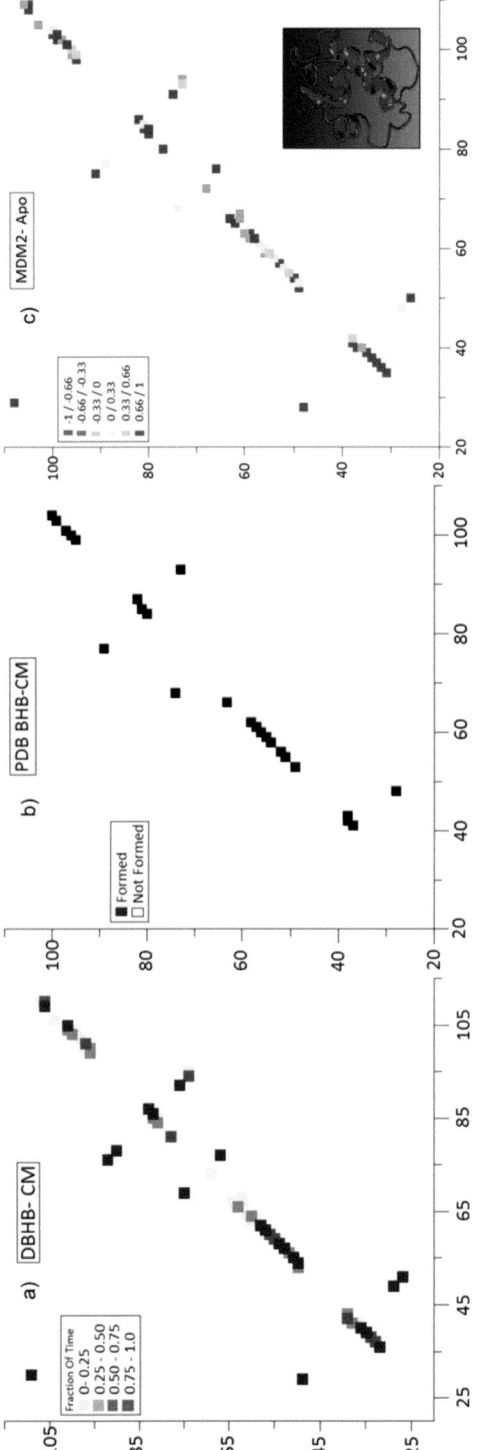

Fig. 5: (a) Dynamic Backbone Hydrogen Bond Contact Matrix (DBHB-CM) for a region containing the binding site of the apo form of protein MDM2; (b) The corresponding PDB BHB Contact Matrix (PDB-BHB-CM); (c) Corresponding distance matrix, the color intensity indicates the size of the distance value, D: intense means large distance, while pale indicates low distance. The insets show the 3D structure.

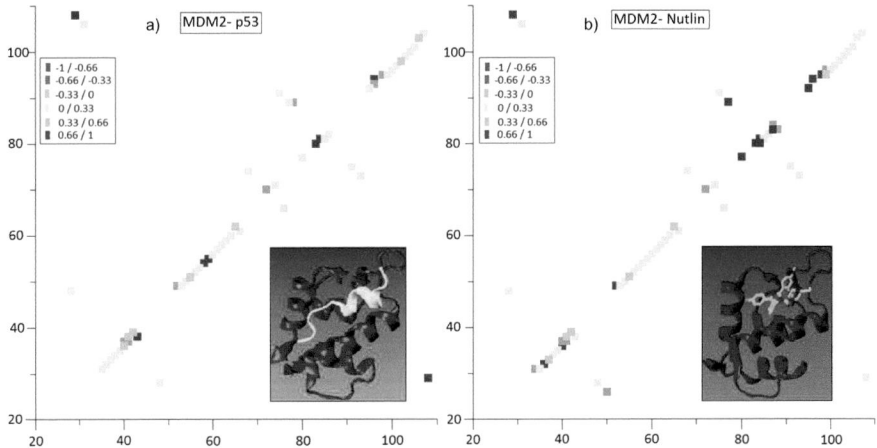

Fig. 6: Distance matrix for MDM2 in complex with p53 (a) and in complex with Nutlin3 (b).

termed as "chameleonic" BHBs (CBHBs). In this sense, the actual dynamical state in solution of such interactions is "hidden" in the PDB structure of the apo protein under an opposite state-value (which might thus confer a misleading dynamical expectation). We note that the determination of CBHBs resorts simply to the PDB structure of the apo protein and a dynamical analysis based on a MD simulation from such a structure (if possible, it might be worthy to employ, instead, experimental dynamical information from techniques like NMR). In turn, when we focus on the DM for the complex of MDM2 with its natural ligand, the MDM2-p53 complex, we can see that the dynamical and the PDB BHB-CMs are more similar, since most of the CBHBs of the binding site have disappeared as a result of the stabilization gained by the binding site upon ligand association. A similar result is found when we study the case of the complex MDM2-Nutlin3, a disruptive drug that acts by mimicking the behavior of p53 and represents a potent inhibitor. It is interesting to note that certain regions of secondary structure are quite disordered in the apo PDB (for example, the region between residues 101 and 107), while they are nicely structured in the complex, as can be learnt from the helical structure in the MDM2-p53 complex. These residues are located in regions of the apo protein with water accessible BHBs, as can be learnt from Fig. 2. However, when in complex with p53 (or with the disruptive molecule Nutlin-3) these BHBs become stabilized in the helical structure since they are now additionally inter-molecularly protected from hydration. Additionally, when we performed a simulation starting from the PDB structure of the apo MDM2 protein but with Nutlin-3 located at the binding site, we found that the secondary structure of this helix is significantly improved during the simulation. The plasticity of the MDM2 binding site, as made evident by the conformational changes that accompany the binding of p53 to MDM2^N, had been already determined experimentally (Uhrinova et al. 2005). In such work (Uhrinova et al. 2005) it was shown that upon binding of p53, the binding cleft of MDM2^N undergoes an expansion, achieved through a rearrangement of its two pseudosymetrically related sub-domains, resulting in the outward displacements of the secondary structural elements that comprise the walls and floor of the p53-binding cleft. Additionally, it has been stated that MDM2^N becomes more rigid and stable upon binding p53 (Uhrinova et al. 2005), also in accord with our results. We then repeated the analysis of Fig. 6 for the other three proteins and their complexes both with their natural protein ligand and with the corresponding disruptive drug or small molecule, IL-2 (PDB: 1M4C) /SP4206 (PDB: 1PY2)/IL-2 receptor alpha-chain (PDB: 1Z92) (Raimundo et al. 2004), BCL-XL (PDB: 1R2D)/ABT-73734 (PDB: 2YXJ)/ BAD-derived peptide (amino acids 100–126) (PDB: 2BZW) (Bruncko et al. 2007) and ZipA (PDB: 1F7W)/Compound 1 (PDB: 1Y2F)/FtsZ-derived peptide (PDB: 1F47) (amino acids 367–383) (Rush et al. 2005), finding in all cases similar results (Menéndez et al. 2015).

Additionally, in Fig. 7 we provide the probability distribution of distance values D (in fact, we use the absolute value of D), of all the matrix elements of the DM of the four apo proteins studied (Menéndez et al. 2015). We distinguish between BHBs at the binding sites of all proteins studied and for the rest ones (BHBs located outside the binding sites studied, indicated as "Rest"). We used criterion 1, but we also include the distribution for the binding site BHBs as determined by criterion 2, which provides similar results. A direct inspection reveals the dominance of two different populations, large or low D values, together with a conspicuous depletion in the region of medium-sized D values. The peak for low D values exhibited by all the curves is obviously

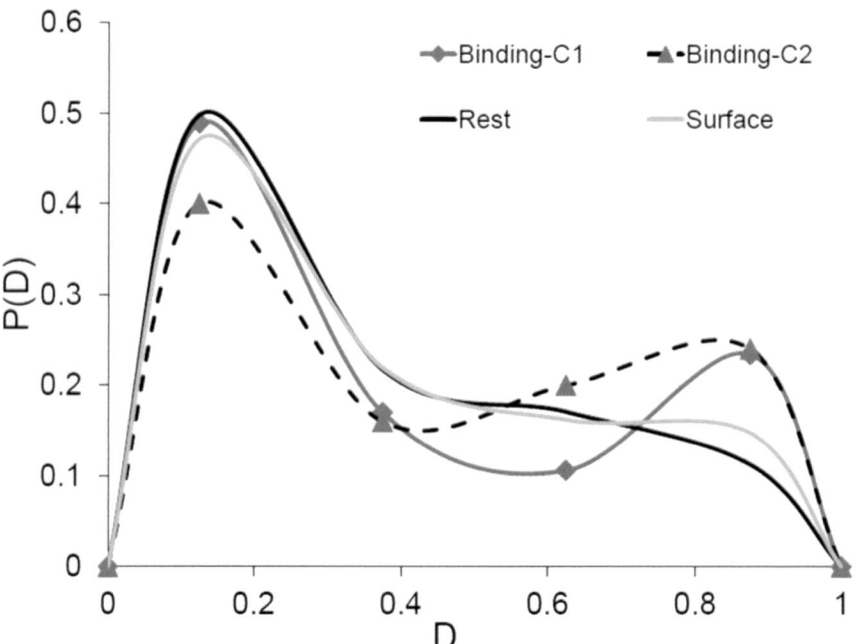

Fig. 7: Probability density distribution of distance values, D, for all the BHBs of the four apo proteins studied. We discriminate between the BHBs located at protein binding sites (criteria 1 and 2) from the rest of the protein BHBs (BHBs outside the binding site). The latter are classified as "Rest" (including all the BHBs outside the binding site, regardless if they are located at the protein surface or buried at the protein interior) or "Surface" (only the ones that are located at the protein surface).

expected, since it speaks of BHBs which are stable in the apo protein. However, the other population (high D values) signals the presence of CBHBs. More interestingly, we can learn that the protein binding site is clearly enriched in CBHBs, as indicated by the right peak that visibly develops for both criteria for the binding site BHBs. To discard that this effect was due to the nature of the binding-site BHBs as surface BHBs which are expected to be more labile than buried BHBs, we also present the curve for the BHBs located outside the binding site but that nonetheless reside at other regions of the protein surface (we call them "Surface" BHBs and identify them with a proximity criterion to water: A surface BHB is one whose distance from any water molecule is less than 6 Å). As expected, from comparison with the curve for all the residues outside the binding site ("Rest" curve), the "Surface" BHBs are a bit more labile than non-surface or buried BHBs. However, the behavior is very different for the clear bimodality and the concurrent enrichment in CBHBs presented by the BHBs of the binding site (Menéndez et al. 2015).

Up to this point, we have shown that CBHBs are motifs that take part in protein binding sites of apo proteins. Additionally, we learnt that these kinds of motifs are not as usual in protein-protein or protein-ligand complexes. To make this statement more quantitative and to make evident the role of CHBs as binding hot spots and drug targets, we now compare the apo protein with the complex with its natural protein partner and with the disrupting drug (small molecule). Direct inspection of the behavior of the protein-protein complex indicates that the binding process removes CBHBs (Menéndez et al. 2015). In fact, if we use a D-value larger than 0.5 in the DM (belonging to the right peak of Fig. 7) as a threshold for CBHB we find that for the four apo proteins, more than 80 percent of their CBHBs disappear upon complex formation (they cease to be CBHBs within the complex). Figure 8 presents such a study. From this figure we can learn that for MDM2, BCL, and Zip proteins, all CBHBs present

Mol	CBHBs		Apo Prot	Complex (Prot.-Prot.)		Complex (Prot.-Mol.)	
M	54	50	0.89	0.12	✓	0.06	✓
D	57	53	0.90	0.16	✓	0.11	✓
M	62	58	0.69	0.09	✓	0.12	✓
2	99	95	0.56	0.29	✓	0.59	✗
	100	96	0.45	0.10	✓	0.05	✓
	103	99	0.85	0.29	✓	0.17	✓
I	39	35	0.84	0.40	✓	Not formed	—
L	41	38	0.87	0.66	✗	0.36	✓
·	61	57	0.56	0.61	✗	0.37	✓
2	68	64	0.77	0.77	✗	0.90	✗
	69	65	0.77	0.41	✓	0.57	✗
B	100	96	0.94	0.09	✓	0.10	✓
C	125	121	0.54	0.29	✓	0.41	✓
L	126	122	0.52	0.39	✓	0.81	✗
Z	40	44	0.58	0.38	✓		
I	44	41	0.45	0.39	✓		
P	64	81	0.85	0.17	✓		

Fig. 8: Distance values, D, for the CBHBs for the four apo proteins studied, indicated by the pairs of residues comprised in the BHB (a value larger than 0.5 corresponds to a CBHB). We also provide the corresponding D-value for the protein-protein and protein-small molecule complexes. Whenever this value falls below 0.5 it indicates a CBHB removal upon complex formation. For the ZipA protein we do not provide the D-values for the complex with the small molecule since its binding affinity is low.

in the corresponding apo form are removed upon complex formation with the partner protein (for IL-2 this CBHB removal is only partial, since three CBHBs still remain as such in the corresponding protein-protein complex). A similar result is obtained when we compare the DMs of the target apo proteins with the DM for their corresponding protein-small molecule complex, albeit with a performance that is a bit suboptimal in terms of CBHB removal.

To further test the validity of our new approach we study the correlation of the parameter D (distance values between DBHB-CM and PDB-BHB-CM) with a quantitative experimental measure of affinity for the interaction between a disruptive molecule and its target protein. In this sense, we study six disruptive molecules (Vassilev et al. 2004; Miyazaki et al. 2013; Fry et al. 2013; Yin et al. 2005; Azevedo et al. 2013) of the MDM2-p53 interaction. These small molecules specifically bind to MDM2 and have been shown to place hydrophobic moieties (aromatic or aliphatic) in regions of the MDM2 targeted by the hot spot hydrophobic residues phe19, trp23, and leu26 of p53 (Vassilev et al. 2004; Miyazaki et al. 2013; Fry et al. 2013; Yin et al. 2005; Azevedo et al. 2013). The experimental values of IC50 (this quantitative measure indicates how much of a particular drug or other substance, inhibitor, is needed to inhibit a given biological process by half) for these six systems are already known from previous results (Vassilev et al. 2004; Miyazaki et al. 2013; Fry et al. 2013; Yin et al. 2005; Azevedo et al. 2013). For this purpose, we calculate the mean value of D, $\langle D \rangle$, of all CBHBs in the MDM2, for a production run time of 40 ns of such protein with each of the disruptive molecules. We calculate D, for each CBHB in the MDM2 protein, as the difference between the value of such CBHB in the DBHB-CM of the complex with the small molecule and the value for the same CBHB in the PDB-BHB-CM of the complex with its natural partner (p53). Then we average all the D values for the entire group of CBHBs. Figure 9(a) shows the correlation between $\langle D \rangle$ with the experimental values of IC50 for the six small molecules studied (for the last 20 ns of the production run). In Fig. 9(b) we also show the correlation between a theoretical estimation of the $\langle \Delta G \rangle$ of binding (calculated by the MMPBSA method (Feig et al. 2004)) and the experimental IC50 values for the same systems.

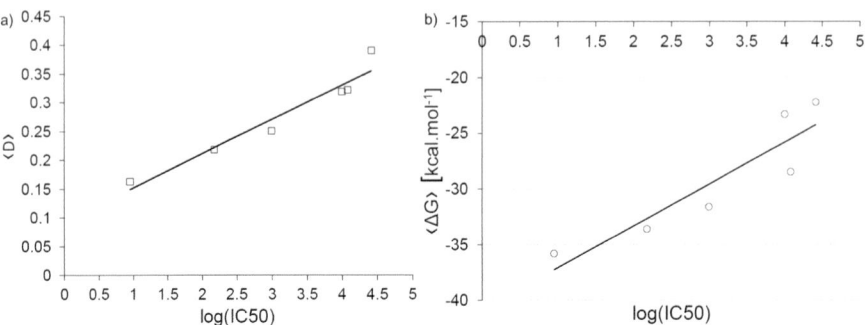

Fig. 9: (a) Correlation between $\langle D \rangle$ (for CBHBs and for the last 20 ns of the production run) with the log(IC50) experimental values for the six systems (MDM2-small molecules) studied. (b) Idem to (a) but for the correlation of the theoretical estimation of the $\langle \Delta G \rangle$ of binding with the log(IC50) experimental values (the mean values $\langle \Delta G \rangle$ were calculated by means of the MMPBSA method (Feig et al. 2004)).

We can see that the correlation with IC50 experimental values is better for the parameter D. We also show in Fig. 10 the correlation between $\langle D \rangle$ and $\langle \Delta G \rangle$.

These facts reveal CBHB-pattern determination as instrumental in defining ligand/ drug targets. In particular, wherever a drug scaffold or lead compound performs a suboptimal CBHB quenching, this method might help as a reengineering tool for drug optimization. As such, it might be easily implemented within existing methods to incorporate a relevant dynamical dimension disregarded by structurally-based approaches. In this sense, our method not only incorporates a dynamical analysis, but also puts the spotlight on a specific dynamical element essential for the binding process: the dynamics of BHBs.

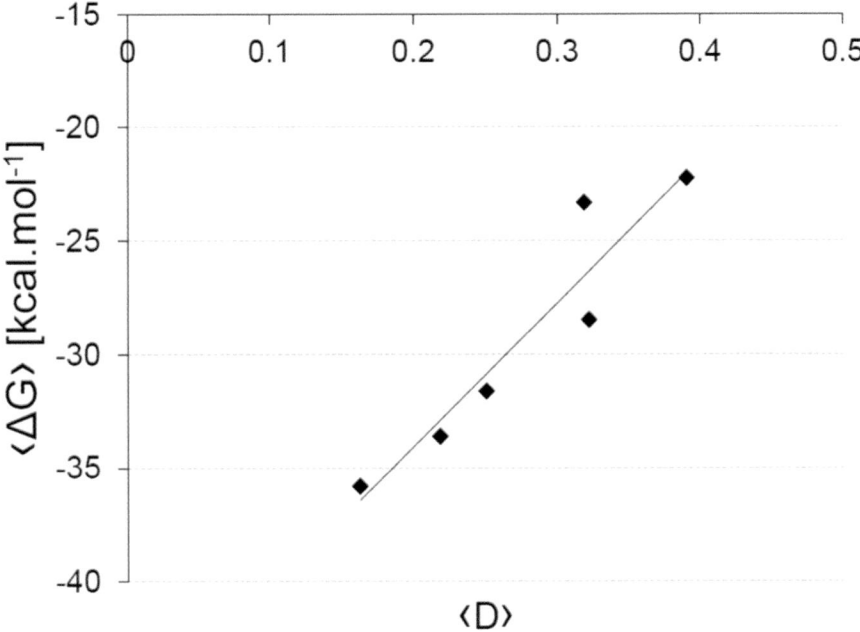

Fig. 10: Correlation between $\langle D \rangle$ and $\langle \Delta G \rangle$ of binding.

Conclusions

Backbone hydrogen bonds (BHBs) are main structural determinants of protein structure. However, being non-covalent interactions, they bare a context-dependent nature. Thus, the stability and dynamics of BHBs at protein binding sites, where they are at least solvent-exposed, are expected to differ from the situation at other, more buried, contexts. In this sense, the static picture of the PDB structure lacks information that might be essential to dynamics and function. In this sense, we have revealed the existence of "chameleonic" protein backbone hydrogen bonds (CBHBs) whose formation propensity during the dynamics in solution significantly differs from their PDB state. We also found that BHBs mainly consist of either CBHBs or stable ones, with a low population of intermediate states. Additionally, the relative abundance of

CBHBs is considerably enhanced at protein binding sites where the protein chain is partially exposed to hydration, thus revealing their role as ligand targets. Upon association, the dehydration of the binding site is completed with the concurrent stabilization and CBHBs removal. Thus, the dynamic analysis of hydrogen bond propensity that determines the pattern of CBHBs might be useful to build protein binding-site predictors and to develop novel design concepts for drug design. In this sense, our approach would be complementary to existing methods since it puts in the picture a novel relevant object, the CBHB, and might enable us to focus on backbone hydrogen bond stabilization as an operational principle to engineer better scaffolds.

Acknowledgments

Financial support from ANPCyT, MinCyT, and CONICET is gratefully acknowledged. SRA thanks CONICET for a fellowship. JARF, DCG, and GAA are research fellows of CONICET.

References

Accordino, S. R., D. C. Malaspina, J. A. Rodriguez Fris and G. A. Appignanesi. 2011. Comment on "Glass transition in biomolecules and the liquid-liquid critical point of water". Phys. Rev. Lett. 106: 029801.
Accordino, S. R., J. A. Rodriguez-Fris, G. A. Appignanesi and A. Fernández. 2012a. A unifying motif of intermolecular cooperativity in protein associations. Eur. Phys. J. E 35: 59.
Accordino, S. R., M. A. Morini, M. B. Sierra, J. A. Rodriguez Fris, G. A. Appignanesi and A. Fernández. 2012b. Wrapping mimicking in drug-like small molecules disruptive of protein-protein interfaces. Proteins: Struct., Funct., Bioinf. 80: 1755.
Accordino, S. R., D. C. Malaspina, J. A. Rodriguez Fris, L. M. Alarcón and G. A. Appignanesi. 2012c. Temperature dependence of the structure of protein hydration water and the liquid-liquid transition. Phys. Rev. E 85: 031503.
Accordino, S. R., J. A. Rodriguez Fris and G. A. Appignanesi. 2013. Wrapping effects within a proposed function-rescue strategy for the Y220C oncogenic mutation of protein p53. PLoS ONE 8: e55123.
Accordino, S. R., J. M. Montes de Oca, J. A. Rodriguez Fris and G. A. Appignanesi. 2015. Hydrophilic behavior of graphene and graphene-based materials. J. Chem. Phys. 143: 154704.
Alarcón, L. M., J. M. Montes de Oca, S. A. Accordino, J. A. Rodriguez Fris and G. A. Appignanesi. 2014. Hydrophobicity and geometry: water at curved graphitic-like surfaces and within model pores in self-assembled monolayers. Fluid Phase Equilibria 362: 81.
Appignanesi, G. A., J. A. Rodriguez-Fris, R. A. Montani and W. Kob. 2006a. Democratic particle motion for metabasin transitions in simple glass formers. Phys. Rev. Lett. 96: 057801.
Appignanesi, G. A., J. A. Rodriguez-Fris and M. A. Frechero. 2006b. Reproducibility of dynamical heterogeneities and metabasin dynamics in glass forming liquids: the influence of structure on dynamics. Phys. Rev. Lett. 96: 237803.
Azevedo, C. M. G., C. M. M. Afonso, J. X. Soares, S. Reis, D. Sousa, R. T. Lima et al. 2013. Pyranoxanthones: synthesis, growth inhibitory activity on human tumor cell lines and determination of their lipophilicity in two membrane models. Eur. J. Med. Chem. 69: 798.
Berne, B. J., J. D. Weeks and R. Zhou. 2009. Dewetting and hydrophobic interaction in physical and biological systems. Annu. Rev. Phys. Chem. 60: 85.
Bizzarri, A. R., A. Paciaroni and S. Cannistraro. 2000. Glasslike dynamical behavior of the plastocyanin hydration water. Phys. Rev. E 62: 3991.
Bizzarri, A. R. and S. Cannistraro. 2002. Molecular dynamics of water at the protein-solvent interface. J. Phys. Chem. B 106: 6617.
Boeckler, F. M., A. C. Joerger, G. Jaggi, T. J. Rutherford, D. B. Veprintsev and A. R. Fersht. 2008. Targeted rescue of a destabilized mutant of p53 by an *in silico* screened drug. Proc. Natl. Acad. Sci. U.S.A. 105: 10360.

Bogan, A. A. and K. S. Thorn. 1998. Anatomy of hot spots in protein interfaces. J. Mol. Biol. 208: 1.

Bruncko, M., T. K. Oost, B. A. Belli, H. Ding, M. K. Joseph, A. Kunzer et al. 2007. Studies leading to potent, dual inhibitors of Bcl-2 and Bcl-xL.J. Med. Chem. 50: 641.

Case, D. A., T. A. Darden, T. E. Cheatham, III, C. L. Simmerling, J. Wang, R. E. Duke et al. 2010. AMBER 11, University of California, San Francisco.

Debenedetti, P. G. 1996. Metastable Liquids. Princeton University Press, Princeton.

Feig, M., A. Onufriev, M. S. Lee, W. Im, D. A. Case and C. Brooks III. 2004. Performance comparison of generalized born and Poisson methods in the calculation of electrostatic solvation energies for protein structures. J. Comp. Chem. 25: 265.

Fernández, A. and R. Scott. 2003. Adherence of Packing Defects in Soluble Proteins. Phys. Rev. Lett. 91: 018102.

Fernández, A. 2010. Transformative Concepts for Drug Design: Target Wrapping Vol. 1. Springer, Heidelberg, pp. 1–224.

Friesner, R. A., R. B. Murphy, M. P. Repasky, L. L. Frye, J. R. Greenwood, T. A. Halgren et al. 2006. Extra precision glide: Docking and scoring incorporating a model of hydrophobic enclosure for protein-ligand complexes. J. Med. Chem. 49: 6177.

Fry, D. C., C. Wartchow, B. Graves, C. Janson, C. Lukacs, U. Kammlott et al. 2013. Deconstruction of a nutlin: dissecting the binding determinants of a potent protein–protein interaction inhibitor. ACS Med. Chem. Lett. 4: 660.

Giovambattista, N., P. G. Debenedetti, C. F. Lopez and P. J. Rossky. 2008. Hydrophobicity of protein surfaces: separating geometry from chemistry. Proc. Natl. Acad. Sci. U.S.A. 105: 2274.

Giovambattista, N., P. J. Rossky and P. G. Debenedetti. 2012. Computational studies of pressure, temperature, and surface effects on the structure and thermodynamics of confined water. Annu. Rev. Phys. Chem. 63: 179.

Jamadagni, S. N., R. Godawat and S. Garde. 2011. Hydrophobicity of proteins and interfaces: insights from density fluctuations. Annu. Rev. Chem. Biomol. Eng. 2: 147.

Jorgensen, W. L., J. Chandrasekhar, J. D. Madura, R. W. Impey and M. L. Klein. 1983. Comparison of simple potential functions for simulating liquid water. J. Chem. Phys. 79: 926.

Kulp, J. L. 3rd, J. L. Kulp, Jr., D. L. Pompliano and F. J. L. Guarnieri. 2011. Diverse fragment clustering and water exclusion identify protein hot spots. J. Am. Chem. Soc. 133: 10740.

Kumar, P., Z. Yan, L. Xu, M. G. Mazza, S. V. Buldyrev, S.-H. Chen et al. 2006. Glass transition in biomolecules and the liquid-liquid critical point of water. Phys. Rev. Lett. 97: 177802.

Li, J. and Q. Liu. 2009. Double water exclusion: a hypothesis refining the O-ring theory for the hot spots at protein interfaces. Bioinformatics 25: 743.

Mahoney, M. W. and W. L. Jorgensen. 2000. A five-site model liquid water and the reproduction of the density anomaly by rigid, non-polarizable models. J. Chem. Phys. 112: 8910.

Malaspina, D. C., E. P. Schulz, L. M. Alarcón, M. A. Frechero and G. A. Appignanesi. 2010. Structural and dynamical aspects of water in contact with a hydrophobic surface. Eur. Phys. J. E 32: 35.

Menéndez, C. A., S. R. Accordino, D. C. Gerbino and G. A. Appignanesi. 2015. "Chameleonic" backbone hydrogen bonds in protein binding and as drug targets. European Physical Journal E 38: 107.

Miyazaki, M., H. Naito, Y. Sugimoto, H. Kawato, T. Okayama, H. Shimizu et al. 2013. Lead optimization of novel p53-MDM2 interaction inhibitors possessing dihydroimidazothiazole scaffold. Bioorg. Med. Chem. Lett. 23: 728.

Qvist, J., M. Davidovic, D. Hamelberg and B. Halle. 2008. A dry ligand-binding cavity in a solvated protein. Proc. Natl. Acad. Sci. U.S.A. 105: 6296.

Raimundo, B. C., J. D. Oslob, A. C. Braisted, J. Hyde, R. S. McDowell, M. Randal et al. 2004. Integrating fragment assembly and biophysical methods in the chemical advancement of small-molecule antagonists of IL-2: an approach for inhibiting protein-protein interactions. J. Med. Chem. 47: 3111.

Rodriguez Fris, J. A., G. A. Appignanesi, E. La Nave and F. Sciortino. 2007. Metabasin dynamics and local structure in supercooled water. Phys. Rev. E 75: 041501.

Rodriguez Fris, J. A., G. A. Appignanesi and E. R. Weeks. 2011. Experimental verification of rapid, sporadic particle motions by direct imaging of glassy colloidal systems. Phys. Rev. Lett. 107: 065704.

Rush, T. S., J. A. Grant, L. Mosyak and A. Nicholls. 2005. A shape-based 3-D scaffold hopping method and its application to a bacterial protein-protein interaction. J. Med. Chem. 48: 1489.

Schulz, E. P., L. M. Alarcón and G. A. Appignanesi. 2011. Behavior of water in contact with model hydrophobic cavities and tunnels and carbon nanotubes. Eur. Phys. J. E 34: 114.

Sierra, M. B., S. R. Accordino, J. A. Rodriguez-Fris, M. A. Morini, G. A. Appignanesi and A. Fernández Stigliano. 2013. Protein packing defects "heat up" interfacial water. Eur. Phys. J. E 36: 62.

Uhrinova, S., D. Uhrin, H. Powers, K. Watt, D. Zheleva, P. Fischer et al. 2005. Structure of free MDM2 N-terminal domain reveals conformational adjustments that accompany p53-binding. J. Mol. Biol. 350: 587.

Vassilev, L. T., B. T. Vu, B. Graves, D. Carvajal, F. Podlaski, Z. Filipovic et al. 2004. *In vivo* activation of the p53 pathway by small-molecule antagonists of MDM2. Science 303: 844.

Wang, G. and A. R. Fersht. 2012. First-order rate-determining aggregation mechanism of p53 and its implications. Proc. Natl. Acad. Sci. U.S.A. 109: 13590.

Wang, L., B. J. Berne and R. A. Friesner. 2011. Ligand binding to protein-binding pockets with wet and dry regions. Proc. Natl. Acad. Sci. U.S.A. 108: 1326.

Wells, J. A. and C. L. McClendon. 2007. Review article reaching for high-hanging fruit in drug discovery at protein–protein interfaces. Nature 450: 1001.

Wilcken, Rainer, Xiangrui Liu, Markus O. Zimmermann, Trevor J. Rutherford, Alan R. Fersht, Andreas C. Joerger et al. 2012a. Halogen-enriched fragment libraries as leads for drug rescue of mutant p53. J. Am. Chem. Soc. 134: 6810.

Wilcken, R., G. Wang, F. M. Boeckler and A. R. Fersht. 2012b. Kinetic mechanism of p53 oncogenic mutant aggregation and its inhibition. Proc. Natl. Acad. Sci. U.S.A. 109: 13584.

Yin, H., G. Lee, H. S. Park, G. A. Payne, J. M. Rodriguez, S. M. Sebti et al. 2005. Terphenyl-based helical mimetics that disrupt the p53/HDM2 interaction. Chem. Int. Ed. 44: 2704.

Young, T., R. Abel, B. Kim, B. J. Berne and R. A. Friesner. 2007. Motifs for molecular recognition exploiting hydrophobic enclosure in protein–ligand binding. Proc. Natl. Acad. Sci. U.S.A. 104: 808.

14

Molecular Dynamics Simulations and Comparison of Two New and High Selective Imprinted Xerogels

Riccardo Concu,[1],* Manuel Azenha[2] and M. Natalia D. S. Cordeiro[1],*

Introduction

Molecular modeling indicates the general process of describing complex chemical systems in terms of a realistic atomic model, with the goal being to understand and predict macroscopic properties based on detailed knowledge on an atomic scale. Often, molecular modeling is used to design new materials, for which the accurate prediction of physical properties of realistic systems is required. These properties could be divided in two main groups: static equilibrium properties, like the binding constant of a drug to a receptor, and dynamic or non-equilibrium properties, like the diffusion of molecules through two phases or reaction kinetics and so on. Due to the great variety of techniques we will carefully choose the most appropriate to our problem. In any case, the most accurate is the so called *ab initio* which uses

[1] REQUIMTE, Department of Chemistry and Biochemistry, Faculty of Sciences, University of Porto, Rua do Campo Alegre, 687, 4169-007 Porto, Portugal.

[2] CIQ-UP, Department of Chemistry and Biochemistry, Faculty of Sciences, University of Porto, Rua do Campo Alegre, 687, 4169-007 Porto, Portugal.

* Corresponding author: riccardo.concu@fc.up.pt; ncordeir@fc.up.pt

the time-dependent Schrödinger equation to describe the properties of molecular systems; however, with the actual technology we are able to simulate systems with few atoms because this method works by computing the forces acting on the nuclei from electronic structure calculations (Marx and Hutter 2000). Due to this, when simulating large systems we have to do approximations using *empirical* parameterization of the model. In this context, the two most famous modeling methods are Molecular Dynamics simulations (MD) and Monte Carlo (MC) simulations. This two methods can be used for the the the generation of a representative equilibrium ensemble while for the generation of non-equilibrium ensembles and for the analysis of dynamic events only MD could be used. The core idea of Monte Carlo is to learn about a system by simulating it with random sampling. This method is used in almost every quantitative subject of study: physical sciences, engineering, statistics, finance, and computing, including machine learning and graphics (Kulkarni et al. 2015; Song et al. 2015; Liang et al. 2016; Yoon et al. 2015; Wilangowski and Stolwijk 2015). On the other hand, MD simulations solve Newton's equations of motion for a system of N interacting atoms and with this calculate the time dependent behavior of a molecular system, thus giving a more realistic image of a simulated system. Due to this MD is the most used technique. The MD method was firstly introduced by Alder and Wainwright in the late 1950's (Alder and Wainwright 1957, 1959) to study the interactions of hard spheres. Briefly, MD simulations generate information at the microscopic level, including atomic positions and velocities. This microscopic information is then transformed to macroscopic observables properties such as pressure, energy, heat capacities, etc. This transformation is done through the use of the statistical mechanic theory (Finkelstein and Reva 1992; Vorob'ev Iu 2003; Molodtsov et al. 2005). These methods are now routinely used to investigate the structure, dynamics, and thermodynamics of biological molecules and their complexes. From those first two papers to now, the MD techniques have greatly expanded and now are widely used to study a great variety of different systems. In fact, at the moment, within pubmed (www.pubmed.org) alone there are more than 13000 papers listed under the term "Molecular Dynamics". At a glance, this technique is widely used to study and simulate proteins or DNA conformation as well as binding affinity between drugs and enzymes, liquid interphase, or even the properties of a pure liquid (DeMarco 2015; Lee et al. 2015; Lang et al. 2015; Wang et al. 2015; Markegard et al. 2015; Guo et al. 2015; Song and Guo 2015; Kachhap and Singh 2015; Tripuraneni and Azam 2015; Verma et al. 2014; Jalkute et al. 2013; Nagayama et al. 2015; Burney et al. 2015; Yang and Laird 2014; Braga et al. 2014; da Silva et al. 2007; Zen et al. 2015; Siberchicot and Clerouin 2012; Bako et al. 2006; Plimpton 1995). Nowadays there are a lot of softwares and computer programs that can perform a MD simulation. The more famous ones are: AMBER, CHARMM, Discovery Studio, GAUSSIAN, GROMACS, GROMOS, and LAMMPS (Case et al. 2015; Brooks et al. 2009; Gao and Huang 2011; Frisch 2009; Van Der Spoel et al. 2005; Van Gunsteren and Berendsen 1987). Some are open source, such as GROMACS or LAMMPS, whether others need a commercial license, GAUSSIAN or Discovery Studio for example. GROMACS is one of the most used softwares to perform MD simulations due to its very fast algorithmic and processor-specific optimization, typically running 3–10 times faster than many simulation programs (Kutzner et al.

2015; Gruber and Pleiss 2011). In addition, with the use of high end GPU instead of a classical large cluster, GROMACS is even faster. Indeed, we can boost our simulations up to 10 times.

On the other hand, sol-gel materials are obtained from the hydrolysis and polycondensation of precursors, usually with a M(OR)4 general structure, which evolve into an inorganic 3D netchapter, built up of -M-O-M- bonds. Most often, M is either Si (the gel is usually called silica) or Ti (titanium dioxide gels). R usually represents an alkyl group that does not link to the netchapter. However, it is possible to produce hybrid organic-inorganic sol-gel netchapters by the co-polycondensation of M(OR)4 and R'-M(OR)3 (or other types of organically modified metal alkoxides), where the non-reactive R' becomes incorporated in the netchapter skeleton. Therefore, it is possible to produce a large diversity of gels bearing some R' functionality. In any case, sol-gel process can be described as follows: in an aqueous solution (in the presence of a co-solvent to prevent immiscibility) metal alkoxides (M-OR) are hydrolized to produce M-OH groups, which will then go under condensation reactions to form a -M-O-M-network that is the foundation of the growing three-dimensional gel structure. Both base- or acid-catalyzed hydrolysis and condensation reactions occur at the same time. During the time required for these reactions to take place the viscosity of the solution gradually increases, and when drying occurs at ambient conditions, the resultant material is denominated xerogel. Books by Brinker and Scherer (Brinker and Scherer 1990) or Wright and Sommerdijk (Wright and Sommerdijk 2001) are recommended for further reading about the physical and chemical principles of sol-gel processing.

Regarding molecular imprinting, this is a new and emerging technique based on natural molecular recognition. Using this technique, we can produce polymers with tailored recognition sites that will specifically interact with template molecules used to produce the sites. In fact, these materials are created through the interaction between the template and complementary functional monomers; this first step is then followed by the polymerization of this conjugate with cross-linkers in an appropriate solvent. Finally, the template molecule is removed from the matrix, usually using a washing procedure, leaving free the binding sites. There are three main methods to produce molecular imprinted materials: covalent, non-covalent, and semi-covalent imprinting. The first one employs reversible covalent bonds between the template molecule and the functional monomer(s) and this linkage needs to be formed before the polymerization step starts. For the rebinding of the template to the imprinted material the same covalent bond is established. Since the functional monomer is associated to the imprinted molecule, it exists only in the imprinted cavity and non-specific binding is reduced. On the other side, non-covalent methodology is an easier process and the most used for the production of molecularly imprinted sol-gel materials. In this case, the bonds between the template and the functional groups of the polymerizable monomer are weaker (hydrogen bonding, ionic interactions, or metal coordination, for example), making the removal of the template simpler and faster. To combine the advantages of both covalent and non-covalent approaches, a hybrid methodology was also developed. The clear-cut nature of covalent imprinting and the fast binding of the guest molecule to the functional monomer of the non-covalent imprinting were combined (polymers are prepared as covalent and the guest binding is based on non-covalent interactions).

Molecularly imprinted sol-gels are obtained during the process of (co-) polycondensation, by inserting inert (usually) templates within the growing netchapter. The purpose of templating is that of occupying a volume inside the gel, which may, subsequently, be converted into a cavity. Since the gel is formed around the template, the cavity left behind is expected to match the size and shape of the template. Moreover, the template is also expected to assemble within the gel, in configurations that reflect the most favorable interactions with the surface groups in the gel backbone. Thus, the cavity originated by the removal of the template is also assumed to possess a chemical complementarity regarding the template. Hence, molecularly imprinted sol-gels are recognitive materials, exhibiting high selectivity for the template (or analogous) molecules, due to the existence of binding sites with matching size, shape and chemical affinity. The chemical affinity is quite often optimized by selecting the appropriate R' functionalities inserted within hybrid sol-gel netchapters.

Due to this, molecular imprinting technology (MIT) has been widely used in recent years in a great variety of areas to prepare the so called molecular imprinted polymers (MIP). With respect to classical techniques, MIT presents several advantages such as physical robustness, long shelf life, simple preparation, great selectivity, etc. For these reasons, MITs are being studied and used in very different fields such as solid phase extraction, enantiomer separations, drug delivery, drug discovery, and ligand binding assays, to prepare synthetic receptors able to recognize and bind or release the template molecules, new HPLC matrix for selective detection and/or separation of drugs. These materials are often based on a silica backbone and on inorganic-organic hybrid materials prepared with organically-modified trialkoxysilanes (ORMOSIL). In this context, MIT is gaining day by day a most relevant role due to the growing demand for sensitive, accurate, and simple methods and materials able to achieve these goals. In fact, MIP mainly has been used to prepare selective materials able to recognize and separate conventional pharmaceuticals and drugs. Regarding the latter, the most tackled molecules are the antibiotics, followed by antidepressives, and NSAID drugs.

Antibiotics are the most studied molecules in this field because they are widely used to control bacterial and virus caused disease in humans as well as in animals. In fact, the presence of trace of antibiotics in food is of major concern because they can generate a growing bacterial resistance to the antibiotics. Nafcillin is a semisynthetic β-lactamic antibiotic employed in the treatment of serious infections caused by penicillinase-producing staphylococci (e.g., septicaemia, osteomyelitis, pneumonia, and endocarditis). This antibiotic is the most studied as a consequence of its extensive use and efficacy; due to this a considerable attention has been paid to the development of systems able to determine and extract this drug from serum, urine, blood, meat, and milk. In this context the paper of Liu et al. (2013) is really relevant because they have developed a novel composite based on core-shell molecularly imprinted polymers combining a surface imprinting technique with a sol-gel process based on carbon nanotubes (CNTs) coated with silica. This new material has shown higher specific recognition ability for nafcillin® over both oxacillin® and mezlocillin®. Another relevant paper in this field was published by Guardia et al. (2012). The authors have used methyltrimethylorthosilicate as precursor to create 22 molecularly imprinted polymers, and the respective control materials, against the nafcillin under different experimental conditions. In addition, they have studied the effect of the increase of the nafcillin concentration in the selectivity of the material. The results clearly shown that the increase of the template in the initial mixture produced imprinted sol-gels with enhanced recognition ability against nafcillin, due to the greater number of active sites present; however, a further increase was deleterious, reducing the number of active sites and the selectivity of the material.

In the case of antidepressives drugs, the most relevant paper was published by Rezaei (Rezaei et al. 2014) in 2013. The authors reported a new sensitive and selective imprinted electrochemical sensor for lorazepam determination; the sensor was based on a pencil graphite electrode (PGE) modified with one-step electropolymerization of the MIP composed from polypyrrole (ppy), sol-gel, gold nanoparticles (AuNPs), and lorazepam. The MIP was produced with TEOS and PTEOS as precursors. To evaluate the selectivity of the prepared sensor some analogues and coexisting substances, which included diazepam, phenobarbital, ascorbic acid, and uric acid were chosen as interference with 20-fold excess of the aforementioned interfering substances. The excellent sensitivity of the polypyrrole@sol-gel@gold nanoparticles MIP/PGE was due to the cavities which matched with the size, shape, and functional group position of the lorazepam. Finally, the capability of the new sensor was examined by determining the lorazepam concentration in tablet, urine, and plasma samples. The authors reported a satisfactory recovery for all samples, between 96% and 108%.

Regarding the NSAID drugs, Ibuprofen® and Naproxen® are the leaders, the most used the most studied. Zhou et al. (Zhou et al. 2013) prepared a new and high selective MIP for the ibuprofen. To evaluate the affinity and the selectivity of MIP towards ibuprofen, the authors had selected similar molecular structures and perform a series of binding tests, the molecules chosen were ketoprofen, naproxen, and aspirin. The results of equilibrium rebinding experiments showed that MIP had a very good adsorption capacity for ibuprofen. In a different work, Kadhirvel et al. (2013) developed a new Naproxen® imprinted polymer that was finally tested against the ibuprofen showing a higher affinity for the template molecule thus, confirming the robustness of the method and the usability of the MIP as a technique to produce new and high selective materials.

Proteins are inspiring the community of molecular imprinters because of their high specificity for specific targets. In molecular imprinting, proteins are also regarded as possible templates for imprints, that is, the preparation of artificial recognitive materials for proteins is an important sub-topic of research. In any case, the most interesting application of imprinted proteins is quantification of proteins in body fluids. However, the preparation of protein imprints is the more challenging task. In fact, the large number of functional groups available is the major complication to the traditional imprinting protocols developed for smaller compounds. This topic has been investigated and reviewed by several authors in the last years such as Hansen, Tao, Li, Zhang, Dickert, and Concu (Hansen 2007; Li et al. 2008; Zhang et al. 2011; Dickert and Hayden 2002; Concu et al. 2015; Tao et al. 2006). In any case, the most used approach in this field is based on the utilization of supporting beads with surficial amine groups, and the conversion of these groups into the aldehyde function, which enables the covalent immobilization of protein by an imide bond. A thin layer of a properly formulated sol-gel film is then deposited onto the bead surface, around the immobilized proteins while creating preferred interaction motifs. The proteins are finally washed out by breaking the labile imide bond. A relevant chapter in this area was published by Crisafulli et al. (2008). Using chitosan beads as starting material, in order to immobilize the bovine serum albumin (BSA) and a binary sol-gel precursor mixture consisting of TEOS and 3-aminopropyltrimethoxysiloxane (APTMOS) they were able to improve the immobilization capacity against a no-imprinted material (15.5 mg g^{-1} I-MIP, 1.6 mg g^{-1} F-MIP, 2.8 mg g^{-1} NIP). Moreover, also the selectivity versus other proteins such as transferrin or cytochrome *c* was tested; they found that the selectivity factors were improved by 4.9 and 25.5. Another relevant chapter was published by Lin et al. (2009). In this case, hybrid bovine hemoglobin (BHb)-imprinted silica beads were tested for the specific removal of BHb from bovine blood. They have incubated a 100-fold diluted bovine blood with the BHb-imprinted polymers. The result was that the blood changed from bright red to brown color suggesting specificity for hemoglobin. This method is a clear clever solution for selective removal of target protein from the biological complex.

As we have seen, MIP materials may represent a new frontier in the development of new and high selective materials able to recognize, bind, and release a great variety of small and big molecules. In the next paragraphs we will present new findings of our group in this area.

Computational Background

The MD simulations were performed with GROMACS 5.0.4 (Van Der Spoel et al. 2005) package applying the OPLS-AA (Jorgensen et al. 1983) force field, including the enhancements proposed by our group for sol-gel reactants in a recent publication (Concu et al. 2014). GROMACS is an open source software package widely used to perform MD simulations to model a great variety of systems; it is one of the best programs to perform MD simulations due to its high speed and reliability, in particular through the new GPU support which is able to speed up a MD simulation up to 10 times (Kutzner et al. 2015). All systems under study contained water, methanol, the anionic form of S-Naproxen (the template, NAP, Fig. 1A), the silica trimer SI3 (Fig. 1D), its anionic form SI$^-$ (Fig. 1E), and the dual cyclic silicate trimer corresponding to a hydrolized and condensed species derived from the cationic dehydroimidazolium ORMOSIL (DHI$^+$, Figs. 1B and 1C), all these structures are reported in the Fig. 1. In a previous chapter, we have presented a DHI$^+$ with a complete –OH hydrolization in the silica rings. In that case the template has shown a good affinity for the MIP; even so, we want to make a step over investigating the affinity of others ORMOSIL species that are likely to be present in the mixture.

Due to this, here we present two new DHI$^+$ molecules; in one case the –OH has been almost completely replaced by –CH$_3$ (Fig. 1B), whether in the second case we represent an intermediate situation with a replacement in a 1:2 ratios (Fig. 1C). These changes have been made in order to study the selectivity of two DHI$^+$ molecules that are likely to be present in the real mixture. Using this kind of representation, we are able to study and simulate the affinity of two new DHI$^+$ molecules for the template, in order to evaluate which one has the better affinity for the template molecule. All the nonstandard parameters were described in a previous report (Azenha et al. 2011; Concu et al. 2014) except those used for the two new DHI$^+$, which were parameterized

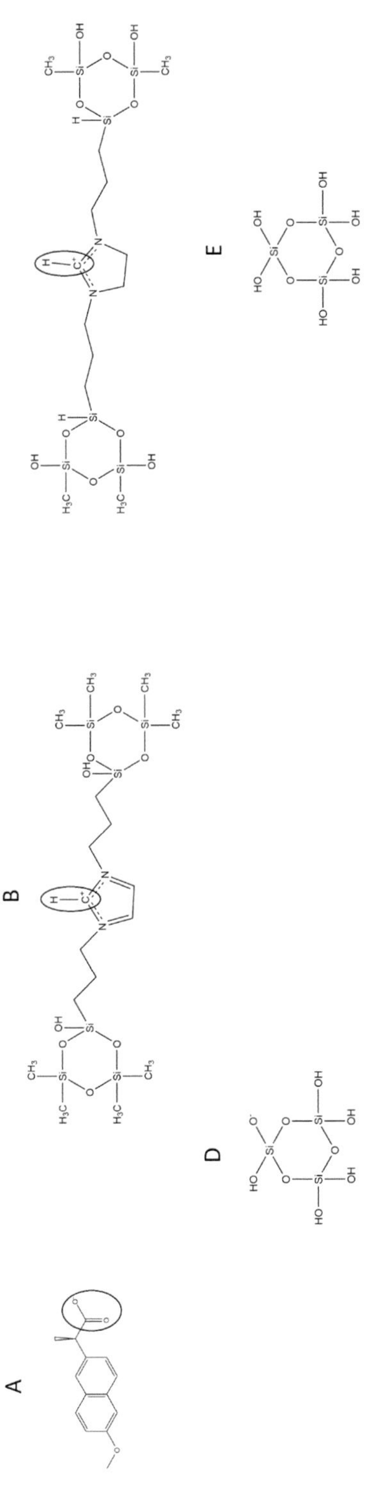

Fig. 1: Structures of the chemical species in the mixtures.

and validated for the first time in this chapter. With regard to the atomic point charges for the DHI$^+$ and NAP species, they were calculated using Gaussian 09 (Frisch 2009) in an OPLS-AA compliant manner; meaning that the geometry was first optimized at HF/6-31G* level, and then partial charges were computed from a single-point run, using the CHelpG scheme (Breneman and Wiberg 1990) at the B3LYP/6-311++G(2d,2p) level of theory; information regarding these molecules is available under request. This approximation was chosen over the standard OPLS-AA force field calculation (MP2/aug-cc-pVTZ//HF/6-31G*) due to a better stability of the DHI$^+$ when using the 6-311++G(2d,2p) basis set. The two studied models are summarized in Table 1. The number of functional silicate (DHI$^+$) units and structural silicate (SI3 plus SI$^-$) units was determined from the experimental concentrations of AO-DHI$^+$ iodide and TMOS. It was assumed that the precursors went through complete hydrolysis and fully condensed to DHI$^+$ or SI3 (or its conjugated bases). On the other hand, the ratios of SI3 to SI$^-$ units and DHI$^+$ were estimated from a species distribution analysis conducted at pH 9, based on the acidity constant of the silanol group, having in mind that pKa decreases by 1–2 units with high methanol contents.

Table 1: Composition of the model.

Molecule	Model A	Model B
NAP	10	10
DHI	10	10
SI3	9	9
SI-	9	9
Na	29	29
I	20	20
WAT	230	230
MET	1130	1130

The initial state of the two systems were obtained using the packmol package which inserts into the boxes the respective number of units at random positions (Martinez et al. 2009). Initial box dimensions were estimated considering the molecular weight and the density of each of the components of the mixture. After energy minimization using steepest-descent methods included in the GROMACS package, a temperature annealing was performed in the *NVT* ensemble for 2 ns, reaching a temperature of 500 K, in order to ensure a proper mixing and gather three random independent initial configurations. These were, subsequently, used as starting configurations for the three independent MD equilibration runs needed to test the reproducibility of the simulations. Before the production stage, ~ 50 ns of simulation time in the *NpT* ensemble were taken to equilibrate the system and reach a stable configuration. Finally, production runs of 50 ns were performed in the *NpT* ensemble for data collection. Observable properties were sampled every 2 ps, from which total averages and standard deviations for each run were computed. The equations of motion were integrated using the Verlet leapfrog algorithm (Hockney et al. 1974), with a time step of 2 fs. Typically, the temperature (*T*) was kept fixed at 298 K by applying the velocity rescaling thermostat

(Bussi et al. 2007), and whenever necessary, the pressure (p) was held constant at 1 bar by using the Parrinello-Rahman scheme (Parrinello and Rahman 1981; Nosé and Klein 1983). The time constant used for the Parrinello-Rahman coupling was set to 1 ps. Periodic boundary conditions were applied in all three Cartesian directions. For the water molecules, the Transferable Intermolecular Potential four-point model (TIP4P) (Jorgensen 1996) was applied. The non-bonded electrostatic interactions were calculated using a sixth-order Particle Mesh Ewald (PME) method (Essmann et al. 1995) beyond a cutoff radius of 1.1 nm. The Lennard−Jones was calculated within a cutoff radius of 1.1 nm with the help of a neighbor list, updated every 10 time steps. A dielectric permittivity, ε_r, equal to 1.0 was used. Statistical and trajectory analysis of the simulations were performed with the utilities included in GROMACS, while visualizations were made with VMD (Humphrey et al. 1996). The analysis consisted essentially in the calculation of radial distribution functions (RDF), diffusion coefficients (D), coordination numbers (N_B), and clustering analysis. The RDF between different types of molecules has been calculated as:

$$g_{AB}(r) = \frac{\langle \rho_B(r) \rangle}{\langle \rho_B \rangle_{loc}},$$

where $\langle \rho_B(r) \rangle$ refers to the average density of particle B at a distance r, around the particle A, and $\langle \rho_B \rangle_{loc}$ refers to the density of the particle B averaged over all spheres around particles A with a maximum radius (r_{max}) which was half of the box length. The RDF function is additionally averaged on all particles of type A present in the system, and also averaged over the trajectory (simulation time). The g_rdf function included in the GROMACS package calculates the RDF in different ways. The normal method is around a (set of) particle(s), the other methods are around the center of mass of a set of particles or to the closest particle in a set. Here the RDFs were calculated using both. The coordination numbers (Nb) of a particle or atom B around another one A were calculated by integrating the radial distribution function $g_{AB}(r)$ between the center of A and the first local minimum, r_m:

$$N_B = 4\pi\rho_B \int_0^{r_m} g_{AB}(r)r^2 dr,$$

Where ρ_B refers to the density of species B (expressed in units of molecules per volume). The cluster analysis was performed using the g_cluster package included in the GROMACS software. This utility can cluster structures using several different methods. We determined structures from the trajectories of the runs using the single linkage which add a structure to a cluster when its distance to any element of the cluster is less than the cutoff. We performed the cluster analysis using cutoff values (i.e., the largest distance to be considered in a cluster) between 0.3 and 1.5 nm. The diffusion coefficient of the mixture components is calculated from the Einstein relation (mean-square displacement, MSD):

$$D = \frac{1}{6t} \langle |\vec{r_i}(t) - \vec{r_i}(0)|^2 \rangle.$$

Where r_i is the centre of mass positions of the molecules. The MSD is averaged over molecules, and in order to improve the statistics, several restarts $r(0)$ were used along the trajectory.

Molecular Dynamics Simulation of Two MIP Systems

In this chapter, we have simulated a rather complex system, comprised by a lot of ionic compounds: NAP, together with SI⁻, DHI⁺, SI3, Na⁺, and I⁻ as well as the solvents water and methanol. When the complexity, variety, and number of species under consideration are increased, the probability of accumulating a significant amount of calculation errors and uncertainties is also increased. Therefore, it was necessary to assess the validity of the potential considered for the simulations. The main limitation for doing it directly is that the real systems present a huge variety of oxysilane species at a certain moment of the process, making really hard to perform exhaustive atomistic simulations to predict experimental properties of a typical silica based sol-gel process. For this reason, the experimental validation of the model had to be partially indirect. We have chosen OPLS-AA potential including fine-tuned parameters by Price et al. (2002) to better describe typical sol-gel reactants. First of all, the accuracy of the OPLS-AA potential is extensively verified over small molecules such as water and methanol, so further testing was considered unnecessary for these substances. This potential was previously studied by our group (Azenha et al. 2011) for the cyclic SI3 in a mixture which included damascenone, tetramethoxysilane (TMOS), water, and methanol.

The two DHI⁺ molecules are the more challenging molecules to simulate in our systems due to the presence at the same time of oxysilane rings and dehydroimidazolium cationic moiety. In a previous chapter, we have validated a DHI⁺ with –OH terminals in the oxysilane rings; however, in this chapter we have partially changed the –OH terminals in the oxysilane rings with some –CH3 because we consider that this specie is likely to be present in the real mixture; thus it is worth investigating in order to understand and uncover the role and the importance of these intermediates in the imprinting process as well as in the formation and stability of the backbone. The validation of these new DHI⁺ has been performed as in our previous work (Concu et al. 2014). For instance, a pure DHI⁺ system was considered and simulated, consisting of 100 ion pairs in a cubic box. The density measured in the laboratory for the DHI⁺ was 1180 ± 40 kg/m3, at 298 K, while the density calculated by MD of these two new DHI⁺ have been 1080 ± 47 kg/m3 and 1430 ± 47 kg/m3 respectively. We consider these values are acceptable according to the modifications thus, we can conclude that the model is good, considering the complexity of the molecule, the potential impurities of the experimental sample (which are not presented in the simulated one) and the inherent limitations of the MD approximation.

Model A

The first model we have simulated contains the DHI⁺ molecule represented in the Fig. 1B. We performed three independent runs for each system, in order to ensure the robustness and the replicability of the simulations. The RDF together with the N_B and the cluster analysis were used to study the affinity between the template and the polymer. As referred in the previous section, the RDF was calculated using a specific atom instead of the centre of the mass of the molecule. The atoms used for the template are the two oxygens of the carboxylic terminal, while for the DHI⁺ the hydrogen and the carbon were chosen in order to evaluate both the affinity and the orientation of the template when interacting with the polymer; these atoms have been circle-marked in the Fig. 1. In Fig. 2, we have reported the RDF analysis calculated using the hydrogen of the DHI^+; as can be seen, in this case the affinity between the template and the DHI^+ doesn't seem to be relevant in two of the three replicas, while in the third one the interaction of the pair NAP/DHI^+ is really good. In order to clarify the interaction in the two replicas, we have calculated the RDF using the carbon atom of the DHI^+ instead of the H atom. As reported in the Fig. 3, in this case the peaks are at a shorter distance in two of the three replicas; in fact, the interaction between the template and the NAP is greater. More in depth, we can see high and sharp peaks at a distance of 0.25–0.3 nM as in the case of the third replica in the Fig. 2, thus confirming that in all the three replicas, a good imprinting effect is occurring. These results are further confirmed by the N_B analysis whose results are reported in the Table 2. Regarding N_B, it is important to underline that this number is calculated using the RDF first global minimum. Thus, it is strictly correlated to the distance at which the minimum is located. In the case of the pair DHI^+/NAP, the first is generally located at 0.5 nm and the N_B calculated is 0.2. In the case of the pairs DHI^+/SI^- and $DHI^+/SI3$, the registered values were 0.01 and 0.12, with the minimum located at 0.35–0.4 nm.

The cluster analysis reported in Fig. 3 is in good agreement with a work of Pereira (Pereira et al. 2002) where the trend of the SI^- to form aggregates were recorded. During the simulation, the typical cluster of the SI^-, SI3 and NAP is formed by two molecules. Also the DHI^+ shows a general trend to form aggregates; however, in this case the cluster is formed by 3 molecules. This result could confirm that the DHI^+ molecules are forming a backbone, which is what really happens during the sol-gel process. Finally, the MSD analysis confirms all the others data; in the Fig. 5 is reported the diffusion of the species included in the simulation. Figure 5A reports the graph of all the species while in Fig. 5B there are the DHI^+, NAP, SI3, and SI^-. The MSD in this case is compatible with the data published by Li (Li et al. 2014).

Overall, the results of this first model can suggest that the simulation was able to mimic the behavior of a real system during an imprinting process.

Model B

Model B represents a mixture with the DHI^+ reported in Fig. 1C. In this system, the –OH groups are more present in the molecule, thus mimicking another molecule which is likely to be present in the real mixture. We have reported the RDF of this system using the hydrogen of the DHI^+ in the Fig. 6. In this case the affinity between the NAP and the DHI^+ is much better than in the previous model. In fact, in all the three replicas the affinity is really clear, which could confirm a better imprinting process. The high and sharp peaks are always located at 0.25 nm which is the optimal in these systems. In addition, it is important to underline that in this case the pairs $SI3/DHI^+$ and $SI-/DHI^+$ have their relative first peaks shifted at a greater distance. In order to confirm these results, as in the previous model we have calculated the RDF using

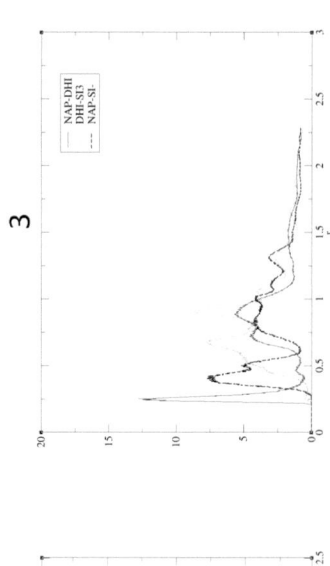

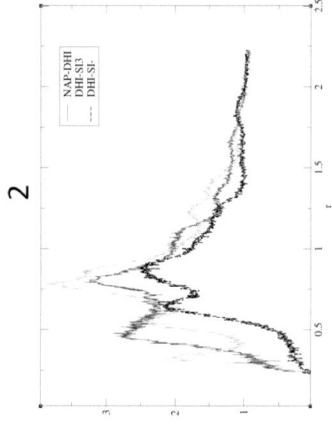

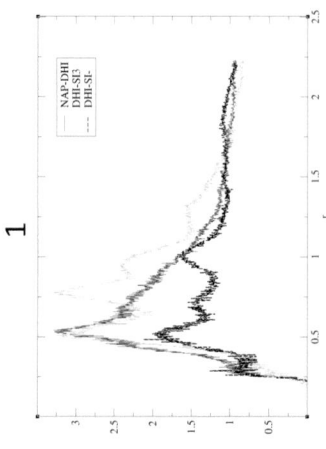

Fig. 2: RDF of the A model calculated using the H of the DHI$^+$.

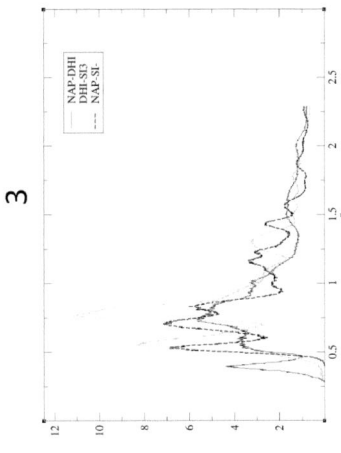

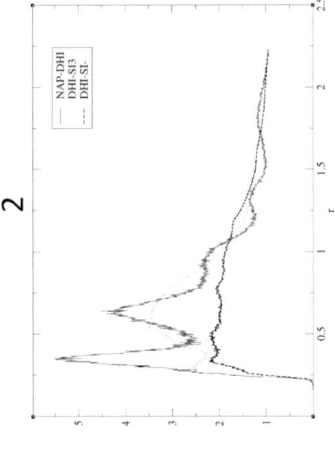

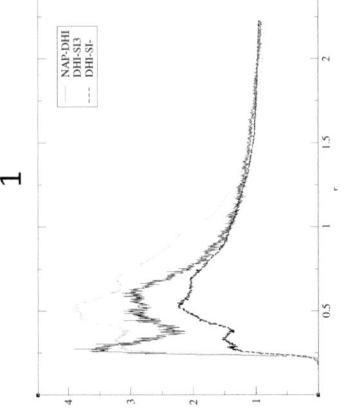

Fig. 3: RDF of the A model calculated using the C of the DHI$^+$.

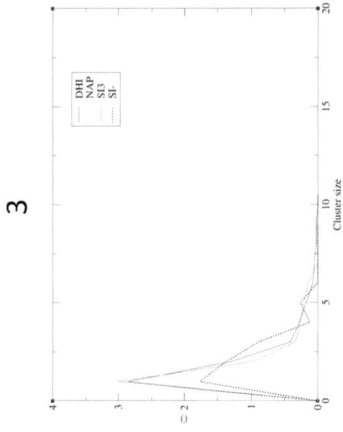
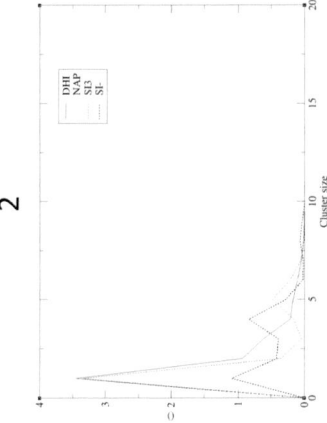
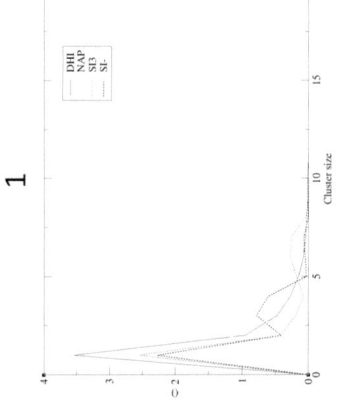

Fig. 4: Cluster analysis of the A model.

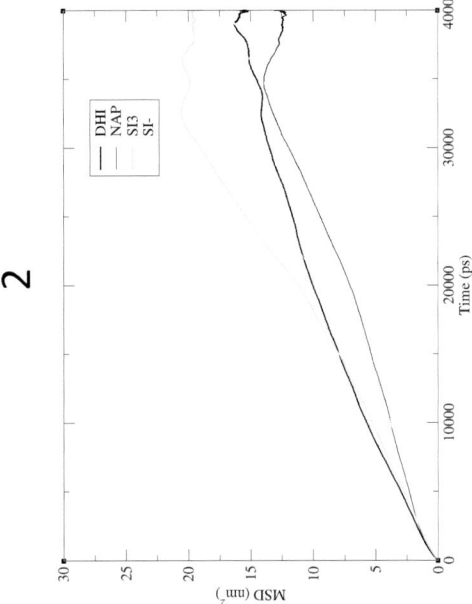

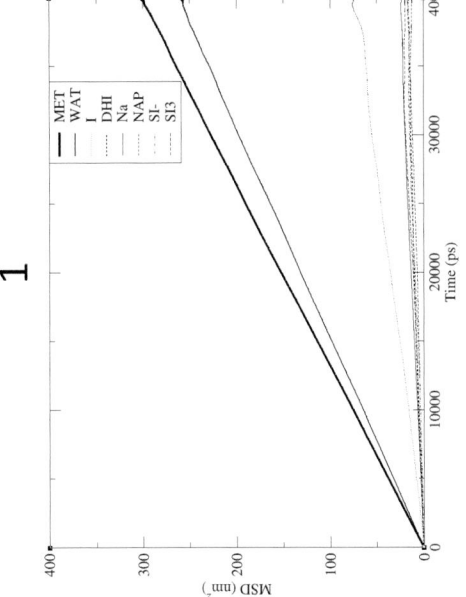

Fig. 5: Diffusion of the species in the A model.

Table 2: Coordination Number.

PAIR	Model A	Model B
NAP/DHI$^+$	0.2	0.12
SI3/DHI$^+$	0.01	0.08
SI$^-$/DHI$^+$	0.12	0.42

the C of the dihydroimidazolium instead of the hydrogen. As shown in Fig. 7, the previous results are further confirmed. Indeed, in all the three replicas the pair NAP/DHI$^+$ is the one with the highest and sharpest peak and at a shorter distance. Only in the third replica the pair DHI/SI3 shows the highest peak; however, it is located at a greater distance. These results are further confirmed by the coordination numbers. The N_B for the pair DHI$^+$/NAP is 0.12 at a very close distance 0.4 nm. For the pairs DHI$^+$/SI3 and DHI$^+$/SI$^-$ are 0.08 and 0.42 respectively and registered at a larger distance, 0.75 and 0.9 for instance.

The cluster analysis confirms and improves the trend shown by the model A of the DHI$^+$ to form large aggregates; indeed, the typical cluster is formed by seven molecules. This result is really important because it endorses that this simulation is capable of reproducing the behavior of this sol-gel system at a stage closer to gelification, where a large and homogenous backbone is presented. Comparing this model with the previous one, we can affirm that the –OH groups in the silica trimers in the DHI$^+$ are essential to simulate the growing of the backbone, as in the real mixture. As well as in the A model SI3 is still forming aggregates of ~ 5 along the three different replicas. On the other hand, the SI$^-$ is still forming small clusters of ~ 2 molecules. All these data are resumed in the Fig. 8. Regarding the MSD, this system shows the same behavior recorded in the A model, thus is not reported.

Summary and Final Remarks

The sol-gel technique has increasingly been employed in the last years for the preparation of molecularly imprinted polymers (MIP) in order to obtain new and high selective materials. In this chapter, we have briefly reviewed recent findings in this area and presented the molecular dynamics (MD) simulation of two new MIPs with a high affinity to a template molecule, the S-Naproxen (NAP). We have simulated two different MIPs that are likely to be present in a sol-gel mixture. These two new MIPs represent the same molecule but in a different state of hydrolization. The two mixtures contain the gel backbone which is a polymer containing the dihydroimidazolium moiety, cyclic trimers, and counter ions; the simulations were performed using an explicit representation of all the ionic species at pH 9 which is essential to have a more realistic representation of the mixture. The main aim of this chapter was to study the affinity between the two different moieties and the template. The MD was performed using GROMACS 5.0 with the GPU support and all the species were parametrized using the OPLS-AA force field. The two MIPs have never been studied before, thus were parametrized and validated in this paper for the first time. The affinity between the MIPs and the template was studied using radial distribution function (RDF),

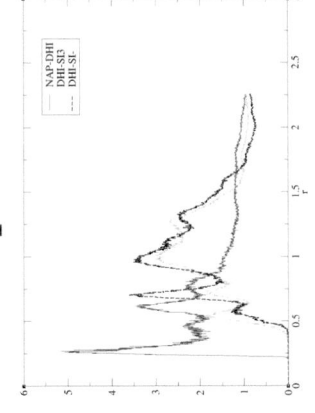

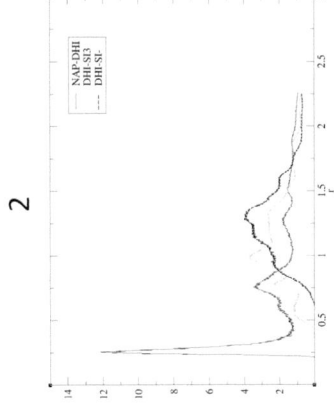

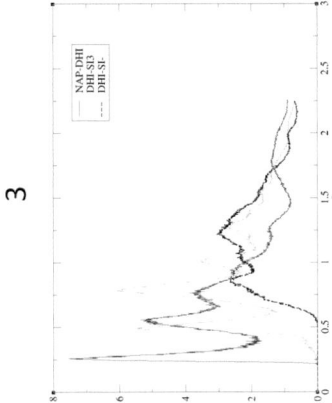

Fig. 6: RDF of the B model calculated using the H of the DHI$^+$.

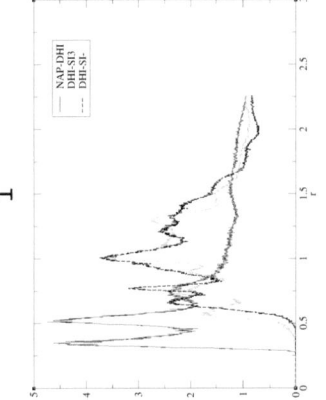

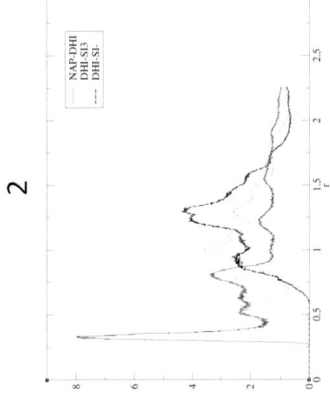

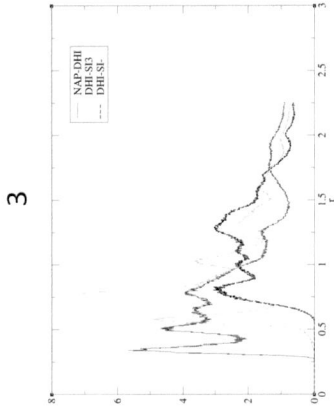

Fig. 7: RDF of the B model calculated using the C of the DHI$^+$.

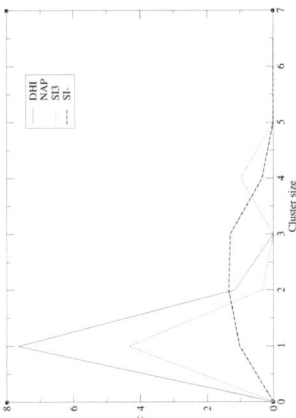

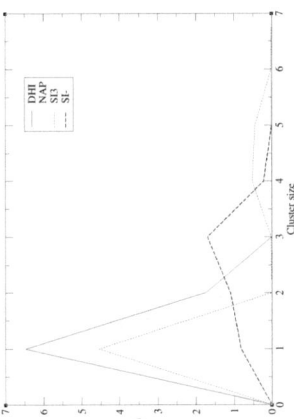

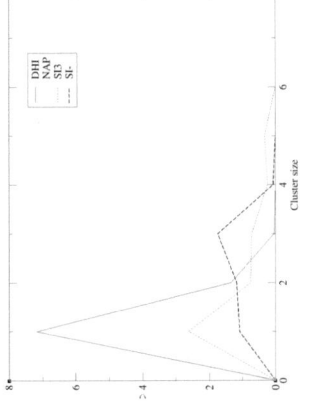

Fig. 8: Cluster analysis of the B model.

coordination number, and cluster analysis. When studying such complex systems, it is essential to have an explicit representation of the ionic species in order to study the molecular imprinting process in a qualitative way; indeed, as we previously have demonstrated, a no-representation of the ionic species may lead to erroneous conclusions or results that are thus not comparable with the behaviour of a real system.

The main aim of this chapter was focused on the study of the affinity of two different dihydroimidazolium moieties against a template in the same sol-gel mixture. Our findings represent a further confirmation of previous studies that we are able to simulate rather complex processes, such as the imprinting process in a sol-gel system, through atomistic MD simulations. The results demonstrate that MD simulations are essential to understand and study the atomistic basis of the interaction occurring during the imprinting process between all the species included in the system, not only between the xerogel and the template molecule. Indeed, in these systems, it is important to evaluate the imprinting factor as well as the formation of the xerogel and which factors are influencing the growing of the backbone. Thus uncovering the molecular level details of these systems is a major goal for the atomistic simulations. In addition, simulating rather complex systems with a high level of ionic species is a key step; however, worthwhile because the results could be compared with data obtained from real systems. In this sense, we have performed two simulations of two different complex systems which included two new functional silicates in its cationic form, DHI$^+$, SI3 with its anionic form, SI$^-$, as well as the anionic form of the Naproxen®. In this context, the main aim of this chapter was focused on the study of the affinity of the two DHI$^+$ with the template molecule. The analysis of the simulations was done by means of RDF, cluster analysis, coordination number, and MSD. Despite the fact that in both models we have recorded a good affinity between the template and the DHI$^+$, the B model was the model with the most remarkable imprinting effect.

The A model represented a system with a low substitution of –OH in the silica trimers of the DHI$^+$ moiety. In this case, all the results obtained show that the template has a good affinity for the DHI$^+$. Even so, all the results obtained from the B model are even better, with a much higher affinity between the template and the xerogel, in fact the affinity between the NAP and DHI$^+$ was always the highest compared with other groups highlighting a successful imprinting process. Furthermore, the results indicate a better formation of the backbone in this system due to the highest number of –OH groups in the silica trimers, remarking their key role in the formation of the xerogel.

Finally, it is important to underline that, the scenarios observed by MD were comparable with the behavior observed for the materials prepared in the lab, namely a good imprinting effect ascertained by an imprinted/non-imprinted adsorption and porosity comparison.

References

Alder, B. J. and T. E. Wainwright. 1957. Phase transition for a hard sphere System. J. Chem. Phys. 27(5): 1208–1209.

Alder, B. J. and T. E. Wainwright. 1959. Studies in molecular dynamics. I. General Method. J. Chem. Phys. 31(2): 459–466.

Azenha, M., B. Szefczyk, D. Loureiro, P. Kathirvel, M. N. Cordeiro and A. Fernando-Silva. 2011. Molecular dynamics simulations of pregelification mixtures for the production of imprinted xerogels. *Langmuir* 27(8): 5062–5070.

Bako, I., J. Hutter and G. Palinkas. 2006. Car-parrinello molecular dynamics simulation of liquid formic acid. J. Phys. Chem. A 110(6): 2188–94.

Braga, C., A. Galindo and E. A. Muller. 2014. Nonequilibrium molecular dynamics simulation of diffusion at the liquid-liquid interface. J. Chem. Phys. 141(15): 154101.

Breneman, Curt M. and Kenneth B. Wiberg. 1990. Determining atom-centered monopoles from molecular electrostatic potentials. The need for high sampling density in formamide conformational analysis. J. Comput. Chem. 11(3): 361–373.

Brinker, C. and George Scherer. 1990. Sol-Gel Science: The Physics and Chemistry of Sol-Gel Processing. Academic Press, Inc., San Diego.

Brooks, B. R., C. L. Brooks, 3rd, A. D. Mackerell, Jr., L. Nilsson, R. J. Petrella, B. Roux et al. 2009. CHARMM: the biomolecular simulation program. J. Comput. Chem. 30(10): 1545–614.

Burney, P. R., E. M. Nordwald, K. Hickman, J. L. Kaar and J. Pfaendtner. 2015. Molecular dynamics investigation of the ionic liquid/enzyme interface: application to engineering enzyme surface charge. Proteins 83(4): 670–80.

Bussi, Giovanni, Davide Donadio and Michele Parrinello. 2007. Canonical sampling through velocity rescaling. J. Chem. Phys. 126 (1): 014101.

Case, D. A., J. T. Berryman, R. M. Betz, D. S. Cerutti, T. E. Cheatham, III, T. A. Darden et al. 2015. AMBER 2015.

Concu, R., M. Perez, M. N. Cordeiro and M. Azenha. 2014. Molecular dynamics simulations of complex mixtures aimed at the preparation of naproxen-imprinted xerogels. J. Chem. Inf. Model. 54(12): 3330–43.

Concu, R., M. Ornelas and M. Azenha. 2015. Molecularly imprinted sol-gel materials for medical applications. Curr. Top. Med. Chem. 15(3): 199–222.

Crisafulli, A., R. Milia, A. Lobina, M. Caddeo, F. Tocco, A. Concu et al. 2008. Haemodynamic effect of metaboreflex activation in men after running above and below the velocity of the anaerobic threshold. Exp. Physiol. 93(4): 447–57.

da Silva, E. F., T. Kuznetsova, B. Kvamme and K. M. Merz, Jr. 2007. Molecular dynamics study of ethanolamine as a pure liquid and in aqueous solution. J. Phys. Chem. B 111(14): 3695–703.

DeMarco, M. L. 2015. Molecular dynamics simulations of membrane- and protein-bound glycolipids using GLYCAM. Methods Mol. Biol. 1273: 379–90.

Dickert, F. L. and O. Hayden. 2002. Bioimprinting of polymers and sol-gel phases. Selective detection of yeasts with imprinted polymers. Analytical Chemistry 74(6): 1302–1306.

Essmann, Ulrich, Lalith Perera, Max L. Berkowitz, Tom Darden, Hsing Lee and Lee G. Pedersen. 1995. A smooth particle mesh Ewald method. The Journal of Chemical Physics 103(19): 8577–8593.

Finkelstein, A. V. and B. A. Reva. 1992. Search for the stable state of a short chain in a molecular field. Protein Eng. 5(7): 617–24.

Frisch, M. J., G. W. Trucks, H. B. Schlegel, G. E. Scuseria, M. A. Robb, J. R. Cheeseman, G. Scalmani, V. Barone, B. Mennucci, G. A. Petersson, H. Nakatsuji, M. Caricato, X. Li, H. P. Hratchian, A. F. Izmaylov, J. Bloino, G. Zheng, J. L. Sonnenberg, M. Hada, M. Ehara, K. Toyota, R. Fukuda, J. Hasegawa, M. Ishida, T. Nakajima, Y. Honda, O. Kitao, H. Nakai, T. Vreven, J. A. Montgomery, Jr., J. E. Peralta, F. Ogliaro, M. Bearpark, J. J. Heyd, E. Brothers, K. N. Kudin, V. N. Staroverov, R. Kobayashi, J. Normand, K. Raghavachari, A. Rendell, J. C. Burant, S. S. Iyengar, J. Tomasi, M. Cossi, N. Rega, J. M. Millam, M. Klene, J. E. Knox, J. B. Cross, V. Bakken, C. Adamo, J. Jaramillo, R. Gomperts, R. E. Stratmann, O. Yazyev, A. J. Austin, R. Cammi, C. Pomelli, J. W. Ochterski, R. L. Martin, K. Morokuma, V. G. Zakrzewski, G. A. Voth, P. Salvador, J. J. Dannenberg, S. Dapprich, A. D. Daniels, Ö. Farkas, J. B. Foresman, J. V. Ortiz, J. Cioslowski and D. J. Fox, Gaussian, Inc., Wallingford CT. 2009. Gaussian 09, Revision E.01.

Gao, Y. D. and J. F. Huang. 2011. An extension strategy of Discovery Studio 2.0 for non-bonded interaction energy automatic calculation at the residue level. Dongwuxue Yanjiu 32(3): 262–6.

Gruber, C. C. and J. Pleiss. 2011. Systematic benchmarking of large molecular dynamics simulations employing GROMACS on massive multiprocessing facilities. J. Comput. Chem. 32(4): 600–6.

Guardia, L., R. Badía, M. Granda-Valdés and M. E. Díaz-García. 2012. Screening of a molecularly imprinted sol-gel library for nafcillin recognition. J. Sol-Gel Sc. Tec. 63(3): 537–545.

Guo, X., Z. Liu, Q. Song, L. Wang and D. Zhong. 2015. Dynamics and mechanism of UV-damaged DNA repair in indole-thymine dimer adduct: molecular origin of low repair quantum efficiency. J. Phys. Chem. B 119(8): 3446–55.

Hansen, D. E. 2007. Recent developments in the molecular imprinting of proteins. Biomaterials 28(29): 4178–4191.

Hockney, R. W., S. P. Goel and J. W. Eastwood. 1974. Quiet high-resolution computer models of a plasma. J. Comp. Physics 14(2): 148–158.

Humphrey, William, Andrew Dalke and Klaus Schulten. 1996. VMD: Visual molecular dynamics. J. Mol. Graphics 14(1): 33–38.

Jalkute, C. B., S. H. Barage, M. J. Dhanavade and K. D. Sonawane. 2013. Molecular dynamics simulation and molecular docking studies of Angiotensin converting enzyme with inhibitor lisinopril and amyloid Beta Peptide. Protein J. 32(5): 356–64.

Jorgensen, William L., Jayaraman Chandrasekhar, Jeffry D. Madura, Roger W. Impey and Michael L. Klein. 1983. Comparison of simple potential functions for simulating liquid water. J. Chem. Phys. 79(2): 926–935.

Jorgensen, William L., David S. Maxwell and Julian Tirado-Rives. 1996. Development and testing of the OPLS all-atom force field on conformational energetics and properties of organic liquids. J. Amer. Chem. Soc. 118 (45): 11225–11236.

Kachhap, S. and B. Singh. 2015. Role of DNA conformation & energetic insights in Msx-1-DNA recognition as revealed by molecular dynamics studies on specific and nonspecific complexes. J. Biomol. Struct. Dyn. 33(10): 2069–82.

Kadhirvel, P., M. Azenha, S. Shinde, E. Schillinger, P. Gomes, B. Sellergren et al. 2013. Imidazolium-based functional monomers for the imprinting of the anti-inflammatory drug naproxen: comparison of acrylic and sol-gel approaches. J. Chrom. A 1314: 115–23.

Kulkarni, M., R. Dendere, F. Nicolls, S. Steiner and T. S. Douglas. 2015. Monte-Carlo simulation of a slot-scanning X-ray imaging system. Phys. Med. 32(1): 284–289.

Kutzner, C., S. Pall, M. Fechner, A. Esztermann, B. L. de Groot and H. Grubmuller. 2015. Best bang for your buck: GPU nodes for GROMACS biomolecular simulations. J. Comput. Chem. 36(26): 1990–2008.

Lang, K. M., J. Kittelmann, C. Durr, A. Osberghaus and J. Hubbuch. 2015. A comprehensive molecular dynamics approach to protein retention modeling in ion exchange chromatography. J. Chromatogr. A 1381: 184–93.

Lee, H. S., Y. Qi and W. Im. 2015. Effects of N-glycosylation on protein conformation and dynamics: Protein Data Bank analysis and molecular dynamics simulation study. Sci. Rep. 5: 8926.

Li, B., J. Xu, A. J. Hall, K. Haupt and B. Tse Sum Bui. 2014. Water-compatible silica sol-gel molecularly imprinted polymer as a potential delivery system for the controlled release of salicylic acid. J. Mol. Recognit. 27(9): 559–65.

Li, F., J. Li and S. S. Zhang. 2008. Molecularly imprinted polymer grafted on polysaccharide microsphere surface by the sol-gel process for protein recognition. Talanta 74(5): 1247–1255.

Liang, Y., G. Yang, F. Liu and Y. Wang. 2016. Monte Carlo simulation of ionizing radiation induced DNA strand breaks utilizing coarse grained high-order chromatin structures. Phys. Med. Biol. 61(1): 445–60.

Lin, Zian, Fan Yang, Xiwen He and Yukui Zhang. 2009. Organic–inorganic hybrid silica as supporting matrices for selective recognition of bovine hemoglobin via covalent immobilization. Journal of Separation Science 32(22): 3980–3987.

Liu, Yu-Xing, Gui-Qin Jian, Xi-Wen He, Lang-Xing Chen and Yu-Kui Zhang. 2013. Preparation and application of core-shell structural carbon nanotubes-molecularly imprinted composite material for determination of nafcillin in egg samples. Chin. J. Anal. Chem. 41(2): 161–166.

Markegard, C. B., A. Mazaheripour, J. M. Jocson, A. M. Burke, M. N. Dickson, A. A. Gorodetsky et al. 2015. Molecular dynamics simulations of perylenediimide DNA base surrogates. J. Phys. Chem. B 119(35): 11459–65.

Martinez, L., R. Andrade, E. G. Birgin and J. M. Martinez. 2009. PACKMOL: a package for building initial configurations for molecular dynamics simulations. J. Comput. Chem. 30(13): 2157–64.

Marx, D. and J. Hutter. 2000. Ab initio molecular dynamics: theory and implementation. pp. 301–449. *In*: Grotendorst, J. (ed.). Modern Methods and Algorithms of Quantum Chemistry, Vol. 1. NIC Series.

Molodtsov, M. I., E. A. Ermakova, E. E. Shnol, E. L. Grishchuk, J. R. McIntosh and F. I. Ataullakhanov. 2005. A molecular-mechanical model of the microtubule. Biophys. J. 88(5): 3167–79.

Nagayama, G., M. Takematsu, H. Mizuguchi and T. Tsuruta. 2015. Molecular dynamics study on condensation/evaporation coefficients of chain molecules at liquid-vapor interface. J. Chem. Phys. 143(1): 014706.

Nosé, Shuichi and M. L. Klein. 1983. Constant pressure molecular dynamics for molecular systems. Mol. Phys. 50(5): 1055–1076.

Parrinello, M. and A. Rahman. 1981. Polymorphic transitions in single crystals: a new molecular dynamics method. J. Appl. Phys. 52(12): 7182–7190.

Pereira, J. C. G., C. R. A. Catlow and G. D. Price. 2002. Molecular dynamics simulation of methanolic and ethanolic silica-based sol-gel solutions at ambient temperature and pressure. J. Phys. Chem. A 106(1): 130–148.

Plimpton, Steve. 1995. Fast parallel algorithms for short-range molecular dynamics. J. Comput. Phys. 117(1): 1–19.

Rezaei, Behzad, Malihe Khalili Boroujeni and Ali A. Ensafi. 2014. A novel electrochemical nanocomposite imprinted sensor for the determination of lorazepam based on modified polypyrrole@sol-gel@gold nanoparticles/pencil graphite electrode. Electrochimica Acta 123(0): 332–339.

Siberchicot, B. and J. Clerouin. 2012. Properties of hot liquid cerium by LDA + U molecular dynamics. J. Phys. Condens. Matter 24(45): 455603.

Song, W. and J. T. Guo. 2015. Investigation of arc repressor DNA-binding specificity by comparative molecular dynamics simulations. J. Biomol. Struct. Dyn. 33(10): 2083–93.

Song, Y., J. Conner, X. Zhang and J. P. Hayward. 2015. Monte Carlo simulation of a very high resolution thermal neutron detector composed of glass scintillator microfibers. Appl. Radiat. Isot. 108: 100–107.

Tao, Zunyu, Elizabeth C. Tehan, Rachel M. Bukowski, Ying Tang, Ellen L. Shughart, William G. Holthoff et al. 2006. Templated xerogels as platforms for biomolecule-less biomolecule sensors. Anal. Chim. Acta 564(1): 59–65.

Tripuraneni, N. S. and M. A. Azam. 2015. A combination of pharmacophore modeling, atom-based 3D-QSAR, molecular docking and molecular dynamics simulation studies on PDE4 enzyme inhibitors. J. Biomol. Struct. Dyn. 12: 1–41.

Van Der Spoel, D., E. Lindahl, B. Hess, G. Groenhof, A. E. Mark and H. J. Berendsen. 2005. GROMACS: fast, flexible, and free. J. Comput. Chem. 26(16): 1701–1718.

van Gunsteren, W. F. and H. J. C. Berendsen. 1987. Groningen Molecular Simulation (GROMOS) Library Manual. Biomos, Groningen, The Netherlands, pp. 1–221.

Verma, S., A. Singh and A. Mishra. 2014. Molecular dynamics investigation on the poor sensitivity of A171T mutant NEDD8-activating enzyme (NAE) for MLN4924. J. Biomol. Struct. Dyn. 32(7): 1064–73.

Vorob'ev Iu, N. 2003. Methods of computer modeling and conformational mobility of DNA duplexes. Mol. Biol. (Mosk) 37(2): 240–54.

Wang, F., H. Wan, J. P. Hu and S. Chang. 2015. Molecular dynamics simulations of wild type and mutants of botulinum neurotoxin A complexed with synaptic vesicle protein 2C. Mol. Biosyst. 11(1): 223–31.

Wilangowski, F. and N. A. Stolwijk. 2015. Monte Carlo simulation of diffusion and ionic conductivity in a simple cubic random alloy via the interstitialcy mechanism. J. Phys. Condens. Matter 27(50): 505401.

Wright, John D. and Nico A. J. M. Sommerdijk. 2001. Sol-Gel Materials, Chemistry and Applications. Taylor & Francis, Great Britain.

Yang, Y. and B. B. Laird. 2014. Thermodynamics and intrinsic structure of the Al-Pb liquid-liquid interface: a molecular dynamics simulation study. J. Phys. Chem. B 118(28): 8373–80.

Yoon, Y., J. Morishita, M. Park, H. Kim, K. Kim and J. Kim. 2015. Monte Carlo simulation-based feasibility study of novel indirect flat panel detector system for removing scatter radiation. Phys. Med. 32(1): 182–187.

Zen, A., Y. Luo, G. Mazzola, L. Guidoni and S. Sorella. 2015. Ab initio molecular dynamics simulation of liquid water by quantum Monte Carlo. J. Chem. Phys. 142(14): 144111.

Zhang, W., X. W. He, Y. Chen, W. Y. Li and Y. K. Zhang. 2011. Composite of CdTe quantum dots and molecularly imprinted polymer as a sensing material for cytochrome c. Biosensors & Bioelectronics 26(5): 2553–2558.

Zhou, Ling, Yanyue Kong, Shian Zhong and Xiaorun Zhou. 2013. Preparation and characterization of molecularly imprinted organic–inorganic hybrid materials by sol-gel processing for selective recognition of ibuprofen. J. Sol-Gel Sc. Tec. 66(1): 59–67.

Index